DISEASES
OF THE CORNEA

DISEASES OF THE CORNEA

MERRILL GRAYSON, M.D.

Distinguished Professor of Ophthalmology,
Department of Ophthalmology,
Indiana University School of Medicine,
Indianapolis, Indiana

Second edition

With **438** illustrations,

including **156** in color

The C. V. Mosby Company

ST. LOUIS • TORONTO • LONDON   1983

MOSBY

A TRADITION OF PUBLISHING EXCELLENCE

Editor: Eugenia A. Klein
Developmental editor: Kathryn H. Falk
Editing supervisor: Lin Dempsey Hallgren
Manuscript editor: Robert A. Kelly
Designer: Jeanne Bush
Production: Linda R. Stalnaker, Judy England

SECOND EDITION

Previous edition copyrighted 1979

Printed in the United States of America

The C.V. Mosby Company
11830 Westline Industrial Drive, St. Louis, Missouri 63141

Library of Congress Cataloging in Publication Data

Grayson, Merrill.
    Diseases of the cornea.

    Bibliography: p.
    Includes index.
    1. Cornea—Diseases. I. Title. [DNLM: 1. Corneal
diseases. WW 220 G784d]
RE336.G76 1983   617.7'19   82-14530
ISBN 0-8016-1973-4

TS/CB/B 9 8 7 6 5 4 3 2 1   01/B/082

To my associates in the
Department of Ophthalmology at Indiana University Medical Center
and to my colleagues
throughout the state of Indiana

whose help and trust made it possible for me to gather
the varied clinical cases presented in this text

Preface

Resident teaching has always been one of the major aims of my academic career. My desire has been to contribute to this dream by preparing and organizing the material of my major interest in ophthalmology so that it can more easily be assimilated by the student. I hope I have done this with *Diseases of the Cornea*.

Because of the close relationship between the conjunctiva and cornea, some diseases affecting both are discussed in the text. Primary corneal diseases and corneal manifestations of systemic diseases are stressed. Throughout the text, tables provide convenient and rapid association for study. *Diseases of the Cornea* is not to be considered an encyclopedia of corneal disease but a thorough aid to help one correlate and organize the large amount of material concerned. Discussion of therapy is included where it is considered necessary and helpful.

Many colleagues in the field have generously given permission to use their illustrations. Dr. Fred M. Wilson II and I took the color photographs of patients who attended the Cornea Service of the Department of Ophthalmology at Indiana University Medical Center. Kenneth Julian and Gene Louden are to be thanked for their generous aid in preparing many of the illustrations.

I greatly appreciate the work of my associate, Dr. Fred M. Wilson II, whose time, help, suggestions regarding the text, and close association in clinical consultation with numerous problems noted in this book were invaluable.

Merrill Grayson

Contents

DISEASES
OF THE CORNEA

1 Anatomy

GROSS ANATOMY

The cornea is the transparent, anterior, avascular tissue corresponding to a watch crystal. It is slightly elliptic horizontally and measures about 12 mm horizontally and 11 mm in the vertical meridian. The cornea is thinner centrally, averaging about 0.58 mm, whereas the periphery measures approximately 1 mm in thickness. The net refractive power of the eye is 43 diopters (D), or 70% of the total refractive power of the eye. The refractive power of the anterior surface of the cornea is +48.8 D and of the posterior surface, −5.8 D. The central one third of the cornea is almost spherical and is the optical zone. The cornea flattens peripherally, contributing to the increased thickness of the edge of the corneal area. In the newborn the cornea is relatively large, averaging 10 mm vertically. It usually reaches adult size in the first year.

MICROSCOPIC ANATOMY

The cornea consists of five layers: epithelium, Bowman's layer, stroma, Descemet's membrane, and endothelium (Fig. 1-1).

Epithelium

Epithelium consists of a five-cell layer with three types of cells: columnal basal, polygonal wing, and flat superficial cells. The deeply situated basal cells comprise the single layer of flat base cells that rest on the basement membrane. These cells are rounded on their anterior surface with oval nuclei arranged perpendicularly to the surface (Fig. 1-2). New cells are constantly being used and migrate superficially to become

1

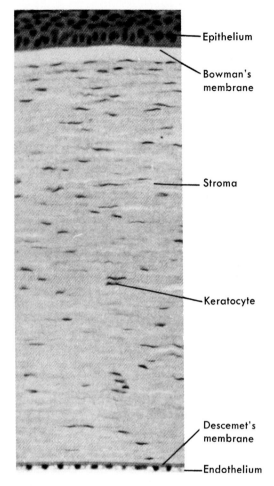

Fig. 1-1. Cross section of human cornea. (From Kuwabara, T.: Fine structure of the eye, ed. 2, Boston, 1970, Howe Laboratory of Ophthalmology, Harvard Medical School.)

wing cells. The wing cells comprise three layers; the more superficial the cell, the flatter its appearance. The nuclei of the wing cells lie parallel to the surface. The superficial cells are flat and lie in two layers, exhibiting microvilli and no keratinization (Fig. 1-3). The epithelial cells of the cornea are interdigitated and firmly attached to each other by many desmosomes. The tight attachment between the cells, together with the fact that the membranes of the basal cells are flat, suggests that the epithelium restricts passage of fluid through this layer.[3]

The cytoplasm of the epithelial cell exhibits a dense matrix in which are found many fine keratofibrils. The microorganelles are sparse in number. Mitochondria are small and not very abundant. Golgi apparatus and rough endoplasmic reticulum (Fig. 1-4) are small in number.

Glycogen particles are seen in the epithelial cells (Fig. 1-4, *B*); the presence of this material varies in clinical pathologic conditions. In disease the epithelial glycogen may be markedly depleted. In addition, the glycogen particles may disappear from epithelial cells during the acute wound-healing process.[12, 16] Desmosomal attachment of epithelial

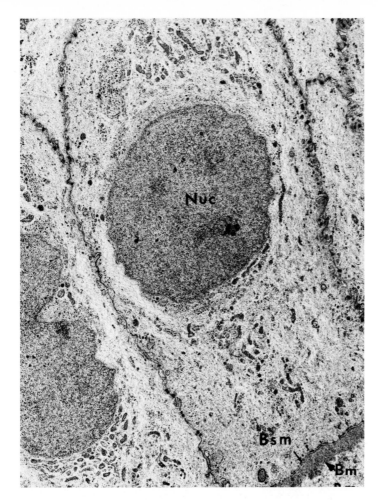

Fig. 1-2. Basal cell of epithelium. Nucleus *(Nuc)* is round, and basement membrane of cell *(Bsm)* borders on Bowman's layer *(Bm)*. (From McTigue, J.W., Goldman, J.N., Fine, B.S., and Kuwabara, T.: Clinical application of electron microscopy of the cornea: a course, Chicago, 1968, American Academy of Ophthalmology and Otolaryngology.)

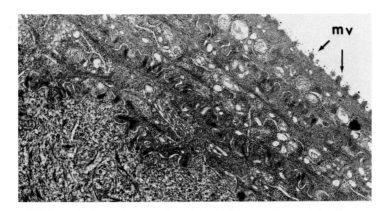

Fig. 1-3. Superficial cells are flat, with microvilli on their surface *(mv)*. (From McTigue, J.W., Goldman, J.N., Fine, B.S., and Kuwabara, T.: Clinical application of electron microscopy of the cornea: a course, Chicago, 1968, American Academy of Ophthalmology and Otolaryngology.)

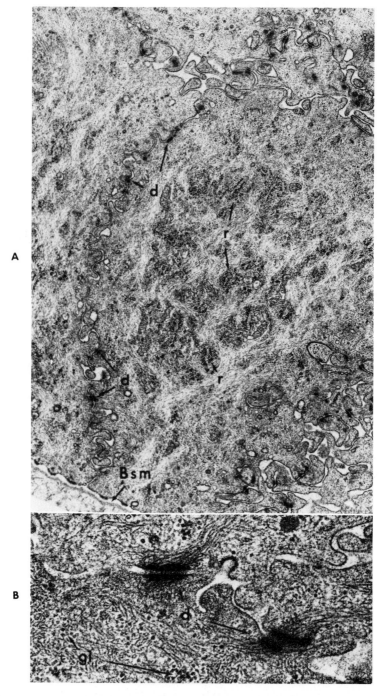

Fig. 1-4. A, Cytoplasm of corneal epithelium contains endoplasmic reticulum *(r)*, glycogen, and keratofibrils. Few mitochondria are seen. Cell membranes are joined by conspicuous desmosomes *(d)*. Basal lamina of epithelial cell is noted *(Bsm)*. **B,** Higher magnification of desmosomal attachments *(d)*, glycogen *(gl)*, and keratofibrils. (From McTigue, J.W., Goldman, J.N., Fine, B.S., and Kuwabara, T.: Clinical application of electron microscopy of the cornea: a course, Chicago, 1968, American Academy of Ophthalmology and Otolaryngology.)

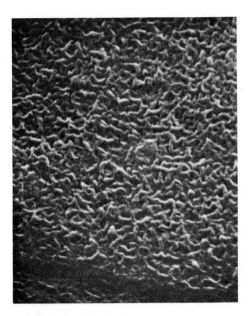

Fig. 1-5. Superficial cell of cornea on scanning electron microscopy exhibits reticulated appearance. (From Kuwabara, T.: Fine structure of the eye, ed. 2, Boston, 1970, Howe Laboratory of Ophthalmology, Harvard Medical School.)

cells becomes very strong in ocular pemphigus; in addition, the number of keratofibrils increases.[1] In epithelial edema, however, the spaces between the epithelial cells enlarge with the accumulation of fluid; nevertheless, in this condition the epithelial cells are shrunken.[4]

Occasionally, one may see small cells with dark nuclei and dendritic processes among the basal cells. In addition, slender basal cells rich in rough endoplasmic reticulum may be seen. Unmyelinated nerve fibers are frequently present in the epithelium. The fibers are usually found among the basal cells but are rare among the wing cells; the nerve appears to end without forming a specific end organ.

On scanning electron microscopy, flat and mostly hexagonal epithelium cells are seen attached to each other by straight cell boundaries.* Grossly the surface of the epithelium looks like a very shiny mirror; however, on scanning electron microscopic examination with high power the surface cell membrane appears finely reticulated (Fig. 1-5). The reticulated surface usually gives a vermiform appearance.[9,10] When drying of the cornea occurs, this vermiform-like surface structure is absent. The application of such drugs as 5% tetracaine can abolish the reticulated structure of the surface epithelium, but when the drug is discontinued and washed off, the flattened surface reforms the fine protuberances.[9] Any number of ophthalmic drug vehicles and preservatives can affect the corneal epithelium; extensive studies along these lines have been performed with the technique of scanning electron microscopy.[14]

The epithelial cells, including the superficial cells, slide toward a wound in an effort to cover a denuded area. This sliding phenomenon of the corneal epithelium and wound

---

*References 5, 7, 9, 10, 13.

healing has been studied by a number of investigators.[12,16] In addition to the entire cell body sliding,[16] one may see thin processes from the epithelial cells extend into fine tissue clefts to fill the defect. New desmosomes are formed as the cytoplasm extends; when the cell reaches the connective tissue surface, rapid differentiation into basal cells begins. When the tip of the extending epithelium meets other epithelial cells, the rapid sliding movement stops, and the epithelium becomes thicker by increasing the volume of cytoplasm and from the addition of more cells over the previously migrated cells[11]; therefore healing of the superficial wounds appears to be completed mainly by filling of the tissue defect by the epithelial cells, making the surface of the cornea optically smooth.

Bowman's layer

Bowman's layer is an acellular zone beneath the epithelium. The anterior margin is limited anteriorly by the basement membrane of the epithelium; the posterior border is formed by collagen fibers. Under the light microscope, Bowman's layer appears homogeneous, but the fine structure of Bowman's layer consists of short collagen fibers and fine fibrils (Fig. 1-6). The collagen fibrils are randomly distributed but are uniform in diameter; these fibers increase and gradually transform into the regular stroma. It appears that the granular basement membrane substance of the basal epithelium forms the previously described fine collagen fibrils that extend posteriorly (Fig. 1-7). Formation of collagen fibers by the epithelium has been observed in developing embryos.[2,6] Poor adhesion of the epithelium to the underlying connective tissue in pathologic problems is caused by the failure in basement membrane formation of the epithelial cells rather than by any abnormality of the basement membrane itself. Destruction of Bowman's layer occurs in keratoconus. Degenerative changes occur in and around Bowman's layer, especially in calcification of the entire thickness of the layer.

Bowman's layer is often said to be resistant to trauma, offering a barrier to invasion of the cornea by microorganisms and tumor cells. The layer cannot be detached from the stroma into which it imperceptibly blends. Bowman's layer is considered to have no regenerative capacity when it is damaged; a thin layer, with a fine structure identical to that of Bowman's membrane, is formed during wound healing. However, this secondary type of layer does not regain its original thickness.

Stroma

The stroma, which constitutes about 90% of the cornea, consists primarily of collagen fibers, stromal cells, and ground substance. It is well known that the bundles of collagen fibers are arranged into lamellae parallel to the tear surface (Fig. 1-8, A). The collagen bundles in the anterior zone are small and neither as clearly defined nor as regular in size and arrangement as those found in the posterior portion of the stroma. Interlacing lamellae cross each other at right angles in a highly regular fashion, and layers of lamellae run parallel to each other and to the surface of the cornea (Fig. 1-8, A). Each lamella runs the full length of the cornea and is made up of a multitude of collagen fibers. The layered arrangement of the fibers facilitates lamellar dissection of the cornea. The collagen fibrils account for about 80% of the dry weight of the cornea; the ground

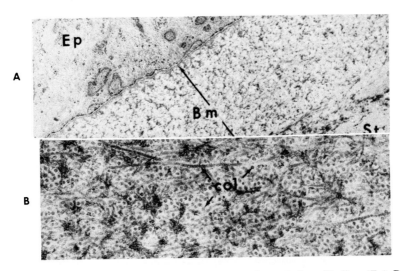

Fig. 1-6. A, Bowman's layer *(Bm)* is noncellular layer seen beneath the epithelium *(Ep)*. **B,** Short and fine collagen fibril material *(col)* intermingling in Bowman's layer. (From McTigue, J.W., Goldman, J.N., Fine, B.S., and Kuwabara, T.: Clinical application of electron microscopy of the cornea: a course, Chicago, 1968, American Academy of Ophthalmology and Otolaryngology.)

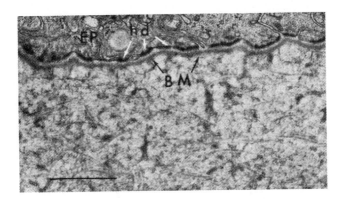

Fig. 1-7. Basement membrane *(BM)* is made up of fine granular material and extends into Bowman's layer to form fine fibrils. Hemidesmosomes *(hd)* are noted. Basal epithelial cell is also seen *(EP)*. (From Kuwabara, T.: Fine structure of the eye, ed. 2, Boston, 1970, Howe Laboratory of Ophthalmology, Harvard Medical School.)

substance, for about 15%; and cellular elements, for only about 5%. The collagen fibers of the corneal stroma are uniform and small, about 250 to 300 Å in length. The fibers show bandings very similar to other collagen fibers. Cross section reveals that the individual fiber is made up of several subunits or extremely fine fibrils (Fig. 1-8, *B*). In addition, one may find filaments that are 15 Å in diameter and about 200 Å in length distributed among the collagen fibers; these filaments appear to be precursors of collagen fiber.

The ground substance surrounding the collagen fibers is rich in mucopolysaccharide. In swollen corneas the volume of the ground substance increases, but the individual collagen fiber size does not change.

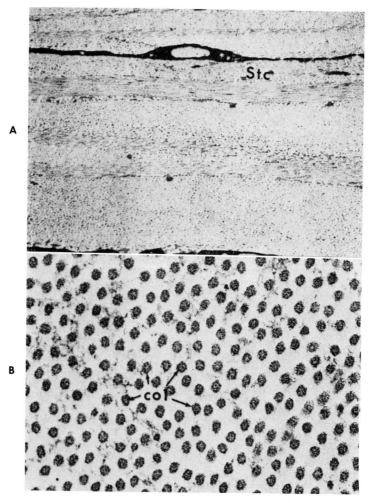

Fig. 1-8. A, Corneal stroma consists of regular arrangement of collagen fibrils parallel to cell surface. **B,** Regularity of 300 Å diameter collagen fiber *(col)* is noted. *Stc,* Stromal cells. (From McTigue, J.W., Goldman, J.N., Fine, B.S., and Kuwabara, T.: Clinical application of electron microscopy of the cornea: a course, Chicago, 1968, American Academy of Ophthalmology and Otolaryngology.)

The keratocyte is a large flat cell with a number of large processes that extend out from beyond the cell body in a satellite fashion (Fig. 1-9). The cells are seen between packed collagen lamellae; the tips of the processes touch neighboring cells. The cytoplasm contains microorganelles, microtubules, some lysosomes, glycogen particles, lipid particles, and various inclusion bodies (Fig. 1-9). The keratocyte, which is believed to be derived from the embryologic mesodermal cells, exhibits certain changes that differentiate it from the fibroblast, which normally contains numerous rough endoplasmic reticula. The cell membrane of the normal keratocyte is usually smooth. However, in some cells there is a specific type of membrane specialization of the keratocyte; thus one may see a hemidesmosome-like structure. Nevertheless, no direct connection exists

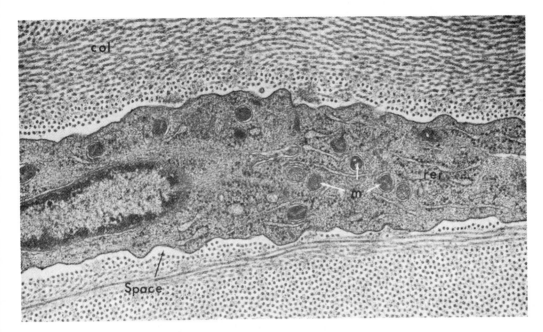

Fig. 1-9. Keratocyte is rich in rough endoplasmic reticulum *(rer)* and mitochondria *(m)*. Small space is seen around keratocyte as it borders stromal collagen *(col)*. (From Kuwabara, T.: Fine structure of the eye, ed. 2, Boston, 1970, Howe Laboratory of Ophthalmology, Harvard Medical School.)

between the plasma cell membrane and collagen fibers. Minute extracellular spaces around the keratocyte are connected to each other along the meshwork of processes of keratocytes; this network is an avenue for tissue fluid and particles within the corneal stroma.

The keratocyte can change its shape on stimulation, producing excess abundant basal lamina in endothelial dystrophy. The keratocyte migrates to a wound area; fibroblast-like cells in fresh stromal wound areas are migrated keratocytes. The migrated cells contribute to the scar formation by proliferation and filament production.[16] In pathologic conditions the keratocyte may exhibit inclusions, such as lipid droplets. The keratocyte accumulates products of defective metabolism in such conditions as cystinosis,[17] multiple myeloma,[15] and diseases of carbohydrate and lipid metabolism, as is noted in mucopolysaccharidosis[8] and sphingolipidosis.

In addition to the keratocyte, wandering cells may be seen when they invade the corneal stroma. Small numbers of invading cells, including polymorphonuclear leukocytes, plasma cells, and histiocytes, are seen in the normal stroma, located between the lamellae of the collagen fibers. Lysosomes for digestion of phagocytosed substances are stored in numerous histiocytes of the stroma rather than in the keratocytes.

Descemet's membrane

Descemet's membrane is 10 μm thick and is a true cuticular membrane that covers the posterior portion of the stroma and separates it from the endothelium (Fig. 1-10). In

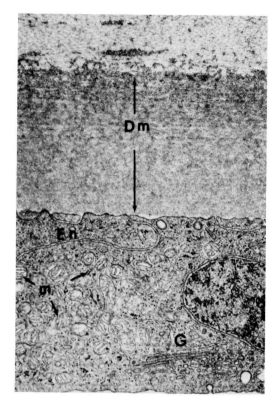

Fig. 1-10. Descemet's membrane *(Dm)* is basement membrane of endothelial cells *(En)*. It is rich in Golgi apparatus *(G)* and mitochondria *(m)*. (From McTigue, J.W., Goldman, J.N., Fine, B.S., and Kuwabara, T.: Clinical application of electron microscopy of the cornea: a course, Chicago, 1968, American Academy of Ophthalmology and Otolaryngology.)

contrast to Bowman's layer, Descemet's membrane is easily detached from the stroma and after injury regenerates readily. It can proliferate over the angle of the anterior chamber and onto the iris and can also form the endothelial warts and hyaline ridges seen in a number of pathologic problems. It generally thickens with age. Schwalbe's ring, an accumulation of circular collagen fibrils, marks the termination of Descemet's membrane. Descemet's membrane is divided into an anterior and a posterior zone. The anterior zone is known as the banded zone; the posterior zone consists of more newly formed basal lamina substance that is homogeneously fine. In some pathologic conditions metallic substances are deposited in Descemet's membrane, for example, copper in Wilson's disease and silver in argyrosis. The endothelial cell, when stimulated by inflammation, trauma, or genetic disturbances, produces excess basal lamina, causing a thickening of Descemet's membrane and Descemet wart formation. Thus the multilayers of Descemet's membrane can be seen and are often demonstrated in the cornea with recurrent disease.

Endothelium

The endothelium is derived from mesoderm; the endothelial cells differentiate from the invading mesodermal cells from the limbal area at the earliest developmental stage.

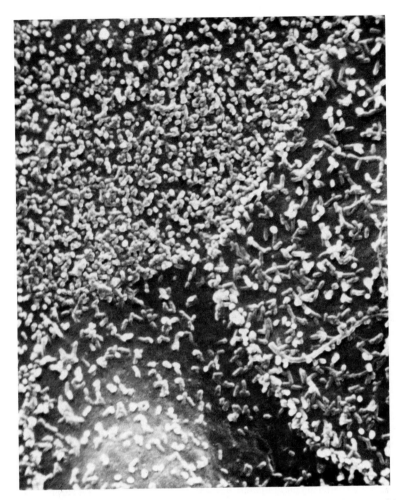

Fig. 1-11. Microvilli noted on endothelial cells in pathologic states. (From Grayson, M.: Trans. Am. Ophthalmol. Soc. **72:**517, 1974.)

A single layer of flat cells borders Descemet's membrane, which is the basement membrane of the endothelial cells. The endothelial cells, more cuboidal in shape and about 10 μm in height at birth, with age average out to about 4 μm. These cells exhibit great metabolic activity, as noted by the fact that the cytoplasm contains numerous large mitochondria, small rough endoplasmic reticula, Golgi apparatus, and free ribosomes (Fig. 1-10). One may occasionally see a microvillus, but usually the microvilli when present denote some pathologic state (Fig. 1-11). The endothelial cell shows great change in response to minor and major pathologic stimulation. The endothelial cells behind the corneal wound area may become swollen and develop numerous protrusions immediately after the injury to the more superficial stroma.

Damaged endothelial cells slide over the injured endothelial area, acting as a reparative element. Generally in the adult stage there is no mitotic activity. Some endothelial cells die throughout life, resulting in a gradual decrease of the endothelial population with age. As this occurs, the neighboring cells use their capability of spreading out to

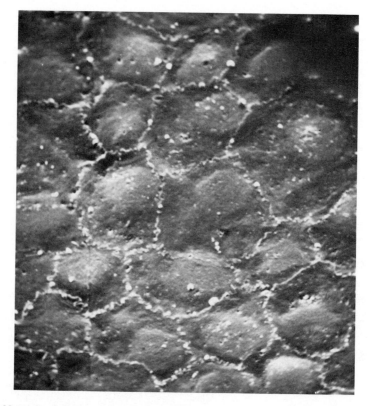

Fig. 1-12. Normal orderly arrangement of endothelium with clear-cut cell borders. (From Grayson, M.: Trans. Am. Ophthalmol. Soc. **72:**517, 1974.)

cover the vacant area. On scanning electron microscopy, one may see the normal flat surface cells with sharply demarcated borders (Fig. 1-12). This appearance is markedly disrupted in pathologic states such as Fuchs' dystrophy (Fig. 1-13), in which the cell has "collapsed," the border is irregular, and the nucleus stands out as a white, raised fluffy structure.

CORNEAL NERVES

The cornea is supplied by the first division of the trigeminal nerve by way of the long and short ciliary, the lacrimal, and the nasal ciliary branches. The anterior ciliary nerves course forward to the limbal area and enter the sclera from the perichoroidal space a few millimeters posterior to the limbus. Here a pericorneal plexus is formed by the anastomosis of the anterior ciliary nerves, made up of both long and short ciliary nerve fibers, and episcleral and conjunctival nerves, which are branches from the lacrimal and nasal ciliary nerves. From the pericorneal plexus about 70 nerve trunks pierce the cornea at the middle one third of its thickness. The nerves lose their myelin sheath after traversing 0.5 mm to 2.5 mm into the cornea and then continue as transparent axis cylinders. The nerves will find their way beneath Bowman's layer and eventually pierce this layer to terminate among the epithelial cells. The nerve trunks, which show dichotomous division in many instances, can proceed into the deep stroma, dividing in a manner similar to

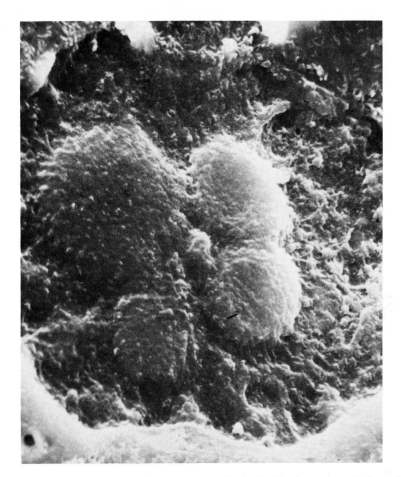

Fig. 1-13. Disorderly arrangement of endothelial cells in Fuch's dystrophy with irregular cell borders. Note "collapse" of cell and irregular fluffy cell nucleus. (From Grayson, M.: Trans. Am. Ophthalmol. Soc. **72:**517, 1974.)

that of the superficial fibers ending among the stromal cells. After sectioning of the nerve trunks at the limbus, there is a migration of neighboring intact nerves into the denervated area; regeneration of damaged fibers usually takes about 9 months.

LIMBUS

The limbus is the semitransparent, vascularized transition zone between the conjunctiva and sclera on one side and the cornea on the other. Clinically the peripheral margin blends inconspicuously with the sclera, and the central extent of the limbus is reasonably defined by a line joining the ends of Bowman's layer and Descemet's membrane.

Several changes occur at the limbus. The epithelium of the cornea is continuous with the respective structures of the conjunctiva but at the limbus becomes thicker, containing about 12 cell layers. The epithelium projects downward between the subepithelial papillae, which appear as white, radially oriented lines crossing the limbus every 1 to 2 mm. These clinically visible projections are known as the *palisades of Vogt*. These

Table 1-1. Precorneal tear film

Layer and structure	Location	Comment
Innermost layer: mucin secretion		
Goblet cells	Conjunctival epithelium	Primary function is lubrication of cornea
Crypts of Henle	In conjunctiva near superior margin of upper tarsus and inferior margin of lower tarsus	
Middle layer: lacrimal secretion		
Lacrimal gland	Lacrimal fossa, superior temporal orbit, orbital and palpebral lobes; ducts enter cul-de-sac in superior temporal area	Measuring tear secretions in anesthetized eye with Schirmer strips gives information concerning glands of Krause and Wolfring, since these are the primary basal secretors; reflex stimulation causes lacrimal gland secretion
Accessory lacrimal glands of Krause	Upper and lower conjunctival fornices	
Accessory lacrimal glands of Wolfring	Adjacent to upper margin of upper tarsus and one below lower tarsus	
Superficial layer: oil secretion		
Meibomian glands	About 25 in upper tarsus, 20 in lower tarsus; empty onto lid margin	Oily secretions prevent escape of lacrimal fluid over lid margins
Glands of Zeis	Palpebral margin of each eyelid; empty directly onto lid margin	
Glands of Moll	Roots of eyelashes; empty into hair follicles	

From Grayson, M., and Keates, R.H.: Manual of diseases of the cornea, Boston, 1969, Little, Brown & Co.

structures may be important in corneal epithelial regeneration. If they are totally destroyed, as in cases of alkali burns, there is a reduced tendency for epithelial regeneration. At the limbus, the stroma of the cornea loses its transparency, and the stromal lamellae lose their orderly arrangement. The individual collagen fibers also become varied in diameter and acquire the characteristics of the sclera. Bowman's layer terminates in a rounded end at the central margin of the limbus and gives rise to fibrous connective tissue, in which the subepithelial papillae develop in the zone of the palisade. The termination of Bowman's layer is clinically demarcated at the apices of the limbal blood vessels.

No lymphatic channels exist in the cornea proper. Channels for passage of fluid, however, are seen around the keratocyte. It has also been observed that in pathologic corneas, such as those which become highly vascularized, lymphatic channels may be established that connect with the lymphatics of the conjunctiva.

PRECORNEAL TEAR FILM

The integrity of the cornea largely depends on the precorneal tear film. This layer, of course, is of great clinical significance and is concerned in maintaining lubrication of the wetting surface of the cornea. The integrity of this particular layer is important to the nature of the epithelial cells, as well as to good visual acuity. Table 1-1 outlines the various layers of the tear film.

REFERENCES

1. Carroll, J.M., and Kuwabara, T.: Ocular pemphigus: an electron microscopic study of conjunctival and corneal epithelium, Arch. Ophthalmol. **80:**683, 1968.
2. Dodson, J.W., and Hay, E.D.: Secretion of collagen by corneal epithelium. II. Effect of the underlying substratum on secretion and polymerization of epithelial products, J. Exp. Zool. **189:**51, 1974.
3. Dohlman, C.H.: The function of the epithelium in health and disease, Invest. Ophthalmol. **10:**383, 1971.
4. Goldman, J., and Kuwabara, T.: Histopathology of corneal edema, Int. Ophthalmol. Clin. **8:**561, 1968.
5. Harding, C.V., Bagchi, M., Weinsieder, A., and Peters, V.: A comparative study of corneal epithelial cell surfaces utilizing the scanning electron microscope, Invest. Ophthalmol. **13:**906, 1974.
6. Hay, E.D., and Dodson, J.W.: Secretion of collagen by corneal epithelium. I. Morphology of the collagenous products produced by isolated epithelia grown on frozen-killed lens, J. Cell Biol. **57:**190, 1973.
7. Hoffman, F.: The surface of epithelial cells of the cornea under the scanning electron microscope, Ophthalmol. Res. **3:**207, 1972.
8. Kenyon, K.R.: Ocular ultrastructure of inherited metabolic disease. In Goldberg, M.F., editor: Genetic and metabolic eye disease, Boston, 1974, Little, Brown & Co.
9. Kuwabara, T.: Structure and function of the superficial corneal epithelium, presented at the Twenty-eighth Annual Meeting of the Electron-microscopy Society of America, 1970.
10. Kuwabara, T.: Surface structure of the eye tissue, presented at the Third Illinois Institute of Technology Research Conference, 1970.
11. Kuwabara, T.: Current concepts in anatomy and histopathology of the cornea: contact and intraocular lens, Med. J. **4:**101, 1978.
12. Kuwabara, T., Perkins, D.G., and Cogan, D.G.: Sliding of the epithelium in experimental corneal wounds, Invest. Ophthalmol. **15:**4, 1976.
13. Pfister, R.R.: The normal surface of corneal epithelium–scanning electron microscopic study, Invest. Ophthalmol. **12:**654, 1973.
14. Pfister, R.R., and Burnstein, N.: The effects of ophthalmic drugs, vehicles, and preservatives on corneal epithelium: a scanning electron microscope study, Invest. Ophthalmol. **15:**246, 1976.
15. Pinkerton, R.M.H., and Robertson, D.M.: Corneal and conjunctival changes in dysproteinemia, Invest. Ophthalmol. **8:**357, 1969.
16. Robb, R.M., and Kuwabara, T.: Corneal wound healing. I. The movement of polymorphonuclear leukocytes into corneal wounds, Arch. Ophthalmol. **68:**632, 1962.
17. Sanderson, P.O., Kuwabara, T., Stark, W.J., Wong, V.G., and Collins, E.M.: Cystinosis: a clinical, histopathologic and ultrastructural study, Arch. Ophthalmol. **91:**270, 1974.

2 History-taking hints and fundamentals of external disease examination

HISTORY TAKING

It is most important for the ophthalmologist to have a comprehensive understanding of external diseases, since persons with these conditions constitute at least one fifth of the patients seen in a private practice.

Well-organized and informative histories afford clues to diagnoses. Specific forms (Figs. 2-1 and 2-2) may be used to facilitate the procedure of comprehensive external disease history taking. The following points will emphasize these concepts.

Complaints

The complaint of decreased vision in the morning, improving in the afternoon, usually connotes intermittent corneal edema.

A sensation of dryness of the eyes, often associated with a dry mouth, may exhibit a keratoconjunctivitis sicca and, with the latter, be part of a collagen or immune disease. The eye complaint is usually worse in the afternoon; in addition, keratoconjunctivitis sicca is aggravated in a dry atmosphere. The dry eye is in essence a compromised one, since there is a decrease in lysozymes and beta lysins, and, in addition, the mechanical flushing of tears is no longer present, which may in itself encourage bacterial growth by stagnation.

Foreign body sensation and pain may be a repetitive complaint and may signal a recur-

WISHARD MEMORIAL HOSPITAL	Indianapolis, Indiana	INDIANA UNIVERSITY HOSPITALS

Revised 1-75	CORNEA - EXTERNAL DISEASE HISTORY	M6322600 WMH61-704

DATE _____ REFERRED BY _____

COMPLAINTS: OD ☐   OS ☐   OU ☐

Decr. Vision	☐	Photophobia	☐	Discharge	☐	Other ☐
Dryness	☐	Itching	☐	Lids Sealed	☐	
F.B. Sensation	☐	Redness	☐	Opacity	☐	
Burning	☐	Tearing	☐	Mass	☐	
Pain	☐	Epiphora	☐	Blepharitis	☐	

☐ In-Patient   ☐ Out-Patient

PRESENT ILLNESS:

Trigger: ☐

Worsened By: ☐

Improved By: ☐

Daily Variation: ☐

Seasonal Variation: ☐

Adenopathy: ☐

MEDICATIONS:

EYE: GENERAL:

PAST HISTORY:

ALLERGY:

FAMILY HISTORY:

_____ M.D.
SIGNATURE

MED. REC. COPY	CORNEA-EXTERNAL DISEASE HISTORY	B—70

B-CLIN. NOTES	E-LAB	G-X-RAY	K-DIAGNOSTIC	M-SURGERY	Q-THERAPY	T-ORDERS	W-NURSING	Y-MISC.

Fig. 2-1. Comprehensive history-taking chart aids in establishing complete background of external disease entity.

MARION COUNTY GENERAL HOSPITAL	Indianapolis, Indiana	INDIANA UNIVERSITY HOSPITALS

Revised 1-75	CORNEA - EXTERNAL DISEASE EXAMINATION	M6322500 MCGH61-705	

DATE:

☐ In-Patient   ☐ Out-Patient

RIGHT EYE | LEFT EYE

VISION SC	
VISION CC	
ADENOPATHY	
LIDS	
DISCHARGE	
CONJUNCTIVA	
CORNEA	

Sensation
R____ L____

Thickness
R____ L____

SCHIRMER	S_____mm C_____mm	S_____mm C_____mm
TEAR FILM	BKUP SEC	BKUP SEC
CHAMBER	
IRIS - PUPIL	
LENS	
I. O. P.	
FUNDUS	
OTHER	
SCRAPING	
DIAGNOSIS	
REC.	

SIGNATURE _____ M.D.

MED. REC. COPY

CORNEA-EXTERNAL DISEASE EXAMINATION B-70

B-CLIN. NOTES	E-LAB	G-X-RAY	K-DIAGNOSTIC	M-SURGERY	Q-THERAPY	T-ORDERS	W-NURSING	Y-MISC.

Fig. 2-2. Complete form for physical examination of external eye allows for thorough coverage of external disease entities.

rent erosion problem of the cornea. The symptoms are usually worse on awakening. A burning sensation is often associated with the drying syndrome, early breakup of the tear film, decreased blinking, and exposure and microerosion of the corneal epithelium.

Photophobia is a prominent complaint seen in phlyctenulosis, exposure to ultraviolet light (sunlamp), severe keratoconjunctivitis, recurrent corneal erosions, and viral, fungal, and bacterial keratitis. It may be observed in some systemic syndromes such as Sjögren's syndrome and Richner-Hanhart syndrome, or it may be seen in some intracranial lesions.

Itching, especially of the inner canthi, is an important complaint to note because of its association with allergic states. Seasonal variation is usually a hallmark of external disease with an allergic etiologic factor.

Redness of the conjunctiva and discharge are always important patient complaints. If the eyelids are sealed in the morning, a polymorphonuclear response should be suspected; watery discharge is suggestive of adenoviral infection; purulent discharge is suggestive of bacterial and chlamydial disease; and a mucous, ropy discharge is highly suggestive of allergic or keratoconjunctivitis sicca factors.

Epiphora is a common complaint; the patient may state that the tears "run down the face," and, of course, it is most annoying because the patient is constantly wiping the eyes, which in itself is irritating to the skin of the lids. Reflex tearing is usually a part of recurrent erosion syndrome, but other irritative agents and conditions should be sought.

If there is a complaint of discharge from the eye and on examination pouting of the canaliculi and swelling in the lacrimal sac area are noted, complete investigation of the lacrimal drainage apparatus is required.

The patient may complain of a lid or conjunctival mass, which can be caused by infection, granulomas, cysts, neoplasms, or foreign bodies.

Observation of a pigmentation of lid, conjunctiva, or cornea should be recorded and inquiry made as to how long the pigmentation has been present. Photographs of these lesions at varying intervals should also be a part of the documentation for increase in size, pigmentation, or vascularization. Changes of unusual intensity may suggest malignant transformation.

The complaint of redness and crusting of the lid margins is common. This can be seen in both the young and the elderly patient. Acute and chronic blepharitis can and often does lead to severe corneal problems.

Pain, as well as its type, distribution, onset, length of duration, frequency, and conditions that aggravate it, should be investigated.

The nutritional status of the patient is important, particularly if associated with deficiency of vitamin A and protein. Faddist and other dietary indiscretions can lead to such conditions. Hypervitaminosis may also cause corneal problems. A good history should include nutritional investigation.

Injury

Injury, present or past, and its nature must be thoroughly investigated. Inquiry as to whether the injury occurred on the job or in the garden is important. If the cornea was struck with vegetable matter and subsequently develops an infiltrate or ulcer, fungal keratitis must be high on the list of suspected etiologic agents.

Trigger mechanisms

When taking the history, one should inquire about trigger mechanisms associated with the patient's complaint. Seasonal variation and even daily variation of symptoms aid in making a diagnosis. Allergic diseases may exhibit seasonal exacerbations. Endothelial dystrophies will produce greater visual complaints in the morning. "Sicca" problems are aggravated in the afternoon. These latter two diseases are also affected by the degree of humidity.

Medications

It is most important to note what medications, both topical and systemic, are used and for how long they have been used. It is also vital to determine if the patient is taking a combination of medications. The preservative present in any one particular medication should be known; for example, thimerosal can cause an allergic conjunctivitis or toxic follicular reaction and epithelial keratitis; benzalkonium chloride can cause a toxic papillary response and epithelial keratitis; phenylmercuric acetate or phenylmercuric nitrate can cause a calcific band keratopathy as well as mercurialentis; and drugs such as idoxuridine, atropine, gentamicin, and miotics can cause follicular responses as well as involve the corneal epithelium. Topical anesthetic agents, if used often and for long periods, may result in several corneal changes. Pigmentation of the conjunctiva and cornea can be caused by epinephrine products, phenothiazines, metallic agents, and systemic diseases. The use of topical and systemic steroids must be thoroughly investigated, since these medications can and do cause serious corneal disease, cataracts, and glaucoma in responders when imprudently used.

Medications such as practolol and miotics may result in scarring and symblepharon formation.

Past history

The patient may have been exposed to therapeutic radiation for some neoplastic problem around the lids and eyes that can contribute to keratinization, cicatrization, and telangiectasia of the conjunctiva as well as to drying of the eye and epithelial keratopathy.

Investigation of past history of systemic disease should include skin, cardiovascular, neurologic, mucous membrane, collagen, lipid, protein, carbohydrate, and immune diseases. Many external disease problems are associated with these entities, as will be seen in the ensuing chapters. Investigation as to whether the host is a compromised one is important. Opportunistic infections, particularly from herpes simplex virus, fungi, and bacteria, should always be kept in mind when one sees a patient with corneal ulceration.

Without doubt, the family history is most important. A number of conditions exhibit external disease on a hereditary basis.

Thus no external ocular problem should be handled without credence given to the patient's general health and known response to infection, family history, and all factors listed previously.

CLINICAL EXAMINATION

Vision should always be taken with and without pinhole test and with correction if the patient wears glasses.

Skin condition

The condition of the patient's skin is vital to a complete external disease examination. It is often helpful in correlating rosacea, eczema, and psoriasis with the external disease of the eye. These diseases are often missed, and problems of the conjunctiva and cornea resulting from them are thus often overlooked.

Lymphadenopathy

Investigation for lymphadenopathy is an important part of the external disease ex-amination. One should look for palpable as well as grossly visible preauricular nodes. Small palpable preauricular nodes are seen in the following conditions:
1. Trachoma
2. Vaccinia
3. Inclusion conjunctivitis
4. Primary herpes simplex
5. Adenoviral conjunctivitis
6. Hyperacute conjunctivitis (*Neisseria* species)
7. Lid conditions such as hordeola, impetigo, and lid cellulitis
8. Dacryoadenitis
9. Toxic reaction to such drugs as idoxuridine
10. Newcastle disease

It is rare for a routine bacterial conjunctivitis to produce a preauricular node. The only exception is hyperacute conjunctivitis.

Grossly visible preauricular nodes are usually associated with localized granulomas or follicular conjunctiva response and may be seen in the following conditions:
1. Leptothrix
2. Syphilis
3. Lymphogranuloma venereum
4. Tularemia
5. Sarcoid
6. Tuberculosis
7. Coccidioidomycosis
8. Foreign body granuloma
9. Mononucleosis

One of the most common causes of grossly visible preauricular nodes is infection of the conjunctival sac with leptothrix. This organism is found in the mouth of cats and frequently in the human mouth *(Leptothrix buccalis)*. The conjunctiva may or may not show a granuloma. Small ulcerations develop on the granuloma. A systemic response occurs with low-grade fever; the organism is located in the subconjunctival area and cannot be cultured. The only way the organism can be seen is by performing biopsy of the granuloma and studying hematoxylin and eosin stains with serial sections. When areas of macrophages and necrosis are encountered, this section is then studied with Verhoeff's leptothrix stain. The biopsy may be curative in itself. The natural course of the disease is usually 3 months, although this may be shortened by the use of broad-band antibiotics and penicillin.

It appears that it is unwise to sleep with cats. The disease is not considered to be transmittable from one person to another in the family. Although the etiologic factors of cat-scratch fever have never really been proved, since the organism has not been isolated, the leptothrix organism may possibly cause cat-scratch disease. Thus it is very important that the physician, in taking the history, ask whether there are pets in the household, especially when seeing conjunctival and corneal conditions with enlarged preauricular glands and correlating all the facts and findings.

Blepharitis

One of the most common causes of chronic red eye is staphylococcal infection of the lids.

A fundamental clinical sign of *staphylococcal blepharitis* is the collarette. Collarettes are composed of fibrin, which is lifted from the lids as the lash grows out. The fibrin sheath is pierced by the lash.

A small ulcerated area around the base of the lash may be seen. Chronic staphylococcal blepharitis, which can cause inferior corneal epithelial keratitis, may exhibit other lid margin problems such as broken lashes, loss of lashes, and thickening of the lid margins. Seborrheic dermatitis may also affect the lid margins, which often are secondarily infected with staphylococcal organisms; of course, under these circumstances the cornea itself can also be affected. An acutely inflamed eye can result from a hypersensitivity reaction to the staphylococcal toxin; marginal infiltrates can occur because of hypersensitivity reaction to this toxin; and small punctate epithelial staining in the inferior of the cornea is frequently seen in staphylococcal blepharitis. A micropannus or a gross pannus can occur in the cornea secondarily to chronic staphylococcal blepharitis. The pannus, of course, is more likely to occur inferiorly; however, superior pannus certainly develops if there is any significant amount of blepharitis on the upper lid. Phlyctenules are commonly associated with staphylococcal blepharitis; phlyctenulosis is discussed at length in Chapter 14.

The ulcerative type of *angular blepharitis* can be caused by *Staphylococcus aureus* and also by the *Moraxella* species. A differential diagnosis of ulcerative blepharitis involves a number of conditions that can cause corneal problems:

1. Candidiasis
2. Herpes zoster
3. Vaccinia
4. Dermatophytes
5. Discoid lupus

The clinical findings of *seborrheic blepharitis* are the large greasy scales (scurf) that stick to the lashes. The lid margins may be erythematous, and there is some seborrhea of the face, chest, and eyebrow region. Budding yeastlike organisms *(Pityrosporum ovale or P. orbiculare)* may be found, the significance of which has not been determined.

Another finding in chronic blepharitis is the presence on the cilium of *Demodex folliculorum,* a microscopic parasite. A thin tubular process, or "sleeve," extends from the skin up over the proximal end of the lash for about 0.5 mm. The diagnosis can be made by removing the lash and placing it on the side with a drop of oil. One can see the parasite as an eight-legged, cigar-shaped organism (Chapter 9). Pediculosis can also affect the lid margins and is caused by the pubic louse *(Phthirus pubis).*

Staphylococcal infection of the sebaceous gland opening into the hair follicles of the cilium (glands of Zeis) is termed an *external hordeolum.* An *internal hordeolum* is an acute infection of the meibomian glands and has often been referred to as an acute chalazion. The causative organism usually is the staphylococcus, although other organisms may be responsible. In contrast to this, a *chalazion* is a granulomatous infection of the meibomian or eyelid glands and is associated not with an infectious process but with an inflammatory process that does not result in any corneal disease.

Chemosis and telangiectasia

Chemosis can occur in the hyperacute infections of gonorrhea and epidemic keratoconjunctivitis. Systemic problems, such as those of Graves' thyroid exophthalmopathy of the conjunctiva, can result in chemosis.

Telangiectasia and sludging of the circulation of the conjunctival vessels can occur in a number of systemic diseases. Telangiectasia of conjunctival vessels is seen in ataxic telangiectasia, in diabetes mellitus, and in late reaction to radiation. Sludging with conjunctival vessels occurs in multiple myeloma and sickle cell disease. Large trunk vessels in the conjunctiva of venous engorgement may be seen in cavernous sinus thrombosis.

Papillae and follicles

Papillae and follicles in the conjunctiva must be identified and differentiated to help solve problems in inflammatory external disease. Papillae can occur in conjunctival inflammation in which the conjunctiva is fastened down to the tarsus (tarsal conjunctiva). Giant papillae result from the breakdown of fine fibrous strands that normally attach the conjunctiva to the tarsus. With the breakdown of the attachments, large papillae develop on the tarsus. Giant papillae can be seen in vernal conjunctivitis and keratoconjunctivitis of atopic dermatitis. Giant papillae of the upper tarsus may also be seen in wearers of soft contact lens.

Follicles may be seen in the normal conjunctiva more often in younger patients with no associated inflammation but in a normal state. In older patients the follicle is less prominent and may not be seen on clinical examination. The follicle represents lymphoid tissue with a germinal center. The newborn is without a follicular response for the first 3 months of life. Follicles are most easily appreciated in the lower cul-de-sac and upper tarsus. The extreme lateral and medial edges of the superior tarsus, and indeed the extreme superior edge of the upper tarsus, should rarely be used to clinically evaluate for follicles. To distinguish papillae from follicles is difficult in this area, in which follicles may be seen anyway. It is extremely important for the ophthalmologist to determine if a significant follicular response is present because the differential diagnosis of acute or chronic follicular response is specific. Differentiation can establish the diagnosis and also may aid in determining the character of the associated corneal problems.

Following are conditions in which acute follicular conjunctivitis occurs:
1. Adenoviral keratoconjunctivitis
2. Adult inclusion conjunctivitis
3. Herpes simplex (primary)
4. Enterovirus
5. Acute hemorrhagic conjunctivitis
6. Newcastle disease
7. Acute trachoma

Chronic follicular conjunctivitis occurs in these conditions:
1. Adult inclusion conjunctivitis
2. Trachoma
3. Toxic reaction to drugs
4. Molluscum
5. *Moraxella* species disease
6. Oculoglandular syndrome
7. Axenfeld's syndrome
8. Merrill-Thygeson syndrome
9. Folliculosis

Most of the preceding conditions do not show a preauricular node except for acute inclusion conjunctivitis and acute trachoma. Rarely will one see a preauricular node from the toxic reaction to drugs such as idoxuridine (IDU).

It is an error to speak of follicles of sarcoid because in effect they are not follicles but yellow-white or opaque granulomas.

It is important to look for and recognize individuals with atopic disease and vernal catarrh. Small white dots (Trantas' dots), which may occur both on the conjunctiva and on the cornea, aid in establishing the diagnosis in the allergic diseases.

Trachoma is a worldwide disease; pathognomonic of trachoma is the presence of Herbert's pits.

Scarring of the conjunctiva can occur and should be sought on the upper lid and on the bulbar conjunctiva itself; when found on the upper lid it is known as Arlt's line, which suggests trachoma. Scarring is seen in mucous membrane diseases and after membranous conjunctivitis and atopic keratoconjunctivitis.

The presence of keratin may be seen in conditions of drying, superior limbic kerato-conjunctivitis, vitamin A deficiency, and squamous neoplasia.

Membranous conjunctivitis

Both membranous and pseudomembranous conjunctivitis are striking clinical signs. Membranes usually form as a result of fibrin on the epithelial surface. Little distinction exists between pseudomembranes and true membranes, except that true membranes might leave a raw surface when peeled off and cause bleeding, thus signifying a more intense conjunctival inflammation. The most common cause of membranous conjunctivitis is probably the β-hemolytic streptococcus. However, adenoviral keratoconjunctivitis, commonly type 8, is seen as a cause of membranous conjunctivitis. Membranes can be seen in systemic disease that affects both the conjunctiva and the cornea, examples of which are Stevens-Johnson syndrome and Lyell's disease. Ligneous conjunctivitis is a special form of membranous disease discussed in Chapter 14.

Gross pannus and micropannus

In examining the cornea one should look for gross pannus or a micropannus. If a gross pannus is seen, one should consider the following:
1. Trachoma
2. Phlyctenulosis
3. Rosacea
4. Keratoconjunctivitis of atopic dermatitis
5. Soft contact lens on pathologic cornea
6. Superficial infections and inflammations

If a micropannus is visible, the following disorders are possibilities:
1. Inclusion conjunctivitis
2. Childhood trachoma
3. Staphylococcal blepharitis
4. Hard contact lens disorder
5. Superlimbic keratoconjunctivitis
6. Vernal conjunctivitis

Filamentary keratitis

Filamentary keratitis is a nonspecific clinical sign, but the specific etiologic factors can be determined when correlated with other clinical findings. Following is a list of the conditions that should be considered when filamentary keratitis occurs:
1. Superlimbic keratoconjunctivitis
2. Ptosis
3. Keratoconjunctivitis sicca
4. Prolonged occlusion in adults
5. Recurrent erosions
6. Posttrauma disorders
7. Neurotrophic keratopathy
8. Herpes simplex keratitis
9. Chronic bullous keratopathy

The filament is actually just a wedge of epithelial cells that has broken away from the cornea on one end and twisted its base and is still attached to the cornea. The pseudofilaments will consist primarily of mucus.

Corneal disease

Corneal disease may reveal interstitial vascularization, epithelial erosions, edema of the corneal epithelium with increased stromal thickness, and increased stromal relucency on slit-lamp examination.

The characteristic findings of the dystrophies and degenerations of the cornea are discussed at length in Chapters 10 and 11.

The cornea should be examined with fluorescein before the corneal sensation is tested, since this testing may leave punctate staining or even linear staining. One should never touch what appears to be an infected area of the cornea and then touch an uninvolved area of the cornea with the same testing device; always use a separate cotton applicator for each eye when there is infection. In herpes simplex keratitis the corneal sensation is decreased.

The opthalmologist should be alert for the presence of epibulbar squamous neoplasms. These may occur either on the conjunctiva or at the limbus and may extend to the corneal surface.

Fluorescein or rose bengal red dyes should be used routinely when diagnosing corneal and conjunctival diseases. Inferior staining is characteristic of staphylococcal blepharitis, exposure, and rosacea. Interpalpebral staining is characteristic of such conditions as keratoconjunctivitis sicca, medicamentosa, exposure, neurotrophic keratitis, and ultraviolet exposure. Staining in the superior portion of the cornea usually occurs in vernal catarrh, in superlimbic keratoconjunctivitis, and in the presence of a foreign body in the upper lid. Sectoral staining may occur in conditions such as trichiasis and trauma.

Tear film

Examination of the tear film is extremely important. The tear meniscus, tear breakup time, and Schirmer's and lysozyme tests may be employed to facilitate a diagnosis.

Lacrimal system

Examination should be focused next on the lacrimal system area; one should determine whether pouting of the punctum exists and also if there is edema, inflammation, and discharge. Swelling, inflammation, and tenderness over the lacrimal sac area will indicate dacryocystitis. Bacterial and fungal organisms may occur in the lacrimal system and occasionally, in the proper setting, result in severe corneal disease.

Following are the organisms most likely to cause canaliculitis:
1. *Actinomyces israelii*
2. *Candida albicans*
3. *Aspergillus niger*

Organisms most likely to cause dacryocystitis follow:

Acute dacryocystitis
  Staphylococcus aureus
  β-Hemolytic streptococcus
Chronic dacryocystitis
  Streptococcus pneumoniae
  Haemophilus influenzae

3   Congenital anomalies

Many of the lesions seen in the cornea and anterior segment are a result of developmental alterations. This chapter describes the more commonly occurring congenital anomalies. It is essential to recognize these problems to separate them from dystrophic and other acquired diseases.

POSTERIOR EMBRYOTOXON[1,2] (Figs. 3-1 and 3-2)

This entity is a thickened and centrally displaced anterior border ring of Schwalbe. Schwalbe's ring consists of collagen and is located on the posterior peripheral portion of the cornea, at the level of Descemet's membrane and just peripheral to its termination, running circumferentially around the cornea. Schwalbe's ring is visible as a relucent irregular ridge, about 0.5 to 2 mm central to the limbus, occurring in about 15% of normal eyes.[11] It is seen more often temporally than nasally. Superiorly and inferiorly the anterior extension of the sclera often hides the ring. Schwalbe's ring may form a complete circle studded with pigment clumps; occasionally it is dislocated and hangs in the angle area. The term *posterior embryotoxon* may be used for variants as well as extremely prominent rings of Schwalbe that are obviously abnormal. Posterior embryotoxon is often transmitted as an autosomal dominant trait; the eye otherwise usually is normal but may be associated with cornea plana, corectopia, and aniridia. It is associated with a number of corneal problems that are, in themselves, part of systemic syndromes.

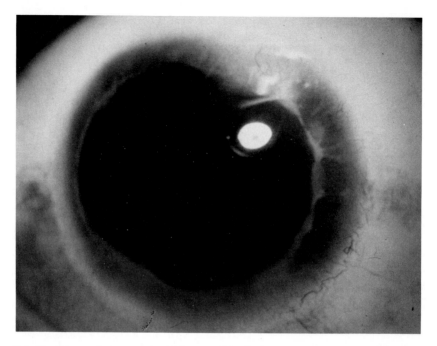

Fig. 3-1. Posterior embryotoxon is thick, centrally displaced anterior border ring of Schwalbe *(arrow)*.

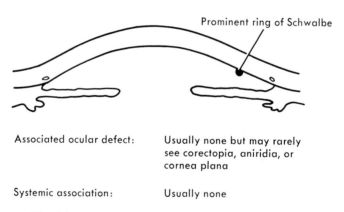

Prominent ring of Schwalbe

Associated ocular defect: Usually none but may rarely see corectopia, aniridia, or cornea plana

Systemic association: Usually none

Fig. 3-2. Posterior embryotoxon in otherwise normal eye.

AXENFELD'S ANOMALY AND SYNDROME (Fig. 3-3)

In this entity, iris strands extend across the angle to insert into a prominent Schwalbe's ring.[34] About 50% of the patients with prominent Schwalbe's ring and attached iris strand develop glaucoma, usually the juvenile type (Axenfeld's syndrome).[18,19] Skeletal anomalies may be present, such as hypertelorism, facial asymmetry, and on occasion hypoplastic shoulder.[8] Prominent iris processes with anterior iris insertions into Schwalbe's ring may be seen in a number of syndromes that are associated with congenital glaucoma, for example, phakomatoses and Marfan's, Lowe's, Turner's, Pierre Robin, Hallermann-Streiff, and Rubinstein-Taybi syndromes.

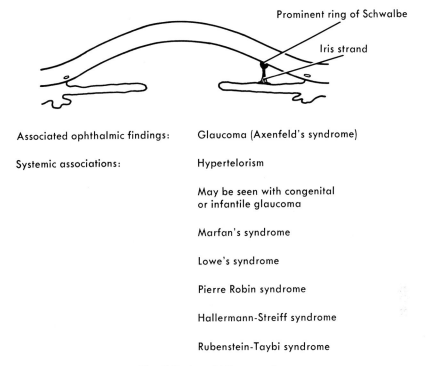

Prominent ring of Schwalbe

Iris strand

Associated ophthalmic findings: Glaucoma (Axenfeld's syndrome)

Systemic associations: Hypertelorism

May be seen with congenital
or infantile glaucoma

Marfan's syndrome

Lowe's syndrome

Pierre Robin syndrome

Hallermann-Streiff syndrome

Rubenstein-Taybi syndrome

Fig. 3-3. Axenfeld's anomaly.

RIEGER'S ANOMALY AND SYNDROME (Fig. 3-4)

This disorder is autosomal dominant in about 75% of cases,[1] with 95% penetrance and extreme variation in expressivity.[18,19] In this condition one will see a prominent Schwalbe's ring, iris strands extending to Schwalbe's ring, and a hypoplasia of the stroma.[18,19,34]

The iris sphincter is easily seen; there are no clear crypts, furrows, or collarettes, and the deep posterior iris stroma seems to be made up of delicate radial fibrils, which give the iris a gray-brown, stringy appearance. An abnormality of the shape of the pupil will be shown by 72% of the cases.[1] Glaucoma occurs in about 60% of these patients and usually begins between 5 and 30 years of age.

Maxillary hypoplasia, a broad flat nasal root, and microdontia or anodontia may occur in Rieger's syndrome (Fig. 3-5). Systemic abnormalities include malformations of the limbs and spine, cerebellohyperplasia, deafness, mental retardation, general heart defects, and Marfan's syndrome.[1] The condition that combines Rieger's anomaly plus the skeletal anomalies previously listed is known as *Rieger's syndrome.*

Rieger's syndrome has been reported in association with a presumptive isochromosome of the long arm of autosome 6.[29] Rieger's syndrome has also been reported in a child with Down's syndrome.[7]

The abnormalities listed previously occur in early development of the embryo. The paraxial mesoderm migrates centrally across the opening of the optic cup in three successive waves. The two anterior waves move beneath the surface ectoderm to form the corneal endothelium and stroma. The third wave passes in front of the lens and forms

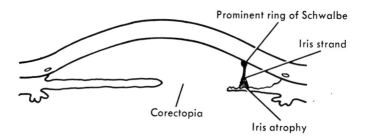

Prominent ring of Schwalbe

Iris strand

Corectopia

Iris atrophy

Associated ocular defects:	Glaucoma, corectopia, pseudopolycoria, hyaline corneal opacities in Descemet's membrane
Systemic associations:	May be present with dental, skull, facial, skeletal anomalies (Rieger's syndrome), chromosomal anomalies, and Down's syndrome

Fig. 3-4. Rieger's syndrome.

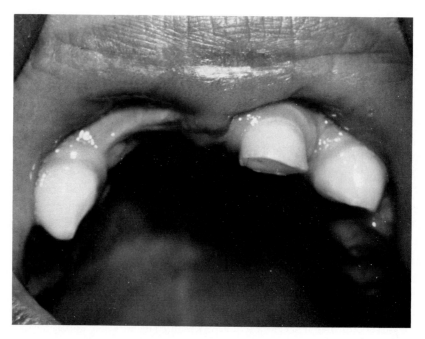

Fig. 3-5. Dental anomalies seen in Rieger's syndrome.

the superficial iris stroma and pupillary membrane. A thin slit is present as the rudimentary chamber recedes. The mesodermal cleavage is responsible for the formation of the chamber[12]; in this particular instance, a differential growth rate of the cornea and the iris and other structures causes a passive pulling apart of mesoderm, creating an anterior chamber in the remaining space.[17] Persistence of the mesodermal tissue in the angle forms the prominent Schwalbe's ring and attached iris strands. If the mesodermal wave that is responsible for the formation of the anterior iris stroma and pupillary membrane does not develop well, hyperplasia of the anterior iris stroma results.

CIRCUMSCRIBED POSTERIOR KERATOCONUS (Fig. 3-6)

Posterior circumscribed keratoconus is a localized crater defect on the posterior corneal surface, with a concavity facing toward the anterior chamber. A rare disorder exhibiting noninflammatory thinning of the cornea, it is also known by the name of keratoconus posticus circumscriptus.[35] One can see a variable stromal haze overlying the involved area. The disease is usually central, unilateral, and sporadic, although familial cases,[16] bilateral cases,[6] and posttraumatic cases have been reported. The anterior corneal surface is normal and nonprotruding. The disorder is unrelated to the usual form of keratoconus. The visual acuity is usually not affected, since the corneal refraction of light is not interfered with. Circumscribed posterior keratoconus may accompany other anterior chamber anomalies, glaucoma, and systemic abnormalities. Associated ocular findings are variable; when present, they may be seen as anterior lenticonus, aniridia, Fleischer's ring, or cleavage anomaly. Associated systemic findings are also variable and may involve hypertelorism, poorly developed nasal bridge, brachydactyly, bull neck, mental retardation, and stunted growth.

Histopathologically, Descemet's membrane and endothelium are present.[35] However, Descemet's membrane may show abnormal anterior banding, a multilayered

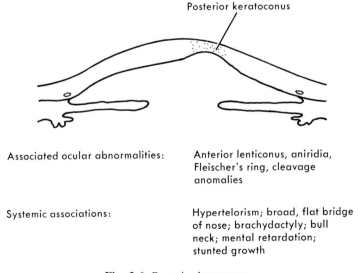

Posterior keratoconus

Associated ocular abnormalities: Anterior lenticonus, aniridia, Fleischer's ring, cleavage anomalies

Systemic associations: Hypertelorism; broad, flat bridge of nose; brachydactyly; bull neck; mental retardation; stunted growth

Fig. 3-6. Posterior keratoconus.

configuration, and posterior excrescences. These alterations suggest an early onset, probably originating prior to the fifth and sixth months of gestation.[22]

PETERS' ANOMALY (Fig. 3-7)

Peters' anomaly must be included here to differentiate it from the preceding condition. Peters' anomaly[26] may show a posterior corneal defect and a leukoma as the only presenting sign. In addition, however, one may see iris adhesions to the leukoma margin. One may also find lens apposition to the leukoma. The anteriorly displaced lens may result in a shallow anterior chamber, and the peripheral anterior synechiae, which are the result of the shallow chamber, may produce secondary glaucoma, aggravating pre-existing goniodysgenesis. Cases that demonstrate lenticular apposition may also be microphthalmic.[31-33] Systemic anomalies such as congenital heart defects, cleft lip and palate,[21] craniofacial dysplasia, and skeletal anomalies are seen.[1]

Histopathologically, a central absence of Descemet's membrane and endothelium appears over the area of the posterior defect. Iris strands, usually from the collarette, extend forward and adhere to the edge of the posterior corneal defect. The lens may be adherent to the corneal stroma with the absence of Descemet's membrane and lens capsule, or the lens may be opposed to the posterior defect and the lens capsule may be retained.[25]

Concerning the etiologic factors of von Hippel's internal corneal ulcer and Peters' anomaly, one may consider the possibilities of intrauterine inflammation for the former and developmental problems in the latter instance. Intrauterine infection may result in the keratitis, with a possible perforation of the cornea by forward movement of the iris and lens, which in turn will result in the posterior corneal defect, leukoma of the cornea, and iris and lens adhesions. Peters' anomaly in all probability results from a developmental abnormality. When studied by the light microscope, the deep stroma was shown to contain abnormal fibroblast and histiocytic cells in the organized stroma, which is more compatible with a developmental cause.

Several suggestions have been made regarding the development of Peters' anomaly. The mesoderm that forms the cornea may not migrate centrally and thus may leave a posterior corneal defect. The iris strands may result if the iris and pupillary membrane and the cornea come in contact in early development. The iris strand may remain adherent to the cornea with poor differentiation of the overlying endothelium and Descemet's membrane.[1,31] Another theory advanced is that, because of improper separation of the lens vesicle from the surface ectoderm, adhesion results between the cornea and lens, which block the ingrowth of corneal mesoderm. The lens may separate from the cornea later, leaving a posterior central defect and cataract. Townsend, Font, and Zimmerman[32] postulated a secondary anterior displacement of the lens iris diaphragm that results in leaving iridocorneal or lenticular corneal attachments or residual pieces of lens and iris on the back surface of the cornea or only isolated posterior cornea defect. Changes can also occur in the endothelium and Descemet's membrane, producing permanent adhesions.

Chromosomal aberrations such as deletion of the short arm of chromosome 4 and syndrome 18Q are associated with anterior chamber cleavage and abnormalities.

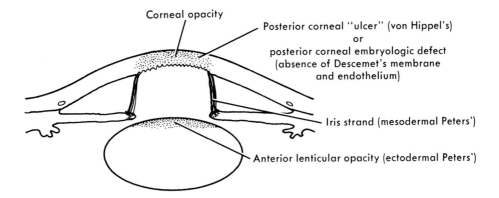

Fig. 3-7. Peters' anomaly.

Associated ocular defects: Glaucoma, microphthalmia

Systemic associations: Cleft palate, congenital heart defects,
skeletal anomalies, craniofacial dysplasia

MEGALOCORNEA

The cornea measures 13 mm or more in this condition. This corneal enlargement is not a result of glaucoma and is nonprogressive. The cornea is clear and is histologically normal. The condition is usually bilateral; in association one may see a deep anterior chamber and enlarged lens and ciliary ring.

Megalocornea may result from the failure of the anterior tips of the optic cup to grow far enough toward each other, with the large remaining space being taken up by the cornea. It might be an exaggeration of the normal tendency for the cornea to be large from embryonic life to age 7, or it may be an atavistic regression. Some investigators believe that megalocornea results from spontaneously arrested congenital glaucoma. It is transmitted as a sex-linked recessive trait; 90% of the patients are male. It is occasionally autosomal dominant and rarely autosomal recessive.

Megalocornea can be associated with ocular abnormalities such as myopia, high astigmatism, anterior embryotoxon, and Krukenberg's spindle. It is interesting that megalocornea and congenital glaucoma may occur in the same family; in addition, although rare, megalocornea may occur in one eye and congenital glaucoma in the other eye of the same patient. When the angle is observed with gonioscopic examination, prominent and anteriorly iris processes and/or a heavily pigmented meshwork is seen.

Often a patient later in life may have an ectopia lentic glaucoma caused by the dislocated lens or angle anomalies. A posterior subcapsular cataract may also be seen.

Systemic associations have been reported in Marfan's and Alport's syndromes.[5]

MICROCORNEA

Corneal diameter in a basically normal-sized eye with this condition is usually less than 10 mm. If the entire eye is small, the term *microphthalmos* applies. The etiologic factor is probably an overgrowth of anterior tips in the optic cup that leaves less than

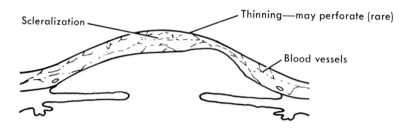

Associated ocular abnormalities: Cornea plana, cleavage anomalies,
                                      perforation of cornea,
                                      aniridia, microphthalmos

Systemic associations: Skull and facial disorders, ear
                                      deformities, deafness, polydactyly,
                                      cerebellar dysfunction,
                                      testicular abnormalities,
                                      hereditary osteo-onychodysplasia
                                      (HOOD syndrome)

Fig. 3-8. Sclerocornea.

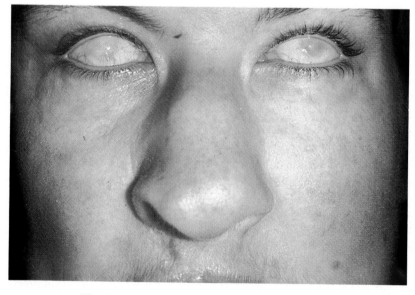

Fig. 3-9. Sclerocornea involving entire corneal area.

normal space for the cornea. The heredity is either recessive or dominant.

Associated ocular abnormalities such as a decreased corneal curvature with resultant hyperopia may occur, but often because of variations in globe length, any refractive error may exist. Glaucoma may occur in 20% of the cases in later life. Occasionally congenital glaucoma may occur in the same or other eye. Coloboma, leukoma, corectopia, microphakia, congenital cataract, microblepharon, and small orbit are present. Systemic associations include Weill-Marchesani and Ehlers-Danlos syndromes and Norrie's disease.

ANTERIOR CHAMBER CLEAVAGE SYNDROME

This entity encompasses the findings of a prominent Schwalbe's ring, iris strands to Schwalbe's ring (Axenfeld's anomaly), hypoplasia of the iris stroma, posterior corneal defect, leukoma, iris adhesions to the leukoma margins, and lens apposition to the leukoma. In addition, one might find pathologic changes in the trabeculum with resultant increased intraocular pressure. Anterior mesodermal dysgenesis has been reported to have occurred in a family of three generations who exhibited posterior polymorphous dystrophy, Rieger's anomaly, central posterior corneal defect, and cataract. In addition, systemic findings were noted in the form of microdontia in one sibling.[15]

SCLEROCORNEA (Figs. 3-8 and 3-9)

Sclerocornea is a congenital anomaly characterized by nonprogressive, noninflammatory, and unilateral or bilateral opacities of the peripheral, central, or entire cornea with deep or superficial vascularization. The disease affects males and females equally. It may be inherited as a dominant or recessive trait. Sclerocornea may be a part of the mesodermal dysgenesis syndrome. Visual acuity may be severely affected, with vision reduced to the level of light perception.

Sclerocornea is an abnormality of the second mesodermal wave, which is normally destined to become corneal stroma but forms tissue resembling sclera instead. The condition may be circumferential (peripheral sclerocornea) or involve the entire cornea (total sclerocornea) (Fig. 3-9). When the condition is total, the central cornea is slightly less opaque than the periphery. Involved areas have fine, superficial, quiet, noninflammatory vessels that are extensions of the normal sclera, episclera, and conjunctival vessels.

Many ocular abnormalities have been described in association with sclerocornea, such as cornea plana, various cleavage anomalies, aniridia, microphthalmos, nystagmus, strabismus, decreased corneal sensation, cataract, elevated intraocular pressure, and enophthalmos.[14] Corneal perforation is a possible hazard in this situation.[20]

In addition, many different systemic abnormalities have been associated with sclerocornea,[14] for example, cases of central nervous system abnormalities involving the cerebellum, brachycephaly with underdevelopment of the maxilla, and facial features seen in Hurler's disease. Cases of sclerocornea have been reported in association with fragile bones; blue sclera and decreased hearing (Lobstein's syndrome); cryptorchidism; deformities of hands and feet with lacunae of parietal bones, occult spina bifida, and trisomy 18[25]; and unbalanced translocation of (17p, 10q) chromosomal defect.[27] Sclero-

Table 3-1. Congenital opacities of the cornea

Peters' anomaly	Sclerocornea	Choristoma (central)[30]	Congenital hereditary stromal dystrophy	Congenital hereditary endothelial dystrophy	Congenital syphilis and rubella	Mucopolysaccharidosis	Congenital glaucoma
Localized, flat avascular opacity	Opacity always begins at the limbus obscuring the junction	Opacity results from replacement of anterior stroma by elevated vascular tissue	Corneal opacity seen at birth	Neonatal corneal opacity	Rarely seen at birth—but is seen much later in childhood	Types IH, IS, IV, and VI are associated with cloudy cornea early in life but are not congenital	May occur at birth but is associated with diffuse edema, increased intraocular pressure, increased corneal diameter, ruptures of Descemet's membrane, buphthalmos, tearing, and photophobia; may be associated with rubella syndrome
Results from absence of endothelium, Descemet's membrane, and Bowman's layer	May remain peripheral or may involve central cornea	Usually corneoscleral junction is preserved; central cornea is involved	Bilateral superficial central corneal clouding	Autosomal recessive disease exhibits bilateral gray-blue ground glass opacity caused by edema	Rubella with opacity of cornea may occur at birth—with or without increased intraocular pressure; in addition, cataracts, pigmentary glaucoma, and iritis may be seen		
Associated with corectopia, iris hypoplasia, anterior lens opacities, iridocorneal adhesions	Usually associated with multiple congenital anomalies (e.g., Mieten's syndrome)		Stroma is not thick and is not vascularized	No vascularization			
			Composed of small-diameter collagen fibers	Collagenous tissue is seen posterior to Descemet's membrane			
				Endothelium is atrophic			
				Dominant disease does not occur at birth			
				Autosomal dominant posterior polymorphous dystrophy with severe edema may be present at birth			

cornea is also seen in hereditary osteo-onychodysplasia (HOOD)[9] and in Hallermann-Streiff syndrome. In the latter, one sees birdlike facies, hypotrichosis, frontal alopecia, and dental anomalies. In addition, congenital glaucoma and buphthalmos have been seen in Hallermann-Streiff syndrome.[28]

Sclerocornea has been described as a part of Mieten's syndrome. The latter exhibits growth failure, dislocation of the head of the radii, abnormally short ulnae and radii, mental retardation, small, pointed nose with a depressed root, low-set ears, flexion contractures of elbows, and extreme flexion of the thumbs.

It has been suggested that during the seventh week of gestation an abnormality develops when the second wave of mesodermal cells grows inward from proliferating mesoderm at the angles of the optic cup. Since cornea plana is so frequently associated with sclerocornea, little development must occur in the cornea after 4 months, the time at which corneal curve increases, creating the corneal scleral sulcus. Attempts at surgical repair have been made, but the results are generally discouraging. In spite of the fact that results are poor, the possible gain of useful eyesight is weighed against the potential loss of a relatively small amount of vision, ranging from deep amblyopia to no light perception; the risk is justified in a young patient, at least unilaterally. Of course, the general status of the eye must be considered before any keratoplasty is performed.

Sclerocornea is compared with other congenital opacities of the cornea in Table 3-1.

CONGENITAL CORNEA GUTTATA

This condition may occur early in life, even congenitally. Sometimes it is familial. Dominant pedigree associated with anterior polar cataract has been described, suggesting some abnormality in the anterior chamber mesoderm that separates the surface epithelium from the lens at about the eighth week.

CONGENITAL HEREDITARY ENDOTHELIAL DYSTROPHY (CHED)

This has been reported with deafness. (For a full description of CHED, see the section on endothelial dystrophies in Chapter 11.)

CONGENITAL HEREDITARY STROMAL DYSTROPHY

See Table 3-1.

EPIBULBAR DERMOIDS (Fig. 3-10)

These lesions are choristomas, which are masses of tissue that have been dislocated from their normal position.[4] This dislocation is in contrast to hamartomas, which are abnormal growths of tissue normally present in the same location, such as that seen in astrocytic hamartoma of the fundus and tuberous sclerosis. Astrocytes are normally present in that location but are not a tumorous growth. Hamartomas are characteristic of the phakomatoses.

Limbal dermoids usually straddle the limbus, overlapping the cornea and sclera. They are often present inferotemporally and may infrequently occur on the conjunctiva, subconjunctivally, or even in the orbit. These tumors contain keratinized epithelium, fibrous tissue, hair, fat, blood vessels, nerves, glands, smooth muscle, cartilage, and

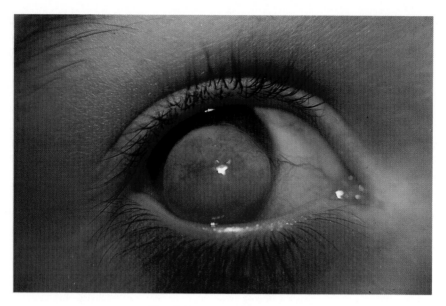

Fig. 3-10. Dermoid of cornea.

even teeth. They are often seen at birth or slightly after birth and may increase in size as the child grows.

Decreased vision may be caused by induced astigmatic error from the tumor. If the dermoid is large enough, it may encroach on the visual axis; often a line of lipid material is seen in front of the tumor on the cornea.

These tumors may be removed; however, although the large tumor mass can be removed, the opacity remains behind. The surgery involves some hazard, since the cornea may be thin under the tumor and can be perforated during dissection of the mass. Subconjunctival and orbital dermoids may extend back into the orbit, with no complete hope of total excision, and if too much dissection is carried out, damage can be done to the structures in the orbit.

DERMISLIKE CHORISTOMA

See Table 3-1, *Choristoma (central)*.

RING DERMOID

An autosomal dominant hereditary syndrome of bilateral ocular dermoids has been reported.[23] They involve the limbus 360° and extend anteriorly on the cornea and extend posteriorly about 5 mm within the conjunctiva for 360°. They cause an irregular astigmatism, amblyopia, and concomitant strabismus. Early surgical intervention may be attempted to improve the visual prognosis and cosmesis. Although bilateral dermoids may be exhibited in Goldenhar's syndrome, they are not seen in an annular display. Ring dermoids lack the anomalies associated with Goldenhar's syndrome. Benjamin-Allen developmental syndrome exhibits bilateral dermoids. The dermoids are usually superiorly limbal, bulbar, and conjunctival. One also sees generalized lymphadenopathy, cutaneous nevoid lesions, alopecia, and growth and mental retardation.[24]

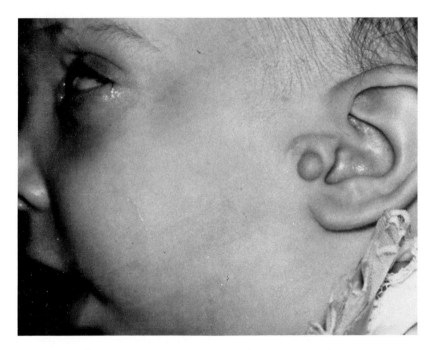

Fig. 3-11. Pretragal appendage in Goldenhar's syndrome.

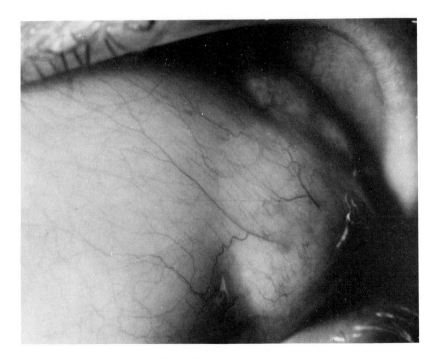

Fig. 3-12. Dermolipoma.

GOLDENHAR'S SYNDROME

The epibulbar dermoid of Goldenhar's syndrome (oculoauriculovertebral dysplasia) has been described with a triad of congenital anomalies consisting of epibulbar dermoids, preauricular appendages, and pretragal fistulas[3] (Fig. 3-11). In addition to these findings, one may see vertebral anomalies, hypoplasia of the mandible, and lid colobomas. Epibulbar dermoids occur in about one third of all patients with Goldenhar's syndrome. The dermoids may occur bilaterally but are more frequently seen unilaterally. There is no sex predilection for epibulbar dermoids. One may also see lipodermoids (dermolipoma), which are frequently located in the superotemporal quadrant and are generally bilateral (Fig. 3-12).

There is usually no difficulty in clinically differentiating a lipodermoid from an epibulbar dermoid, aside from the difference in location. Lipodermoids are often subconjunctival and soft, sliding easily under the palpating finger. Their color is usually that of the normal conjunctiva or slightly yellowish. They are frequently found extending back from the site between the eyeball and the globe.

Epibulbar osteomas and epibulbar ectopic lacrimal gland must be kept in mind as differential points when a diagnosis of epibulbar dermoids is being made.

Other ocular abnormalities associated with Goldenhar's syndrome are microphthalmos, coloboma of the iris or lid (upper outer lid), aniridia, Duane's retraction syndrome, and miliary aneurysms of the retina.

Systemic abnormalities may be associated with Goldenhar's syndrome, such as mandibulofacial dysostosis, cri du chat syndrome (deletion of the short arm of chromosome 5), incontinentia pigmenti (Bloch-Sulzberger syndrome), linear sebaceous nevus syndrome, and encephalocraniocutaneous lipomatosis. Skull, limb, facial, skeletal, and fistula abnormalities may be found.

CORNEA PLANA (FLAT CORNEA)[8, 10]

Cornea plana is usually seen in association with sclerocornea or microcornea and is often associated with diffuse opacities of the cornea stroma. One may see a shallow anterior chamber caused by the flat cornea, and since the cornea is flat, it should produce a hyperopia, but the globe varies in size so that any type of refractive error may exist. Often one may find other anomalies of the eye with cornea plana, such as coloboma of the iris, congenital cataract, ectopia lentis, retinal and macular aplasia, blue sclera, microphthalmos, glaucoma, and pseudoptosis. The condition is transmitted as a dominant or recessive trait.

Systemic association has been seen with osteogenesis imperfecta.

Cornea plana might be caused by a deep developmental arrest in the fourth month, at which time the cornea begins to increase its curvature relative to the sclera.

VERTICAL OVAL CORNEA

Luetic interstitial keratitis, when congenital, may produce a vertically oval cornea. In addition, Turner's syndrome often presents a vertical oval cornea as a typical finding. Iris coloboma may be associated with vertical oval cornea.

Table 3-2. Conditions with cloudy cornea at birth or in infancy

Edema	Malformation	Inflammations	Dystrophy	Neurologic disease	Systemic disease	Syndromes
Congenital glaucoma	Sclerocornea	Rubella	Congenital hereditary endothelial dystrophy	Riley-Day syndrome	Cystinosis	Trisomy 13 and 18
Birth trauma (forceps delivery)	Anterior mesodermal dysgenesis	Lues	Congenital hereditary stromal dystrophy	Congenital alacrima	Lowe's syndrome	Turner's syndrome
Congenital hereditary endothelial dystrophy	Dermoid	Gonorrhea			Soluble tyrosine amino-transferase (STAT) deficiency	Phenylketonuria
Posterior polymorphous dystrophy with mesodermal dysgenesis	Aniridia (peripheral or complete corneal opacity)	Intrauterine			Juvenile arcus	Chédiak-Higashi syndrome
	Dermislike choristoma				Schnyder's crystalline dystrophy	Norrie's disease
	Congenital anterior staphyloma				Tangier disease	
	Peters' anomaly				Familial plasma lecithin cholesterol-acyltransferase deficiency	
					Mucopolysaccharidosis (Hurler's syndrome [IH], Scheie's syndrome [IS], Morquio's syndrome [IV], Maroteaux-Lamy syndrome [VI])	
					Gangliosidosis	

CRYPTOPHTHALMOS (ABSENCE OF THE CORNEA)[13]

Cryptophthalmos is a condition in which the lid folds fail to form and the cornea undergoes metaplasia to skin. There are no lashes and no brows, and the skin is actually in front of the eye so that an incision enters the eyeball. The eye often has other deformities. In addition, systemic problems such as facial and genitourinary abnormalities, dental anomalies, and syndactyly are commonly seen. Cryptophthalmos may occur unilaterally or bilaterally, and it is autosomal recessive.

CLOUDY CORNEA

As seen, a number of the preceding problems exhibit a total or partial cloudy cornea at birth or in infancy. In Table 3-2 a complete differential diagnosis is listed.

REFERENCES

1. Alkemade, P.P.H.: Dysgenesis mesodermalis of the iris and the cornea, Springfield, Ill., 1969, Charles C Thomas, Publishers.
2. Axenfeld, T.: Embryotoxon cornea posterius, Dtsch. Ophthalmol. Gesamte **42**:301, 1920.
3. Baum, J.L., and Feingold, M.: Ocular aspects of Goldenhar's syndrome, Am. J. Ophthalmol. **75**:250, 1973.
4. Benjamin, S.N., and Allen, F.: Classification of limbal dermoid choristomas and branch arch anomalies, Arch. Ophthalmol. **87**:305, 1927.
5. Calamandrei, D.: Megalocornea in due pazienticon syndrome craniosinotoscia, Q. Ital. Ophthalmol. **3**:278, 1950.
6. Collier, J.: Le kératocône posterieur, Arch. Ophthalmol. (Paris) **22**:376, 475, 1962.
7. Dark, A.J., and Kirkham, T.H.: Congenital opacities: patient with Rieger's anomaly and Down's syndrome, Br. J. Ophthalmol. **52**:631, 1968.
8. Desvignes, P., Pouliquen, Y., Legras, M., and Giyot, J.D.: Aspect iconographique d'une cornea plana dans une maladie de Lobstein, Arch. Ophtalmol. (Paris) **27**:585, 1967.
9. Fenske, H.D., and Spitalny, L.A.: Hereditary osteo-onychodysplasia, Am. J. Ophthalmol. **70**:604, 1970.
10. Fishman, A.J., Ackerman, J., Kanarek, I., Novetsky, A., Ackerman, E., and Schiowitz, S.: Cornea plana: a Case Report, Ann. Ophthalmol. **14**:47, 1982.
11. Forsius, H., Eriksson, A., and Fellman, J.: Embryotoxon corneae posterius in an isolated population, Acta Ophthalmol. **42**:42, 1964.
12. François, J., Berger, E., and Saraux, H.: 79th Congress of the French Society of Ophthalmology, Arch. Ophthalmol. **89**:437, 1973.
13. Goldhammer, Y., and Smith, J.L.: Cryptophthalmos syndrome with basal encephaloceles, Am. J. Ophthalmol. **80**:146, 1975.
14. Goldstein, J.E., and Cogan, D.G.: Sclerocornea and associated congenital anomalies, Arch. Ophthalmol. **67**:761, 1962.
15. Grayson, M.: The nature of hereditary deep polymorphous dystrophy of the cornea: its association with iris and anterior chamber dysgenesis, Trans. Am. Ophthalmol. Soc. **72**:516, 1974.
16. Haney, W.P., and Falls, H.F.: The occurrence of congenital keratoconus posticus circumscriptus in two siblings presenting a previously unrecognized syndrome, Am. J. Ophthalmol. **52**:53, 1961.
17. Hansson, H., and Jerndal, T.: Scanning electron microscopic studies on the development of the iridocorneal angle in human eyes, Invest. Ophthalmol. **10**:252, 1971.
18. Henkind, P., and Friedman, A.H.: Iridogoniodysgenesis with cataract, Am. J. Ophthalmol. **72**:949, 1971.
19. Henkind, P., Siegel, I.M., and Carr, R.E.: Mesodermal dysgenesis of the anterior segment: Rieger's anomaly, Arch. Ophthalmol. **73**:810, 1965.
20. Ide, C.H., Landhuis, L.R., and Wilson, R.J.: Spontaneous perforation of congenital sclerocornea, Arch. Ophthalmol. **88**:204, 1972.
21. Ide, C.H., Matta, C., Holt, J.E., and Felker, G.V.: Dysgenesis mesodermalis of the cornea (Peters' anomaly): associated cleft lip and palate, Ann. Ophthalmol. **7**:841, 1975.
22. Krachmer, J., and Rodrigues, M.M.: Posterior keratoconus, Arch. Ophthalmol. **96**:1867, 1978.
23. Mattos, J., Contreras, F., and O'Donnell, F.E.: Ring dermoid syndrome: a new syndrome of autosomal dominantly inherited bilateral, annular limbal dermoids with corneal and conjunctival extension, Arch. Ophthalmol. **98**:1059, 1980.
24. Mackman, G., Brightbill, F.S., and Opitz, J.B.: Corneal changes in aniridia, Am. J. Ophthalmol. **87**:497, 1979.

25. Nakaniski, I., and Brown, S.I.: The histopathology and ultrastructure of congenital central corneal opacity (Peters' anomaly), Am. J. Ophthalmol. **72**:801, 1971.

26. Peters, A.: Über angeborene Defektbildung der Descemetschen Membran, Klin. Monatsbl. Augenheilkd. **44**:27, 105, 1906.

27. Rodrigues, M.M., Calhoun, J., and Weinreb, S.: Sclerocornea with unbalanced translocation (17p, 10q), Am. J. Ophthalmol. **78**:49, 1974.

28. Schanzlin, D.J., Goldberg, D.B., and Brown, S.I.: Hallerman-Streiff syndrome associated with sclerocornea, aniridia and a chromosomal abnormality, Am. J. Ophthalmol. **90**:411, 1980.

29. Tabbara, K.F., Khouri, F.P., and Kaloustian, V.M. der: Rieger's syndrome with chromosomal anomaly: report of a case, Can. J. Ophthalmol. **8**:488, 1973.

30. Topilow, H.W., Cykiert, R.C., Goldman, K., et al.: Bilateral corneal dermis-like choristomas: an X chromosome-linked disorder, Arch. Ophthalmol. **99**:1387, 1981.

31. Townsend, W.M.: Congenital corneal leukomas. I. Central defect in Descemet's membrane, Am. J. Ophthalmol. **77**:80, 1974.

32. Townsend, W.M., Font, R.L., and Zimmerman, L.E.: Congenital corneal leukomas. II. Histopathologic findings in 19 eyes with central defect in Descemet's membrane, Am. J. Ophthalmol. **77**:192, 1974.

33. Townsend, W.M., Font, R.L., and Zimmerman, L.E.: Congenital corneal leukomas. III. Histopathologic findings in 13 eyes with paracentral defect in Descemet's membrane, Am. J. Ophthalmol. **77**:400, 1974.

34. Waring, G.O., III, Rodrigues, M.M., and Laibson, P.R.: Anterior chamber cleavage syndrome. A stepladder classification, Surv. Ophthalmol. **20**:3, 1975.

35. Wolter, J.R., and Haney, W.P.: Histopathology of keratoconus posticus circumscriptus, Arch. Ophthalmol. **69**:357, 1963.

ADDITIONAL READING

Hittner, H.M., Kretzer, F.L., Antoszyk, J.H., Ferrell, R.E., and Mehta, R.S.: Variable expressivity of autosomal dominant anterior segment mesenchymal dysgenesis in six generations, Am. J. Ophthalmol. **93**:57, 1982.

Jacobs, H.B.: Posterior conical cornea, Br. J. Ophthalmol. **41**:31, 1957.

Jacobs, H.B.: Traumatic keratoconus posticus, Br. J. Ophthalmol. **41**:40, 1957.

Jerndal, T.: Goniodysgenesis and hereditary juvenile glaucoma: a clinical study of a Swedish pedigree, Acta Ophthalmol. **107**:1, 1970.

Kanai, A., Wood, T.C., Polack, F.M., et al.: The fine structure of sclerocornea, Invest. Ophthalmol. **10**:687, 1971.

Reese, A.B., and Ellsworth, R.M.: The anterior chamber cleavage syndrome, Arch. Ophthalmol. **75**:307, 1966.

Scheie, H.G., and Yanoff, M.: Peters' anomaly and total posterior coloboma or retinal pigment epithelium and choroid, Arch. Ophthalmol. **87**:525, 1972.

Speakman, J.S., and Crawford, J.S.: Congenital opacities of the cornea, Br. J. Ophthalmol. **50**:68, 1965.

Sugar, H.S.: Juvenile glaucoma with Axenfeld's syndrome: a histologic report, Am. J. Ophthalmol. **59**:1012, 1965.

von Hippel, E.: Über Hydrophthalmus congenitus nebst Bemerkungen über die Verfarbung der Cornea durch Blutfarbstoff. Pathologisch-anatomische Untersuchungen, Albrecht von Graefes Arch. Ophthalmol. **44**:539, 1897.

4 Keratitis

Bacterial keratitis

Central corneal ulcers, whether peripheral or central, at the onset will tend to progress toward the central cornea away from the vascularized limbus. These ulcers represent an infection of the cornea by virus, bacteria, or fungi. Herpes simplex infections of the cornea are by far the most common in the developed countries of the world. Bacterial corneal ulcers are less frequent and fungal corneal ulcers the least frequent in the developed areas, but they have become more important numerically in the past two decades. However, one should suspect a bacterial or fungal etiologic factor in any central corneal ulcer that is not obviously herpes simplex. Immediate laboratory studies and therapy should be instituted. A central corneal ulcer represents a threat to vision and to the eye; therefore it is a true ocular emergency.

The corneal epithelium serves as a natural barrier to all bacterial and fungal organisms that infect the cornea except for *Neisseria gonorrhoeae, Corynebacterium diphtheriae,* and *Listeria* species. Thus an abrasion, foreign body, erosion, or ruptured corneal epithelial bulla may precede a central corneal ulcer; such a lesion is a greater potential source of danger in individuals with decreased resistance, as seen in debilitated, elderly, alcoholic, and diabetic individuals and patients with keratoconjunctivitis sicca. Drugs that tend to decrease the immune mechanisms or further compromise the cornea, such as corticosteroids, idoxuridine, and topical anesthetics, may also play an important role.

Following are the most common organisms seen in bacterial corneal ulcers in an uncompromised cornea (that is, without herpetic infection, keratoconjunctivitis sicca, or the use of immunosuppressive drugs):

1. *Pseudomonas aeruginosa*
2. *Streptococcus pneumoniae*
3. *Moraxella* species
4. β-Hemolytic streptococcus
5. *Klebsiella pneumoniae*
6. Many other organisms that have been isolated but are more infrequently seen (for example, *Escherichia coli, Proteus* species, *Mycobacterium fortuitum,* and *Nocardia* species)

In the compromised cornea, especially with the use of immunosuppressive drugs or occurring as a secondary infection arising in a herpes simplex keratitis, *Staphylococcus aureus* is an important cause of central corneal ulcers; however, such an infection in an otherwise uncompromised cornea is unusual.

Opportunistic pathogens are microbic agents that have been regarded as contaminants or harmless inhabitants but that, in the compromised host, can multiply and produce corneal disease.[33] In severely compromised tissue a wide range of microorganisms, such as the following, can produce serious disease:

1. *Staphylococcus aureus*
2. *Staphylococcus epidermidis*
3. α-Hemolytic streptococcus
4. β-Hemolytic streptococcus
5. *Pseudomonas aeruginosa*
6. *Proteus* species

7. *Enterobacter aerogenes*
8. Others such as *Escherichia* and *Nocardia* species

Bacterial organisms that may cause keratitis are classified according to type, Gram's stain, and desire for oxygen:

Gram-positive organisms

A. Aerobes
   1. Micrococci
      a. *S. aureus*
      b. *S. epidermidis*
   2. Streptococci
      a. α-Hemolytic streptococcus
      b. β-Hemolytic streptococcus
      c. *S. pneumoniae*
   3. Bacilli
      a. Spore-forming: *Bacillus* species, including *B. cereus*
      b. Non-spore-forming
         (1) *Corynebacterium* species
         (2) *Listeria* species
B. Anaerobes
   1. Cocci: *Peptostreptococcus* species
   2. Bacilli (rods)
      a. Spore-forming: *Clostridium* species
      b. Non-spore-forming
         (1) *Actinomyces israelii*
         (2) *Propionibacterium acnes*
C. Acid-fast bacillus (gram-positive rod)
   1. *Mycobacterium fortuitum* (banded)
   2. *Nocardia* species

Gram-negative organisms

A. Aerobes
   1. Diplococcus: *Neisseria* gonococcus
   2. Rods: family Enterobacteriaceae
      a. *Escherichia coli*
      b. *Klebsiella pneumoniae*
      c. *Enterobacter aerogenes*
      d. *Proteus mirabilis*
      e. *Pseudomonas* species
      f. *Serratia marcescens*
   3. Diplobacillus: *Moraxella* species
   4. Coccobacillus: *Haemophilus influenzae*
B. Anaerobes
   1. Rods (non-spore-forming): *Fusobacterium* species

Intact skin and mucous membranes are important factors because they are the first line of defense against infection. In the eye the mechanical flushing action of the tears is important as a defense against infection, as is the presence of lysozymes, betalysins, and natural antibodies, principally IgA. In addition, the acute nonspecific inflammatory reactions to injury through phagocytosis of the invaders by neutrophils and, later, macrophages helps the uncompromised host to live with or destroy the opportunists whether they are bacteria or fungi. After a delay of 5 to 8 days, unless there has been previous exposure to the invading microbic agent, specific humoral and cellular reactions also come to the defense of the uncompromised host to confront the opportunists. The inflammatory reaction ordinarily takes care of all opportunists that have breached the skin and mucous membranes; the specific humoral and cellular reactions are needed by the uncompromised host only if the microbic inoculum is overwhelming. The physician should recognize these natural defense mechanisms, using them to advantage and refraining from thwarting them.

Many conditions, some of which follow, are considered compromising situations of a local nature:

1. Ocular burns
2. Dry eye status
3. Topical drug abuse with such agents as antibiotics, anesthetics, and IDU
4. Contact lens abuse
5. Cauterizing agents

In addition to locally compromising conditions, a number of systemic conditions can result in a compromised host and thus[1,2,31] can contribute to the enhancement of corneal infection:

1. Immunosuppressive drugs
2. Extensive body burns
3. Pregnancy (last trimester)
4. Chronic alcoholism
5. Severe malnutrition
6. Infancy
7. Old age
8. Immunodeficiency syndromes such as Wiskott-Aldrich syndrome
9. Drug addiction

It appears that the most common causes of the compromised host are the use of systemic corticosteroids and immunosuppressive drugs in autoimmune diseases. Antibiotics have played a role in the frequency of opportunistic involvement of the cornea. Abuse of antibiotics can contribute to a compromising situation by shifting the normal gram-positive flora of the conjunctival sac to abnormal negative flora. In the newborn the cellular immune system is slow to develop and therefore is subject to opportunistic infection. In old age there is a decline in the ability of the body to react to opportunistic agents by inflammatory and cellular mechanisms. Malnutrition, debilitating disease, and drug addiction are commonly seen in modern society and play a prominent role in opportunistic infections. Contact lenses, since they deprive the cornea of oxygen and interfere with protective tear flow, may result in the conjunctiva and cornea becoming a compromised area. The dry eye has a poor flushing mechanism and a decreased tear lysozyme content, which affords the opportunistic organisms a chance to contribute to the possibility of keratitis.

Pseudomonas aeruginosa may contaminate ophthalmic preparations, eye cosmetics such as mascara,[46] and contact lens cases.[13] Heavy inocula are obtained in this fashion; thus the normal defenses of an eye may be overcome if the corneal epithelium has been abraded or if the eye has been opened for intraocular surgery. As with most opportunists, small inocula may be managed reasonably well by the defenses of the normal eye so that only in the immunologically compromised eye will they produce disease. The corneal epithelial barrier may be damaged in vitamin A deficiency, and cellular immunity is often suppressed in conditions of protein-calorie deficiency. It is understandable then why severe nutritional corneal ulcers are seen with greater frequency in some parts of the world in which malnutrition plays a role.

DIFFERENTIAL DIAGNOSIS

The most common causes of bacterial keratitis are the Micrococcaceae *(Staphylococcus, Micrococcus), Streptococcus* species, *Pseudomonas* species, and the Enterobacteriaceae *(Citrobacter, Enterobacter, Klebsiella, Proteus,* and *Serratia).*

It is most important to make an etiologic diagnosis in dealing with bacterial keratitis,[14] but in doing so herpes simplex hominis indolent ulceration, marginal infiltrative and ulcerative keratitis, trophic keratopathy, and toxic keratopathy should be kept in mind as differential diagnostic conditions.

If one is confronted with what may be a herpes simplex hominis indolent ulceration, various aids can be employed to differentiate it from a bacterial ulcer. In the herpetic infection, the cornea sensitivity is decreased, scrapings may show the presence of multinucleated giant cells, the absence of bacteria is noted, and the fluorescent antibody test is positive. A history of previous herpes keratitis infection or herpes labialis may be elicited and will alert the physician to the problem.

The limbal corneal ulcers and infiltrates may grow out pathogens, and this should always be considered. For instance, the *Alternaria* organism has been seen in marginal infiltrates that resemble an immune infiltrate, and occasionally gram-negative organisms may be seen in ocular pemphigoid with corneal ulcers. It is necessary therefore to pursue the laboratory diagnosis in spite of the fact that one may have a high index of suspicion for immune etiologic or other factors as the primary problem.

Trophic keratopathy, especially when it is associated with keratitis sicca, may lead to stromal lysis and even perforation in the absence of cellular infiltration. The lack of cellular infiltration should put one on the alert, since this may help distinguish it from a bacterial cause. Toxic keratopathy is often seen from abuse of such drugs as amphotericin B, idoxuridine, Neosporin, gentamicin, and topical anesthetics. If these drugs are used for 10 or more days, one may see areas of multiple focal stromal infiltration.

Bacterial corneal ulcers,[9] by active invasion of proliferating bacteria, can be a result of staphylococcic disease. A large number of such cases are caused by the *S. epidermidis* strain (perhaps more so than the *S. aureus* strain). Larger numbers of the *S. aureus* strains are penicillinase producers. The staphylococcus organism is a rare cause of keratitis in healthy eyes but may be seen specifically in posttrauma situations.[18] *Streptococcus* and *Pseudomonas* species, *Proteus mirabilis, Serratia* and *Klebsiella* organisms, and *Escherichia coli* are offenders and can cause corneal ulcers. In addition, but less commonly seen, are *Moraxella* species infection, gram-negative diplococci, and, on occasion, gram-negative or gram-positive anaerobic infections.[20] Rarely, *Propionibacterium acnes,* an anaerobe, has been noted as a cause of corneal ulcers.[20]

Bacillus species includes *B. cereus,* which has emerged as the most important ocular pathogen in this genus and possibly one of the most destructive organisms to affect the eye. Most cases of *B. cereus* infection have occurred as a result of hematogenous dissemination, usually in intravenous drug abusers. Panophthalmitis may follow penetrating trauma by a metallic foreign body. Characteristically, severe pain develops within 24 hours of the injury and is followed rapidly by chemosis, periorbital swelling, and extreme proptosis. Shortly thereafter, low-grade fever may occur accompanied by a moderate polymorphonuclear leukocytosis. Invariably a ring of edema forms in the peripheral cornea followed by the rapid development of a circumferential corneal abscess.

There are certain situations in which *B. cereus* infection must be suspected. Most important is a penetration injury caused by a metallic foreign body and occurring in an environment in which contamination with soil is a likelihood. Ring abscess of the cornea is an uncommon finding in ocular infectious disease. Its occurrence is an indication of the devastating nature of the inflammatory reaction and usually foretells a grave prognosis for the eye. Although a variety of microorganisms, including *Pseudomonas aeruginosa* and *Proteus* species, have been implicated in causing ring abscess, *Bacillus* species have been isolated most frequently.[28]

It appears that the staphylococcus ulcer is seen more frequently in the eastern and northeastern areas of the United States, whereas the *Pseudomonas* organism is found more often in the more temperate climates of the country. *Streptococcus pneumoniae* as the cause is more frequent in the eastern and western areas of the nation. The *S. pneumoniae* and *Pseudomonas* organism infections are the main pathogens of previously healthy eyes, but the latter is often seen with steroid abuse. *Moraxella* species infection of the cornea usually involves a debilitated host.

Acanthomeba can cause a purulent keratitis and should be kept in mind in severely resistant ulcers.

CLINICAL APPEARANCE

When a corneal ulcer of bacterial cause develops, the conjunctiva and lid become injected and edematous, and there may be a purulent discharge. The corneal epithelium becomes ulcerated, and the stroma exhibits infiltration and may be gray-white and necrotic. Infiltration and edema of the cornea may even be observed in areas away from the site of the ulcer. Stromal abscesses may be evident as small and deep infiltrates, and fibrin plaques may be observed on the endothelium. In addition, a fibrinoid aqueous and hypopyon may be seen. The hypopyon is caused by the toxic effects of the organism on the vessels of the iris and ciliary body with resultant outpouring of fibrin and polymorphonuclear leukocytes. Usually the hypopyon is sterile as long as Descemet's mem-

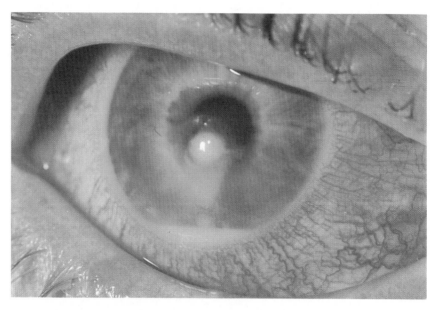

Fig. 4-1. Hypopyon ulcer resulting from staphylococcal infection. Area is round and is localized with more or less distinct borders.

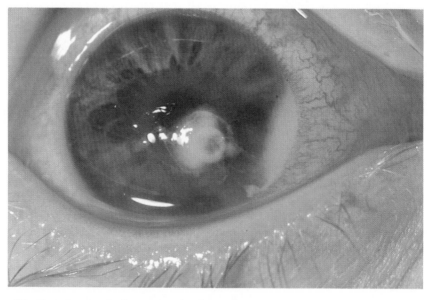

Fig. 4-2. Central corneal ulcer as result of *Streptococcus pneumoniae*. Eccentric location of hypopyon was caused by patient lying on side.

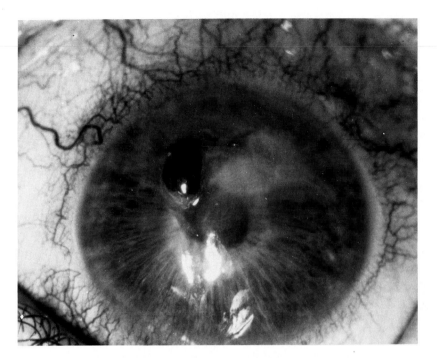

Fig. 4-3. Perforated corneal ulcer with iris prolapse.

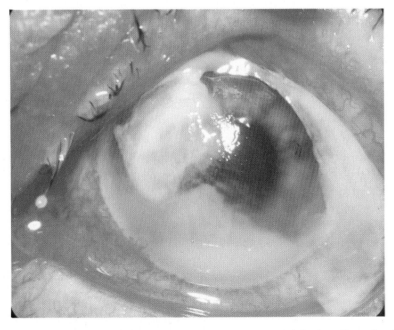

Fig. 4-4. Hypopyon ulcer as result of *Pseudomonas aeruginosa* infection. Extensive lysis of collagen structure has taken place.

brane is intact. A hypopyon can be seen with staphylococcic infection (Fig. 4-1), *Strepto-coccus pneumoniae* (Fig. 4-2), and *Pseudomonas* organism corneal ulcers (Fig. 4-3). It should be remembered that hypopyons are also seen with viral and fungal corneal ulcers. Nonbacterial or nonfungal problems such as Behçet's syndrome, abuse of the use of topical anesthetic agents, and severe lye burns may also result in hypopyon formation. The presence of white blood cells on the endothelium and in the corneal stroma can be a serious problem, since the cells can cause extensive damage to the endothelial structure by virtue of their lysosomal enzymes and thus result in permanent corneal edema.

It is most important to carefully follow the corneal ulcer progress.[18,19] The immediate suppuration and infiltration are extremely important to observe; perhaps this is even more important than the hypopyon. Many danger signs alert one to further trouble: pain, change in ulcer surface area, increase in cellular stromal infiltration, increase in suppuration, increase in anterior chamber reaction, lysis of corneal stroma (Fig. 4-3), and at times lysis of sclera.

The severe inflammatory reaction from virulent bacterial ulcers of the cornea may lead to permanent changes such as anterior polar cataracts, posterior and anterior synechiae, increased intraocular pressure, descemetocele or perforation (Fig. 4-4),[18] stromal scars, and edema of the cornea.

LABORATORY WORK

The mere clinical appearance of the ulcer is inadequate in making a specific etiologic diagnosis. Every ophthalmologist should be equipped to take adequate scrapings of the ulcer and should know how to interpret the findings. In an adult, the specimen should be obtained with the aid of the slit lamp and 0.5% proparacaine hydrochloride as a topical anesthetic. This anesthetic agent is less bactericidal than cocaine or tetracaine. Obtaining a specimen from children may require a general anesthetic and the operating microscope. The ulcer margins and base should be thoroughly scraped with a Kimura spatula and not with cotton-tipped applicators. The scrapings may serve as a form of débridement and may enhance topical antibiotic activity. Multiple specimens and multiple areas of the ulcer should be sampled.[14,18] Sometimes as many as five to ten scrapings are necessary because any given area may not contain the organism, and it may be necessary to scrape deeply to obtain the proper material. The common causes for lack of positive scrapings are insufficient material, failure to examine the entire slide, and previous therapy. All these factors must be kept in mind when the laboratory work is being done, as well as the fact that purulent exudate and necrotic surface material are of no value for laboratory organism diagnosis.

Superficially spreading ulcers may be a result of *Streptococcus pneumoniae;* when spreading corneal ulceration is seen, one should be on guard for this organism when the stained material is being examined. Deep corneal abscesses often are caused by the *Moraxella* organism, and one should be on the alert for this organism's characteristics when the Gram stain is being examined. This type of correlation may be useful.

Slides should be prepared for Gram's and Giemsa's stains. In general Gram's stain will demonstrate bacteria and yeast, whereas the Giemsa stain demonstrates hyphae crosswalls, multinucleated giant cells, intracytoplasmic inclusions, and cellular morphologic characteristics.[24] Intranuclear inclusions can be demonstrated by Papanicolaou's stain with an acid fixative. However, the latter stain must be done in the clinical laboratory. Several additional slides should be kept in reserve for later special stains if they prove to be necessary. A small area of the slide should be outlined with a glass marker, and the material obtained spread within the confines of this outlined area. The slide is then fixed with 95% alcohol instead of heat, since heat may result in gram-positive organisms staining gram negative.

The samples should be plated onto or injected into one of the following types of culture media:

1. Blood agar
2. Sabouraud's agar
3. Beef heart medium
4. Chocolate agar
5. Thayer-Martin medium
6. Para-aminobenzoic acid (PABA)
7. Thioglycolate broth
8. Löwenstein-Jensen medium

The blood agar plate is most important to use in culturing the scrapings from corneal ulcers, since it will allow growth of most aerobic pathogens and some fungi.

Chocolate agar will grow *Neisseria, Haemophilus,* and *Moraxella* species.

Thioglycolate broth is a liquid medium that contains a reducing agent and will grow both aerobic and anaerobic organisms (*Actinomyces* species). The aerobes will grow near the surface, and anaerobes will grow below the surface.

Löwenstein-Jensen medium may be used for isolation of *Mycobacterium* and *Nocardia* species.

Thayer-Martin medium is an enriched chocolate agar containing antibiotics and is the medium of choice for *Neisseria* organisms. It must be incubated in 5% to 10% carbon dioxide (candle jar).

Fungal organisms may grow at room temperature; one plate should be prepared for this purpose. Fresh blood agar plates should be used at all times, since they dry out; any plate older than 2 weeks should be discarded.

Sabouraud's medium without cycloheximide (an inhibitor of saprophytic fungi) is selective for fungi. It has a low pH, which inhibits bacterial growth. It is incubated at room temperature (26° C). Fastidious fungi will also grow on beef heart media containing gentamicin.

The minimum laboratory work should consist of Gram's stain and culture on blood agar. If a fungus is suspected, an additional culture on Sabouraud's agar is needed. If sufficient material is available, an additional scraping for Giemsa's stain and perhaps thioglycolate broth may be desirable.

When doing a Gram stain, one should remember that organisms may look gram negative on the slide when in fact they may be gram positive because of increased decolorization from previous antibiotic treatment, leukocytic destruction, or heat. These latter facts must be considered when there are contradictory findings.

It is most necessary that the bacteriologic report be followed up and the laboratory contacted as early as 12 to 18 hours for a report so that positive and effective treatment can be undertaken. Sensitivity tests may be obtained even before the organism is isolated.

Negative cultures in 3 to 11 days may indicate that the ulcer is not caused by bacteria, that previous antibiotic therapy may have prevented the recovery of the organism, or that inadequate specimens and culture techniques may have been performed. As an example of inadequate techniques, some *Streptococcus pneumoniae* organisms require— and some *Neisseria* and *Streptococcus* species may grow better in—increased carbon dioxide concentration. Anaerobic organisms may be present in the ulcer, but in this example no anaerobic culture had been used for them to grow out.

Anaerobic cultures should be taken when infection persists; in addition, one should look for parasites.

If the ulcer is suspected to be caused by a slow-growing organism such as *Mycobacterium fortuitum,* acid-fast stains should be done. The ulcer may be the result of a virus, in which case no bacterial organisms are recovered unless they are secondary invaders. This should always be kept in mind.

Suggestions for laboratory work and analysis of conjunctival and corneal smears and scrapings are given in the Appendix.

The limulus endotoxin assay, which is used for early detection of certain gram-negative corneal infections, is based on the specific activation of clottable problems that are derived from the amebocytes of the horseshoe crab, *Limulus polyphemus.* The natural response of this organism to gram-negative bacterial infection is disseminated intravascular coagulation. This endotoxin activation of the coagulation pathway has been adapted as a sensitive in vitro assay for the presence of bacterial lipopolysaccharide. It is a sensitive method for the detection of gram-negative bacterial endotoxin, even in slight quantities, during an inactivation period of 1 hour or less. It becomes positive earlier than bacterial cultures. The limulus assay is unaffected by the presence of antibiotics and therefore allows accurate diagnosis of partially treated patients with gram-negative corneal infections. The test is not used to assess the effectiveness of antibacterial therapy since endotoxin persists in the corneal debris for several days despite negative cultures taken from ulcer areas.[43]

SPECIFIC CORNEAL ULCERS
Staphylococcus species

S. aureus. This organism appears as an irregular group of clusters of spheres that may vary in size and staining qualities. The older organisms may stain gram negative. The pathogenicity of *S. aureus* is determined by mannitol fermentation and the production of coagulase, an enzyme that clots blood. Coagulase is perhaps the best single test for identifying pathogenic staphylococci.

S. aureus is found on the skin, nose, and conjunctiva and is an opportunistic pathogen. The corneal ulcer resulting from this organism tends to be round or oval and may remain localized (Fig. 4-1) with distinct borders; however, on occasion the ulcer may be diffuse, demonstrating microabscesses in the anterior stroma that are connected by stromal infiltrates.

S. epidermidis. The *S. epidermidis* strain is a frequent cause of keratitis in a cornea with previous disease and may be seen in individuals who do not use proper contact lens hygiene. *S. epidermidis* is an opportunist and an unlikely cause of infection in a healthy cornea. The two species, *S. epidermidis* and *S. aureus,* cannot be distinguished from each other by Gram's stain. *S. aureus* is more virulent, but antibiotic resistance may be more common among strains of *S. epidermidis*. It must be emphasized that the *S. epidermidis* strain is toxicogenic and pathogenic.[41] The corneal ulcer of *S. epidermidis*, nevertheless, has a similar clinical appearance to the corneal ulcer caused by the *S. aureus* strain.

Streptococcus organisms

S. pneumoniae is found in the upper respiratory tract in 50% of the population; its proximity to the eye may account for the frequency of problems associated with it, such as keratitis, dacryocystitis, and postoperative endophthalmitis. Dacryocystitis, which can be chronic, may be a causative factor of keratitis associated with minor corneal trauma. It may occur as a saprophyte on the lid or in the conjunctival sac.

This end-to-end paired organism is encapsulated, gram positive, and lancet shaped. It occurs in coccus or chain form in culture and may require 5% to 10% carbon dioxide for the recovery. It may stain gram negative in older cultures. *S. pneumoniae* is α-hemolytic and shows umbilicated colonies after 48 hours; it is not raised in the same manner as the other streptococci.

The ulcer of the cornea may be localized or have a tendency to spread in one direction, usually centrally. The edge may be undermined and covered by the overhanging tissue. The pneumococcal ulcers have a tendency to form hypopyons (Fig. 4-2) and may perforate[29] (Fig. 4-3).

S. pyogenes (beta streptococcus) is an infrequent cause of corneal infection. Marginal corneal ulcers resulting from this organism may be associated with dacryocystitis.[23] α-Hemolytic streptococcus is present in the upper respiratory tract and the mouth. This organism is relatively nonvirulent and causes infections mainly in corneas with previous chronic disease. *S. faecalis* may cause an ulcer of the cornea in the presence of severely impaired host resistance or after epithelial injury. The beta strain causes total hemolysis of blood cells, whereas the alpha strain causes partial hemolysis; the surrounding area is green because of reduction of the hemoglobin.

Other gram-positive organisms

Gram-positive rods, an infrequent cause of keratitis, usually involve only the cornea when host resistance is impaired.

Anaerobic gram-positive cocci commonly reside in the skin and mucous membranes and are seen in the fecal flora. *Peptostreptococcus* organisms and other strains have been reported as a cause of corneal ulcers[21,31] and should always be kept in mind when one is dealing with recalcitrant corneal ulcers.

Pseudomonas aeruginosa

This organism is one of the most important corneal pathogens and is perhaps the most common gram-negative organism[7,9,17] causing corneal ulcers. *P. aeruginosa* is a slender, motile, gram-negative rod and is found on skin, in saliva, and in the gastrointestinal tract and occurs ubiquitously in the environment. *P. aeruginosa* exhibits a sweet odor in the culture plates. The virulency of this pathogen is probably related to its motility and production of calcium-dependent collagenase, which is inhibited by disodium ethylenediamine tetraacetic acid (EDTA) but not by cysteine.

P. aeruginosa causes a rapidly spreading ulcer, which can follow minor corneal trauma. Most strains of *Pseudomonas* species contain proteolytic enzymes that break down the collagen fibers of the stroma and cause rapid destruction of the cornea. In 24 hours the ulcer may extend to twice its size (Fig. 4-4), with a copious mucopurulent discharge that may have a greenish color. The ulcer may be central or paracentral, and dense stromal infiltrates and necrosis are characteristic. Edema of the surrounding cornea, posterior corneal stromal folds, and endothelial plaques are seen. Hypopyon is usual (Fig. 4-4). Early descemetocele formation, melting, and perforation are not infrequent. The infection may smolder for a long time and may recur many days after therapy has been discontinued. Thus therapy should be continued for several weeks after apparent clinical cure.

P. aeruginosa is to be considered as a cause of scleritis. *Pseudomonas* corneal infection can extend into the sclera, and then medical treatment is in most cases difficult.[34]

Perforated *Pseudomonas* corneal ulcers with scleral extension have been treated successfully with keratoplasty and cryotherapy, the latter applied to the remaining cornea and corneoscleral limbus. Since *Pseudomonas* organisms seem to be susceptible to cryotherapy in vivo, this may be considered a mode of therapy as an adjunct to medical and surgical treatment of *Pseudomonas* scleral abscesses.[10] A ring-shaped keratitis from *P. aeruginosa* may occur. The *P. aeruginosa* endotoxin may go through an epithelial break into the superficial stroma, lending to ring formation via endotoxin-initiated, properdin-mediated, antibody-independent complement activation.[5]

P. aeruginosa has been found as a contaminant in hospitals, in fluorescein solutions,[42] in eye mascara,[46] and in poorly cared-for contact lens cases. It has been seen as a source of infection in young healthy patients who wear contact lenses and who institute poor contact lens hygiene.[13] It is also observed as a cause of keratitis in comatose patients[16] and has been cultured from patients with tracheostomies.

P. fluorescens has produced an ulcerative keratitis in eyes predisposed to previous abnormalities. However, this organism is less destructive than *P. aeruginosa* because of the absence of collagenase.

Moraxella species

This group consists of gram-negative diplobacilli and are plump, paired rods arranged end to end but without capsules. They are the largest gram-negative organisms causing corneal disease. Polar staining with rounded or rectangular ends is a characteristic feature of these species. These characteristics aid the physician in recognizing the organism with routine Gram's stain.

Moraxella species grow on desquamated epithelial cells and need enriched media and an alkaline pH. *M. liquifaciens* has been eliminated in taxonomy; *M. lacunata* is probably responsible for angular conjunctivitis and corneal ulcers. These organisms are opportunistic pathogens and grow on chocolate agar and blood agar. They may on occasion appear as gram-positive rods since they may retain the crystal violet on Gram's stain.

The corneal ulcer is an indolent paracentral or peripheral one that is usually oval in shape and localized with an undermined necrotic edge centrally. It progresses deep into the stroma over days or weeks. Hypopyon is variable. The organism is present in the depths of the crater, and untreated ulcers may perforate. The anterior segment is highly inflamed, and host resistance is usually low.

Family Enterobacteriaceae

Enterobacteriaceae species such as *Escherichia coli* and *Aerobacter* and *Proteus*[30] organisms have remained reasonably uncommon in bacterial keratitis despite their increase in urinary tract infection. *Proteus vulgaris* causes most eye infections, and the keratitis may be severe (Fig. 4-5). Perforation and ring ulcer have been seen. *Serratia marcescens,* one of this group, is an opportunistic organism. It is a gram-negative rod or oval coccobacillus, will grow on simple media, and is found in soil but not in normal conjunctiva. It has been observed growing in contact lens cases. It contains an endotoxin and proteinase that can cause a severe ulcer, resulting in perforation.[25] The cornea may also show peripheral infiltrates and paracentral ulcers.

The *Klebsiella* organism is a gram-negative diplobacillus. It is a short, fat organism with a capsule and causes corneal ulcers in debilitated hosts.

Neisseria species

The gram-negative cocci such as *N. gonorrhoeae* and *N. meningitidis* may invade the cornea after conjunctivitis. The organisms are kidney-shaped diplococci and are found intracellularly. The organism may be distorted after antibiotic exposure, may not decolorize well, and thus will stain poorly. It requires special media with an increased atmosphere of carbon dioxide. The *N. gonorrhoeae* may invade the cornea through an intact epithelium and cause an ulcer. These ulcers are extremely dangerous, particularly in the newborn, since they may lead to corneal perforation. *N. gonorrhoeae* ferments glucose but not maltose or sucrose. *N. meningitidis* ferments glucose and maltose but not sucrose. *N. catarrhalis* ferments none of these agents.

Haemophilus influenzae

This organism requires hemin and VAD for growth. These properties are present in chocolate agar or by a combination of blood agar and staphylococci. The blood supplies the hemin and the staphylococci supply the VAD. The *Haemophilus* organism will grow around the staphylococcus colonies; this is called *satellitism. H. influenzae* has been observed recently to develop an increasing resistance to ampicillin.

The corneal ulcers, although infrequently found, may be difficult to treat, particularly if the disease is seen in children.

Acid-fast organisms: Mycobacterium fortuitum

Corneal ulcers caused by the *M. fortuitum* organism may simulate those caused by *Moraxella* species in that they are indolent, progressing slowly over a period of weeks or months.[26] Often minimal anterior chamber reaction occurs with little or no hypopyon. These are harbored in the soil. The ulcer most frequently occurs after trauma to the cornea.

M. fortuitum is best isolated in Löwenstein-Jensen media. It requires an enriched

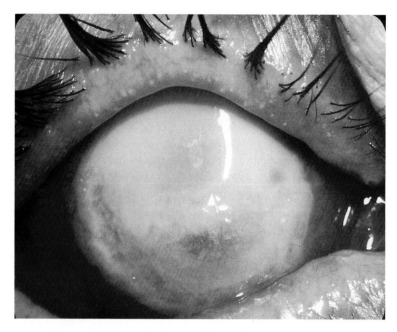

Fig. 4-5. Severe keratitis resulting from *Proteus mirabilis*.

medium, an aerobic atmosphere, and an increased amount of carbon dioxide. Any recalcitrant ulcer should cause one to suspect a *Mycobacterium* species etiologic factor and to order an acid-fast stain. Growth in blood agar may not appear for 3 to 5 days.

Mycobacterium and *Nocardia* organisms appear very much alike both on scraping and culture. They are gram-positive, slender, and variable-sized rods and variable acid-fast organisms.

M. fortuitum responds poorly to all medication and minimally to therapy, although supportive treatment appears to be the treatment of choice. Rifampicin has been reported to be of value in therapy.[32]

Norcardia species

Corneal ulcers caused by the *Nocardia* organisms are usually indolent in type and may simulate the indolent ulcers of *Moraxella* species and *M. fortuitum* origin. In these cases, there is usually minimal anterior chamber reaction. Nocardial corneal ulcers may simulate mycotic corneal ulcers because of the presence of "hyphate edges," satellite lesions, and, occasionally, elevated lesions. Such ulcers are usually considered with fungal corneal ulcers.[35] The organisms are found in the soil and are intertwining, branching filaments with or without clubs or coccoid and diphtheroid forms. Some filaments stain positively with the acid-fast stain. The organism is an obligate anaerobe and will grow on blood agar or Sabouraud's dextrose agar. On prolonged incubation it develops a yellow-to-orange color.

Nocardia species respond to topical sulfacetamide, 15%, and tetracycline, 5 mg/ml. Systemic medication may occasionally be necessary; sulfonamides or tetracyclines are employed in this instance.

Actinomyces israelii

This obligate anaerobe grows well on blood agar enriched with vitamin K. One may use freshly boiled thioglycolate broth supplemented with serum and vitamin K–hemin. A. *israelii* is gram positive; the stain reveals intertwining, branching filaments with or without clubs and diphtheroid forms.

ANTIBIOTICS

The following section contains information concerning antibiotic drugs used in the treatment of corneal ulcers. A number of tables are provided. Tables 4-2 and 4-3 outline a general attitude and medical approach to treatment of corneal ulcers that have been fostered by Dan B. Jones. Table 4-4 lists a general survey of microbial organisms with antibiotic agents suitable for their treatment. Table 4-5 lists the infectious organisms for which penicillins are effective antimicrobial agents. Table 4-6 compiles facts concerning the most-used agents and classifies them according to their effectiveness and penetration into the eye. Tables 4-7 to 4-9 are concerned with methods of preparation for various modes of administration and proper dosages of the usual antibiotics for use in treatment of bacterial keratitis, which is summarized in Table 4-10.

The initial decision should be based on the interpretation of the corneal smears, the assessment of the severity of the keratitis, and the clinical impression (Table 4-1).

A plan for initial therapy of nonsevere keratitis is based on the interpretation of the smears and the clinical impression (Table 4-2).

Antibacterial drops should be administered at 15-minute intervals. Subconjunctival antibiotics may be given every 12 hours during the initial 24 to 48 hours of therapy, but some investigators think that the concentrated and frequent topical drops are better and just as effective. Systemic therapy should be reserved for scleral suppuration or impending or existing corneal perforation.[20]

The cephalosporin antibiotics are generally more active in vitro against penicillinase-producing staphylcocci and the streptococci than bacitracin, erythromycin, and lincomycin (Table 4-11). Cefazolin (50 mg/ml) is less toxic than bacitracin (10,000 units/ml) to the conjunctiva and cornea following topical application and less irritating than methicillin or other semisynthetic penicillins following subconjunctival infection of equal doses (100 mg). Cefazolin has a low degree of serum binding and produces less pain following injection than other cephalosporin derivatives.

Gentamicin and tobramycin remain the initial antibiotics of choice in suspected gram-negative rod keratitis on the basis of stability, corneal and intraocular penetration, and bactericidal activity against *Pseudomonas, Enterobacter, Klebsiella,* and other aerobic gram-negative organisms. Tobramycin is two to four times more active by weight than gentamicin against *Klebsiella, Enterobacter, Serratia,* and *Proteus.* Some strains of *Pseudomonas* organisms resistant to gentamicin are also resistant to tobramycin. Since amikacin is less susceptible to inactivation by bacterial enzymes than either gentamicin or tobramycin, strains of gram-negative bacteria resistant to gentamicin and tobramycin may be sensitive to amikacin. Tobramycin may be less nephrotoxic than gentamicin.

Strict guidelines cannot be provided for the decision to reduce or terminate antibiotics in keratitis improving with therapy. The duration of viable organisms in the cornea must

Table 4-1. Severity grade of microbial keratitis

Feature	Severity grade	
	Nonsevere	Severe
Rate of progression	Slow, moderate	Rapid
Suppuration		
Area	< 6 mm diameter	> 6 mm diameter
Depth	Superficial two thirds	Inner one third
Depth of ulceration	Superficial one third	Inner one third
Perforation	Unlikely to occur	Present, imminent
Scleral suppuration	Absent	Present

From Jones, D.B.: Ophthalmology **88:**814, 1981.

Table 4-2. Initial therapy of nonsevere keratitis

Result of smears	Selection of agent(s)
One type of bacterium	One antibacterial agent
Two or more types of bacteria	Multiple, specific antibacterial agents
Hyphal fragments, yeasts, or pseudohyphae	Natamycin
No microorganisms	Clinical impression: bacterial keratitis—combined (broad) antibacterial therapy*; fungal keratitis—defer therapy; noninfectious keratitis—defer therapy

From Jones, D.B.: Ophthalmology **88:**814, 1981.
*"Combined (broad) antibacterial therapy" implies the use of a cephalosporin antibiotic (cefazolin or cephaloridine) and gentamicin.

Table 4-3. Initial therapy of severe keratitis

Result of smears	Selection of agent(s)
One type of bacterium	Antecedent therapy: none—one antibacterial agent; received—combined (broad) antibacterial agent
Two or more bacteria	Combined (broad) antibacterial therapy

From Jones, D.B.: Ophthalmology **88:**814, 1981.

Table 4-4. General survey of antimicrobial coverage

Organism	Effective antibiotic
Gram-positive cocci	
Staphylococcus aureus	Oxacillin, methicillin, or cephalosporin, if penicillinase producer
	Penicillin G, if nonpenicillinase producer
Streptococcus species	Penicillin G
S. pneumoniae	Penicillin G
	Erythromycin
Anaerobic streptococcus	Penicillin G
Gram-negative cocci	
Neisseria gonorrhoeae	Aqueous penicillin (with probenecid)
	Ampicillin (with probenecid)
	Tetracycline
	Spectinomycin
	Bacitracin (topically)
Gram-positive bacilli	
Clostridium species	Penicillin G
Bacillus species	Penicillin G
Corynebacterium diphtheriae	Erythromycin
	Penicillin G
Listeria monocytogenes	Ampicillin
Gram-negative bacilli	
(Family Enterobacteriaceae)	
Escherichia coli	Ampicillin
Klebsiella pneumoniae	Gentamicin
	Cephalosporin
Proteus mirabilis	Ampicillin
Serratia marcescens	Gentamicin
Haemophilus influenzae	Penicillin
	Sulfonamides
	Tetracyclines
	Spectinomycin
Pseudomonas aeruginosa	Ticarcillin
	Gentamicin
	Carbenicillin
	Tobramycin
	Colistin
	Polymyxin B
	Amikacin
Moraxella species	Cephaloridine
	Penicillin G
	Ampicillin
	Colistin
	Neomycin
	Gentamicin (response is variable)
Acinetobacter (formerly Mimeae) species	Gentamicin
	Colistin
Miscellaneous organisms	
Actinomyces israelii	Penicillin G
	Clindamycin
Nocardia species	Ampicillin
	Sulfonamides

Table 4-5. Infectious organisms for which penicillins are effective antimicrobial agents

Drug	Organism
Penicillin G	*Streptococcus pneumoniae*
	Streptococcus pyogenes
	α-Hemolytic streptococcus
	Staphylococcus aureus (nonpenicillinase producing)
	Neisseria gonorrhoeae (nonpenicillinase producing)
	Corynebacterium diphtheriae
	Actinomyces israelii
Methicillin	*Staphylococcus aureus* (penicillinase producing)
Oxacillin	
Cloxacillin	
Dicloxacillin	
Ampicillin	Nonpenicillinase-producing staphylococcus
	Proteus mirabilis
	Haemophilus influenzae
	Escherichia coli
	Listeria myogenes
Amoxicillin*	Same as for ampicillin
Carbenicillin	*Pseudomonas aeruginosa*
Ticarcillin†	*Pseudomonas* species
	Indole-positive and -negative *Proteus* species
	E. coli
	Enterobacter species

*Same as ampicillin but absorbed better.
†Similar in structure and antimicrobial activity to carbenicillin.

vary by the responsible bacterium or fungus, duration of infection, severity of the suppuration, and other factors.

Repeat corneal cultures during therapy are not reliable. Tissue destruction may occur by mechanisms other than replication of microorganisms. The objectives of this stage of management are to halt additional structural alteration, promote stromal healing and re-epithelialization, and prevent drug toxicity.[21]

The decision to ease up on or discontinue therapy should be based on daily slit-lamp examinations. The most helpful signs of improvement are blunting of the perimeter of the stromal suppuration, reduction in the cellular infiltrate and edema in the transition zone in the adjacent stroma, and progressive epithelialization. Fibrin exudate on the endothelium and hypopyon may resolve slowly and do not necessarily reflect the degree of improvement of the corneal process.[20]

Following discharge from the hospital, the patient should be alert to the danger signs of resurgent keratitis and promptly report increased pain, decreased vision, or purulent discharge. Epithelialization does not indicate the completion of therapy because any of these antibiotics may deter epithelial healing and produce other toxic and allergic reactions.

Penicillin G[45] (Tables 4-5 and 4-6)

These compounds penetrate into the aqueous humor of the normal eye. Intraocular inflammation reduces the effect of blood-aqueous humor barrier; thus high levels of penicillin are found in the intraocular fluids of inflamed eyes.

Benzyl penicillin (penicillin G) is absorbed poorly from the gastrointestinal tract; the drug is therefore given intravenously or intramuscularly. It is bactericidal by virtue of inhibiting the biosynthesis of cell wall mucopeptide. It is effective against penicillin-sensitive staphylococci, *Streptococcus pneumoniae, S. pyogenes, Neisseria gonorrhoeae,* and *N. meningitidis.* It is the most active agent against the majority of gram-positive and gram-negative anaerobes, excluding *Bacteroides fragilis.*[19]

Although the penicillins are considered bactericidal drugs, the presence of penicillin in the medium is not directly lethal to the organism. If the bacterial protoplast is protected against osmotic destruction by an artificial hypertonic medium or is in a loculated accumulation of protein-rich exudate (abscess), renewed growth of bacteria occurs when penicillin is removed from the environment.[45] The penicillins are effective only against active, growing bacteria and have little effect on vegetating organisms not synthesizing new cell wall material.

The systemic dose is 2 to 6 megaunits every 4 hours, to be given intravenously (Table 4-9). The subconjunctival injection is 0.5 to 1 megaunit[3,21,36] (Table 4-8).

The rapid secretory mechanism from the kidney and clearance of the drug can be blocked by probenecid, 500 mg orally every 6 hours. If this is given, the level of penicillin will be raised two to four times the normal systemic dose.

The adverse reactions to penicillin G are hypersensitivity reactions, including skin rash, drug fever, urticaria, and occasionally an anaphylactic reaction that may be fatal.

Carbenicillin (Table 4-6)

This drug is a semisynthetic penicillin with a range against gram-positive and gram-negative organisms.[6,14,15,19] It is useful in *Pseudomonas aeruginosa* and indole-positive *Proteus* species infections. Carbenicillin is not useful in managing ulcers caused by gram-positive cocci, since it is not penicillinase resistant. It should not be used if the patient has a history of sensitivity to penicillin. Its subconjunctival dose is 100 to 125 mg (Table 4-8); the systemic dose is listed in Table 4-9.

Ticarcillin (Table 4-6)

Ticarcillin is similar in structure and antimicrobial activity to carbenicillin. It exhibits broad activity against indole-positive and -negative *Proteus* organisms, *E. coli,* and *Enterobacter* species. It is not active against penicillinase-producing staphylococci. Subconjunctival injection of 100 mg (Table 4-8) produces high concentrations. Intravenous injection of 200 mg/kg in three divided doses for systemic administration is recommended (Table 4-9). The main indication for parenteral ticarcillin would be in combination with gentamicin or tobramycin in keratitis and endophthalmitis caused by *Pseudomonas* organisms. In other gram-negative infections one is guided by the sensitivities. Ticarcillin may have an effect against some anaerobes.

Ampicillin (Table 4-6)

Ampicillin, like penicillin G, is destroyed by bacterial penicillinase. It is less active than penicillin G against streptococci, staphylococci, and pneumococci. The spectrum of action against gram-negative organisms includes action against *Haemophilus influenzae,*

Table 4-6. Spectrum, penetration, and action of principal antibiotics used in treatment of bacterial corneal ulcers

Drug	Spectrum		Penetration	Action	Important facts
	Gram-positive organisms	Gram-negative organisms			
Ampicillin	+	+	Good	Bactericidal	Not effective against penicillinase-producing staphylococci or *Proteus* or *Pseudomonas* organisms
Amoxicillin (oral use only)	+	+	Good	Bactericidal	Like ampicillin, but more completely absorbed
Cephalosporins (similar in action to penicillins)	+	±	Good	Bactericidal	Effective against penicillinase staphylococci and streptococci (except enterococci) and isolates of *E. coli*, *Klebsiella* organisms, and indole-positive *Proteus* species; not good against *Pseudomonas* or indole-positive *Proteus* organisms or *H. influenzae* Nephrotoxic
Colistin (polymyxin E, polymyxin B)	−	+	Poor	Bactericidal	Effective against *Pseudomonas* organisms but not against *Proteus vulgaris* Nephrotoxic
Gentamicin	+	+	Poor[38]	Bactericidal	Effective against *Pseudomonas* species and some staphylococci Renal toxicity
Chloramphenicol	+	+	Good	Bacteriostatic	Serious blood dyscrasias
Methicillin	+	−	Poor	Bactericidal	Effective against penicillinase-producing staphylococci Nephrotoxic; depresses bone marrow
Penicillin G	+	−	Good in inflamed eye	Bactericidal	
Vancomycin	+	−	Fair	Bactericidal	Very toxic—not used extensively in ophthalmology Ototoxic (nephrotoxic)

Drug	Gram (+)	Gram (−)	Activity	Type	Remarks
Erythromycin	+	−		Bacteriostatic	Topical ointment is used. Subconjunctival injection is also given. May be employed in cases of allergy to penicillin
Carbenicillin	+	+	Fair	Bactericidal	Works well in combination with gentamicin in severe *Pseudomonas*, *Proteus* species, and *E. coli* infections; not effective against penicillinase-producing staphylococcus, as well as *Klebsiella* and *Serratia* organisms
Ticarcillin	+	+	Good	Bactericidal	Same as for carbenicillin
Oxacillin	+	+	Poor	Bactericidal	Penicillinase resistant
Cloxacillin	+	+		Bactericidal	Penicillinase resistant
Dicloxacillin	+	+	Good	Bactericidal	Penicillinase resistant
Bacitracin	+	±		Bactericidal	Allergy is rare; not to be given systemically because of toxicity
Tobramycin	Some +	+		Bactericidal	Effective against penicillinase-producing *Staphylococcus*, *Pseudomonas*, *Enterobacter*, *Klebsiella*, *Serratia* and *Escherichia* organisms; resistant strains of these organisms may show up. Ototoxic and nephrotoxic, with some neuromuscular toxicity. Should be currently reserved for infections caused by resistant strains of *P. aeruginosa* of family Enterobacteriacea. IV dose: 3 to 5 mg/kg IM or slow IV. Subconjunctival injections: 5 to 10 mg
Amikacin	−	+		Bactericidal	Active against large number of gram-negative bacteria. Resistant to gentamicin and kanamycin. Tobramycin are sensitive to amikacin. Activity against *Mycobacterium fortuitum*. Cochlear toxicity. Dose: 15 mg/kg IM or slow IV
Spectinomycin	−	+		Bacteriostatic	May be used in penicillin-sensitive individuals with gonorrheal infection

Table 4-7. Preparation of principal topical antibiotics commonly used for treatment of bacterial corneal ulcers

Antibiotic	Remove	Add	Replace	Content	Final concentration
Bacitracin	9 ml from 15 ml tear substitute vial	3 ml tears to each of 3 vials	All 3 ml from each of 3 vials (total, 9 ml) to original tear substitute	9 ml reconstituted bacitracin and 6 ml tears	10,000 units/ml
Neomycin	1 ml from 15 ml tear substitute vial	1 ml tears to 1 vial neomycin (500 mg)	1 ml reconstituted neomycin into tear squeeze bottle	1 ml neomycin and 14 ml tears	8 mg/ml
Kanamycin		1 vial (500 mg in 2 ml) kanamycin to full vial tears		2 ml kanamycin and 15 ml tears	30 mg/ml
Penicillin G	3 ml tears from 15 ml tear substitute bottle	3 ml tears to 1 vial penicillin G (5 megaunits)	3 ml reconstituted penicillin into tear bottle	3 ml penicillin G and 12 ml tears	110,000 units/ml
Carbenicillin		1 ml carbenicillin (prepared according to instructions) to 15 ml tear substitute		1 ml carbenicillin and 15 ml tears	6 mg/ml
Vancomycin	2 ml tears from 15 ml tear substitute bottle	2 ml tears to 1 vial vancomycin (500 mg)	2 ml reconstituted vancomycin into tear bottle	2 ml vancomycin and 13 ml tears	30 to 33 mg/ml
Gentamicin		1 ml parenteral solution to 5 ml bottle ophthalmic gentamicin			8 to 10 mg/ml
Cephazolin		5 ml of sterile water to 1 g vial of cephazolin		Add this to 15 ml bottle of artificial tears	50 mg/ml
Tobramycin		2 ml of tobramycin (systemic) to bottle of 5 ml ophthalmic preparation			13 mg/ml fortified

Proteus mirabilis, E. coli, Salmonella and *Moraxella* organisms, and some strains of *Aerobacter* species and *Alcaligenes faecalis*. It is not effective against *Pseudomonas aeruginosa*.[19,45]

The systemic dose of 2 to 4 g every 4 hours intravenously (Table 4-9) and subconjunctival dose of 100 mg in 0.33 ml of sterile water are advised[3,19] (Table 4-8). Ampicillin is used against *N. gonorrhoeae* in a dose of 3.5 g orally with probenecid (0.5 g to 1 g).

Allergic phenomena occurring with ampicillin are similar to those reported from penicillin G, but in addition, there may be a transient increase in the serum glutamic-oxaloacetic transaminase (SGOT) level.[45]

Amoxicillin (Table 4-6)

Amoxicillin is similar in structure, spectrum, and activity to ampicillin. It is effective against nonpenicillin-producing staphylococci, streptococci, a majority of isolates of *H. influenzae, E. coli*, and *P. mirabilis*. Blood levels are usually higher than those with ampicillin. Oral doses produce high levels (500 mg to 1 g every 8 hours is recommended) (Table 4-9).

Isoxazolyl penicillins (Table 4-6)

This group includes oxacillin, cloxacillin, and dicloxacillin. They differ from each other by the presence and number of chlorine atoms: one chlorine atom is absent in oxacillin, one in cloxacillin, and two in dicloxacillin. Isoxazolyl penicillins are bactericidal.

These drugs are strongly resistant to destruction by bacterial penicillinase. In vitro they are less effective against non-penicillinase-producing, gram-positive microorganisms than is penicillin G and should be reserved to treat infections known to be produced by penicillinase-producing staphylococci.[19,45] Of these three drugs, dicloxacillin penetrates the inflamed eye best. The agent of choice of these penicillins appears to be dicloxacillin. It should be noted that penicillin G is more effective than these drugs against gram-positive cocci and rods and gram-negative cocci. Isoxazolyl penicillins are ineffective against *Streptococcus faecalis*. Ampicillin is more effective than oxacillin against certain gram-negative bacilli. The subconjunctival dose (Table 4-8) of 50 to 100 mg in 0.5 ml of distilled water may be given daily.[3] The systemic dose (Table 4-9) is 2 to 2.5 g orally every 4 hours.

Hypersensitivity phenomena include skin rash, drug fever, urticaria, and anaphylaxis. Occasionally disturbances in the gastrointestinal system and in SGOT levels may be seen; other systemic problems, such as hemorrhagic nephritis, are occasionally encountered in infants.

Methicillin (Table 4-6)

This drug is the preferred semisynthetic penicillin used against unidentified gram-positive organisms and is bactericidal. Compared with oxacillin and cloxacillin, methicillin is less active by weight against penicillinase-producing staphylococci, but this difference is insignificant because of adjusted doses and degree of serum binding. Methicillin has relatively low serum binding; theoretically there is greater availability

Table 4-8. Subconjunctival antibiotic preparation and dosage of commonly used drugs for treatment of bacterial corneal ulcers

Antibiotic	Dose per vial	Diluent volume	Concentration	Injection	Total dose
Carbenicillin	1 g	5 ml	200 mg/ml	0.5 ml	100 mg
Colistin*	150 mg	2 ml	75 mg/ml	0.3 ml	25 mg
Gentamicin	80 mg	—	40 mg/ml	0.5 ml	20 to 40 mg
Methicillin	1 g	5 ml	200 mg/ml	0.5 ml	100 mg
Ampicillin	1 g	5 ml	200 mg/ml	0.5 ml	100 mg
Cephaloridine	500 mg	2.5 ml	200 mg/ml	0.5 ml	100 mg
Cephazolin	500 mg	2.5 ml	200 mg/ml	0.5 ml	100 mg
Neomycin	500 mg	1 ml	500 mg/ml	0.5 ml	250 to 500 mg
Penicillin G*	5 megaunits	2.5 ml	2 megaunits/ml	0.5 ml	0.5 to 1 megaunit
Vancomycin	500 mg	5 ml	100 mg/ml	0.25 ml	25 mg
Bacitracin	50,000 units	2.5 ml	20,000 units/ml	0.5 ml	10,000 units
Polymyxin B*	50 mg	5 ml	10 mg/ml	0.5 ml	5 mg
Erythromycin	50 mg	5 ml	10 mg/ml	0.5 ml	5 mg
Tobramycin	80 mg	—	20 mg/cc	0.25 ml	20 mg
Ticarcillin	—	—	—	—	100 mg

*Painful subconjunctival injection can be avoided if tetracaine is applied topically before injection. To reenforce this, one may apply 4% cocaine with a cotton type of applicator to the area of the intended injection. Use a tuberculin syringe with a 27-gauge needle, and inject 0.5 ml 1% lidocaine. This may be given before the injection of the drug or with the drug. Colistimethate sodium (Coly-Mycin M) parenteral is the generic name for colistin to be used for subconjunctival injection.

for antimicrobial action. As with other penicillinase-resistant penicillins, methicillin is not as effective as penicillin G against nonpenicillinase organisms.[45]

The indicated use is primarily against infection caused by penicillinase-producing staphylococci.

The adult dose is 4 to 6 g intravenously in divided doses (Table 4-8). Pulse-dose injection of the proper dose of methicillin dissolved in a small amount of fluid is the best method of administration. Subconjunctival injection of 100 mg can be given daily[3, 18, 19, 36] (Table 4-8).

With the use of methicillin, one may see skin rashes, urticaria, and bone marrow depression with reversible neutropenia. In some individuals renal function is impaired.

Bacitracin (Table 4-6)

The action of bacitracin, which is similar to that of penicillin and is bactericidal, is by interfering with cell wall synthesis and binding to cell membranes to produce false pores and flux of ions. Bacitracin is effective against gram-negative coccus (*Neisseria*

Table 4-9. Antibiotic dosages for principal antibiotics used in treatment of bacterial keratitis

Drug	Subconjunctival dose	Parenteral dose
Carbenicillin (Geopen)	100 mg	2 to 6 g every 4 hours IV with 0.5 g probenecid orally four times a day
Cephaloridine (Loridine)	100 mg	1 g every 4 hours IV (maximum is 4 g every 24 hours, since it is nephrotoxic)
Cephalothin (Keflin)	Too irritating	1 to 2 g every 3 to 4 hours IV
Methicillin (Staphcillin)	75 to 100 mg	2 g every 4 hours IV with 0.5 g probenecid orally four times a day
Erythromycin	5 to 10 mg	2 to 4 g daily orally in divided dose or 1 g every 6 hours IV
Oxacillin (Prostaphlin)	75 to 100 mg	2 to 2.5 g every 4 hours IV with 0.5 g probenecid orally four times a day
Gentamicin (Garamycin)	20 to 40 mg	3 to 5 mg/kg/day IM
Ampicillin	100 mg	2 to 4 g every 4 hours IV
Colistimethate sodium (Coly-Mycin M)	25 mg	5 mg/kg/day IM in two to four doses
Penicillin G	500,000 to 1 million units (300 to 600 mg)	2 to 6 megaunits every 4 hours IV with 0.5 g probenecid orally four times a day
Tobramycin	5 to 10 mg	3 to 5 mg/kg IM or slow IV
Ticarcillin	100 mg	200 mg/kg IV in three divided doses
Amoxicillin		500 mg to 1 g every 8 hours orally
Amikacin		15 mg/kg IM or slow IV
Spectinomycin		2 g IM
Bacitracin*	10,000 units/ml	—
Neomycin* (Mycifradin)	250 to 500 mg	—
Vancomycin* (Vancocin)	25 mg	—
Kanamycin* (Kantrex)	30 mg	—

*Bacitracin, neomycin, vancomycin, and kanamycin should be used topically and should not be used parenterally, since they are all extremely toxic. The latter two are both nephrotoxic and ototoxic.

species) infection, gram-positive coccus infection, and some gram-positive bacillus infections, including those caused by *Corynebacterium diphtheriae* and *Clostridium* and *Actinomyces* organisms. It may also have an effect on the gram-negative bacillus of *Haemophilus*. Bacitracin is effective against penicillinase-producing staphylococci.[18, 19]

The use of bacitracin in ophthalmology should be restricted to topical administration by drops, ointment (Table 4-7), and subconjunctival injections (Table 4-8). In severe infections the concentration can be increased so that the dose of the ophthalmic drops is 10,000 units/ml[18] (Table 4-7).

Allergic sensitization or primary irritation is rare.

Gentamicin (Table 4-6)

In the last decade the aminoglycoside gentamicin has proved effective in the treatment of *P. aeruginosa* keratitis and has replaced polymyxin B and colistin in the initial management. Although carbenicillin may act synergistically with gentamicin in vitro and has been recommended for use along with gentamicin, no synergism was seen in pseudomonas keratitis experiments.

Gentamicin is bactericidal[38] (Table 4-6). Its activity is associated with its ability to inhibit bacterial protein synthesis. It is effective against *Pseudomonas aeruginosa; E. coli; Serratia marcescens;* and *Proteus, Klebsiella, Aerobacter,* and *Moraxella* species. Gentamicin is active in vitro against penicillinase and nonpenicillinase staphylococci and has been clinically effective in serious staphylococcal infections.[37] It is neither a suitable antibiotic against diplococcus or streptococcus infections nor recommended for continued therapy against *Staphylococcus aureus* corneal ulcers, but it may be employed in such diagnosed cases with one of the synthetic penicillinase-resistant penicillins.[19, 37]

It shares some of the toxic effects of other aminoglycosides and is ototoxic and nephrotoxic. Gentamicin should never be administered systemically unless the renal function is known to be adequate; it is never to be given concurrently with other ototoxic agents.[19]

It can be given subconjunctivally 20 mg/ml (Table 4-8) and topically via drops with concentrations of 8 to 13.6 mg/ml (Table 4-7), depending on the severity of the infection. If it is found necessary to give gentamicin systemically, it may be given intramuscularly, 3 to 5 mg/kg daily in divided doses; careful monitoring of kidney function is necessary (Table 4-7).

Tobramycin[39] (Table 4-6)

Tobramycin, a new aminoglycoside, has also proved extremely effective in the treatment of *P. aeruginosa* keratitis. Tobramycin is similar to gentamicin in antimicrobial activity and toxicity and is reported to be two to four times more active in vitro by weight, as compared with gentamicin, against *P. aeruginosa*. It has been shown to be effective against some gentamicin-resistant strains, and approximately 50% of *P. aeruginosa* organisms resistant to gentamicin remain sensitive to tobramycin. However, there has been no evidence to date that tobramycin has been significantly superior clinically to gentamicin in the treatment of *Pseudomonas* keratitis.

The current preferred drugs for the initial treatment of suspected gram-negative rod keratitis and *Pseudomonas* keratitis are either gentamicin or tobramycin.[12] When a

Table 4-10. Initial antibiotic selection based on smear morphology

Smear morphology	Antibiotic		
	Topical	Subconjunctival	Intravenous*
Gram-positive cocci	Cephaloridine or cefazolin (50 mg/ml)	Cephaloridine or cefazolin (100 mg)	Methicillin (200 mg/kg/day)
Gram-positive rods	Gentamicin (14 mg/ml)	Gentamicin (20 mg)	Gentamicin (3.0-7.0 mg/kg/day)
Gram-positive filaments	Penicillin G (100,000 units/ml)	Penicillin G (500,000 units/ml)	Penicillin G (2.0-6.0 M units/4 hr)
Gram-negative cocci	Penicillin G (10,000 units/ml)	Penicillin G (500,000 units/ml)	Penicillin G (2.0-6.0 M units/4 hr)
Gram-negative rods	Gentamicin (14 mg/ml) Tobramycin (14 mg/ml)	Gentamicin (20 mg) Tobramycin (10-20 mg)	Gentamicin (3.0-7.0 Tobramycin (3.0-5.0 mg/kg of body weight IM)
Acid-fast bacilli†	Amikacin (10 mg/ml)	Amikacin (25 mg)	Amikacin (5 mg/kg/day)
Two or more bacteria	Cephaloridine or cefazolin (50 mg/ml) and gentamicin (14 mg/ml)	Cephaloridine or cefazolin (100 mg) and gentamicin (20 mg)	Methicillin (200 mg/kg/day) and Gentamicin (3.0-7.0 mg/kg/day)

From Jones, D.B.: Ophthalmology **88**:814, 1981.
*Reserve for scleral suppuration or corneal perforation (impending or existing).
†Reserve for suppurative *Mycobacterium* species (atypical complex).

strain is resistant to gentamicin and tobramycin, amikacin may be tried. Most acquired resistance to aminoglycosides has occurred from acquired microbial enzymatic inactivation in the bacterial membrane or near the site of drug transport. Amikacin is a new semisynthetic aminoglycoside that is resistant to inactivation by most bacterial enzymes and has had a good therapeutic effect against *P. aeruginosa* keratitis. Colistin or polymyxin B may also be useful therapeutic alternatives.

Doses for tobramycin are as follows: subconjunctival, 10 to 20 mg (Table 4-8); intramuscular, 3 to 5 mg/kg of body weight (Table 4-10); and intravenous, 3 to 5 mg/kg in slow intravenous drip (Table 4-9).

Fortified topical drops may be prepared by adding 2 ml of the systemic preparation (Nebcin) to 5 ml of ophthalmic tobramycin. Tobramycin should be used in ocular infections presently for gentamicin-resistant strains of *P. aeruginosa* or the family Enterobacteriaceae and for other gram-negative infections as indicated by sensitivity tests.

Amikacin (Table 4-6)

This semisynthetic aminoglycoside is similar in structure to kanamycin. It is resistant to enzymes that render kanamycin, gentamicin, and tobramycin inactive. Therefore some gram-negative bacteria resistant to these aminoglycosides are sensitive to amikacin. However, organisms resistant to amikacin are usually resistant to gentamicin,

Table 4-11. Modified antibiotic therapy based on preliminary identification of selected organisms

Organism	Antibiotic		
	Topical	Subconjunctival	Intravenous*
Micrococcaceae sensitivities unknown	Cephaloridine or cefazolin (50 mg/ml)	Cephaloridine or cefazolin (100 mg)	Methicillin (200 mg/kg/day)
Micrococcus, Staphylococcus; penicillin-resistant	Cephaloridine or cefazolin (50 mg/ml)	Cephaloridine or cefazolin (100 mg)	Methicillin (200 mg/kg/day)
Micrococcus, Staphylococcus; penicillin-sensitive	Penicillin G (100,000 units/ml)	Penicillin G (500,000 units)	Penicillin G (2.0-6.0 M units/4 hr)
Streptococcus†, Pneumococcus	Penicillin G (100,000 units/ml)	Penicillin G (500,000 units)	Penicillin G (2.0-6.0 M units/4 hr)
Anaerobic gram-positive coccus	Penicillin G (100,000 units/ml)	Penicillin G (500,000 units)	Penicillin G (2.0-6.0 M units/4 hr)
Corynebacterium species	Penicillin G (100,000 units/ml)	Penicillin G (500,000 units)	Penicillin G (2.0-6.0 M units /4 hr)
Azotobacter species	Gentamicin (14 mg/ml)	Gentamicin (20 mg)	Gentamicin (3.0-7.0 mg/kg/day)
Mycobacterium species	Amikacin (10 mg/ml)	Amikacin (20 mg)	Amikacin (5 mg/kg/day)
Neisseria gonorrhoeae, N. meningitidis	Penicillin G (100,000 units/ml)	Penicillin G (500,000 units)	Penicillin G (2.0-6.0 M units/4 hr)
Enterobacteriaceae	Gentamicin (14 mg/ml)	Gentamicin (20 mg)	Gentamicin (3.0-7.0 mg/kg/day)
Pseudomonas species	Gentamicin (14 mg/ml), tobramycin	Gentamicin (20 mg), tobramycin (5-10 mg)	Gentamicin (3.0-7.0 mg/kg/day)
Other aerobic, gram-negative rod	Gentamicin (14 mg/ml)	Gentamicin (20 mg)	Gentamicin (3.0-7.0 mg/kg/day)
Anaerobic gram-negative rod	Penicillin G (100,000 units/ml)	Penicillin G (500,000 units)	Penicillin G (2.0-6.0 M units/4 hr)

From Jones, D.B.: Ophthalmology **88**:814, 1981.
*Reserve for scleral suppuration or corneal perforation (impending or existing).
†Excludes *S. faecalis;* requires combined therapy (e.g., penicillin G or gentamicin).

tobramycin, and kanamycin. Like other aminoglycosides, amikacin possesses toxicity to the cochleovestibular apparatus. It is given in doses of 15 mg/kg by slow intravenous drip (Table 4-9). It is a second-order drug to be used in infections caused by susceptible strains of *P. aeruginosa* or other gram-negative organisms known to be resistant to kanamycin, gentamicin, and tobramycin.

Erythromycin (Table 4-6)

Bacteriostatic (Table 4-6) in low concentrations and bactericidal in high concentrations, erythromycin is effective against gram-positive cocci and gram-positive bacilli.[18,19] It is also effective against chlamydial infection in the newborn, especially since a propensity to pneumonitis exists in these cases.

Erythromycin is used as either a topical solution or an ointment in a concentration of 5 mg/ml. It is well tolerated by the conjunctiva and the cornea. Subconjunctival injections of 5 to 10 mg in a small volume of distilled water may be used (Table 4-8). The drug may be employed in cases of allergy to the penicillins or cephalosporins or when antibiotic sensitivity specific to erythromycin only is encountered.

Cephalosporins[27,40]

These drugs are effective against penicillinase-producing staphylococci, pneumococci and streptococci, as well as many strains of gram-negative bacilli, particularly *E. coli, Proteus mirabilis,* and *Klebsiella* organisms. They are bactericidal (Table 4-6) but are ineffective against *Pseudomonas aeruginosa.* Cephalosporins have been proposed as an alternative antibiotic for use in cases of known penicillin allergy.[22,36] Many patients known to be sensitive to penicillin have been given cephalosporin without difficulty, but the cephalosporins should be administered with caution to any patient known to be allergic to penicillin.[36]

The primary indication for the use of *cephalothin* in ophthalmology is severe bacterial infection of the cornea, orbit, or globe in a patient who has a sensitivity to penicillin or when the causative organism is thought to be a species sensitive to cephalothin.

Cephalothin is less sensitive to penicillinase-producing staphylococci than other of this group and is preferred for staphylococcal infections. It may be given 1 g in 10 ml of sterile water injection intravenously over a 5-minute period, with the dose to be repeated every 4 to 6 hours.[18,19] It is painful on intramuscular injection. A subconjunctival injection of 50 mg is used and may be repeated daily as needed.[18]

Cephaloridine penetrates the intact and inflamed eye easily to produce effective levels in the intraocular fluids. The antibacterial spectrum of cephaloridine is similar to cephalothin. Nephrotoxicity limits its systemic usage and should be used with utmost caution if at all by way of systemic routes. Subconjunctival injections of cephaloridine, which are nonirritating,[3] can be given in 50 to 100 mg doses (Table 4-8). The systemic adult dosage is 3 to 4 g daily given in 1 g divided doses. Usually 1 g is dissolved in 10 ml of sterile distilled water and given intravenously every 6 to 8 hours (Table 4-9).

Cephazolin is another cephalosporin that can be given as an alternative to penicillin. Its systemic dose is 1 g intravenously four times a day. It is less painful on intramuscular injection and is therefore preferred for this method. It has greater accumulation in renal problems than does cephalothin. It is given topically (50 mg/ml) and subconjunctivally (100 mg/ml). It is used with gentamicin as initial treatment when the bacterium is not yet identified.

In general, the indication for the cephalosporins are gram-positive infections and a long history of nonsevere penicillin reaction and certain gram-negative infections as directed by sensitivity reactions.

Chloramphenicol (Table 4-6)

This drug is bacteriostatic (Table 4-6) with good activity against *Haemophilus influenzae*. Chloramphenicol penetrates into aqueous and vitreous along parenteral or oral routes. Topical administration also results in detectable antibiotic levels in the cornea. The wide spectrum and excellent penetration plus the convenience should have made this a reasonably desirable drug; however, it should be used only in severe infections in which there is known sensitivity of the organism to chloramphenicol and to no other drug. It is better to use other safer antibiotics such as penicillin G, semisynthetic penicillins, and cephalosporins. Chloramphenicol should not be administered to children or adolescent girls or to any person at all for longer than 7 days. Adverse reactions, which include skin rash, optic neuritis, "gray illness" in premature infants, and blood dyscrasias, are either idiosyncratic, not dose related or toxic dose related. The patients should receive a reticulocyte count and complete blood count repeated in four 8-hour periods. Chloramphenicol should be discontinued if granulocyte, platelet, red cell, or reticulocyte counts decline. Some persons develop severe bone marrow depression even after the drug has been discontinued.[14,19] The dose is 50 mg/kg given daily in a divided dose. The oral route is indicated. Topical preparations are available.

Polymyxin B (Aerosporin)

This antibiotic is effective only against gram-negative bacteria, is bactericidal, and penetrates the cornea poorly. It binds to plasma membranes to produce altered cell permeability. Organisms resistant to polymyxin are also resistant to colistin. Polymyxin B is used in *Pseudomonas* species and Enterobacteriaceae infections, but not in *Proteus* organism infections. Corneal epithelial deficiency enhances the absorption and penetration of the drug.

Polymyxin B is nephrotoxic in doses exceeding 2.2 mg/kg daily; in view of its toxicity, it should only be used topically.

Colistin

In structure colistin is similar to polymyxin and is thought to be the same as polymyxin. This drug is bactericidal (Table 4-6) and is active against gram-negative bacilli, including the *Pseudomonas* and *Moraxella* species.[14,18,19] Some strains of *Proteus* are resistant to colistin, as are most gram-positive organisms. Colistin may be obtained as a sulphate or a methane sulphate salt. For local and topical use in ophthalmology the sulphate is the preparation of choice. Colistimethate sodium (Coly-Mycin M) can be used for subconjunctival injection (25 mg)[19] (Table 4-8).

These preparations are nephrotoxic.

•   •   •

Systemic antibiotics have not been routinely recommended in the treatment of infected corneal ulcers. Even in inflamed eyes, only low concentrations of gentamicin can usually be achieved in the cornea and aqueous after systemic administration, and this has been true with other antibiotics. Systemic antibiotics should be used as concomitant therapy along with local antibiotics in corneal infections caused by *Neisseria gonorrhoeae* and *Haemophilus* organisms in which other noncorneal tissues are frequently involved, in imminent or perforated corneal ulcers, in corneal ulcers with associated scleral infiltration or endophthalmitis, and in some cases as adjunctive therapy when an ideal local antibiotic regimen cannot be used.

Sloan and associates[38] demonstrated that topical aminoglycosides provided high therapeutic levels of antibiotic in the aqueous of infected eyes when high topical concentrations of antibiotics were given at 15-minute intervals. The authors of this study compared frequent topical administration of the fortified gentamicin solution (20 mg/ml) with subconjunctival gentamicin and continuous-lavage gentamicin. Extremely high therapeutic levels of gentamicin were attained by all routes. They concluded that since similarly high concentrations of gentamicin can be attained in the infected eye by the less traumatic means of frequent topical drops, topical medication may prove more logical and just as effective a form of therapy as subconjunctival antibiotics. This is important, especially since subconjunctival antibiotic therapy has certain disadvantages: patient apprehension, more ocular inflammation, more pain than topical therapy, and a risk of intraocular administration (although rare, important). Recently Davis and associates[11] reported in a comparative study of experimental *Pseudomonas* keratitis in rabbits and guinea pigs that a highly concentrated dose of topical tobramycin (20 mg/ml) administered every 30 minutes was significantly more effective than subconjunctival therapy with tobramycin (20 mg) in eliminating *Pseudomonas* organisms from the cornea. Also, in a therapy trial with combined topical tobramycin and subconjunctival tobramycin, subconjunctival therapy did not improve the efficacy of intensive topical tobramycin in killing organisms in the treatment of *Pseudomonas* keratitis.

OTHER DRUGS
Rifampicin

This oral antibiotic is effective against chlamydial agents and some viruses. Bacteria resistant to other antibiotics may be sensitive to rifampicin, and its activity extends to *Mycobacterium fortuitum*. Rifampicin inhibits bacterial growth by binding the DNA-dependent, RNA-polymerase therapy, preventing the formation of initiation complex and subsequent replication. The range of activity extends to gram-positive cocci and some gram-negative organisms.[44]

Neomycin

In *Moraxella* species infections, neomycin may be given topically. Occasionally it may be given subconjunctivally, 250 mg/ml (Table 4-7).

Since subconjunctival injections may be quite painful, it is advisable to first instill a topical tetracaine anesthetic agent, followed by an injection of 0.5 ml of 1% lidocaine. Injection of the neomycin should be given slowly after the lidocaine is administered. The material should be allowed to diffuse; then the medication desired for antibacterial use should be slowly and carefully injected.

Spectinomycin (Table 4-6)

This drug is different in structure and action from the other aminoglycosides. It has a broad in vitro action against gram-positive and gram-negative aerobic organisms. Spectinomycin is primarily used for treatment of penicillin-sensitive persons with gonorrheal infections. The recommended dose is 2 to 4 g by intramuscular injection (Table 4-9).

CORTICOSTEROIDS[11]

The use of corticosteroids in the initial and subsequent management of microbial keratitis remains controversial. Corticosteroids are the most effective agents for suppression of the harmful effects of the inflammatory response, and there is ample evidence that topically applied corticosteroids suppress corneal inflammation. Animal studies of *S. aureus* and *P. aeruginosa* keratitis have implied that topical corticosteroids do not interfere with the bactericidal activity of antibiotics to which the organisms are sensitive. Other experimental studies have suggested that corticosteroids prolong replication of the responsible organisms and would delay healing despite concurrent antibacterial therapy. The safety and efficacy of corticosteroids in human microbial keratitis have not been established by controlled clinical trials.[20]

Fungal keratitis

The problem of fungal keratitis causes great concern for many ophthalmologists.[69] It is necessary therefore to be promptly aware of the possibility of such infection and to introduce proper laboratory investigation to establish a diagnosis and to treat with the necessary drugs. The morbidity of fungal infections tends to be greater than that of bacterial keratitis because of the delay in diagnosis.

Fungal keratitis is more prevalent in the southern and southwestern parts of the United States. The fact that there has been an increase in the number of cases in the United States since 1960 suggests that there is an increase not only in the incidence but perhaps in the recognition of fungal keratitis as well.[66] Some evidence suggests that the extensive use of corticosteroids may possibly have contributed to the increase in incidence. Seasonal incidence of fungal keratitis, particularly the forms caused by filamentous fungi, is most likely a result of environmental factors. Of course, endogenous fungal endophthalmitis offers no seasonal variation.

The most virulent fungal infections occur in persons with no apparent deficiency in resistance. These cases are usually associated with injury to the cornea from twigs or other plant matter. Less virulent organisms such as *Candida albicans* pick out immune deficient individuals. In Sjögren's syndrome; erythema multiforme; conditions in which there is a defect in macrophage and neutrophil leukocytic function or deficiencies in the cell-mediated immune response and antibody production, especially IgA; and in endocrinopathy,[75] *C. albicans* may play an important etiologic role in fungal keratitis. Diabetes mellitus and alcoholism, which may contribute to reduced systemic resistance, may also be factors, as may hypovitaminosis A in association with generalized mucocutaneous candidiasis.[68]

CLASSIFICATION OF FUNGI

A brief classification of fungi important as a cause of ocular disease may be tabulated as follows.[76]

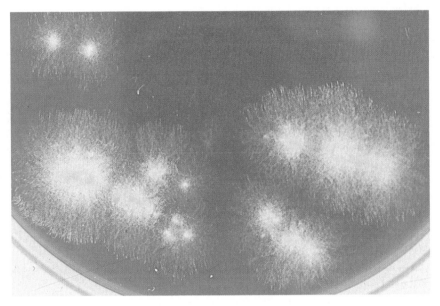

Fig. 4-6. Blood agar plate incubated at room temperature showing *Aspergillus fumigatus* growth.

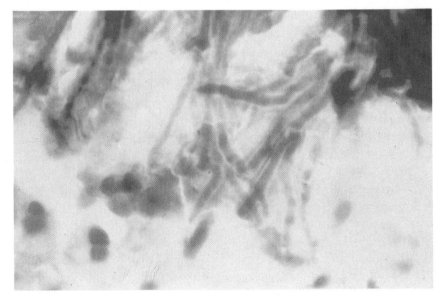

Fig. 4-7. Giemsa's stain from corneal ulcer exhibiting septated hyphae.

Filamentous fungi

The hyphae of these multicellular fungi branch, forming a tangled mass on the culture medium called *mycelium* (Fig. 4-6).

Septate organisms. The hyphae are divided by cell walls into cellular compartments that contain one or more than one nucleus (Fig. 4-7). The fungi in this group are of interest:
1. *Fusarium* species
2. *Acremonium* species[52]
3. *Aspergillus* species[51]
4. *Cladosporium* species
5. *Penicillium* species
6. *Paecilomyces* species[54]
7. Others such as *Phialophora, Curvularia,* and *Alternaria* species

The filamentous organisms in the class of Fungi Imperfecti, such as *Fusarium* and *Cephalosporium* species, may affect normal eyes after corneal abrasion or trauma, which occurs most often in farm workers or people who have been injured with some kind of vegetable matter. Infections with these fungi occur more frequently in the temperate zones of the country.

Topical steroids may enhance replication by these inocula. No convincing evidence exists that antibiotics after trauma contribute significantly to the development of the fungal ulcers.

The most common cause of fungal keratitis is the hyphate group of filamentous fungi, which includes *Aspergillus, Acremonium, Curvularia,* and *Fusarium. Candida albicans* is the most frequently isolated yeast. The free-living amoeba, *Acanthamoeba,* is a newly recognized cause of suppurative keratitis, which is clinically indistinguishable from bacterial and fungal infections.

Fusarium solanae is the major cause of fungal keratitis in Florida and certainly occurs in other areas of the United States. The *Acremonium* organism is capable of producing corneal ulceration and opacification by virtue of a proteolytic enzyme. In addition, *Cephalosporium* species is reported as a cause of fungal endophthalmitis and canalicular and lacrimal sac infections. *Aspergillus* species is a ubiquitous organism and is responsible for endophthalmitis, orbital cellulitis, lacrimal sac infections, and keratitis.

Nonseptate organisms. There is no division of hyphae, but long tubes with numerous nuclei are scattered throughout. This group, Phycomycetes, is the cause of hematogenous endophthalmitis; the more commonly occurring organisms follow:
1. *Mucor* species
2. *Rhizopus* species
3. *Absidia* species

Yeasts

These are fungi with usual and dominant growth as unicellular organisms that may develop pseudohyphae and buds. In this group one may see the following organisms:
1. *Candida albicans* (in worldwide distribution)
2. *Cryptococcus* species
3. *Rhodotorula* species

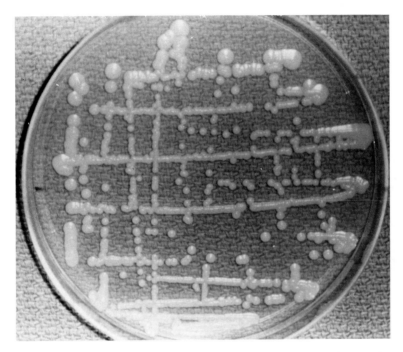

Fig. 4-8. Colonies of *Candida albicans* growing on Sabouraud's medium. They can be mistaken for colonies of staphylococci.

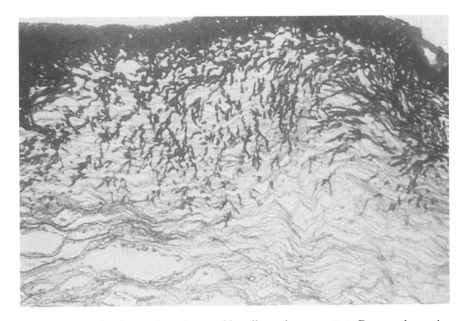

Fig. 4-9. Fungus makes its way through corneal lamellae and may penetrate Descemet's membrane.

The corneal ulcers caused by the *Candida* organism usually occur in eyes where there is some predisposing factor. Some of these factors have already been mentioned, but one may include herpes simplex keratitis and chronic use of corticosteroids as well. Agricultural exposure and trauma occurring outdoors are usually not factors in the pathogenesis of fungal keratitis with yeasts. They have been found in the lacrimal passages and on the lids, conjunctiva, and cornea as ocular pathogens. Their growth on Sabouraud's media may be mistaken for staphylococcal colonies (Fig. 4-8).

Diphasic fungi

These fungi possess two distinct morphologic forms: the yeast phase, occurring in tissues, and the mycelial phase, occurring on media. Diphasic fungi, although not too important in exogenous infections, are more important in endogenous disease. Following are the more common fungi:

1. *Blastomyces* species[77]
2. *Coccidioides* species
3. *Histoplasma* species
4. *Sporothrix* species

Many fungal ulcers are caused by fungi that are commonly considered to be saprophytes. About 7% of normal healthy eyes have fungi on the lids at one time or other, but no fungi are primary indigenous microflora of the conjunctival sac.

CLINICAL APPEARANCE

Severe inflammation of the cornea occurs as a result of fungal infection in the form of replicating and nonreplicating fungi, mycotoxins, proteolytic enzymes, and soluble fungal antigens.[48] These agents can result in necrosis of the corneal lamellae, acute inflammation, antigenic response with immune ring formation, hypopyon, and severe uveitis.[54] In general, the virulence of the filamentous fungi of environmental origin ranges from the rapidly destructive *Fusarium solanae* down through many species, including those of *Cephalosporium, Aspergillus,* and *Penicillium,* to the more leisurely pathogens such as *Phialophora* organisms, which may grow indolently in the cornea over a period of months. Multiple microabscesses may surround the main lesion of central ulceration and infiltration; a tendency exists for the hyphae to penetrate the stromal lamellae (Fig. 4-9), attack Descemet's membrane, and spread into the anterior chamber. Fungi may be absent near the surface and the superficial stroma, which may explain the difficulty in obtaining scrapings for study as well as recovery of the organism. Some *Fusarium* species infections have a predilection for the posterior chamber, which results in severe glaucoma and adds to the severity of the disease.

The corneal ulcer caused by filamentous fungi may show grayish-white infiltration exhibiting a rough texture, with areas elevated above the plane of the uninvolved cornea (Fig. 4-10). The margins, which are irregular and extend into the adjacent stroma (Fig. 4-11), may exhibit a feathery outline. Satellite lesions occur that are separate from the area of involvement (Fig. 4-12) and correspond to stroma microabscesses. An endothelial plaque may be seen paralleling the ulcer. An immune ring may surround the primary lesion, representing an antibody response between fungal antigen and host-antibody response. In addition, a hypopyon and purulent discharge may occur (Fig.

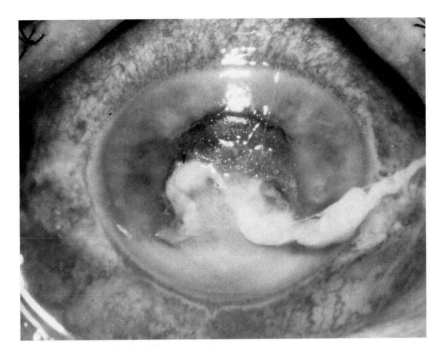

Fig. 4-10. Stromal infiltration and hypopyon. Raised edge and extensive amount of purulent discharge.

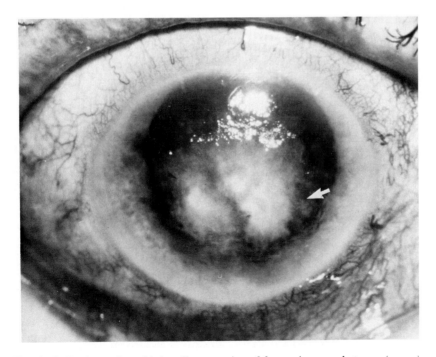

Fig. 4-11. Feathery edge with lamellar extension of fungus in corneal stroma *(arrow)*.

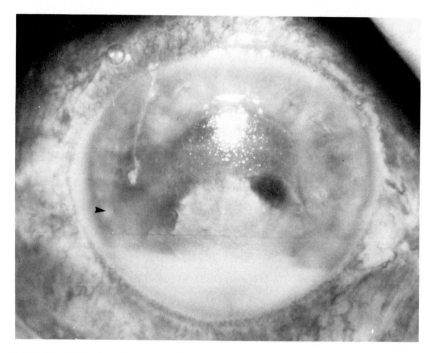

Fig. 4-12. Satellite lesion *(arrow)* in fungal ulcer with large hypopyon and extensive stromal necrosis.

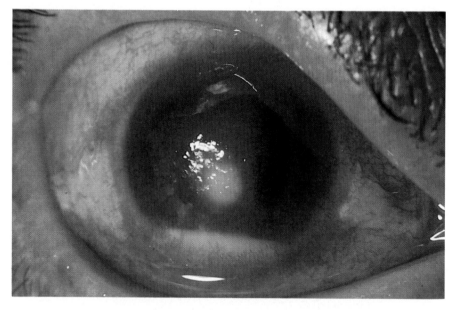

Fig. 4-13. *Candida albicans* corneal infection.

4-10). Conjunctival injection and anterior chamber reaction may be quite severe.

Actually a typical appearance of fungal ulcers does not exist. Early infections may resemble staphylococcal infiltrative disease, especially near the limbus, as may herpes. A large ulcer may resemble a severe bacterial infection.

Candida albicans ulcers usually exhibit an oval, plaquelike, elevated lesion that is reasonably well outlined and may resemble a bacterial keratitis (Fig. 4-13).

Although it is difficult to distinguish filamentous fungal keratitis from yeast *(C. albicans)* keratitis, the findings listed in Table 4-12 may enable one to do so.

Corneal scrapings of the ulcer, under slit-lamp magnification, must be done. Multiple (five to ten) samples should be taken and observed. All staining material and all media should be fresh.[67,83,84] A stain of direct smear is done immediately and fixed with methyl alcohol. Two slides are fixed for Giemsa stain, two for Gram's stain, and two for special stain. Gram's stain will enable the fungus to be seen directly; the Giemsa stain may show ghosting of fungal walls but will also stain the fungus. In addition, budding yeast may also be noted. Although one cannot make a diagnosis of specific fungi on Giemsa- or gram-stained hyphal fragments, one can definitely say that a hyphal organism or a yeast is present. If these steps are followed, it is possible to obtain positive results in about 75% of cases. The best tissue stain for fungi is the Gomori methenamine silver technique. This stain delineates the hyphae as sharp black structures against a pale green background. The next step is to inoculate the proper medium, such as one of the following:

1. Blood agar plate incubated at 25° and 37° C. *Fusarium solanae* grows well at 37° C.
2. Sabouraud's medium incubated at 25° C (no additives).
3. Beef heart infusion broth at 25° C (gentamicin added). With this medium, which may be put on a platform shaker, the isolates may be obtained by 3 days.

Table 4-12. Comparison of characteristics of keratitis caused by filamentous yeast organisms

Filamentous keratitis	Yeast *(Candida albicans)* keratitis
Occurs more frequently in young people (occupational and outdoor activity)	Usually occurs in compromised host; there may be preexisting corneal disease; preexisting steroid treatment on long-term basis may be evident in history
Signs may be present 24 to 48 hours after injury; no priming factor essential, such as application of steroids or antibiotics	May be more focal and suppurative and may penetrate stroma in localized area even to point of perforation and thus resemble bacterial keratitis
Area involved can be localized; a defect may or may not be evident in epithelium; by the time patient is seen, epithelium may have healed over, indicating that inflammatory process is not severe	Edges usually not feathery, and satellitism not usually seen
Hyphal fragments spread in lamellae; feathery edge appearance and infiltrate; satellite phenomenon	
Inflammation can be severe with hypopyon and endothelial plaque; may be quite suppurative and thus resemble bacterial keratitis	

Table 4-13. Drugs and their actions

Organism	Flucytosine	Amphotericin B	Pimaricin
Candida species	+	+	+
Aspergillus species	0	+	+
Fusarium species	0	±	+

Table 4-14. Antifungal drugs and their actions

	Miconazole	Econazole	Clotrimazole	Ketaconazole	Flucytosine
Candida	+ (Ten times better than econazole)	±	+	+ (More active than miconazole)	+
Aspergillus	±	+	Active +	—	—
Fusarium	±	±	—	—	—
Gram-positive cocci and bacilli	+	No activity	—	—	—
Oral, IV, or topical administration	IV and topical in arachnis oil Has been given orally in cutaneous fungal infection Subconjunctivally 10 mg/day	Has been given IV Topical in arachnis oil	Hepatic degradation enzymes limit oral effectiveness Topical 1% solution	It is absorbed well orally	Topical drops 1%

PRINCIPLES OF TREATMENT[57,65]

Following are the main drugs used for treatment of filamentous and yeast infection of the cornea:

1. Flucytosine[49,50,61]
2. Pimaricin[61,64]
3. Amphotericin B[50,61]

Tables 4-13 and 4-14 illustrate the actions of these drugs.

The drug selected should be the one that best inhibits fungal growth. The treatment should be carried on long enough so that the normal body defenses are capable of coping with remaining organisms. Tables 4-15, 4-16, and 4-17 tabulate selection of antibiotics for treatment.

Table 4-15. Selection of initial drug based on smear morphology

Smear	Topical antibiotic	Subconjunctival	Intravenous
Hyphal fragments	Natamycin (50 mg/ml)	None*	None†
Yeasts, pseudohyphae	Natamycin (50 mg/ml)	None*	None‡

From Jones, D.B.: Ophthalmology **88**:814, 1981.
*Consider miconazole in the presence of scleral suppuration, corneal perforation, or intraocular extension of suppuration (5 mg).
†Consider intravenous miconazole in the presence of scleral suppuration, corneal perforation, or intraocular extension of suppuration (1200 to 3600 mg/day).
‡Consider oral flucytosine in the presence of scleral suppuration, corneal perforation, or intraocular extension of suppuration (150 mg/kg/day).

Table 4-16. Severe keratitis

Results of smears	Selection of antibiotic
Hyphal fragments, yeasts, or pseudohyphae	Natamycin and/or miconazole

From Jones, D.B.: Ophthalmology **88**:814, 1981.

Table 4-17. Treatment based on organism

Organism	Topical	Subconjunctival	Intravenous
Fusarium species	Natamycin (50 mg/ml)	None	None
Other filamentous fungi	Natamycin (50 mg/ml)	None*	None†
Candida species	Natamycin (50 mg/ml)	None*	None‡

From Jones, D.B.: Ophthalmology **88**:814, 1981.
*Consider miconazole (5 mg) in the presence of scleral suppuration, corneal perforation, or intraocular extension of suppuration.
†Consider intravenous miconazole (1200 to 3600 mg/day) in the presence of scleral suppuration, corneal perforation, or intraocular extension of suppuration caused by susceptible strains.
‡Consider oral flucytosine (150 mg/kg/day) in the presence of scleral suppuration, corneal perforation, or intraocular extension of suppuration.

Available drugs

Amphotericin B, a heptane polyene,[47,57,60] is active against *Candida* and *Aspergillus* organisms but possesses a variable activity against *Fusarium* species. It binds to the membrane of the fungal cell and increases its permeability. Amphotericin B is fungistatic, insoluble, and, by virtue of its ability to bind to the sterol moiety of human renal tubular cells and erythrocytes, toxic. It is unstable in light, water, heat, and pH extremes. Cell membrane changes that it induces are reversible. The drug is applied as topical medication in concentrations of 2 mg/ml and should not be given as a subconjunctival injection. Topical medication may be given every half hour at first in severe infections and then every hour if the clinical condition improves. Amphotericin B is quite toxic to the conjunctiva and corneal epithelium: it may take the resulting necrotic conjunctiva 6 weeks to recover from a single subconjunctival injection and therefore should not be used by this route.

Amphotericin B is to be prepared in distilled water for eye drops since it precipitates in sodium chloride solution. Amphotericin B can be esterified; the compound thus formed is 10 times less toxic to the cornea and much more water soluble. The methyl ester compound also reduces toxicity to kidney and red blood cells.

Natamycin (pimaricin 5%)[64,71,74] is a tetraene polyene antibiotic. It produces irreversible alterations in the cell membrane but is insoluble and lacks stability. It has a broad spectrum against filamentous fungi and *Candida albicans* and is at present the drug of choice for these organisms.[61] Natamycin is more effective than amphotericin B against *Fusarium* organisms and is useful against *Candida* and *Aspergillus* species. A 5% suspension is applied topically and with excessive use may cause some epithelial toxicity to the cornea. It may be used every 2 to 4 hours. Since natamycin is a suspension, it "adheres" to the ulcer site. It is more stable than amphotericin B.

Flucytosine[80,82] (5-fluorocytosine, or Ancobon) is a fluorinated pyrimidine and is fungistatic. Antifungal activity is related to deamination to fluorouracil by susceptible fungi, thus blocking thymidine synthesis. It is not metabolized by human cells, and 95% is excreted. Flucytosine is effective against *Candida* organisms and only certain strains of *Aspergillus, Penicillium,* and *Cladosporium* species, but is not effective against *Fusarium* or *Cephalosporium* organisms. *Candida* species resistance reduces its effectiveness; this phenomenon should be watched for if flucytosine is employed. In general, the results have been disappointing when flucytosine is used alone. Topically it is used as drops in a 1% solution (10 mg/ml) every hour. The combination of flucytosine and amphotericin B may be of value in systemic candidiasis. The suggested oral dose is 50 to 150 mg/kg/day in four divided doses.

Other drugs

Other drugs included are imidazole compounds:
1. Clotrimazole[53,61,63]
2. Miconazole[58,61,81,82]
3. Econazole[61]
4. Ketonazole

Flucytosine, miconazole, and ketoconazole did not retard the closure of corneal epithelial defects in rabbits. However, amphotericin B produced dramatic pathologic changes. Ketoconazole produced modest biomicroscopic and histologic changes in regenerating corneal epithelium; flucytosine and miconazole did not produce changes.[58]

Selection of proper medication may be based on identification of fungi in proper culture media and sensitivity determination, but if the patient is doing well on one drug, treatment should not be changed unless toxicity to the drug develops. Long-term therapy in fungal keratitis should be anticipated.

Signs of improvement of a fungal ulcer are decrease in the size of the central corneal infiltrate, disappearance of the satellite lesions, and rounding out of the feathery margins. Persistent epithelial staining may be noticed, but often this indicates toxicity to the medications. Negative scrapings during treatment are not indicative of eradication of the fungal agent, and great care should be exercised in continuing treatment, using one's clinical judgment in evaluating the signs of improvement just mentioned.

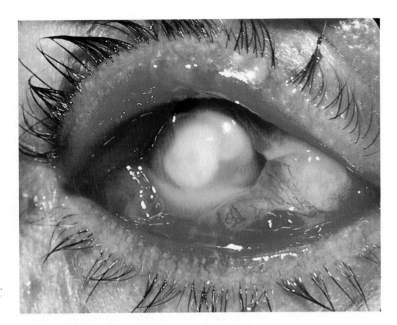

Fig. 4-14. Perforated *Fusarium solani* corneal ulcer.

Corticosteroids

The aim of giving corticosteroids in conjunction with the proper antifungal agent[70,72] is the control of active inflammation to minimize or eliminate structural alteration. If steroids are given for this reason, they should be given only when antifungal treatment has resulted in clinical improvement. It is most important that *no* systemic steroids be given, that effective antifungal agents be given before topical steroids are introduced, and that the patient be observed carefully. One must be prepared to cope with any emergency that may arise and to determine if the patient is immunologically competent. Some investigators believe that steroids do not cause melting but that the thinning may come about after the inflammation subsides. Abrupt cessation of steroids may be dangerous, since it causes a rebound response, and perforation may follow.

Corticosteroids remove leukocytic elements, and, when the treatment is stopped, white cell proliferation occurs. The reaction is characterized by proliferation of immature cells, which produce antibodies to residual antigen in the stroma. Therefore abrupt cessation of steroids will cause an explosive reaction of immunologic nature and polymorphonuclear reaction. Under these circumstances the cornea may perforate (Fig. 4-14).

Severe corneal damage occurs rapidly as a result of replicating fungus, mycotoxins, and enzymes, and the battle may be lost, particularly if a *Fusarium* organism is the etiologic agent. The cornea may perforate (Fig. 4-14), or a descematocele may develop. If no response to medication occurs, the corneal infiltration and ulceration expand, and a descematocele or perforation occurs, a keratoplasty is indicated (Figs. 4-15 and 4-16).* Of course, if a large residual corneal scar results from the ravages of the disease, a

---

*References 56, 61, 62, 73, 78, 79.

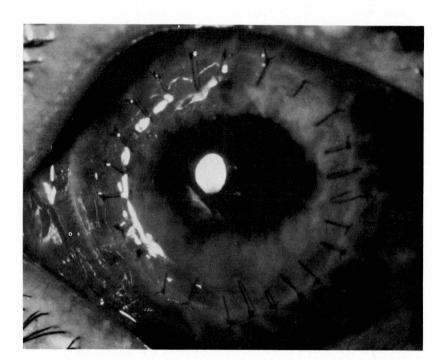

Fig. 4-15. Penetrating keratoplasty, 8.5 mm, for perforated fungal ulcer in Fig. 4-12.

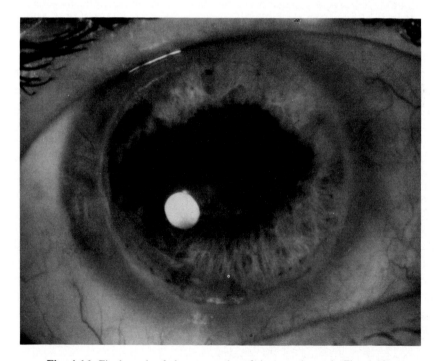

Fig. 4-16. Final result of clear corneal graft in case shown in Fig. 4-12.

corneal transplant can be performed at a planned date. Posterior chamber glaucoma is a fearful complication, and vitrectomy may have to be performed.

In fungal infections, invasion of the cornea is aided by alteration of the host. One of the ways to alter host defenses to weigh against the host at the time of inoculation of the fungal organism is to interject the use of steroid medication. Fungal keratitis can occur without steroids; however, many cases show some kind of epithelial abrasion after trauma with vegetable matter, and, with subsequent steroid therapy, a fungal ulcer may come about. Steroids aid replication of fungal filamentous organisms and should be avoided.

Interstitial keratitis and nummular keratitis

INTERSTITIAL KERATITIS

The term *interstitial keratitis* refers to vascularization and nonsuppurative infiltration affecting the corneal stroma, usually associated with a systemic disease. Interstitial keratitis may involve the whole cornea or only a section, or it may even be localized to the peripheral areas of the cornea.

Nonsuppurative, nondisciform interstitial keratitis may be caused by the following pathologic conditions, the first 10 of which are the most common:

1. Congenital syphilis
2. Acquired syphilis
3. Tuberculosis
4. Leprosy
5. Onchocerciasis
6. Mumps
7. Lymphogranuloma venereum
8. Cogan's syndrome
9. Gold toxicity
10. Herpes simplex
11. Herpes zoster
12. Rubeola
13. Trypanosomiasis
14. Leishmaniasis[98]
15. Influenza (rare)
16. Hodgkin's disease (rare)
17. Kaposi's sarcoma (rare)
18. Mycosis fungoides (rare)
19. Sarcoid (rare)
20. Incontinentia pigmenti (rare)
21. Toxicity to drugs such as arsenicals

Nonsystemic conditions that may result in interstitial keratitis are chemical burns of the eye and chromium deficiency in laboratory animals on a low-chromium diet.[94]

Disciform keratitis can be seen in herpes zoster, herpes simplex, mumps, varicella, variola, and vaccinia.

Congenital and acquired syphilis

In general terms, 90% of interstitial keratitis is caused by syphilis, with 87% resulting from congenital lues and 3% to 4% from acquired lues.

Indirect evidence, largely in the form of clinical observations, is used to invoke allergy as an explanation. The body of this evidence comprises several pieces of information:

1. Interstitial keratitis rarely develops in early congenital syphilis when *Treponema pallidum* abounds.

2. Treponemes are rarely found in the corneas of patients with active interstitial keratitis.

3. A delay occurs between the onset of active congenital syphilis and interstitial keratitis. The body takes a while to recognize that the organism is foreign.

4. Interstitial keratitis responds to neither penicillin nor heavy metal therapy.

5. Interstitial keratitis has a tendency to commence or relapse during active treatment when other syphilitic lesions are responding.

6. The cornea often shows prompt clinical improvement with corticosteroids.

Presumably antibodies are formed in the cornea that react with antigen to produce a more widespread reaction.

Interstitial keratitis seems to have a higher incidence in females[88]; about two thirds of the cases resulting from congenital syphilis occur between the age of 5 and the late teens. It is rare to find any cases after 30 years of age. The congenital form of disease is usually bilateral (80%) with the second eye becoming involved within a year in 75% of the cases. As time passes, the second eye has less tendency to be involved, since it is involved after five years in only 2% of cases.

The interstitial keratitis secondary to acquired syphilis may occur within months after the onset of the infection but generally occurs 10 years later. The clinical course closely resembles that in congenital syphilis except that interstitial keratitis in acquired syphilis is usually uniocular (60% of cases), frequently milder, limited to a sector of cornea, and occasionally more amenable to treatment.

Clinical course. The first signs of congenital luetic interstitial keratitis, which may precede symptoms by as much as several weeks, consist of an indistinct cellular infiltrate and edema in the endothelium followed by keratic precipitates and tiny opacities of the stroma. These changes are thought to be caused by an incipient iridocyclitis. With the beginning of symptoms, the untreated disease exhibits a progressive, a florid, and a retrogressive stage. A wrinkling or folding of Descemet's membrane usually occurs. In severe cases, the endothelium may be destroyed or damaged; this can result in permanent bullous corneal disease.

The progressive stage, which usually lasts 2 weeks, begins with severe symptoms of pain, lacrimation, photophobia, and blepharospasm occurring with circumcorneal vascular injection. The cornea becomes cloudy rapidly and extensively over a period of a few days, and then blood vessels appear. An iridocyclitis and anterior choroiditis occur during this stage.

In the florid stage the changes that began in the progressive stage become more evident. The acute inflammation of the eye and heavy deep vascularization of the cornea persist about 2 to 4 months. Bilateral extensive edema and cellular infiltration of the stroma with deep vascularization should be considered as lues until proved otherwise.

During the retrogressive stage the symptoms abate, and the corneal cloudiness and vascularization decrease. This stage lasts from 1 to 2 years.

The corneal cloudiness that begins in the progressive stage is a result of changes in all corneal layers. It imparts to the cornea a ground-glass appearance and reduces vision to light perception. Epithelial edema occurs and may progress to vesicle and bullae formation. Stromal cellular and vascular infiltration usually appear as faint gray, soft-edged opacities that increase in number and coalesce to form a general haze. In other cases, the process starts from the upper periphery and advances centrally.

Vascular invasion follows the corneal cloudiness and starts from the periphery. The

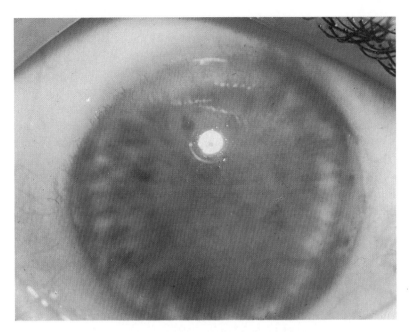

Fig. 4-17. Diffuse opacity of cornea from luetic interstitial keratitis.

vessels arise from conjunctival vessels and anterior ciliary vessels. Superficial vascularization can occur in the opacities mentioned and comes from the conjunctival vasculature. These vessels extend 4 mm into the cornea and are characterized as epaulet-like vascularization. Those arising from the ciliary vessels invade the deeper tissue, running between the lamellae in long, wavy, parallel lines. Vessels are usually brushlike. If the opacities begin in one sector, the vascularization is also a sector. The extent of vascular invasion can vary widely. Extensive invasion by the deeper vessels produces a mass of vessels that causes the cornea to appear a dull reddish pink, the so-called salmon patch. The vascular invasion continues for 4 to 5 weeks, and finally the whole cornea becomes intensely red. Complete corneal vascularization seems to be the crisis in the course of the disease because, after it occurs, the inflammation and symptoms begin to subside, and clearing starts.

In most cases, clearing begins peripherally and proceeds centrally after the vascular invasion and is accompanied by thinning of the cornea as a result of stromal collagen destruction and inflammation. Even though remarkable clearing may occur, especially in young people, usually some opacity is left centrally as a diffuse haze (Fig. 4-17). The blood vessels, which tend to persist as fine opaque lines, are not obliterated, although thinner branches of larger open vessels might be closed. In some the lumen is so small that a red blood cell is able only occasionally to pass through. These vessels were called "ghost vessels" in the past, since they persisted but were not thought to carry blood.

There are many variations from the typical course of the disease. The disease may remain in the periphery of the cornea, be confined to one sector only, and be of short duration, or it may have more than one separate center of inflammation with its own vascular invasion existing simultaneously.

Diagnosis. The diagnosis of interstitial keratitis at any stage is a clinical one. To see the acute attack is rare; most cases now seen are in adults with residuals of previous disease diagnosed by careful examination. The hallmark is stromal scarring, opacification, and residual deep vascularization. In the late cases, deep stromal opacities, usually with a metallic sheen reflex in front of Descemet's membrane, are seen. Stromal "ghost" vessels become evident by direct illumination or retroillumination. Linear formations of cornea guttata are seen. There may be splits in Descemet's membrane,[104] hyaline ridges and networks attached to the endothelium, band keratopathy, corneal thinning, lipid keratopathy, and Salzmann's degeneration.[103] Astigmatism occurs because of corneal irregularity and thinning. Late glaucoma[89,91,93,101] is a problem that may occur as a result of hypertrophy of Descemet's membrane over the chamber angle,[104] inflammatory sclerosis of the meshwork, synechiae, or narrow anterior chamber angles.

Iridocyclitis is the most common form of uveal involvement associated with interstitial keratitis. Anterior choroiditis is evidenced by vitreous opacities. After the attack has passed, changes frequently occur because of preceding uveal involvement caused by the general luetic involvement, including atrophy of the iris stroma, posterior synechia, salt-pepper fundus, large pigmentary patches in the periphery, a picture resembling retinitis pigmentosa, retinal scars, vascular atresia, and increased pigment or a white patch surrounded by pigment in the macula. Sclerokeratitis may be a part of the picture.

More than 90% of interstitial keratitis cases as determined by slit-lamp diagnosis are caused by syphilis, either congenital or acquired. To establish the diagnosis more firmly, one should seek help from the history in the form of an ocular inflammation in childhood that lasted several months; a positive serologic finding or previous treatment for venereal disease; or positive serologic findings (positive fluorescent treponemal antibody absorption [FTA-ABS] test), abortions, or stillbirths in the family history. Following are procedures and diagnostic information to be obtained in interstitial keratitis:

1. FTA-ABS test: most sensitive and specific
2. Venereal Disease Research Laboratories (VDRL) test: measures ABS reagins that are not specific for lues; not a treponemal test
3. Intermediate-strength purified protein derivative (PPD) skin test
4. Examination for evidence of phlyctenular scarring and pannus
5. History of vestibuloauditory disturbance (Cogan's syndrome)
6. Exposure to and/or history of tuberculosis
7. Evidence of congenital lues in history, for instance, frontal bossing, overgrowth of maxillary bones, Hutchinson's teeth, early loss of teeth, saddle nose, rhagades, saber shins, and deafness

Other stigmata of the later stage (beyond 2 years of age) of congenital syphilis are frontal bossing, saber shin, saddle nose, scaphoid scapulae, high palatine arch, epiphyseal enlargement, congenital eighth nerve deafness, rhagades, and perforation of palate or nasal septum. Hutchinson's teeth in congenital lues refers to small, barrel-shaped central permanent incisors, frequently with a central notch in the thickened biting edge caused by *T. pallidum* attacking the middle group of dental cells of the developing tooth. Hutchinson's triad is classic: characteristic appearance of the teeth, deafness, and interstitial keratitis. Loss of teeth early in life also occurs.[88] The FTA-ABS test will be positive even after treatment, whereas the VDRL probably will be negative.[99,100]

Medical treatment can be tried; however, if medications are ineffective, filtering surgery may be employed.

The prognosis in terms of resultant visual acuity is good.

Treatment. Late burned-out interstitial keratitis needs no local treatment other than keratoplasty, as indicated[97] (Fig. 4-18).

Since steroids merely suppress the disease process, they sometimes must be continued one and a half to two years. Some ophthalmologists believe that interstitial keratitis should run its course with no steroids. Others believe that the end result will be better with steroids, although the steroid may prolong the disease.

Without treatment or with heavy metal treatment, 25% to 50% of eyes recover to 20/30 or better vision and 70% to 20/60 or better; with steroid treatment, 85% to 90% recover to 20/30 vision or better. Topical steroids and cycloplegia are also employed; atropine may be too strong—the pupil should be kept moving.[95] Atropine is generally used during the active stages of the disease.

Antimicrobial therapy should be given not for the eyes but for the systemic problem. Penicillin[99] (2.4 megaunits of benzathine penicillin G weekly for two to three doses) is employed in the treatment of late congenital syphilis to prevent or treat cardiovascular, central nervous system, visceral, and osseous lesions. It does not seem to have any dramatic effect on the course of interstitial keratitis except that it may cause a flare-up, probably from liberation of antigen as in the systemic Herxheimer's reaction. Also, treatment of congenital syphilis does not prevent the onset of keratitis later, and penicillin treatment during the first attack of keratitis does not prevent subsequent involvement of the other eye.

Generally recurrences are transient and slight; about 9% of cases may be associated with mild trauma (Fig. 4-19), laceration, or impairment of general health.

Glaucoma[89,91,93,101] can occur years after congenital interstitial keratitis, or it may occur during the active phase, at which time it is not considered to be a serious problem. More than one mechanism may be involved in the production of late glaucoma in interstitial keratitis, at least in the few cases reported. Glaucoma appears to be secondary to extensive peripheral anterior synechiae from previous iritis. Acute angle-closure glaucoma can occur from multiple intraepithelial uveal cysts, which seem to be present in some cases of interstitial keratitis.

Cogan's syndrome

Cogan's syndrome of nonsyphilitic interstitial keratitis is bilateral and painful. It exhibits photophobia, fever, periorbital edema, and unilateral proptosis. It is associated with acquired vestibuloauditory symptoms, which may progress despite steroid treatment. Cogan's syndrome is characterized by deep yellow nodular corneal stromal opacities (Fig. 4-20). Deep corneal vascularization, and mild uveitis are noted, as are episcleral nodules and skin nodules. Vertigo, tinnitus, and acquired eighth-nerve deafness sometimes precede or rapidly follow the ocular changes. The etiologic factors are unknown but may be part of a general hypersensitivity reaction. Approximately 25% of patients with this syndrome have had clinical or tissue findings consistent with a polyarteritis-like condition.[85,86]

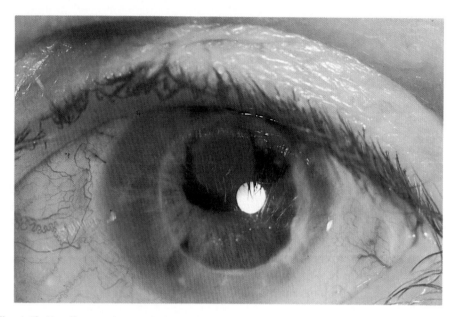

Fig. 4-18. Excellent results are obtained with penetrating keratoplasty when scarring of interstitial keratitis is sufficient to cause decreased vision.

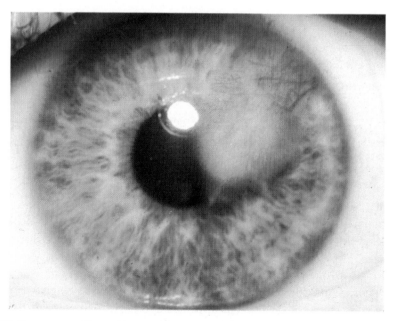

Fig. 4-19. Recurrence of interstitial keratitis because of trauma. Note sectoral response. (Courtesy F. Wilson II, M.D., Indianapolis, Ind.)

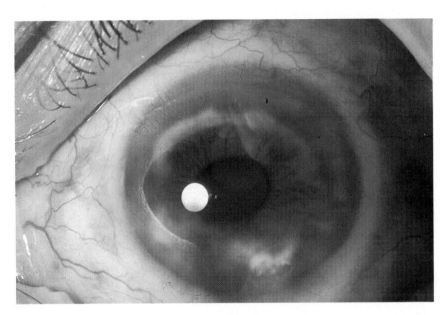

Fig. 4-20. Cogan's interstitial keratitis. (From Grayson, M.: The cornea in systemic disease. In Duane, T.D. [ed.]: Clinical Ophthalmology. Hagerstown, Md.: Harper & Row, 1976, vol. 4, chap. 15.)

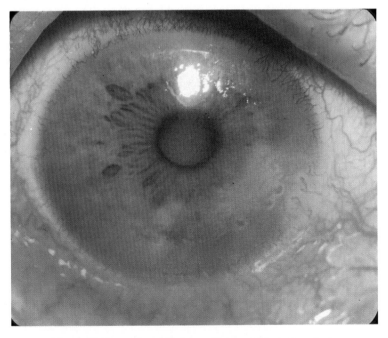

Fig. 4-21. Sector interstitial keratitis caused by tuberculosis.

Cogan's interstitial keratitis responds to topical steroid therapy. A negative reaction to hepatitis B antigen has been found.

Tuberculosis

Tuberculous interstitial keratitis is probably an allergic reaction to tuberculoprotein occurring in individuals with a focus of tuberculous disease elsewhere in the body. This disease is acquired, is often unilateral, and may show findings similar to luetic interstitial keratitis. However, in tuberculosis, infiltration occurs in the middle and deep layers of the cornea; if a phlyctenular component is present, it will be a positive factor in making a diagnosis of tuberculous keratitis. In tuberculous keratitis the cornea is often involved in the peripheral inferior sector only (Fig. 4-21), where it becomes a dense, abscesslike, nodular opacity, similar to a ring in shape. The central cornea is relatively spared. The clearing is less rapid and less complete than that of the syphilitic variety, leaving a dense, sectorlike scar. In lues, more diffuse corneal involvement is seen, and the blood vessels are deeper and clear from the periphery. A sector-shaped sclerokeratitis may also be seen.

A positive tuberculin skin test and a negative FTA-ABS test aid in diagnosis.

A combination of rifampin and isoniazid therapy may be helpful.

Leprosy

In leprosy, ocular involvement is more common and more severe in the lepromatous type. Granulomatous inflammation occurs in the form of giant leproma foam cells that contain the leprosy bacilli, for which a negative skin test suggests little or no immunity.

Ocular involvement with superficial and subepithelial neovascular keratitis spreads from the upper outer margin of the cornea like grains of chalk. The keratitis may extend over the entire cornea with formation of pannus, exposure keratitis, glaucoma, chronic conjunctivitis, lid nodules, thickened corneal nerves with beading opacification, and corneal anesthesia. In addition, loss of eyebrows and eyelashes, distortion of the lids, and scleritis may be found. The conjunctiva can be scraped, and an acid-fast stain done. One may see acid-fast–positive, beaded lepra bacilli. Sclerokeratitis may also occur.

Interstitial keratitis, which is a deep infiltration extending centrally from the periphery as a sequela of involvement of the ciliary body or a limbal nodule, is bilateral, occurs in 6% of the cases, and is seen late in the disease. Primary leprous keratitis results from invasion of the cornea by lepra bacilli.

Avascular keratitis (superficial stromal keratitis) begins in the superior temporal quadrant as discrete white opacities near the limbus. It can spread inferiorly and centrally. These chalk-dust opacities are phagocytosed lepra bacilli that form small lepromas on the superficial stroma. Avascular keratitis is usually preceded by iritis.

In lepromatous leprosy the cellular immunity is poor. In this type the clinical findings are severe. If the cellular immunity is intact, the tuberculoid type of leprosy is seen. There is a marked involvement of nerve tissue. Here there is loss of corneal sensation. Epithelioid cells and granulomas are seen in pathologic slides. Acid-fast stain must be employed; biopsies of cutaneous lesions stained with Fite-Faraco acid-fast stain may be employed. Treatment involves clofazimine, rifampin, and dapsone.

Viral interstitial keratitis

Although viral stromal keratitis is usually of a discoid type, it sometimes appears as a diffuse type of interstitial keratitis. This has been known to occur in mumps, lymphogranuloma venereum, influenza, herpes, measles, and vaccinia. In mumps, for example, the corneal involvement appears shortly after the parotitis and is usually unilateral, consisting of a transient, mild, interstitial keratitis. On occasion severe keratitis profunda may develop, appearing as a gray opacity with white interlacing fibrillae. No permanent vascularization, however, is generally seen with a mumps keratitis. Vaccinia keratitis may either be disciform or exhibit superficial ulcers. Frequently it has been reported to be recurrent.

Filariasis

Another form of stromal keratitis is exemplified by ocular onchocerciasis, a filarial disease that is a major cause of blindness seen in Central and Equatorial Africa and Central America. The disease is caused by *Onchocerca volvulus,* which produces subcutaneous nodules from which filariae discharge and spread to the eye, causing chronic conjunctivitis and keratitis. Onchocerciasis is spread by the *Simulium* fly species vector.

Limbal swelling is seen. Opacities may lie on either side of Bowman's layer. One corneal form of filarial keratitis occurs with a subepithelial pannus resembling a pterygium. The pannus has the appearance of invading tongues in the 3 to 9 o'clock meridian, leaving the superior portion of the cornea clear. These opacities may eventually wind up as densely scarred and vascularized cornea. A second form of filarial keratitis is fluffy, nummular,* and subepithelial. These areas are supposedly associated with, or reactions in the cornea from, dead microfilariae. Living microfilariae have been reported in the anterior chamber. The opacities are usually permanent and cause decreased visual acuity if sufficient in number. Sclerokeratitis may also be seen.

Levamisole solution, 3%, and 0.03% diethylcarbamazine citrate are filaricidal and, when applied to the cornea, rapidly cause entry of the microfilariae, the straightening out of previously curled microfilariae with formation of limbal globular infiltrates, and the subsequent formation of fluffy opacities around the microfilariae.[90]

In addition to the aforementioned findings, optic atrophy and chorioretinitis may occur in filarial keratitis.

Drug-induced interstitial keratitis

Systemic medications such as arsenic and gold over rather long periods of time have been associated with severe corneal infiltration and vascularization, probably on an allergic basis.

NUMMULAR KERATITIS

Nummular keratitis has been described[87] as a slowly developing, benign keratitis usually occurring unilaterally in young land workers and characterized by disc-shaped

---

*Other causes of nummular keratitis are listed on p. 101.

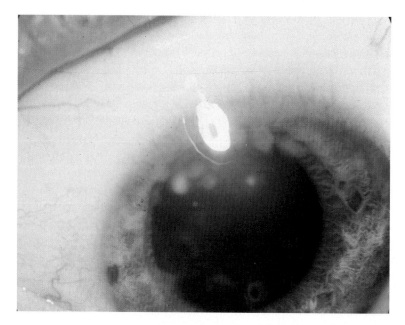

Fig. 4-22. Dimmer's nummular keratitis.

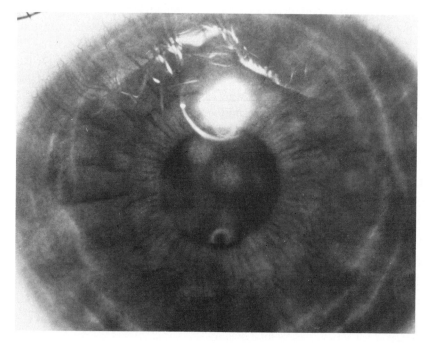

Fig. 4-23. Typical coin-shaped lesions in nummular keratitis.

infiltrates in the superficial stroma that later develop facets. This keratitis, characterized by these coin-shaped opacities and not associated with any conjunctivitis, is now known as Dimmer's nummular keratitis (Fig. 4-22). Related conditions have been described by Westhoff[105] and Lagraulet.[92] Recently, it has been observed in the Far East, where the disease is more commonly seen, and has been called "*padi* keratitis." (*Padi* means "unhusked rice" in the Malayan language.)

The disease is usually seen in rice-field workers with foreign body sensation, tearing, photophobia, blurred vision, and some degree of ciliary injection unassociated with any conjunctival discharge. Most patients have a history of trauma. One will see a keratitis without an associated conjunctivitis. The keratitis is characterized by coin-shaped opacities in the cornea numbering from 10 to 50 (Fig. 4-23).

Clinical course

During the first few weeks of involvement the corneal infiltrates show a nondiscrete, round configuration and a dull-white opacification that tends to spread and fade off into the surrounding cornea in edematous haze. Up until about 3 months, the epithelium over the discoid infiltrates remains smooth, but it may exhibit some edema and roughness and will exhibit a faint degree of fluorescein punctate staining. Beneath the edematous epithelium, one can see the stromal infiltrates, which are slightly subepithelial in depth. Peripheral lesions may develop superficial vascularization and will rarely proceed to ulceration. During the first 2 or 3 months some of the nummular lesions may develop a necrosis centrally, which appears clinically as central dense nuclei. However, after about the fourth month these dense nuclei of corneal opacities absorb and may result in annular forms with much clearer, slightly translucent centers and more opaque, dense rims, usually without the central depression or facet formation, although in some cases of nummular keratitis, facets are noted. These lesions are usually in one plane of the cornea but may be seen at all levels.[87] The patient by this time is much more comfortable, although vision may still be blurred.

Central lesions may coalesce and may form a disciform keratitis.[102]

A deep stromal involvement with edema and infiltration of the stroma is seen. To a more severe degree, one may observe an interstitial vascularization and edema in addition to stromal necrosis; in a few cases one may find a ring infiltration forming around the central discoid lesion.[102] Epithelial bullae may be seen as a result of Descemet's and endothelial edema. Corneal sensation is intact in all these patients. The deep central stromal infiltrate and edema usually start clearing during the fourth month, although some stromal haze may persist for a couple of years.

Etiologic factors

The cause of nummular keratitis is probably viral in nature; however, this has not definitely been proven. In regard to the possible mechanism of production of the deep stromal keratitis and nummular opacities with stromal infiltrates, it has been suggested that the mechanism is similar to that which is seen in herpes simplex virus disciform keratitis. The suggestion is that the virus may replicate in the epithelial cells; when these cells die, the antigen is liberated, and the underlying stroma soaks up the antigen, leading to stromal opacities that probably are a hypersensitivity reaction resulting from the combination of viral antigens with host antibodies. The beneficial effect of steroids on these infiltrates further substantiates the possibility of an immunologic reaction. Of course, another mechanism to explain the deep involvement is the direct viral invasion of the tissue and damage by toxins.

Differential diagnosis

Herpes simplex and herpes zoster may present a picture with subepithelial lesions. In herpes simplex, round subepithelial lesions in the anterior stroma may occur, particularly if steroid medications were employed. The lesions are nebulous in nature and may appear at any level of the corneal stroma. In herpes zoster the lesion may be a round subepithelial one and is usually in one level of the corneal stroma, appearing after the epithelial keratitis.

Other viral diseases with subepithelial lesions are epidemic keratoconjunctivitis types 8 and 19 and pharyngoconjunctival fever due to adenoviruses 3, 4, and 7. In the former instance the lesions are usually seen by the fifteenth day and may be present for 2 years. These coin-shaped lesions, which have no tendency to vascularize, are generally seen in the superficial layers of the cornea. In pharyngoconjunctival fever the lesions are transitory and are usually gone by the sixth to eighth week.

Bilateral interstitial and nummular keratitis associated with infectious mononucleosis confirmed by positive heterophil antibody test and rising titer to the Epstein-Barr virus does occur. Differentiation from zoster and herpes simplex must be made. In mononucleosis the opacities are bilateral in all levels of the stroma and confined to the peripheral cornea. In addition, with mononucleosis the corneal sensation is normal, and there are no epithelial defects. No anterior chamber reaction is seen and there are no rising viral titers to herpes simplex.[96]

Trachoma and inclusion disease may exhibit subepithelial lesions and must be considered in the differential diagnosis. However, in trachoma a gross pannus and conjunctival scarring may be present, whereas in adult inclusion disease one may see a micropannus and no conjunctival scarring. The subepithelial lesions in trachoma may be as large as 2 mm, and they may scar. They have a superficial and a superior corneal location. Brucellosis has also been reported as a clinical entity causing nummular keratitis.[106]

In syphilis the subepithelial opacities may precede the interstitial keratitis and may be deep, round, and scattered.

In onchocerciasis peripheral, coin-shaped corneal lesions occur in the interpalpebral area and may form large, triangular-shaped lesions with an advancing zone of gray opacities. One may also see large amounts of pigment entering the cornea from the limbal area. Band-shaped keratopathy is not uncommon. The microfilaria may be seen on occasion in the anterior chamber with careful slit-lamp examination. It may also be seen on examination of skin biopsy. Diethylcarbamazine citrate has been used for the microfilarial therapy. The adult worm is attacked with sodium suramin.

The following conditions may elicit a picture with subepithelial and nummular lesions:

1. Sarcoid
2. Tuberculosis
3. *Padi* keratitis
4. Dimmer's nummular keratitis
5. Herpes zoster
6. Herpes simplex

7. Leprosy
8. Lues
9. Onchocerciasis
10. Epidemic keratoconjunctivitis
11. Brucellosis
12. Epstein-Barr infection

REFERENCES
Bacterial keratitis

1. Allen, H.F.: Current status of prevention, diagnosis and management of bacterial corneal ulcers, Ann. Ophthalmol. **3:**235, 1971.
2. Allen, J.C.: Infection and the compromised hosts, Baltimore, 1976, The Williams & Wilkins Co.
3. Baum, J.L., Barza, M., and Weinstein, L.: Preferred routes of antibiotic administration in treatment of bacterial ulcers of the cornea, Int. Ophthalmol. Clin. **13:**31, 1973.
4. Baum, J.L., Barza, M., Shushan, D., et al.: Concentration of gentamicin in experimental corneal ulcers: topical vs. subconjunctival therapy, Arch. Ophthalmol. **92:**315, 1974.
5. Belmont, J.B., Ostler, H.B., Chandler, R.D., and Schwab, I.: Noninfectious ring-shaped keratitis associated with *Pseudomonas aeruginosa*, Am. J. Ophthalmol. **93:**338, 1982.
6. Bodey, G.P., Whitecar, J.P., Jr., Middleman, E., et al.: Carbenicillin therapy for *pseudomonas* infection, JAMA **218:**62, 1971.
7. Bohigian, G.M., and Escapini, H.: Corneal ulcer due to *Pseudomonas aeruginosa:* a comparison of the disease in California and El Salvador, Arch. Ophthalmol. **85:**405, 1971.
8. Brown, S.I., Bloomfield, S.E., and Wai-fong, I.T.: The cornea destroying enzyme of *Pseudomonas aeruginosa*, Invest. Ophthalmol. **11:**174, 1974.
9. Burns, R.P.: Laboratory methods in diagnosis of eye infections. In Infectious diseases of the conjunctiva and cornea: Symposium of the New Orleans Academy of Ophthalmology, St. Louis, 1963, The C.V. Mosby Co.
10. Codére, F., Brownstein, S., and Jackson, B.: *Pseudomonas aeruginosa* scleritis, Am. J. Ophthalmol. **91:**706, 1981.
11. Davis, S.D., Sarff, L.D., and Hyndiuk, R.A.: Corticosteroid in experimentally induced *Pseudomonas* keratitis: failure of prednisolone to impair the efficacy of tobramycin and carbenicillin therapy, Arch. Ophthalmol. **96:**126, 1978.
12. Fugiuell, F.P., Smith, J.P., and Baron, J.G.: Tobramycin levels in human eyes, Am. J. Ophthalmol. **85:**121, 1978.
13. Golden, B., Fingerman, L., and Allen, H.F.: Pseudomonas corneal ulcers in contact lens wearers: epidemiology and treatment, Arch. Ophthalmol. **85:**543, 1971.
14. Herman, P.E.: General principles of antimicrobial therapy, Mayo Clin. Proc. **52:**603, 1977.
15. Hoffman, T.A., and Bulloch, W.E.: Carbenicillin therapy of *Pseudomonas* and other gram-negative bacillary infections, Ann. Intern. Med. **73:**165, 1970.
16. Hutton, W.L., and Sexton, R.R.: Atypical *Pseudomonas* corneal ulcers in semicomatose patients, Am. J. Ophthalmol. **73:**37, 1972.
17. Hyndiuk, R.A.: Experimental *Pseudomonas* keratitis, Trans. Am. Ophthalmol. Soc. **79:**541, 1981.
18. Jones, D.B.: Early diagnosis and therapy of bacterial corneal ulcers, Int. Ophthalmol. Clin. **13:**1, 1973.
19. Jones, D.B.: A plan for antimicrobial therapy in bacterial keratitis, Trans. Am. Acad. Ophthalmol. Otolaryngol. **79:**95, 1975.
20. Jones, D.B.: Decision-making in the management of microbial keratitis, Ophthalmology **88:**814, 1981.
21. Jones, D.B., and Robinson, N.M.: Anaerobic ocular infections, Trans. Am. Acad. Ophthalmol. Otolaryngol. **83:**309, 1977.
22. Kaplan, K., Reisberg, B., and Weinstein, L.: Cephaloridine studies of therapeutic activity and untoward effects, Arch. Intern. Med. **121:**17, 1968.
23. Kim, H.B., and Ostler, H.B.: Marginal corneal ulcer due to beta-streptococcus, Arch. Ophthalmol. **95:**454, 1977.
24. Kimura, S.J., and Thygeson, P.: The cytology of external ocular disease, Am. J. Ophthalmol. **39:**127, 1955.
25. Kreger, A.S., and Griffin, Q.K.: Cornea damaging proteases of *Serratia marcescens*, Invest. Ophthalmol. **14:**190, 1975.
26. Lazar, M., Nemet, P., Bracha, R., and Campus, A.: *Mycobacterium fortuitum* keratitis, Am. J. Ophthalmol. **78:**530, 1974.
27. Moellering, R.C., Jr., and Swartz, M.N.: The newer cephalosporins, N. Engl. J. Med. **294:**24, 1976.

28. O'Day, D.M., Smith, R.S., Gregg, C.R., Turnbull, P.C.B., Head, W.S., Ives, J.A., and Ho, P.C.: The problem of Bacillus species infection with special emphasis on the virulence of *Bacillus cereus*, Ophthalmology **88**:833, 1981.

29. Okumoto, M., and Smolin, G.: Pneumococcal infections of the eye, Am. J. Ophthalmol. **77:** 346, 1974.

30. Okumoto, M., Smolin, G., Belfort, A., Jr., Kim, H.B., and Siverio, C.E.: *Proteus* species isolated from human eyes, Am. J. Ophthalmol. **81:**495, 1976.

31. Ostler, H.B., and Okumoto, M.: Anaerobic streptococcal corneal ulcer, Am. J. Ophthalmol. **81:**518, 1976.

32. Polascek, M., and Golden, B.: Rifampicin, Ann. Ophthalmol. **3:**877, 1971.

33. Prier, J.E.: Opportunistic pathogens, Baltimore, 1974, University Park Press.

34. Raber, I.M., Laibson, P.R., Kruz, G.H., et al.: *Pseudomonas* corneal-scleral ulcers, Paper presented at the annual meeting of the Ocular Microbiology and Immunology Group, San Francisco, Nov. 3, 1979.

35. Ralph, R.A., Lemp, M.A., and Liss, G.: *Nocardia asteroides* keratitis: a case report, Br. J. Ophthalmol. **60:**104, 1976.

36. Records, R.E.: Antimicrobial therapy in ophthalmology, Int. Ophthalmol. Clin. **10:**473, 1970.

37. Richards, F., McCall, D., and Cox, C.: Gentamicin treatment of staphylococcal infections, JAMA **215:**1297, 1971.

38. Sloan, S.H., Pettit, T.H., and Letwach, K.D.: Gentamicin penetration in aqueous humor of eyes with corneal ulcers, Am. J. Ophthalmol. **73:**750, 1972.

39. Stewart, R.H., Smith, R.E., Cagle, G.D., and Rosenthal, A.L.: Tobramycin in the treatment of external ocular infections: a clinical study, Ocular Ther. Surg. January-February 1982, p. 72.

40. Thompson, R.L.: The cephalosporins, Mayo Clin. Proc. **52:**625, 1977.

41. Valenton, M.J., and Okumoto, M.: Toxin producing strains of *Staphylococcus epidermidis*, Arch. Ophthalmol. **89:**186, 1973.

42. Vaughan, D.G.: Contamination of fluorescein solutions, Am. J. Ophthalmol. **39:**55, 1955.

43. Walters, R.W., Jorgensen, J.H., and Calzado, E.: Limulus lipate assay for early detection of certain gram-negative corneal infections, Arch. Ophthalmol. **97:**875, 1979.

44. Wilkie, J., Smolin, G., and Okumoto, M.: The effect of rifampicin on *Pseudomonas* keratitis, Can. J. Ophthalmol. **7:**309, 1972.

45. Wilkowske, C.J.: The penicillins, Mayo Clin. Proc. **52:**616, 1977.

46. Wilson, L.A., and Ahearn, D.C.: *Pseudomonas* induced corneal ulcers amorrated with contaminated eye mascara, Am. J. Ophthalmol. **84:**112, 1977.

Fungal keratitis

47. Anderson, B., and Chick, E.W.: Treatment of corneal fungal ulcers with amphotericin B and mechanical debridement, South. Med. J. **56:** 270, 1963.

48. Aronson, S.B., and Elliott, J.H.: Ocular inflammation, St. Louis, 1972, The C.V. Mosby Co.

49. Bennett, J.E.: Flucytosine, Ann. Intern. Med. **86:**319, 1977.

50. Block, E., and Bennett, J.: Pharmacologic studies with 5-fluorocytosine, Antimicrob. Agents Chemother. **1:**476, 1972.

51. Brightbill, F.S., and Fraser, L.K.: Unilateral keratoconjunctivitis with canalicular obstruction by *Aspergillus fumigatus*, Arch. Ophthalmol. **91:**421, 1974.

52. Burda, C.D., and Fisher, E., Jr.: Corneal destruction by extracts of *Cephalosporium mycelium*, Am. J. Ophthalmol. **50:**926, 1960.

53. Burgess, M.A., and Body, C.P.: Clotrimazole (Bay b 5097) in vitro and pharmacological studies, Antimicrob. Agents Chemother. **2:**423, 1972.

54. Dudley, M.A., and Chick, E.W.: Corneal lesions produced in rabbits by an extract of *Fusarium moniliforme*, Arch. Ophthalmol. **72:**346, 1964.

55. Forster, R.K., and Rebell, G.: The diagnosis and management of keratomycoses. I. Cause and diagnosis, Arch. Ophthalmol. **93:**975, 1975.

56. Forster, R.K., and Rebell, G.: Therapeutic surgery in failures of medical treatment of fungal keratitis, Br. J. Ophthalmol. **59:**366, 1975.

57. Forster, R.K., Rebell, G., and Wilson, L.A.: Dematiaceous fungal keratitis. Clinical isolates and management, Br. J. Ophthalmol. **59:**372, 1975.

58. Foster, C.S.: Miconazole therapy for keratomycosis, Am. J. Ophthalmol. **91:**622, 1981.

59. Foster, C.S., Lass, J.H., Moran-Wallace, E., et al.: Ocular toxicity of topical antifungal agents, Arch. Ophthalmol. **99:**1081, 1981.

60. Green, W.R., Bennett, J.E., and Goos, R.D.: Ocular penetration of amphotericin B, Arch. Ophthalmol. **73:**769, 1965.

61. Jones, B.R.: Principles in the management of oculomycosis: XXXI Edward Jackson memorial lecture, Am. J. Ophthalmol. **79:**15, 1975.

62. Jones, B.R., Jones, D.B., and Richards, A.B.: Surgery in the management of keratomycosis, Trans. Ophthalmol. Soc. U.K. **89:**887, 1976.

63. Jones, B.R., Richards, A.B., and Clayton, Y.N.: Clotrimazole, in the treatment of ocular

infections by *Aspergillus fumigatus,* Postgrad. Med. J. (suppl.) 39, July, 1974.

64. Jones, D.B., Forster, R.K., and Rebell, G.: *Fusarium solani* keratitis treated with natamycin (pimaricin): 18 consecutive cases, Arch. Ophthalmol. **88:**147, 1972.

65. Jones, D.B., and O'Day, D.M.: Diagnosis and management of ocular fungal infections, presented at the meeting of the American Academy of Ophthalmology and Otolaryngology, Dallas, Oct., 1977.

66. Jones, D.B., Sexton, R.R., and Rebell, G.: Mycotic keratitis in South Florida: a review of thirty-eight cases, Trans. Ophthalmol. Soc. U.K. **89:**781, 1969.

67. Jones, D.B., Wilson, L.A., Sexton, R.R., and Rebell, G.: Early diagnosis of mycotic keratitis, Trans. Ophthalmol. Soc. U.K. **89:**805, 1969.

68. Montes, L.F., Krumdiek, C., and Cornwell, P.E.: Hypovitaminosis in patients with mucocutaneous candidiasis, J. Infect. Dis. **128:**227, 1973.

69. Naumann, G., Green, W.R., and Zimmerman, L.E.: Mycotic keratitis, Am. J. Ophthalmol. **64:**668, 1969.

70. Newmark, E., Ellison, A.C., and Kaufman, H.E.: Combined pimaricin and dexamethasone therapy of keratomycosis, Am. J. Ophthalmol. **71:**718, 1971.

71. Newmark, E., Kaufman, H.E., Polack, F.M., and Ellison, A.C.: Clinical experience with pimaricin therapy in fungal keratitis, South. Med. J. **64:**935, 1971.

72. O'Day, D.M., Moore, T., and Aronson, S.: Deep fungal corneal abscess: combined corticosteroid therapy, Arch. Ophthalmol. **86:**414, 1971.

73. Polack, F.M., Kaufman, H.E., and Newmark, E.: Keratomycosis, medical and surgical treatment, Arch., Ophthalmol. **85:**410, 1971.

74. Raab, W.P.: Natamycin (pimaricin): its properties and possibilities in medicine, Stuttgart, 1972, Georg Thieme Verlag.

75. Richman, R.A., Rosenthal, I.M., Solomon, L.M., and Karachorlu, K.V.: Candidiasis and multiple endocrinopathy with oral squamous cell carcinoma complications, Arch. Dermatol. **111:**625, 1975.

76. Rippon, J.W.: Medical mycology: the pathogenic fungi and actinomycetes, Philadelphia, 1974, W.B. Saunders Co.

77. Rodrigues, M.M., and Laibson, P.: Exogenous mycotic keratitis caused by blastomyces dermatitidis, Am. J. Ophthalmol. **75:**782, 1973.

78. Sanders, N.: Penetrating keratoplasty in treatment of fungus keratitis, Am. J. Ophthalmol. **70:**24, 1970.

79. Singh, G., and Malik, S.R.K.: Therapeutic keratoplasty in fungal corneal ulcers, Br. J. Ophthalmol. **65:**41, 1972.

80. Steer, P.L., Marks, M.I., Klite, P.D., et al.: 5-Fluorocytosine: an oral antifungal compound: a report on clinical and laboratory experience, Ann. Intern. Med. **76:**15, 1972.

81. Stevens, D.A., Levine, H.B., and Deresinski, S.C.: Miconazole in coccidioidomycosis. II. Therapeutic and pharmacologic studies in man, Am. J. Med. **80:**191, 1976.

82. Symoens, J.: Clinical and experimental evidence on miconazole for the treatment of systemic mycoses: a review, Proc. R. Soc. Med. **70:**4, 1977.

83. Wilson, L.A., and Sexton, R.R.: Laboratory diagnosis in fungal keratitis, Am. J. Ophthalmol. **66:**646, 1968.

84. Wilson, L.A., and Sexton, R.R.: Laboratory aids in diagnosis. In Duane, T., editor: Clinical ophthalmology, vol. 4, New York, 1976, Harper & Row, Publishers.

Interstitial keratitis

85. Char, D.H., Cogan, D.G., and Sullivan, W.R., Jr.: Immunologic study of nonsyphilitic interstitial keratitis with vestibuloauditory symptoms, Am. J. Ophthalmol. **80:**491, 1975.

86. Cheson, B.D., Bluming, A.Z., and Alroy, J.: Cogan's syndrome: a systemic vasculitis, Am. J. Med. **60:**549, 1976.

87. Dimmer, F.: A type of corneal inflammation closely related to keratitis nummularis, Z. Augenheilkd. **13:**621, 1905.

88. Duke-Elder, S., and Leigh, A.G.: Interstitial keratitis; Deep keratitis. In System of ophthalmology, vol. 8, Diseases of the outer eye. Pt. 2, Cornea and sclera, St. Louis, 1965, The C.V. Mosby Co.

89. Grant, M.W.: Late glaucoma with interstitial keratitis, Am. J. Ophthalmol. **79:**87, 1975.

90. Jones, B.R., Anderson, J., Fuglsang, H.: Evaluation of microfilaricidal effects in the cornea from topically applied drugs in ocular onchocerciasis: trials with levamisole and mebendazole, Br. J. Ophthalmol. **62:**440, 1978.

91. Knox, D.L.: Glaucoma following inactive syphilitic interstitial keratitis, Arch. Ophthalmol. **66:**18, 1961.

92. Lagraulet, J.: La kératite ponctuée "en volcan" des pays tropicaux, Arch. Ophthalmol. Rev. Gen. Ophthalmol. (Paris) **24:**15, 1964.

93. Lichter, P.R., and Shaffer, R.N.: Interstitial keratitis and glaucoma, Am. J. Ophthalmol. **68:**241, 1969.

94. Martin, G.D., Stanley, J.A., and Davidson, I.W.: Corneal lesions in squirrel monkeys

maintained on a low chromium diet, Invest. Ophthalmol. **2:**153, 1972.

95. Oksala, A.: Interstitial keratitis: its treatment by mydriatics and hydrocortisone and its recurrence, Am. J. Ophthalmol. **44:**217, 1957.

96. Pinnolis, M., McCulley, J.P., and Urman, J.D.: Keratitis associated with infectious mononucleosis, Am. J. Ophthalmol. **89:**791, 1980.

97. Rabb, M.F., and Fine, M.: Penetrating keratoplasty in interstitial keratitis, Am. J. Ophthalmol. **67:**907, 1969.

98. Roisenblatt, J.: Interstitial keratitis caused by American (mucocutaneous) leishmaniasis, Am. J. Ophthalmol. **87:**175, 1979.

99. Ryan, S.J., Hardy, P.H., Hardy, J.M., and Oppenheimer, E.H.: Persistence of virulent *Treponema pallidum* despite penicillin therapy in congenital syphilis, Am. J. Ophthalmol. **73:**258, 1972.

100. Smith, J.L.: Testing for congenital syphilis in interstitial keratitis, Am. J. Ophthalmol. **72:** 816, 1971.

101. Sugar, H.S.: Late glaucoma associated with inactive syphilitic interstitial keratitis, Am. J. Ophthalmol. **53:**602, 1962.

102. Valenton, M.J.: Deep stromal involvement in Dimmer's nummular keratitis, Am. J. Ophthalmol. **78:**897, 1974.

103. Vannas, A., Hogan, M.J., and Wood, I.: Salzmann's nodular degeneration of the cornea, Am. J. Ophthalmol. **79:**211, 1975.

104. Waring, G.O., Font, R.L., Rodrigues, M.M., and Mulberger, R.D.: Alterations of Descemet's membrane in interstitial keratitis, Am. J. Ophthalmol. **81:**773, 1976.

105. Westhoff, C.H.A.: Keratitis punctata tropica (Sawah-keratitis), Geneesk, T. Ned. Ind. **52:** 419, 1912.

106. Woods, A.C.: Nummular keratitis and ocular brucellosis, Arch. Ophthalmol. **34:**490, 1946.

ADDITIONAL READING
Bacterial keratitis

Aronson, S.B., Elliott, J.H., and Moore, T.E.: The cornea. In Aronson, S.B., and Elliott, J.H.: Ocular inflammation, St. Louis, 1972, The C.V. Mosby Co.

Barza, M., and Baum, J.: Penetration of ocular compartments by penicillins, Surv. Ophthalmol. **18:**71, 1973.

Barza, M., Baum, J., Birkby, B., et al.: Intraocular penetration of carbenicillin in the rabbit, Am. J. Ophthalmol. **75:**307, 1973.

Benson, H.: Permeability of the cornea to topically applied drugs, Arch. Ophthalmol. **91:**313, 1974.

Brightbill, F.S.: Central corneal ulcers, Ann. Ophthalmol. **4:**331, 1972.

Burns, R.P.: *Pseudomonas aeruginosa.* In Franfelder, F.T., and Ray, F.H., editors: Current ocular therapy, Philadelphia, 1980, W.B. Saunders Co.

Chandler, J.W., and Milam, F.: Diptheria ulcers, Am. J. Ophthalmol. **96:**53, 1968.

Cox, C.E.: Gentamicin, Med. Clin. North. Am. **54:**1305, 1970.

Davis, S.D.: Bacteriologic cure of experimental *Pseudomonas* keratitis, Invest. Ophthalmol. Vis. Sci. **17:**916, 1978.

Davis, S.D., Sarff, L.D., and Hyndiuk, R.A.: Topical tobramycin therapy of experimental *Pseudomonas* keratitis: an evaluation of some factors that potentially enhance efficacy, Arch. Ophthalmol. **96:**123, 1978.

Duke-Elder, S., and Leigh, A.G.: System of ophthalmology, vol. 8, Diseases of the outer eye. Pt. 1. The conjunctiva. Pt. 2. Cornea and sclera, St. Louis, 1965, The C.V. Mosby Co.

Finegold, S.M., and Martin, W.J.: Diagnostic microbiology, ed. 6, St. Louis, 1982, The C.V. Mosby Co.

Hyman, B.N.: *Shigella sonnei* corneal ulcer, Am. J. Ophthalmol. **69:**873, 1970.

Jawetz, E., Melnick, J.L., and Adelberg, E.A.: Review of medical microbiology, ed. 10, Los Altos, Calif., 1972, Lange Medical Publications.

Jones, D.B.: Pathogenesis of bacterial and fungal keratitis, Trans. Ophthalmol. Soc. U.K. **98:**367, 1978.

Kim, H., and Ostler, H.B.: Marginal ulcer due to beta-streptococcus, Arch. Ophthalmol. **95:**454, 1977.

Klein, J.O., Sabaith, L.D., and Finland, M.: Laboratory studies on oxacillin, Am. J. Med. Sci. **245:**399, 1963.

Krachmer, J.H., and Purcell, J.J.: Bacterial corneal ulcers in cosmetic soft contact lens wearers, Arch. Ophthalmol. **96:**57, 1978.

Leibowitz, H.M.: Management of inflammation in the cornea and conjunctiva, Ophthalmology **87:** 753, 1980.

Leibowitz, H.M., and Kupferman, A.: Bioavailability and therapeutic effectiveness of topically administered corticosteroids, Trans. Am. Acad. Ophthalmol. Otolaryngol. **79:**78, 1975.

Locatcher-Khorazo, D., and Seegal, B.C.: Microbiology of the eye, St. Louis, 1972, The C.V. Mosby Co.

Presley, G.D., and Hale, L.M.: Corneal ulcer due to *Bacterium anitratum,* Am. J. Ophthalmol. **65:**571, 1968.

Raber, I.M., Laibson, P.R., Kruz, G.H., and Bernardino, V.B.: *Pseudomonas* corneoscleral ulcers, Am. J. Ophthalmol. **92:**353, 1981.

Records, R.E.: Intraocular penetration of cephalo-thin, Am. J. Ophthalmol. **66:**436, 1968.

Records, R.E., and Ellis, P.P.: The intraocular penetration of ampicillin, methicillin, and oxacillin, Am. J. Ophthalmol. **64:**135, 1967.

Sande, M.A., and Mandell, G.L.: Antimicrobial agents: the aminoglycosides. In Goodman, A.G., Goodman, L.S., and Gilman, A., editors: The pharmacological bases of therapeutics, ed. 6, New York, 1980, Macmillan Publishing Co., Inc.

Simon, H.J.: Chemotherapy of bacterial infections. IV. The penicillins. In Drill, V.A., editor: Drill's pharmacology in medicine, edited by J.R. Di-Palma, ed. 3, New York, 1965, McGraw-Hill Book Co.

Smith, C.R., Lipsky, J.J., Laskin, O.L., et al.: Double-blind comparison of the nephrotoxicity and auditory toxicity of gentamicin and tobramycin, N. Engl. J. Med. **302:**1106, 1980.

Smolin, G., Okumoto, M., and Leong-Sit, L.: Combined gentamicin-tobramycin-corticosteroid treatment. II. Effect on gentamicin-resistant *Pseudomonas* keratitis, Arch. Ophthalmol. **98:**474, 1980.

Smolin, G., Okumoto, M., and Wilson, F.M.: The effect of tobramycin on *Pseudomonas* keratitis, Am. J. Ophthalmol. **76:**555, 1973.

Troub, W.H., and Raymond, E.A.: Evaluation of the in vitro activity of tobramycin as compared with that of gentamicin sulfate, Appl. Environ. Microbiol. **23:**4, 1972.

Wilson, L.A.: Bacterial corneal ulcers. In Duane, T.D., editor: Clinical ophthalmology, vol. 4, Hagerstown, Md., 1976, Harper & Row, Publishers, Inc.

Fungal keratitis

Azar, P., Aquevella, J.V., and Smith, R.S.: Keratomycosis due to an *Alternaria* species, Am. J. Ophthalmol. **79:**881, 1975.

Chin, G.N., Hyndiuk, R.A., Kwasny, G.P., and Schultz, R.O.: Keratomycosis in Wisconsin, Am. J. Ophthalmol. **79:**121, 1975.

Forster, R.K., Wirta, M.G., Solis, M., and Rebell, G.: Methenamine-silver-stained corneal scrapings in keratomycosis, Am. J. Ophthalmol. **82:**261, 1976.

Jones, F.R., and Christensen, G.R.: *Pullalaria* corneal ulcer, Arch. Ophthalmol. **92:**529, 1974.

Kapoor, S., Sood, G.C., Mahableshwar, I., and Sood, M.: Rhinosporidiosis in children, J. Pediatr. Ophthalmol. **13:**103, 1976.

Palmer, E., Ferry, A.P., and Safir, A.: Fungal invasion of a soft (Griffin-Bionite) contact lens, Arch. Ophthalmol. **93:**278, 1975.

Polack, F.M., Sivirio, C., and Bresky, R.H.: Corneal chromomycosis: double infection by *Phialophora verrucosa* (Medlar) and *Cladosporium cladosporioides* (Frescenius), Ann. Ophthalmol. **8:**139, 1976.

Interstitial keratitis

Britten, M.J.A., and Palmer, C.A.L.: Glaucoma and inactive syphilitic interstitial keratitis, Br. J. Ophthalmol. **48:**181, 1964.

Drews, L.C., Barton, G.D., and Mikkelsen, W.M.: The treatment of acute syphilitic interstitial keratitis with topical cortisone, Am. J. Ophthalmol. **36:**90, 1953.

Gilbert, W.S., and Talbot, F.J.: Cogan's syndrome: signs of periarteritis and central venous thrombosis, Arch. Ophthalmol. **82:**633, 1969.

Golden, B., Watzke, R.C., Lindell, S.S., and McKee, A.P.: Treponemal-like organisms in the aqueous of nonsyphilitic patients, Arch. Ophthalmol. **80:**727, 1968.

Goldman, J.N., and Girard, K.F.: Intraocular treponemes in treated congenital syphilis, Arch. Ophthalmol. **78:**47, 1967.

Hardy, J.B., Hardy, P.H., Oppenheimer, E.H., et al.: Failure of penicillin in a newborn with congenital syphilis, JAMA **212:**1345, 1970.

Heinemann, M.H., Soloway, S.M., and Lesser, R.L.: Cogan's syndrome, Ann. Ophthalmol. **12:**667, 1980.

Horne, G.O.: Topical cortisone in syphilitic interstitial keratitis: review of twenty-three cases, Br. J. Vener. Dis. **31:**9, 1955.

Israel, C.W.: The fluorescent antibody tissue stain for *Treponema pallidum*. In Smith, J.L., editor: Neuro-ophthalmology: Symposium of the University of Miami and the Bascom Palmer Eye Institute, vol. 4, St. Louis, 1968, The C.V. Mosby Co.

Oksala, A.: Studies on interstitial keratitis associated with congenital syphilis occurring in Finland, Acta Ophthalmol. Suppl. 38, 1952.

Patterson, A.: Interstitial keratitis, Br. J. Ophthalmol. **50:**612, 1966.

Ryan, S.J., Nell, E.E., and Hardy, P.H.: A study of aqueous humor for the presence of spirochetes, Am. J. Ophthalmol. **73:**250, 1972.

Smith, J.L.: Spirochetes in late seronegative syphilis despite penicillin therapy. In Smith, J.L., editor: Neuro-ophthalmology: Symposium of the University of Miami and the Bascom Palmer Eye Institute, vol. 4, St. Louis, 1968, The C.V. Mosby Co.

Smith, J.L., and Israel, C.W.: Treponemes in aqueous humor in late seronegative syphilis, Trans. Am. Acad. Ophthalmol. Otolaryngol. **72:**63, 1968.

Syphilis—CDC recommended treatment schedules, 1976, J. Infect. Dis. **134:**97, 1976.

5 Superior limbic keratoconjunctivitis

Superior limbic keratoconjunctivitis (SLK) is a frequently unrecognized cause of chronic, recurrent keratoconjunctivitis.[3,7,12] Because it is a distinct clinical entity, SLK usually can be diagnosed readily if the clinician is familiar with the condition. Accurate diagnosis, in turn, enables initiation of the proper therapy and avoidance of harmful or ineffective measures. Often the patient has been using topical antibiotic, antiviral, or corticosteroid medications to which the entity does not respond. Such medications are likely to produce toxic or allergic reactions that can obscure the signs of the original disease. A high index of suspicion must be maintained by the ophthalmologist since misdiagnosis of SLK is common.

Superior limbic keratoconjunctivitis is a chronic, inflammatory condition of the eye that can produce considerable ocular irritation.[3] It occurs most commonly between 20 and 60 years of age.[8] Cases have been reported in 4- to 81-year-old patients; the mean age of patients with SLK is 49 years. At least 75% of the cases occur in females.[1] There appears to be no racial predilection. The disease occurs nationwide in the United States; the cases occur sporadically and are nonfamilial. Seasonal variation is not a factor.

Superior limbic keratoconjunctivitis may be bilateral, but there is an equal chance that it can occur unilaterally. If bilateral, one eye is often more severely involved than the other. If one considers cases in which the two eyes are involved at different times, bilateral involvement is slightly more common.

ETIOLOGIC FACTORS

The cause of SLK is unknown. Viral and fungal cultures have been negative. Reports of the finding of nontoxic staphylococci have been made but are not considered significant. Eosinophils, basophils, and inclusions have not been found. Giemsa-stained scrapings from the superior bulbar conjunctiva show marked keratinization of the epithelial cells (Fig. 5-1) and polymorphonuclear leukocytes.[11] Keratinized epithelial

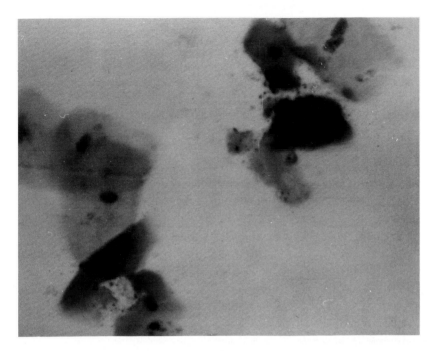

Fig. 5-1. Keratinized epithelial cells.

cells reveal keratohyaline granules. The cytoplasm of the epithelial cell takes on a purplish hue, and a loss of nuclear cytoplasm difference occurs. Some epithelial cells may demonstrate degenerated nuclei that appear pyknotic and shrunken. Scrapings of the palpebral conjunctiva reveal normal epithelium and a polymorphonuclear response.[11] Biopsy specimens of the bulbar conjunctival epithelium exhibit keratinization, acanthosis, and mild dyskeratosis. Cytoplasmic edema, nuclear pyknosis (balloon degeneration), and neovascularization of the stroma are seen. Biopsy specimens of the epithelium and stroma of the palpebral conjunctiva demonstrate an inflammatory infiltration consisting of neutrophils, lymphocytes, and plasma cells with a preponderance of neutrophils. An inflammatory exudate of similar cellular makeup may be present, overlying the thickened conjunctiva.[11] Staining with the periodic acid–Schiff or alcian blue stain does not occur. The laboratory test of consistent value seems to be the finding of keratinized cells.

No evidence exists that the disease occurs on an immunologic basis, but the frequent association with thyroid disease may suggest some immunologic connection in which autoantibody reactions are involved. Reports mentioning thyroid disease in association with SLK have been published.[1,4,6,9]

The finding of thickened and keratinized conjunctiva may suggest an association with a defect of cyclic 3':5'adenosine monophosphate (cyclic AMP).[13] Epidermal cell division appears to be slowed by beta-adrenergic stimulation. The latter, in association with increased cyclic AMP, decreases the rate of epidermal cell division. If adenyl cyclase is deficient, a decrease in, or lack of, cyclic AMP will occur; this may account for the accelerated rate of cell division such as that seen in psoriasis and perhaps in SLK.

SYMPTOMS

The symptoms of SLK are usually more severe than objective findings would suggest. One of the foremost complaints is the sensation of burning. In addition, patients almost always complain of foreign body sensation, pain, and photophobia and may exhibit blepharospasm.

Visual impairment and discharge or itching of the eyes are not usually encountered. The disease is quite unpredictable as to duration and recurrence. It may last for several weeks to 10 years or perhaps even longer. Periods of remission and exacerbation occur; remissions are observed within a few weeks to several years.

Decreased tear production does not appear to be related to SLK, although it is occasionally seen. Theodore[7] saw only one dry eye in 80 cases of SLK. He reported a case of SLK with superior corneal filaments and Sjögren's syndrome with inferior filaments. Canalicular occlusion resulted in resolution of inferior filaments but had no effect on the superior ones. Areas of localized dryness of the involved superior bulbar conjunctiva may be present, but tear production is normal.

CLINICAL FINDINGS

Papillary hypertrophy and marked inflammation occur on the superior tarsal conjunctiva (Fig. 5-2); in severe cases this area may have a diffusely velvety appearance. The severity of involvement of the superior tarsus usually parallels that of the superior limbal involvement. In extremely severe cases, a pseudomembrane is occasionally seen on the superior tarsus.[8] The conjunctiva of the lower lid is not involved.

The superior limbus is almost always involved by papillary hypertrophy and hyperemia. A fleshy, gray thickening of epithelium occurs in the superior limbal area (Fig. 5-3). A boggy apron of conjunctiva, folding over the superior limbus, is occasionally seen. In severe cases, edema or even bullous keratopathy in the superior cornea occurs. Filaments in the superior limbal areas are present in a third of the cases (Fig. 5-4) and may also occur on the bulbar and tarsal conjunctiva.[7] Appearance of the filaments usually is accompanied by an acute worsening of the symptoms; desquamation of filaments may lead to epithelial loss. When filaments occur, they may overshadow the picture of the underlying disease, and the condition may be diagnosed simply as filamentary keratitis. A micropannus is occasionally noted but is an inconsistent finding.

Hyperemia of the superior bulbar conjunctiva arranged in "corridor" fashion is a constant finding and is most evident when the gaze is directed downward (Fig. 5-5). This injection is most intense at the limbal area and fades as it approaches the superior fornix. The remaining conjunctiva exhibits a mild hyperemia.

Other findings include the presence of mucus, pseudoptosis, and edema of the superior limbal and superior bulbar conjunctiva.[7] Loss of luster of the superior bulbar conjunctiva may be seen and is caused by keratinization of surface epithelium. Decreased corneal sensation and decreased vision caused by induced astigmatism occur rarely.

The instillation of fluorescein and rose bengal reveals rather characteristic involvement of the cornea, limbus, and conjunctiva.[10] Fine and uniform areas of epithelial staining are found immediately above and below the superior limbus. Superficial, punctate staining of the bulbar conjunctiva usually involves the 10:30 to 1:30 area and extends

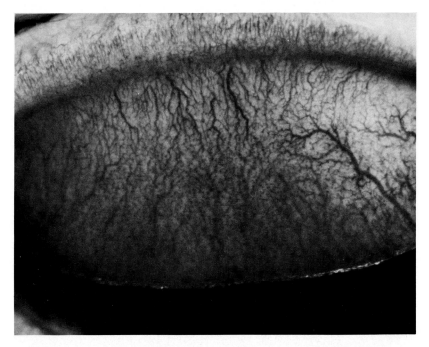

Fig. 5-2. Papillary hypertrophy of superior tarsal conjunctiva. (From Grayson, M.: In Duane, T. D., editor: Perspectives in ophthalmology, vol. 1, Hagerstown, Md., 1976, Ankho International Co.)

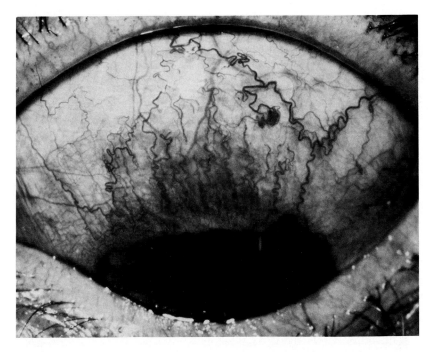

Fig. 5-3. Thickening and graying of epithelium in superior limbal area, associated with characteristic vessel injection of bulbar conjunctiva. (From Grayson, M.: In Duane, T. D., editor: Perspectives in ophthalmology, vol. 1, Hagerstown, Md., 1976, Ankho International Co.)

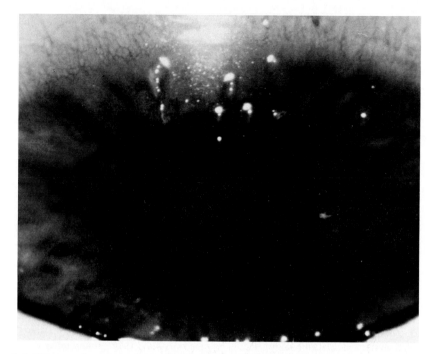

Fig. 5-4. Filaments in superior limbal areas. (From Grayson, M.: In Duane, T. D., editor: Perspectives in ophthalmology, vol. 1, Hagerstown, Md., 1976, Ankho International Co.)

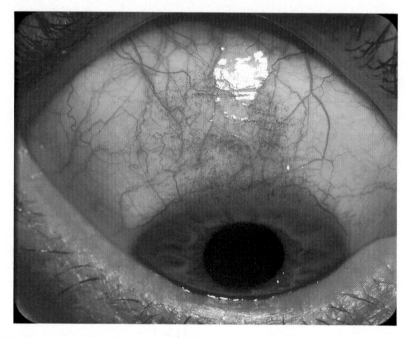

Fig. 5-5. Rose bengal red stain of superior bulbar conjunctiva showing corridor type of injection and stain.

about 4 to 5 mm above the limbus. Corneal staining often occupies a zone of 1 to 2 mm at the limbus. Fine and uniform infiltrates may be seen best with the cobalt-blue filter of the slit lamp but are often visible with ordinary illumination. Similar selective staining of the involved bulbar conjunctiva and adjacent limbic cornea is noted with the use of rose bengal red. Fine rose bengal red staining may also involve the superior limbic area of the cornea (Fig. 5-5). These rose bengal red lesions become visible with green light and are purple-blue, punctate lesions, even when obscured by severe conjunctiva injection.

DIFFERENTIAL DIAGNOSIS

Differential diagnosis can be approached by considering conditions with or without filaments:

Conditions without filaments
Trachoma
Marginal infiltrates at superior corneal location
Limbal vernal keratoconjunctivitis
Phlyctenulosis
Staphylococcal keratoconjunctivitis
Conditions with filaments
Keratoconjunctivitis sicca
Ocular occlusion (including ptosis)
Recurrent corneal erosion (anterior basement membrane disease)
Superficial punctate keratitis (Thygeson)
Bullous keratopathy
Herpetic keratitis
Superior limbic keratoconjunctivitis

In none of the nonfilamentous conditions listed is there significant bulbar conjunctival staining. Corneal staining, follicles, and scarring on the upper tarsal conjunctiva, Herbert's pits, and gross pannus help differentiate trachoma. The presence of basophilic intracytoplasmic inclusions and response to specific treatment for trachoma aid in the differentiation. Limbal vernal disease may be differentiated by the presence of fragmented eosinophils on scrapings, the gelatinous appearance of the limbal lesion and the presence of Trantas' dots, and giant papillae on the upper tarsal plate. In addition, the seasonal nature and response of vernal disease to steroids and cromolyn sodium are important clues. The limbal phlyctenule has a characteristic clinical picture. The raised yellow-white, self-limited, conjunctival limbal lesion is primarily associated with a sensitivity to the tubercle bacillus. A positive tuberculin skin test will aid in the identification of the problem. Other causes of phlyctenular disease such as candidiasis and staphylococcal disease should be kept in mind. Staphylococcal keratoconjunctivitis is characterized by the presence of epithelial corneal staining with fluorescein on the lower third of the cornea.

When one considers the filamentous conditions, it should be remembered that the corneal and conjunctival staining of keratoconjunctivitis sicca is mainly in the interpalpebral zone. Schirmer's test is markedly reduced, and the precorneal tear film is usually

Table 5-1. Differentiating features of GPC and SLK

Clinical features	GPC	SLK
Decreased vision (from punctate keratopathy) correctable with contact lenses but not glasses	Yes*	No
Exacerbations and remissions unrelated to contact lens wear	No	Yes
Itching	Yes	No
Medium or giant papillae	Yes*	No
More than minimal hyperemia of nasal temporal and inferior bulbar conjunctiva	Yes*	No
Punctate keratopathy extending more than 3 mm below upper limbus	Yes*	No
Gelatinous papillary hypertrophy of limbus	Yes*	No
Gross pannus (more than 2 mm)	Yes*	No
Corneal filaments	No†	Yes*
Eosinophils in conjunctival scrapings	Yes*	No
Response to cessation of contact lens wear	Yes	No

Reproduced with permission from Wilson, F.M., II: Differential Diagnosis of Superior Limbic Kerato-conjunctivitis and Papillary Keratoconjunctivitis and Papillary Keratoconjunctivitis Associated With Contact Lenses, in Hughes, W.F. (ed.): THE YEARBOOK OF OPHTHALMOLOGY 1981. Copyright © September 1981 by Year Book Medical Publishers, Inc., Chicago.
*This feature is not always present but is of diagnostic value when found.
†This feature has not been seen or reported to date.

filled with debris. A loss of luster occurs on the corneal surface. Scrapings may reveal goblet cells.

Superficial punctate keratitis of Thygeson exhibits a fine epithelial stain. The punctate epithelial aggregates are characteristic. No bulbar conjunctival staining occurs, and there is a dramatic response to steroids.

Bullous keratopathy may exhibit filaments because of the presence of epithelial disease and corneal edema. The condition can be readily recognized on biomicroscopic examination. The presence of epithelial bedewing, epithelial bullae, stromal edema, and endothelial pathologic conditions help differentiate the entity. Recurrent corneal erosion syndrome presents a typical history of severe pain, especially in the morning, and often reveals a history of injury to the corneal epithelium. As noted, ocular occlusion can be the cause of filaments, and of course, the history of use of an occluder is the clue.

It has been noted that giant papillary conjunctivitis and superior limbic keratocon-junctivitis may offer some problems in diagnosis in contact lens wearers. Table 5-1 aids in this differential diagnosis.

TREATMENT

The therapy of SLK involves the use of silver nitrate solution.[1] The condition of the majority of patients improves, and some achieve complete remission. Filaments often disappear, and the symptoms and clinical findings are usually reduced by the next day. Limbal staining is most resistant to treatment and may take several weeks to disappear. As mentioned, however, recurrences are not uncommon. A cotton-tipped applicator that has been impregnated with a 0.25% to 0.5% solution of silver nitrate is used. Strong concentrations of silver nitrate cause chemical burns and silver staining of the cornea. Solid-tipped silver nitrate applicators must be avoided. Their use may result in a severe burn and opacification of the cornea that may necessitate penetrating keratoplasty.[2]

My practice has been to treat the upper tarsal conjunctiva. On occasion in resistant cases the upper bulbar conjunctiva is treated in addition with 0.5% silver nitrate solution. In a few cases topical decongestants, zinc salts, and artificial tears may bring about some temporary, symptomatic relief but will have no effect on the progress of the disease.

Recession of the conjunctiva was effective in two cases that had not responded to application of 1% silver nitrate to the superior limbus.[5] A superior forniceal flap was made from the 10:30 to 1:30 positions at the limbus, and the conjunctiva was recessed 4 mm and sutured to the sclera with the interrupted 7-0 chromic sutures. This procedure resulted in the elimination of the patient's symptoms in both cases. Excision of thickened and redundant conjunctiva at the superior limbus will produce similar results.

REFERENCES

1. Cher, I.: Clinical features of superior limbic keratoconjunctivitis in Australia: a probable association with thyrotoxicosis, Arch. Ophthalmol. **82:**580, 1969.
2. Grayson, M., and Pieroni, D.: Severe silver nitrate injury to the eye, Am. J. Ophthalmol. **70:**227, 1970.
3. Grayson, M., and Wilson, F.M., II: Superior limbic keratoconjunctivitis, Perspect. Ophthalmol. **1:**234, 1977.
4. Sutherland, A.L.: Superior limbic keratoconjunctivitis, Trans. Ophthalmol. Soc. N.Z. **21:**89, 1969.
5. Tenzel, K.: Resistant superior limbic keratoconjunctivitis, Arch. Ophthalmol. **89:**439, 1973.
6. Tenzel, R.R.: Comments on superior limbic filamentous keratitis, Arch. Ophthalmol. **79:**508, 1968.
7. Theodore, F.H.: Superior limbic keratoconjunctivitis, Eye Ear Nose Throat Mon. **42:**25, 1963.
8. Theodore, F.H.: Further observations on superior limbic keratoconjunctivitis, Trans. Am. Acad. Ophthalmol. Otolaryngol. **71:**341, 1967.
9. Theodore, F.H.: Comments on findings of elevated protein-bound iodine in superior limbic keratoconjunctivitis, Arch. Ophthalmol. **79:**508, 1968.
10. Theodore, F.H.: Diagnostic dyes in superior limbic keratoconjunctivitis and other superficial entities. In Turtz, A.I., editor: Proceedings of the Centennial Symposium: Manhattan Eye, Ear and Throat Hospital, vol. 1. Ophthalmology, St. Louis, 1969, The C.V. Mosby Co.
11. Theodore, F.H., and Ferry, A.P.: Superior limbic keratoconjunctivitis: clinical and pathological correlations, Arch. Ophthalmol. **84:**481, 1970.
12. Thygeson, P.: Observations on filamentary keratitis, transactions of the one-hundred second annual meeting of the American Medical Association Section of Ophthalmology, 1963.
13. Voorhees, J.J., and Duell, E.A.: Psoriasis as a possible defect of the adenyl cyclase cyclic AMP cascade: a defective chalone mechanism? Arch. Dermatol. **104:**352, 1971.

6 Acute and chronic follicular conjunctivitis

Acute follicular conjunctivitis
Subacute and chronic follicular conjunctivitis

The following sections on acute and chronic follicular conjunctivitis will show some overlap in the classification; however, in each instance the entities are presented in a different light.

Follicular conjunctivitis may be divided into three main sections:

1. Acute follicular conjunctivitis
2. Chronic follicular conjunctivitis
3. Folliculosis

The clinical and histologic appearance of the conjunctival follicle is important to observe. Clinically, follicles appear as elevated lesions of the conjunctiva that are yellowish white to grayish white in color and approximately 0.5 to 2 mm in diameter, with small blood vessels only at their periphery. Histologically, these lesions consist of

Table 6-1. Characteristics of follicles and papillae

Follicle	Papilla
Discrete, round, elevated lesion of conjunctiva	Elevated polygonal hyperemic areas separated by paler areas
Diameter of 0.5 to 5 mm	
Vascular network grows around follicle	Central fibrovascular core is noted in each papilla with central blood vessel, which, when reaching surface, forms arborized vascular figure
Vessels disappear toward center of follicle	
Represents new formation of lymphoid tissue	
Histopathologically lymphoid in response, which probably correlates with cellular antibody production	
Composed of lymphocytes, macrophages, and plasma cells; true lymph follicles are not present in normal conjunctiva; on prolonged irritation lymphocytes in adventitia aggregate into follicles	Composed of polymorphonuclear leukocytes and other acute inflammatory cells; hypertrophy of epithelium of mucous membrane; connective tissue septae are anchored into deeper tissues, resulting in polygonal outline; giant papillae occur when these septae rupture
No histologic difference in follicles in irritants, folliculosis, or infections such as trachoma	
Usually located in inferior palpebral conjunctiva, although they can be seen superiorly	

single lymphoid germinal centers. Follicles caused by idoxuridine and eserine toxication have true germinal centers. Atropine may cause follicles, also.

Follicles must be differentiated from papillae, as illustrated in Table 6-1. Granulomatous lesions must also be differentiated. Fig. 6-5 demonstrates the solitary, solid, raised, rounded, opaque lesion characteristic of sarcoid granuloma.

Laboratory procedures useful in the diagnosis of follicular conjunctivitis include the following:

1. Bacterial cultures to rule out a primary or secondary bacterial infection
2. Scrapings of the conjunctiva, to reveal cytologic characteristics, which are frequently useful in the classification of follicular conjunctivitis
3. Fluorescent-antibody studies in adenoviral and chlamydial disease[6,15,17]

ACUTE FOLLICULAR CONJUNCTIVITIS (Table 6-2)

Acute follicular conjunctivitis, usually of rapid onset, is often unilateral early in the infection, with involvement of the second eye within a week's time. It is frequently accompanied by preauricular lymphadenopathy. Following are some of the diseases considered in this category:

1. Epidemic keratoconjunctivitis (EKC) (adenovirus type 8, rarely type 19)[*]
2. Pharyngoconjunctival fever (PCF) (adenovirus types 3, 5, 7, and others)[11]
3. Primary herpes simplex hominis keratoconjunctivitis (herpesvirus hominis type I, rarely type II)
4. Adult inclusion conjunctivitis *(Chlamydia oculogenitalis)*[†]
5. Epidemic hemorrhagic keratoconjunctivitis (picornavirus)[‡]
6. Newcastle disease conjunctivitis (Newcastle disease virus)[5]
7. Acute trachoma *(C. trachomatis)*
8. Neonatal inclusion conjunctivitis[†]

SUBACUTE AND CHRONIC FOLLICULAR CONJUNCTIVITIS (Table 6-3)

Subacute and chronic follicular conjunctivitis can be diagnosed in cases that continue for more than 15 days. These patients may have an acute onset with persistent disease or may develop disease insidiously. The conjunctivitis may continue for months or years. The following diseases and related conditions should be considered:

1. Trachoma *(C. trachomatis)*
2. Inclusion conjunctivitis *(C. oculogenitalis)*[†]

---

[*]References 1, 4, 6, 7, 9, 13, 15, 17.
[†]A difference of opinion exists concerning the classification of chlamydiae. Some believe that the agents causing inclusion conjunctivitis and trachoma are one and the same and thus refer to the agent as *C. trachomatis*. Others think that there are two distinct etiologic agents, *C. trachomatis* (trachoma) and *C. oculogenitalis* (inclusion conjunctivitis and genital disease). The latter term will be used throughout this text in describing inclusion conjunctivitis. Other chlamydial agents that affect humans are *C. lymphogranulomatis* (lymphogranuloma venereum) and *C. psittaci* (psittacosis and ornithosis). In this text *C. lymphogranulomatis* will be used to designate the etiologic agent of lymphogranuloma, keeping in mind the dispute regarding the naming and classification of chlamydiae.
[‡]References 8, 10, 12, 19-21.   *Text continued on p. 128.*

Table 6-2. Diagnostic features of acute follicular conjunctivitis*

Disease	Discharge and conjunctival appearance	Cornea
Epidemic keratoconjunctivitis (EKC)	Watery discharge Hyperemia and chemosis Pseudomembranes in one third of cases, which may result in scars (Fig. 6-1) Course of 7 to 14 days Subconjunctival hemorrhages in types 8 and 19 Follicular response in upper and lower fornices—mostly lower (Fig. 6-2) Case of chronic papillary conjunctivitis resulting from type 19 occurs[3]	Fine, diffuse, slightly elevated epithelial punctate keratitis early; persists 3 more weeks in types 8 and 19; affects entire cornea Focal epithelial keratitis on seventh to thirtieth day Subepithelial opacities (fourteenth to twentieth day) at sites of epithelial lesions in 50% of cases; may last 3 months (Fig. 6-3) (usually) or years, especially types 8 and 19 May have stromal infiltration and edema, severe keratitis No pannus (no vascularization)
Pharyngoconjunctival fever	Scanty, watery discharge Hyperemia chemosis Follicular—may have papillary reaction in upper and lower fornices (Fig. 6-5) No scars Lasts for 7 to 14 days	Fine epithelial keratitis affecting entire cornea Occasionally same as EKC (especially types 3, 4, and 7) but milder and lasts only 1 to 3 weeks; subepithelial opacities smaller than in EKC No pannus
Acute trachoma† (occurs usually in young adults)	Follicles typically prominent on upper tarsal plate; trachoma follicles soft, necrotic, and often seen on semilunar fold and limbus Conjunctival scarring, especially of upper lid Arlt's line: horizontally linear scar at junction of posterior two thirds and anterior one third of tarsal conjunctiva Pain, discharge, photophobia Papillary hypertrophy	Fine epithelial keratitis; fine punctate, subepithelial infiltrate; fine keratitis may last until disease subsides Gross superior pannus Marginal corneal infiltrates Occasionally dense focus of cellular infiltrates (trachoma pustule) Cicatrized limbal follicles (Herbert's pits) May end up with markedly scarred and vascularized cornea

*Coxsackieviruses A and B have been reported to cause follicular conjunctivitis, as has Asian influenza.
†These entities can be classified also with chronic follicular conjunctivitis.

Laboratory	Etiologic factors	Epidemiologic and other characteristics
Mononuclear response (Fig. 6-4) except for polymorphonuclear leukocytes with pseudomembranes Fluorescent-antibody (FA) staining of conjunctival smears produces rapid and simple method for detection of adenoviral infection[1,18] Fourfold increase of antibody titer between acute and convalescent sera[1] Adenovirus 8 or 19 can be recovered on HeLa cells	Adenovirus types 8 and 19 Transmission from respiratory tract to eye is responsible for sporadic outbreaks Eye-to-eye transmission causes outbreaks Isolation of virus up to 2 weeks after onset Virus was isolated from chronic papillary conjunctivitis[3] Incubation period is 7 to 9 days Other eye involved usually in 2 to 7 days	Age group: 20 to 40 years[3] Incidence in men greater than in women Eye is infectious up to 14 days Transmission from hand (or instrument) to eye Acute systemic symptoms only in children; hyperacute eye involvement Lymph nodes: prominent, palpable, tender, and occasionally visible (90% of cases) Unrecognized presence of adenovirus type 19 in chronic papillary conjunctivitis provides source of infection to initiate further outbreaks of hospital transmission[3] Vision may be decreased if subepithelial corneal infiltrates are pupillary in location
Mononuclear response (Fig. 6-4) FA studies of conjunctival smears detect adenovirus The virus can be cultivated in HeLa cells A rising neutralizing antibody titer is useful	Adenovirus types 3, 4, 5, 7, and others Incubation 7 to 9 days Types 5 and 7 may be severe	Acute systemic symptoms Lymph nodes small and palpable but not visible or tender (90% of cases) Occurs in schools and swimming pools (virus not killed by chlorine) Adenovirus 7 may be more frequent in summer[3] No sequelae

Basophilic, cytoplasmic, epithelial inclusions‡ (infrequent)
Mainly polymorphonuclear response; may have equal numbers of polymorphonuclear and mononuclear cells in chronic phase
Cytologic findings of expressed follicle:
  1. Leber's cell (macrophages)
  2. Plasma cells
  3. Lymphoblasts
	C. trachomatis
	Secondary bacterial infection common in endemic areas
		Well described since 1500 BC
		Other complications are trichiasis, distichiasis, keratitis sicca
		Some heal spontaneously; thus some relation to immunity may exist
		Preauricular nodes: palpable, rarely tender or visible
		Antibody in tears to *C. trachomatis* correlates with presence of infectious agent in eye and not intensity of conjunctional inflation (trachoma inclusion conjunctivitis [TRIC] serotype A)

"Follicles" of sarcoid are actually granulomas. They are yellow-white and opaque and are not follicles.

Continued.

Table 6-2. Diagnostic features of acute follicular conjunctivitis—cont'd

Disease	Discharge and conjunctival appearance	Cornea
Adult oculogenital disease† (inclusion conjunctivitis)	Mild-to-moderate mucopurulent discharge Never membranous in adults Worse below No conjunctival cicatrization Redness, chemosis Follicular reaction	Superficial punctate to slightly coarse epithelial and peripheral subepithelial infiltrates (smaller than in EKC), which may leave scars Superior micropannus
Neonatal inclusion conjunctivitis	Purulent discharge Papillary hypertrophy and pseudomembranes are main features in infants (nonfollicular) May become follicular if duration is longer than 6 weeks May cause mild conjunctival scarring, as can trachoma, because of pseudomembrane formation Usually 4 to 12 days postpartum	May have fine superficial epithelial keratitis Superior micropannus
Herpes simplex hominis (primary)	Usually unilateral Scantly watery unless pseudomembranous (50% of cases) Follicles often masked by membrane May have conjunctival scars caused by membrane formation Pain, photophobia, mucoid discharge	Fine epithelial keratitis (punctate, stellate) Dendrites after 7 days Decreased corneal sensitivity Stromal disease Pannus extremely uncommon
Newcastle disease	Watery discharge: scanty Primarily affects inferior conjunctiva May have papillary or follicular conjunctivitis Follicles are prominent on lower lid Usually unilateral Pain, redness, tearing	Cornea rarely affected, but fine punctate epithelial keratitis and occasionally small subepithelial infiltrates can be seen No pannus

‡Inclusion bodies cap the nucleus. The infectious particle is the elementary body. It stains purple with latter stains blue with Giemsa's stain. The initial body divides by binary fusion and forms new elementary

Laboratory	Etiologic factors	Epidemiologic and other characteristics
Polymorphonuclear response May have 50% polymorpho-nuclear and 50% mono-nuclear cells in chronic phase Basophilic, intracytoplasmic, epithelial inclusions‡ FA-stained conjunctival cells	C. trachomatis (oculogenital strains)	Venereal hand-to-eye trans-mission Persists for 3 to 12 months in untreated cases in contradis-tinction to adenoviral infection Lymph nodes: palpable, sometimes tender or visible Otitis media in 15% of cases Rarely swimming pool (chlorine inhibits agent)
Early (first 2 days) one may see mononuclear cells, which change to poly-morphonuclear cells Can have equal number of polymorphonuclear and mononuclear cells in chronic phase Large number of basophilic, intracytoplasmic, epithelial inclusions on Giemsa's stain FA-stained conjunctival scrap-ings in 95% of cases	C. trachomatis (oculogenital strains)	Untreated cases last 3 to 12 months Neonate contracts disease from mother's birth canal May have node late in disease Pneumonitis may be a compli-cation; therefore erythromy-cin (systemically) may be choice
Mononuclear cells, except for polymorphonuclear leuko-cytes when pseudomem-branes are present Multinucleated giant cells FA stain	Herpesvirus hominis, usually type 1	Usually occurs in children but can occur in adults Type I: direct transfer from relatives and friends, that is, blister to eye Type II: transfer from birth canal in neonate Vesicles on lid Ulcerative blepharitis Lymph nodes: small, palpable, occasionally tender or visible Duration: 2 weeks
Mononuclear response	Newcastle disease virus (para-myxovirus)	Droplet (finger-to-eye) trans-mission from poultry to human Occurs only with occupational exposure (poultry workers, veterinarians, virologic workers) Lymph nodes: palpable, small, sometimes tender No sequelae Duration: 7 to 10 days

Giemsa's stain. The elementary body is phagocytosed by the host cell and forms the initial body. The bodies. Clumps of particles form the inclusion body, which caps the nucleus. *Continued.*

Table 6-2. Diagnostic features of acute follicular conjunctivitis—cont'd

Disease	Discharge and conjunctival appearance	Cornea
Hemorrhagic keratocon-junctivitis (acute hemorrhagic [Apollo] conjunctivitis)	Serous to mucoid discharge; chemosis—early in first 24 hours Bilateral subconjunctival pinpoint hemorrhages in upper palpebral or bulbar conjunctiva; becomes more profuse temporally on bulbar conjunctiva; takes 1 to 2 weeks to absorb Follicles, but not prominent No pseudomembranes Pain, photophobia, redness Lasts 10 days or less	May have fine superficial epithelial keratitis[8] Subepithelial infiltrates may last for 18 months No pannus
Infectious mononucleosis (Epstein-Barr)	Acute conjunctivitis Membranous or follicular conjunctivitis[2] Subconjunctival hemorrhage[14]	Epithelial keratitis Nummular keratitis (lesions are on the peripheral cornea and at all levels)

Table 6-3. Diagnostic features of chronic follicular conjunctivitis and related conditions

Disease	Conjunctiva	Cornea
Molluscum contagiosum	Pseudotrachomatous reaction Conjunctival scarring Follicular conjunctivitis Occlusion of punctum May have molluscum on conjunctiva	Find epithelial keratitis superiorly Pannus that is visible superiorly Pseudodendrite Keratinization
Drug-induced follicular conjunctivitis	Pseudotrachomatous picture (Fig. 6-7) Keratinization Drying	Fine or blotchy epithelial keratitis Pseudodendrite Keratinization Pannus (Fig. 6-7) Limbal follicles can occur with IDU No Herbert's pits, as in trachoma

Laboratory	Etiologic factors	Epidemiologic and other characteristics
Mononuclear response in early stages, polymorphonuclear in later stage	Picornavirus (enterovirus)	First appeared in Ghana in 1969 Massive epidemics in Asia and Africa Hand-to-eye transmission; short incubation period (2 to 10 days); possible droplet infection Small preauricular node (sometimes absent) No sequelae except for neurologic complications with elevated antibody titer after acute hemorrhagic conjunctivitis[6] Anterior uveitis
Epstein-Barr virus	Epstein-Barr virus	Uveitis and episcleritis and may have retinal hemorrhages, papillitis, and retinal edema[16]

Cytologic findings	Etiologic factors	Remarks
Molluscum bodies (Fig. 6-6) (eosinophilic, cytoplasmic inclusions) in biopsy of lid margin nodule Mononuclear	Molluscum contagiosum virus	Molluscum of lid should be eradicated by curetting of lesion Often in adolescents and young adults with molluscum on other parts of body as well as lids; may spread venereally Self-limited unless cellular immunity is depressed, but ocular disease may persist for months and can result in visual loss No lymph node enlargement
Polymorphonuclear leukocytes and lymphocytes	"Toxic" reaction Agents causing epithelial keratitis include IDU, adenine arabinoside, Neosporin, gentamicin, topical broadband antibiotics, and preservatives	Seen after prolonged use of miotics (e.g., eserine and diisopropyl fluorophosphate [DFP]) and IDU May see follicles without germinal centers with atropine Palpable preauricular adenopathy occurs rarely (IDU) Epithelial keratitis may last several weeks after stopping of medication

Continued.

Table 6-3. Diagnostic features of chronic follicular conjunctivitis and related conditions

Disease	Conjunctiva	Cornea
Axenfeld's chronic follicular conjunctivitis	No bulbar conjunctival follicles Follicles mainly on lower fornix and tarsus, but also on upper tarsus Heals in 1 to 2 years without scars	No keratitis No pannus
Merrill-Thygeson chronic follicular conjunctivitis	Follicles mainly on lower fornix and tarsus, but also on upper tarsus Heals in 4 to 5 months without scars	Epithelial keratitis, mainly above Micropannus in some cases
Oculoglandular (Parinaud's) syndrome	Focal granulomatous conjunctivitis (Fig. 6-8) Granulomas may be surrounded by follicles May have conjunctival ulcers	Usually no involvement; however, it depends on etiology
Moraxella species	Tarsal follicles Subacute conjunctivitis with moderate discharge Angular blepharoconjunctivitis	Occasionally, marginal (catarrhal) infiltrate
Eye makeup–induced follicular conjunctivitis	Insidious or asymptomatic Pigment (mascara) in "follicles" on tarsal and fornicate conjunctiva	No keratitis
Folliculosis of childhood	No inflammation Upper lid can be mildly involved Semilunar fold is spared Follicles tend to be prominent in fornix and fade out toward lid margins	No corneal disease

*Serum studies include (1) tularemia agglutination titer, (2) FTA-ABS and VDRL, (3) angiotensin-converting for mononucleosis.
Skin tests include (1) PPD, (2) coccidioidin, and (3) blastomycin.
The granuloma requires a biopsy.

—cont'd

Cytologic findings	Etiologic factors	Remarks
Mononuclear	May be a slow virus	Seen in orphanages No symptoms Trachoma in children is often mild No lymph node enlargement
Mononuclear No inclusions	Unknown	Cannot transfer to monkeys or rabbits May be transmitted by sharing of eye makeup No lymph node enlargement
Mixed mononuclear and polymorphonuclear leukocytes	*Leptothrix buccalis* (cat mouth, 100%; human mouth, 5%) Tuberculosis Tularemia Sarcoid (node rarely enlarged) Coccidiomycosis Blastomycosis Lues Mononucleosis	Leptothrix patients usually have history of sleeping with pet cat Lymph node visibly enlarged May have fever Serum and skin tests* plus anaerobic and aerobic cultures (Gram's, Giemsa's and acid-fast stains) Chest x-ray
Gram-negative diplobacilli on smear Much fibrin and only scant polymorphonuclear leukocytes	*M. lacunata*	Adolescent patient Most common in southwestern United States Other bacteria, especially those in lacrimal system (i.e., *Streptococcus* and *Haemophilus* organisms), occasionally cause follicular conjunctivitis No lymph node enlargement
Pigment granules only	Incorporation of makeup granules in conjunctival cysts; uncertain whether true follicles develop	In user of cosmetics No lymph node enlargement
Mononuclear cells occasionally	Physiologic change of childhood and adolescence	Seen in children and associated with generalized lymphoid hyperplasia Newborn cannot have follicles until 3 months of age Lymph nodes may be enlarged as part of generalized folliculosis

enzyme, (4) complement fixation titer for blastomycosis and coccidiomycosis, and (5) heterophile agglutinins

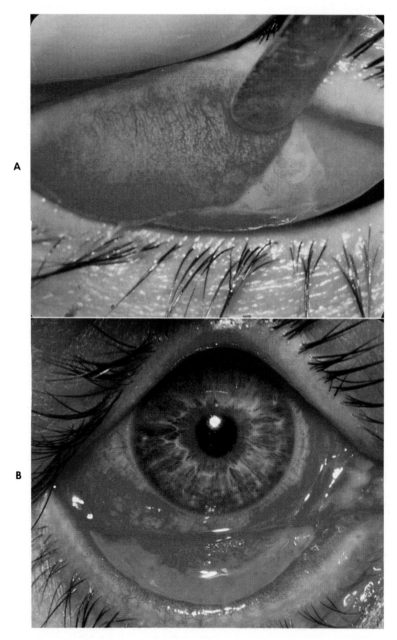

Fig. 6-1. Membrane formation of tarsal conjunctiva in case of epidemic keratoconjunctivitis. **A,** Upper lid. **B,** Lower lid.

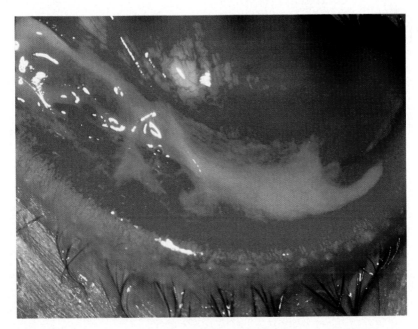

Fig. 6-2. Severe conjunctival hyperemia, follicular response, and membrane formation in EKC.

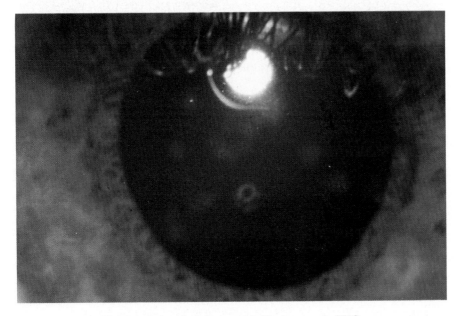

Fig. 6-3. Subepithelial corneal infiltrates seen in EKC.

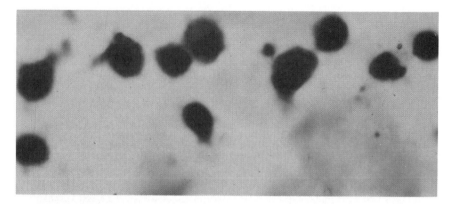

Fig. 6-4. Mononuclear cell response in EKC and other adenovirus infections.

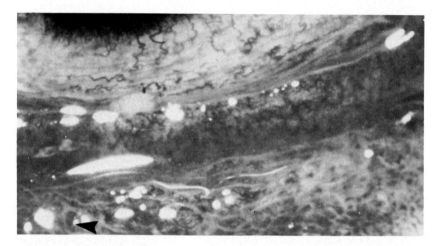

Fig. 6-5. Large follicles in lower tarsal conjunctiva in pharyngoconjunctival fever.

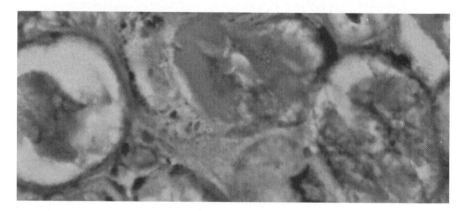

Fig. 6-6. Molluscum bodies.

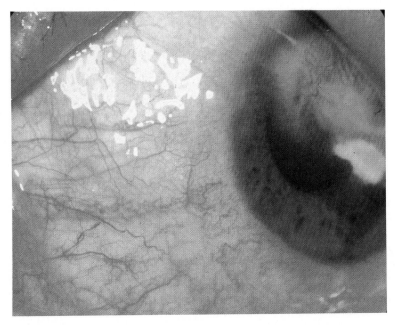

Fig. 6-7. Limbal follicles and pannus resulting from idoxuridine toxicity, giving pseudotrachomatous picture. (From Wilson, F.M., II: Surv. Ophthalmol. **24:**57, 1979.)

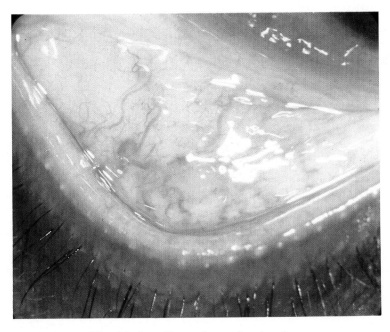

Fig. 6-8. Sarcoid granuloma of conjunctiva.

3. Molluscum contagiosum
4. Drug-induced conjunctivitis (eserine, idoxuridine, and eye cosmetics)
5. Bacterial conjunctivitis (*Moraxella* organisms and rarely other bacteria in adolescents *only*)
6. Axenfeld's chronic follicular conjunctivitis (orphan conjunctivitis)
7. Chronic follicular conjunctivitis of Merrill-Thygeson type
8. Parinaud's oculoglandular syndrome (cat-scratch fever and others)
9. Folliculosis of childhood

Tables 6-2 and 6-3 offer the pertinent details of the diseases just listed. The conditions are outlined in this manner so that an overall view of these diseases is achieved.

REFERENCES

1. Adenovirus keratoconjunctivitis (editorial), Br. J. Ophthalmol. **61:**73, 1977.
2. Bernstein, A.: Infectious mononucleosis, Medicine **19:**85, 1940.
3. Darougar, S., Quinlan, M.P., Gibson, J.A., and Jones, B.R.: Epidemic keratoconjunctivitis and chronic papillary conjunctivitis in London due to adenovirus type 19, Br. J. Ophthalmol. **61:**76, 1977.
4. Dawson, C.R., Hanna, L., and Tagni, B.: Adenovirus type 8 infections in the United States: ten observations on the pathogenesis of lesions in severe eye disease, Arch. Ophthalmol. **87:**258, 1972.
5. Hales, R.H., and Ostler, B.H.: Newcastle disease conjunctivitis with subepithelial infiltrates, Br. J. Ophthalmol. **57:**694, 1973.
6. Hart, J.C.D., Barnard, D.L., Clark, S.R.R., and Marmion, V.J.: Epidemic keratoconjunctivitis: a virological and clinical study, Trans. Ophthalmol. Soc. U.K. **92:**795, 1972.
7. Hierholzer, J.C., Guyer, B., O'Day, D., and Shaffner, W.: Adenovirus type 19 keratoconjunctivitis, N. Engl. J. Med. **290:**1436, 1974.
8. Hung, P.T., and Sung, S.M.: Neurologic complications with elevated antibody titer after subacute hemorrhagic conjunctivitis, Am. J. Ophthalmol. **80:**832, 1975.
9. Jawetz, E., Thygeson, P., Hanna, L., Nichols, A., and Kimura, S.J.: The etiology of epidemic keratoconjunctivitis, Am. J. Ophthalmol. **43:**79, 1957.
10. Jones, B.R.: Epidemic hemorrhagic conjunctivitis in London, 1971, Trans. Ophthalmol. Soc. U.K. **92:**625, 1972.
11. Kimura, S.J., Hanna, L., Nichols, A., Thygeson, P., and Jawetz, E.: Sporadic cases of pharyngoconjunctival fever in northern California, Am. J. Ophthalmol. **43:**14, 1957.
12. Kono, R., Mujamura, K., Tajiri, E., et al.: Neurologic complications associated with acute hemorrhagic conjunctivitis virus infection and its serologic complication, J. Infect. Dis. **129:**590, 1974.
13. Laibson, P.R., Ortolan, G., and Dupré-Strachan, S.: Community and hospital outbreak of epidemic keratoconjunctivitis, Arch. Ophthalmol. **80:**467, 1968.
14. Librach, I.M. Ocular symptoms in glandular fever, Br. J. Ophthalmol. **40:**619, 1956.
15. O'Day, D.M., Guyer, B., Hierholzer, J.C., Rosing, K.J., and Schaffner, W.: Clinical and laboratory evaluation of epidemic keratoconjunctivitis due to adenovirus types 8 and 19, Am. J. Ophthalmol. **81:**207, 1976.
16. Piel, J.J., Thelander, H.E., and Shur, E.B.: Infectious mononucleosis of the central nervous system with bilateral papilledema, J. Pediatr. **37:**661, 1950.
17. Schwartz, H.S., Vastine, D.W., Yamashiroya, H., and West, C.: Immunofluorescent detection of adenovirus antigen in epidemic keratoconjunctivitis, Invest. Ophthalmol. **15:**199, 1976.
18. Vastine, D.W., Schwartz, H.S., Yamashiroya, H.M., Smith, R.F., et al.: Cytologic diagnosis of adenoviral epidemic keratoconjunctivitis by direct immunofluorescence, Invest. Ophthalmol. Visual Sci. **16:**195, 1977.
19. Whitcher, J.P., Schmidt, N.J., Mabronk, R., Messadi, M., Daghfons, T., Hoshiwara, I., and Dawson, C.K.: Acute hemorrhagic conjunctivitis in Tunisia, Arch. Ophthalmol. **94:**51, 1976.
20. Wolken, S.H.: Acute hemorrhagic conjunctivitis, Surv. Ophthalmol. **19:**71, 1974.
21. Yang, Y.F., Hung, P.T., Lin, L.K., et al.: Epidemic hemorrhagic keratoconjunctivitis, Am. J. Ophthalmol. **80:**192, 1975.

7 Oculogenital disease and related conditions

In this chapter the oculogenital diseases of the infant as well as the adult will be discussed. In addition, a differential diagnosis of this group of diseases will be covered; as a result some nongenital conditions are considered.

The chlamydiae have been classified as members of the order Chlamydiales. Like bacteria, they contain both DNA and RNA, divide by binary fission, are inhibited by sulfonamides and antibiotics, and contain muramic acid in their cell walls; like true viruses, they are obligate intracellular parasites. Two large subgroups exist: subgroup A includes the clinical condition of trachoma, inclusion conjunctivitis, and lymphogranuloma venereum; subgroup B contains feline pneumonitis and psittacosis.

OPHTHALMIA NEONATORUM
Inclusion conjunctivitis of the newborn (inclusion blennorrhea)

The etiologic agent of this condition is *Chlamydia oculogenitalis,* which is closely related to *C. trachomatis,* the organism that causes trachoma. It should be emphasized, however, that these two agents are distinct entities, since the agent of inclusion conjunctivitis can cause acute or subacute disease in the conjunctivae of primates, which does not occur with the trachoma agent. The diseases these agents cause are two distinct entities; the agents can be separated into immunologic types (A to C for trachoma

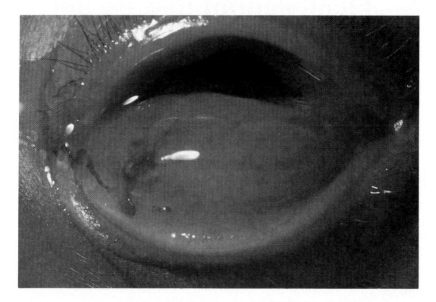

Fig. 7-1. Infantile inclusion conjunctivitis.

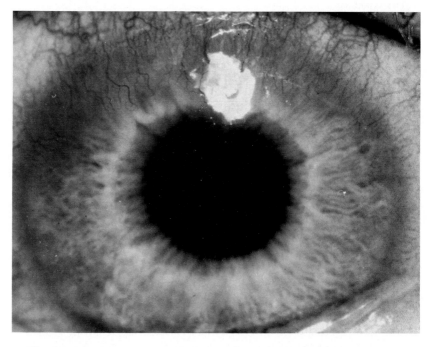

Fig. 7-2. Micropannus in untreated case of inclusion conjunctivitis of newborn.

agent and D to F for inclusion conjunctivitis agent) by the microimmunofluorescence test.[14, 32]

The reservoir of infection with *C. oculogenitalis* is in the urethra or cervix; the disease is transmitted venereally. The infant is infected during its passage through the birth canal.[25, 29, 31] Inclusion conjunctivitis is the result of contamination of the eye by genital secretion. The disease may be transmitted by fingers or fomites and may occur in those who harbor the genital infection. Eye-to-eye transmission is extremely rare.

Inclusion conjunctivitis of the newborn is the most common infectious type of ophthalmia neonatorum and appears as a purulent or mucopurulent papillary conjunctivitis[1, 18] (Fig. 7-1). No follicles appear in the newborn state, since there is immature lymphoid tissue in the newborn conjunctiva. Follicles may occur if the disease persists and may become apparent between 6 weeks and 3 months of age. Swelling of the lids and conjunctiva is common. A conjunctival pseudomembrane consisting of fibrin may be present, revealing conjunctival scars.[9] No preauricular adenopathy exists. Superficial vascularization of the cornea as a micropannus can be seen, as well as a fine epithelial keratitis and, on occasion, underlying areas of stromal haze and infiltrate. Although these areas may occur anywhere in the cornea, they are seen more numerously in the peripheral areas. The disease may resolve in 3 to 4 weeks or longer, but the longer it is left untreated, the greater the possibility that the patient may be left with a micropannus (Fig. 7-2) and subepithelial corneal scar. Mild scarring of the conjunctiva is seen if conjunctival disease has been membranous.[9, 11] Pneumonitis,[27] rhinitis,[17] otitis, vaginitis,[17] and hearing loss[10] have been reported.

Scrapings of the conjunctival epithelium with Giemsa's or Wright's stain are of immense value.[35] The predominant inflammatory cells are polymorphonuclear leukocytes. Inclusions can be seen both in Giemsa's stain and fluorescent antibody–stained conjunctival scrapings. One does not usually find bacteria on these scrapings. The inclusions, which are basophilic and are located in the cytoplasm of the epithelial cells, are similar to the inclusions (Halberstaedter-Prowazek bodies) that are found in trachoma. The inclusion bodies are located immediately above the nucleus and form a small cap that sits on the nucleus. The inclusion consists of infectious chlamydial particles called *elementary bodies*. The elementary bodies are round, appear to be equal in size, have sharp-edged cell walls, and are light purple when stained with Giemsa's stain. One must make sure when viewing the slide that true inclusion bodies are not mistaken for pseudo-inclusions such as bacteria, extrusions of nuclear chromatin granules, or other pigment granules. In addition to the elementary bodies, *initial bodies* may be found. The initial body is the metabolically active particle into which the elementary body transforms after entering the host cell. The initial body is larger than the elementary body and stains dark blue, often in a bipolar fashion. Inclusion bodies are seen much more frequently in the chlamydial oculoglandular infection of infancy; they may be difficult to find in adults.

Although the incidence of chlamydial infection in the newborn is frequent (3% of all newborn, according to some publications),[4, 11] one must rule out infection caused by the gonococcus or meningococcus and other bacteria.

Scrapings, cultures, and biochemical tests are imperative. *Neisseria gonorrhoeae* ferments glucose but not maltose, whereas *N. meningitidis* ferments both. As was stated

Table 7-1. Differential diagnosis and treatment of ophthalmia neonatorum

Agents	Day of onset after exposure	Laboratory findings	Types of discharge	Presence of membrane	Presence of follicles	Corneal involvement	Recommended treatment
Neonatal inclusion disease	5 to 10 days	Polymorpho-nuclear cells Basophilic Cytoplasmic inclusions Positive FA test	Purulent	+ May result in conjunctival scars	None in new-born; may develop in 6 weeks Response may be papillary early	Superior micropannus in nonrelated cases Fine epithelial keratopathy	1% Tetracycline in oil six times a day for 2 weeks Topical sulfonamides six times a day for 2 weeks
Silver nitrate irritation (Credé's method)	24 hours	Polymorpho-nuclear cells	Purulent in severe cases	+ In severe cases	—	If severe, may have epithelial keratopathy Corneal scarring	Proper administration of drug (1%) Clear discharge away Do not use stock bottles of silver nitrate—concentration of drug may be 90%
Neisseria gonor-rhoeae*	3 to 5 days or shorter if very severe After 5 days indicates exposure after birth	Epithelial parasitism with gram-negative diplococci	Mucopurulent	—	—	Marginal or central ulcer or ring abscess Perforation	Topical: bacitracin or aqueous penicillin G in normal saline, 10,000 to 20,000 units/ml every minute for 45 minutes, then hourly for 2 or 3 days Systemic: 500,000 units of aqueous penicillin daily IM with probenecid (also may use with ampicillin, spectinomycin, or tetracyclines)
Staphylococcus aureus	5+ days	Gram-positive cocci among polymorpho-nuclear cells	Catarrhal to mucopurulent	—	—	Fine epithelial keratopathy	Erythromycin ointment (0.5%) six times daily for 2 or 3 weeks
Streptococcus pneumoniae	5+ days	Gram-positive cocci in chains and polymorpho-nuclear cells	Purulent	—	—	Ulcer may develop or fine epithelial keratopathy resembling staphylococcal keratitis	Erythromycin ointment (0.5%) or sulfacetamide sodium (Sulamyd) (10%) every 2 hours

Organism	Incubation period	Laboratory findings	Discharge	Pseudomembrane	Systemic involvement	Corneal complications	Treatment
Haemophilus species	5+ days	*H. aegyptius*: gram-negative with epithelial parasitism; *H. influenzae*: no epithelial parasitism; gram-negative coccobacillus	Catarrhal in severe cases Purulent	—	—	Rare, but may develop fine epithelial keratopathy, especially with *H. aegyptius* (Koch-Weeks conjunctivitis)	*H. aegyptius* and *H. influenzae*: 10% sulfacetamide or erythromycin ointment (0.5%) six times every 2 hours
Coliform species	5+ days	Gram-negative noncapsulated rods in and among polymorphonuclear cells	Copious Purulent	—	—	Rare	Irrigation of conjunctival sac Neomycin (0.5%) or tetracycline in oil every hour for 24 hours, then six times daily for 2 weeks
Primary herpes type II	3 to 15 days	Multinucleated giant cells Positive FA test	Nonpurulent Watery	+	— In newborn may develop in 6 to 12 weeks	Dendritic or stromal disease	Débridement and patching Idoxuridine (IDU) drops every 4 hours during day and IDU ointment every 4 hours at night; vidarabine may be used if no response to IDU; trifluorothymidine may also be used
Candida species conjunctivitis	5+ days	Pseudohyphal Budding yeast forms Polymorphonuclear cells	Sometimes conjunctival necrosis	—	—	Occasional marginal corneal ulcer	5% Primaricin ophthalmic drops or 1% flucytosine drops

*Some strains may produce the enzyme β-lactamase, which destroys the penicillin nucleus, rendering the drug ineffective; these strains are mutant and occur rarely.

in Chapter 4, one should employ Thayer-Martin or chocolate agar media, as well as blood agar media, to grow *Neisseria* gonococcus. It is absolutely imperative to rule out *N. gonorrhoeae* and *N. meningitidis;* the preceding laboratory hints aid in this differentiation.

Staphylococcal conjunctivitis

Staphylococcal conjunctivitis resulting from *S. aureus* is a rather common finding and may become serious because of the immature immunity in infants. Usually the disease occurs initially as a mild catarrhal conjunctivitis with hyperemia and mucopurulent secretion. There may be some edema of the lids. Scrapings will show gram-positive cocci with polymorphonuclear cells. Staphylococcal conjunctivitis does not become chronic in the newborn. This is usually not the case in the older child or adult, in whom it often becomes chronic by invading the follicles of the eyelashes or the meibomian glands. This chronicity may result in severe corneal disease.

E. coli conjunctivitis

Neonatal conjunctivitis caused by coliform organisms is most frequently a result of *E. coli;* the disease in the newborn is usually an acute, purulent conjunctivitis with severe chemosis of the conjunctiva, swelling of the lids, and copious purulent secretion.

Streptococcus pneumoniae and streptococcal conjunctivitis in newborns exhibit a similar picture. Cultural and Gram's stains will facilitate the diagnosis so that proper therapy may be introduced.

Haemophilus influenzae conjunctivitis

The conjunctivitis caused by *H. influenzae* is usually a severe one with much purulent conjunctivitis and edema of the lid, in contrast to the conjunctivitis caused by *H. aegyptius,* which is a mild disease with only a small amount of mucoid exudate. On scrapings and Gram's stains, *H. influenzae* shows no epithelial parasitism and appears as a tiny, gram-negative coccobacillus, whereas *H. aegyptius* shows epithelial parasitism and appears as a long, fine, gram-negative bacillus.

Gonorrheal conjunctivitis

In every case of ophthalmia neonatorum, gonococcal infection must absolutely be ruled out. The incubation period for this infection is usually 3 to 5 days. However, if premature rupture of the membranes occurs, the infant can be infected in utero, and the infection may show up earlier. Edema of the lids with severe chemosis and watery or serosanguineous exudate may occur. In addition, if untreated, this exudate is followed by large amounts of puslike discharge. The more severe the conjunctivitis, the more likely the cornea is to be affected: the cornea may break down with ulceration either centrally or marginally. Multiple peripheral ulcers may become confluent and form a ring abscess.

Pneumococcal conjunctivitis can occur in the newborn and can simulate gonorrheal conjunctivitis; therefore it is mandatory for the organism to be cultured and proper fermentation studies to be performed, as already noted.

Herpes simplex hominis virus type II

Herpes simplex hominis type II conjunctivitis is associated with vesicular blepharitis or disseminated infection. In addition, iris atrophy, chorioretinitis, and corneal dendrites may be observed. A nonpurulent exudate with a mononuclear response occurs; however, if a membrane is present, polymorphonuclear leukocytes are seen in numbers. If one strongly suspects a herpetic infection, examination of the scrapings for multinucleated epithelial cells and FA studies may be performed. The finding of typical herpetic corneal involvement is also an aid in the diagnosis. The conjunctival inflammation of herpes simplex and nearly all other nonchlamydial causes of ophthalmia neonatorum resolves spontaneously in 2 or 3 weeks, although corneal complications can persist longer. It is important to remember that, if scrapings and cultures from the untreated patient are negative for bacteria and if there is no evidence to suggest herpetic infection, one must presume the presence of chlamydial infection.

Chemical conjunctivitis

Chemical conjunctivitis is mild and of only a few days' duration. It appears within 24 hours after instillation of the silver nitrate. In high concentrations, of course, silver nitrate can be most irritating and might cause a purulent discharge and ulceration of the conjunctival membranes.

Table 7-1 records the treatment of various entities that are responsible for ophthalmia neonatorum.

ADOLESCENT AND ADULT OCULOGENITAL AND CHLAMYDIAL INFECTIONS AND RELATED CONDITIONS (Table 7-2)

Infection after the newborn period may spread from the genitalia to the fingers to the eyes, from the genitalia directly to the eye, or from the genitalia to fomites to the eye. Eye-to-eye transmission is unusual. Inclusion conjunctivitis can be transmitted in swimming pools with inadequately prepared chlorination.[16] Most conjunctivitis from swimming pools is caused by the chlorine-resistant adenoviruses.

Inclusion conjunctivitis of the adolescent and adult (Table 7-2)

This acute follicular conjunctivitis usually persists for 2 to 3 months; when a conjunctivitis persists for this length of time in a person of the sexually active age group, one should be suspicious of the possibility of inclusion conjunctivitis.

In the adult, a mucopurulent discharge occurs, with follicular hypertrophy more marked in the lower tarsal conjunctiva (Fig. 7-3). No pseudomembranes are present, but a small, preauricular, tender node may occur. A pseudoptosis is often seen, but this is also observed at times in acute adenoviral conditions. Epithelial keratitis with peripheral subepithelial infiltrates and a superior corneal micropannus are seen. The follicular conjunctivitis persists for a long time, much longer than that seen in adenoviral infection.

Scrapings will reveal a preponderance of polymorphonuclear leukocytes. Routine bacteriologic findings are negative. Chlamydial inclusion bodies are difficult to find and are much less numerous than those found in the infantile form of inclusion conjunctivitis. Positive FA-stained conjunctival scrapings are found.

Table 7-2. Differential diagnosis of adult inclusion disease

Disease	Laboratory findings	Types of discharge	Presence of follicles	Corneal involvement	Systemic signs	Treatment
Inclusion conjunctivitis	Polymorphonuclear leukocytes Rare inclusions (basophilic and cytoplasmic) Positive FA-stained conjunctival scraping	Mucopurulent No membrane	+ Lower lid	Superior micropannus Fine epithelial keratitis Subepithelial infiltrates (mostly peripheral)	Preauricular node on occasion	Tetracycline, 500 mg orally three times a day for 3 weeks Do not prescribe for pregnant women or children under 2 months old Give three trisulfapyrimidine tablets* (70 mg/kg) daily, not to exceed 40 g/day for 3 to 4 weeks
Neisseria species infection with gonococcus	Polymorphonuclear leukocytes Gram-negative diplococci (intracellular)	Purulent or mucopurulent Pseudomembrane on occasion	−	May be severe with peripheral and marginal ulcers Perforation may result	Iridocyclitis Urinary symptoms Urethritis Preauricular glands	4,800,000 units of aqueous penicillin IM in two doses daily with probenecid, 1 g, 30 minutes before (only in adults) Spectinomycin IM, tetracycline, and ampicillin may also be given orally
Phthiriasis pubis	Nits and adult organisms	Watery	+ Severe, resulting from toxicity of parasites' feces	—	Parasite found in axillary, body, chest, and perianal hair	Remove nits manually Smother parasites with bland ointment Shampoo with Kwell 20% fluorescein solution
Reiter's syndrome	Some cases associated with chlamydial disease, as noted by positive complement-fixation titers and positive FA staining Others may be associated with dysentery (*Shigella* organisms)	Mucopurulent	− Papillary response	Epithelial keratitis Subepithelial keratitis with infiltration Loss of central epithelium	Urethritis Arthritis Keratoderma blennorrhagica Nongranulomatous iritis	Systemic tetracyclines may be of some help Same dose as for inclusion conjunctivitis

Venereal wart	Mononuclear reaction	−	Papillary response	Fine epithelial keratitis	Pedunculated lobular skin lesion	Lid lesions can be removed; cauterize base. Conjunctival ones are best left alone; will regress in time. If removing them, use −80° C cryo-application for 1 minute; repeat
Molluscum contagiosum	Mononuclear response	−	+	"Pseudotrachoma" Superior micropannus with follicular conjunctivitis and fine epithelial keratitis. Macropannus can be seen rarely	Umbilicated, raised, white, noninflammatory nodule on lid or conjunctiva	Curettage of central core of molluscum
Lymphogranuloma venereum	May see typical chlamydial inclusions in macrophages	−	Papillary response	May have severe corneal scarring	Granulomatous reaction to conjunctiva Preauricular gland enlargement Elephantiasis of lids Neuritis Uveitis Episcleritis Sclerokeratitis	Tetracyline, 1 to 1.5 g orally every day for 3 to 4 weeks

*Adult dose of trisulfapyrimidines (triple sulfa): 2 to 4 g immediate loading dose followed by maintenance dose of 2 to 4 g (about 70 mg/kg) four times a day for at least 3 weeks. Do not use in pregnancy or for nursing mothers. Trisulfapyrimidines (Terfonyl) tablets contain equal amounts of sulfadiazine, sulfamerazine, and sulfamethazine.

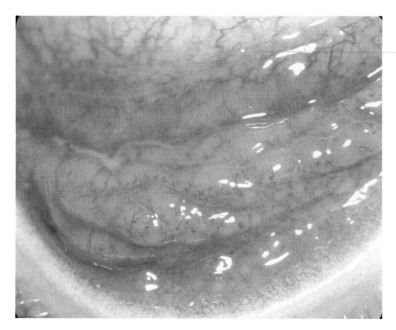

Fig. 7-3. Marked follicular response in lower conjunctival area in adult inclusion conjunctivitis. (Courtesy F. Wilson II, M.D., Indianapolis, Ind.)

Reiter's syndrome[12]

Some cases occur after epidemics of bacillary dysentery[20]; others appear to follow or relate to chlamydial infection.[33] Inclusion disease is a major cause of nonbacterial and so-called nonspecific urethritis and cervicitis and may well be the most prevalent venereal disease.[13, 26, 33]

The diagnostic criteria for Reiter's syndrome are nonspecific urethritis; arthritis, usually of the large joints; and conjunctivitis or iridocyclitis.[8] Keratoderma blennor-rhagica is also seen. Some individuals will manifest periostitis and other systemic problems, including cardiac involvement.

The conjunctivitis is papillary in nature, with mucopurulent discharge (Fig. 7-4). The iridocyclitis is a nongranulomatous one, and posterior synechiae are rare. The corneal complications consist of punctate epithelial lesions, central erosive corneal lesions, and peripheral subepithelial infiltrations.[19]

As stated, some cases are associated with chlamydial infections, as indicated by the presence of positive complement-fixation titers and positive FA staining to chlamydiae. Positive isolation of the agent from the eyes, genital tract, and joints has been made. Interestingly, more than 95% of patients with Reiter's syndrome have the HL-A W27 histocompatibility antigen; the normal incidence of such an antigen is less than 10%. Reiter's syndrome has been associated with *Campylobacter jejuni*[23] and *Salmonella enteritis*.[24]

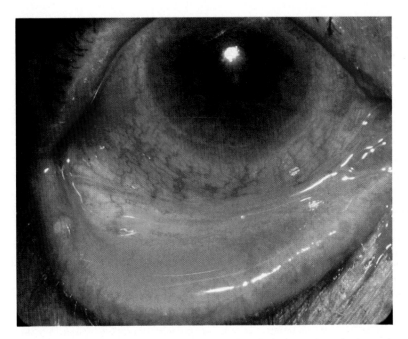

Fig. 7-4. Mucopurulent papillary hypertrophy conjunctival disease in Reiter's syndrome.

Phthiriasis pubis

The adult organism is transparent and can be missed in an eyelash examination. The pubic louse prefers eyelashes and pubic hair. Intimate contact is required for transmission of the parasite since it does not survive when separated from its host for any length of time. Nits, which are oval and cemented to the eyelashes, are easier to see than the adult organism.

The lid margins are red and swollen, probably as a result of inflammation caused by the parasite taking its blood meal. A severe blepharoconjunctivitis occurs particularly in children, probably because of toxicity of the parasite's feces. A follicular reaction is seen.

An application of 20% fluorescein to the lashes has been advised for phthiriasis palpebrarum.[15] The louse is dislodged from the cilia root by the fluorescein, which is nontoxic. The procedure, which requires no anesthetic or sedative is effective as an outpatient treatment.

Neisseria gonococcus conjunctivitis

Most cases of ocular *Neisseria* species infection in the younger age group occur in girls as the result of vaginal disease. In adults, gonorrheal conjunctivitis may manifest itself as a pseudomembranous conjunctivitis or a mild catarrhal conjunctivitis. Most persons, however, exhibit a rather severe purulent discharge with marked chemosis and swelling of the lids. The cornea has a great tendency to become involved with both marginal and central corneal ulceration.

As in the newborn, scrapings will show gram-negative intracellular diplococci.

Lymphogranuloma venereum (LGV)

This disease, transmitted venereally, is a granulomatous reaction of the conjunctiva associated with periauricular adenopathy. It can result in elephantiasis of the lids. Episcleritis and sclerokeratitis are seen. An infiltration of the superficial cornea becomes deep and vascular. Interstitial keratitis is also associated with lymphogranuloma. Optic neuritis and anterior uveitis are occasionally seen.[28] The orbit may also be involved.[7] The conjunctiva and the cornea become diffusely scarred. Chlamydial agents are found on conjunctival scrapings. The Frei test is positive in 50% of patients.

Verrucal conjunctivitis (venereal wart)

Verruca and condylomata acuminatum are caused by the same virus, but the site of infection is different.[22,34] Verrucae of the lid are multilobular lesions that may be papillary or broad based.

A verruca of the lid margin may result in a mild papillary conjunctivitis and a fine epithelial keratitis. The conjunctiva can be affected; here the lesion is frondlike and has a predunculated base.

Conjunctival scrapings from a verrucal conjunctivitis usually show a mononuclear type of reaction.

Molluscum contagiosum

Molluscum contagiosum can occur by genital spread.[5] The molluscum nodule is a pearly-white, raised, round, noninflammatory lesion with a craterous center. It may occur on the lid margin or on the conjunctiva. It may be obvious (Fig. 7-5) or subtle (Fig. 7-6). Chronic follicular conjunctivitis is seen in molluscum contagiosum. In long-standing cases, one may find a chronic conjunctivitis with a superior micropannus and a fine epithelial keratitis in the superior corneal quadrants (Fig. 7-7) that can simulate trachoma. However, follicular conjunctivitis and micropannus suggest inclusion conjunctivitis.

A scraping from the conjunctiva reveals mononuclear cells. Molluscum bodies are seen in microscopic section of the lesion (Fig. 7-8).

Other conditions to be considered in differential diagnosis

Other diseases that may rarely result in an oculogenital[6] infection are diphtheria, listeriosis,[3] Mimeae conjunctivitis,[4] and chancroid *(Haemophilus ducreyi).*

It is most important in any of these oculogenital infections to examine the patient's sexual partner.

● ● ●

Table 7-2 lists the classification and therapeutic measures used to treat the preceding oculogenital infections.

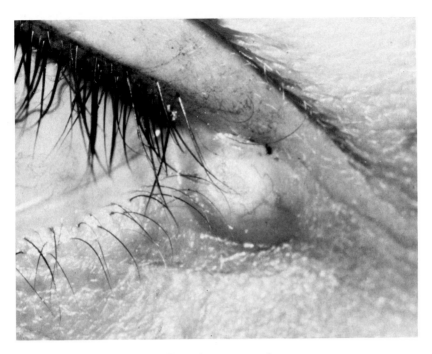

Fig. 7-5. Molluscum contagiosum.

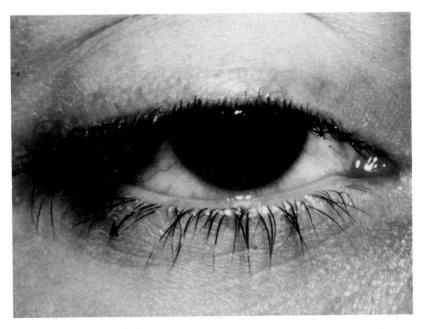

Fig. 7-6. Inconspicuous molluscum contagiosum lesion hidden by cilia *(arrow)*, causing persistent injection of eye with follicular conjunctivitis.

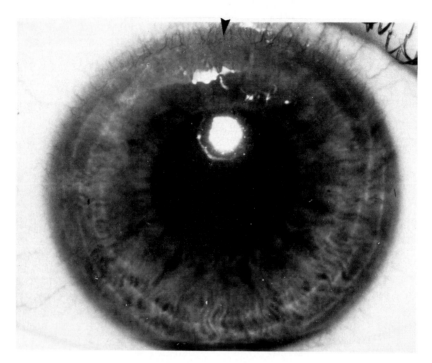

Fig. 7-7 Untreated molluscum contagiosum may cause pannus *(arrow)*.

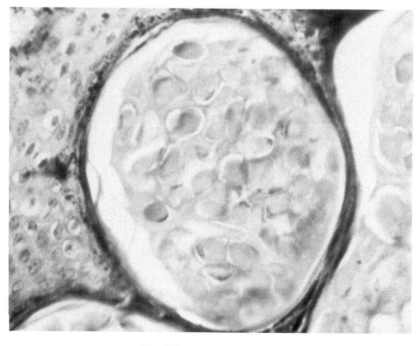

Fig. 7-8. Molluscum bodies.

OTHER CHLAMYDIAL OCULAR INFECTIONS[21] (Table 7-3)

The chlamydial ocular infections of subgroup A include (1) trachoma *(C. trachomatis)*, (2) inclusion conjunctivitis of newborn and adults *(C. oculogenitalis)*, (3) lymphogranuloma venereum *(C. lymphogranulomatis)*, (4) psittacosis *(C. psittaci)*, (5) feline pneumonitis, and (6) Reiter's syndrome.

Trachoma

This disease has been around for 3000 years, if not longer, and has ravaged a good part of the world. Even today it is a major cause of preventable blindness in the world. Around the world, 700 million cases are estimated, about 200 million of which involve blindness or a significantly decreased visual acuity.

Table 7-3. Correlation of features of chlamydial infections of the eye

| Characteristics | Subgroup A | | | Subgroup B | |
	Trachoma	Inclusion conjunctivitis	Lympho-granuloma venereum	Feline pneumonitis	Psittacosis (parakeet)
Onset	Insidious in childhood, acute in adults	Subacute or acute	Insidious	Subacute	Subacute
Duration	Years	3 to 4 months	Years	3 months	3 to 4 months
Palpable pre-auricular node	Small	Small	Very large (bubo)	Small	Very small
Conjunctivitis	Follicular; mainly superior	Papillary in newborn, follicular in adult; mainly inferior	Papillary	Follicular	Follicular (minimal)
Pannus	Gross	Micropannus occasionally	Severe	None	None
Epithelial lesions	Mainly superior	Mainly superior	Minimal	Mainly central	Severe, diffuse
Subepithelial infiltrates	Rare; "trachoma pustules	Rare	Severe, diffuse	Moderately superior	Severe, diffuse
Limbal follicles or Herbert's pits	Common	Absent	Absent	Absent	Absent
Sequelae	Stellate scars, flat scars, Arlt's line, trichiasis, corneal scars	Minor flat scars in newborn; none in adult	Total pannus; obliteration of fornices	None	None
Transmission	Eye to eye	Oculogenital	Oculogenital	Cat to human	Laboratory infection

Trachoma is prevalent among the American Indians of the southwestern part of the United States. Many cases are located in the "trachoma belt" of Arkansas, Missouri, Oklahoma, West Virginia, and Kentucky.

The disease is spread from eye to eye by way of fingers, fomites, and water; its highest incidence is in unhealthy, dirty, crowded conditions, primarily in the low socio-economic stratum of society. In a number of instances trachoma is associated with secondary bacterial conjunctivitis. This association is a circumstance under which the disease is worsened.

Clinical features. The clinical features of trachoma have been divided into the four stages described by MacCallan. In this classification stage I is characterized by the presence in the upper tarsal conjunctiva of immature follicles with poor germinal centers. These follicles are soft and are easily expressible, unlike those of non-trachomatous follicular conjunctivitis. Follicles can also be seen at the limbus and on the caruncle. A minimal exudate usually occurs; however, if a secondary infection is present, a greater exudation is seen. Intense cellular infiltration of the conjunctiva can occur; the subepithelial tissue of the conjunctiva is edematous and infiltrated with round inflammatory cells, mainly lymphocytes and plasma cells. Papillary hypertrophy also occurs, and the follicles may be buried as a result. In this stage of early formation of conjunctival follicles, one may see a diffuse punctate keratitis and early superior corneal pannus formation. Fibrovascular tissue may grow into the cornea underneath the epithelium and destroy Bowman's layer.

In MacCallan's stage IIa, mature follicles appear in the upper tarsus in addition to papillary hypertrophy (Fig. 7-9); in stage IIb follicles are seen but may be obscured by a rather intense papillary response. This stage is primarily a florid inflammation of the upper tarsal conjunctiva; the follicles give the appearance of "sago" grains. The corneal pannus as well as the subepithelial edema and round cell infiltration may increase. Large macrophages with phagocytosed debris (Leber's cells) appear in the conjunctival substantia propria. At this stage, the follicles cannot be differentiated histologically from lymphoid follicles secondary to other causes.

Stage III brings about variable amounts of scarring and cicatrization (Fig. 7-10). The limbal corneal follicles, if present, cicatrize, and the area is covered with thickened transparent epithelium (Herbert's pits) (Fig. 7-11). These pits are 100% diagnostic of trachoma. Scarring occurs in the palpebral conjunctiva and is manifest clinically by the appearance of fine linear scars on the tarsal conjunctiva and sometimes in the bulbar conjunctiva. The horizontal linear scars that are noted in the upper tarsal conjunctiva are known as Arlt's line. Cicatrization of the lids and symblepharon trichiasis and other lid distortions are added problems, as seen in stage IV. In this stage no further inflammation occurs, and the corneal inflammation as well as the pannus has subsided.

These described findings may occur with a gross pannus of the upper portion of the cornea, epithelial and subepithelial keratitis, and corneal ulceration. Corneal scarring, opacification, and vascularization may be so severe that vision is severely impaired (Fig. 7-12). Most of the findings are aggravated in the superior portions of the cornea, and the condition may last for years.

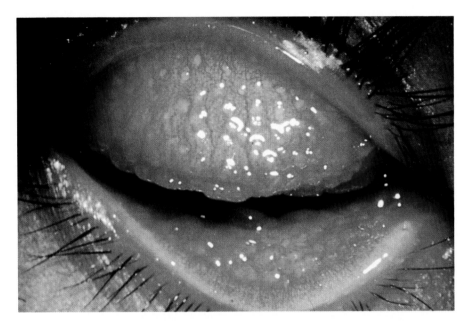

Fig. 7-9. Stage IIa trachoma.

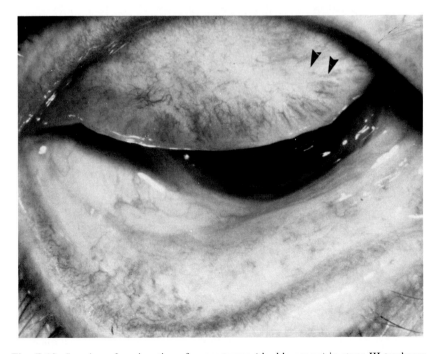

Fig. 7-10. Scarring of conjunctiva of upper tarsus *(double arrow)* in stage III trachoma.

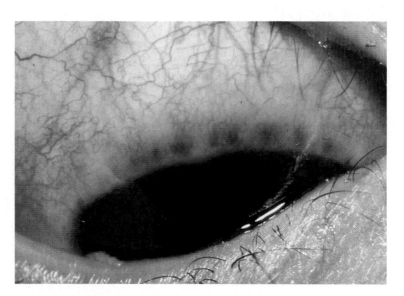

Fig. 7-11. Herbert's pits in stage III trachoma.

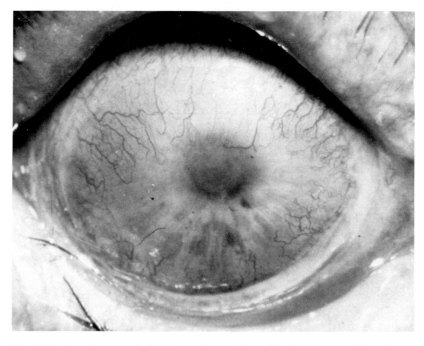

Fig. 7-12. Scarring, vascularization, and corneal opacification in stage IV trachoma.

Secondary complication in addition to corneal opacifications and lid and lash distortions includes "drying" of the conjunctiva and the cornea.

Lacrimal complications such as punctal phimosis, punctal occlusion, canalicular occlusion, nasolacrimal obstruction, dacryocystitis, and fistulae in the skin have been reported in trachoma.[29]

The primary inflammatory reaction may be a polymorphonuclear response with a mucopurulent discharge and preauricular adenopathy; however, lymphocytes, plasma cells, lymphoblasts, necrotic epithelial cells, and multinucleated giant epithelial cells may be seen. Basophilic, intracytoplastic, epithelial inclusion bodies (Halberstraedter-Prowazek bodies) similar to those described in inclusion conjunctivitis are seen in this disease.

Epidemiologic factors. Childhood trachoma is often missed or confused with folliculosis or follicular conjunctivitis. It is the childhood form that is important in the spread of disease in both family and community. Trachoma acquired in adulthood usually has an acute onset. A failure to induce immunity in trachoma may occur and may account for a long duration of the disease and for the reinfections that are so common among schoolchildren who have been treated successfully during the school year. The epidemiology is also affected by the characteristic association of trachoma virus with conjunctivitis-producing bacteria such as *H. aegyptius* that may increase the activity of the agent.

Treatment. The ideal treatment is with a full, oral dose of tetracycline, sulfonamide, or erythromycin for at least 3 weeks. If tetracycline is the drug given, one should use 500 mg orally three times a day for at least 3 weeks. This medication should be taken 1 hour before or 2 hours after meals with water or juice but no milk. This systemic treatment is most effective in trachoma therapy in communities in which seasonal bacterial conjunctivitis is not a problem. However, in hyperendemic areas in which 50% or more of the children have active disease and seasonal epidemics of bacterial conjunctivitis are present, the aim of the therapy is to prevent blindness. Topical tetracycline given as a continuous 6-week course twice a day appears to reduce or eliminate blinding complications. Similar results with a 5-day course of topical tetracycline repeated once monthly for 6 months seems to be effective. Topical medication may act by reducing the ocular bacterial flora and seasonal conjunctivitis that contribute to the gravity of trachoma in these areas. Therefore one may have to add topical medication together with oral medication. Tetracycline is not to be used in pregnant women or in children younger than 7 years.

Trisulfapyrimidines (triple sulfa) may be used. In adults the dose is 2 to 4 g immediately followed by a maintenance dose of 2 to 4 g daily three times a day or four times a day for at least 3 weeks. In children a loading dose of one half of the 24-hour dose is followed by a maintenance dose of 150 mg/kg for 24 hours in three to four dosages for at least 3 weeks. The maximum 6 g per 24 hours is to be given. Trisulfapyrimidines are not to be used in pregnant women, nursing mothers, or infants younger than 2 months.

In subgroup B psittacosis (ornithosis) and feline pneumonitis are included.

Psittacosis

Psittacosis exhibits a subacute onset with a mild preauricular adenopathy and follicular conjunctivitis, which is minimal. A mucupurulent discharge can be seen; however, no pannus is noted. A severe, rather diffuse, epithelial keratitis and subepithelial infiltration occur. There is no scarring of the conjunctiva; no inclusions can be found on scrapings. There are no sequelae of any importance, and the disease apparently responds to tetracycline. Psittacosis appears to be a laboratory infection that can be transmitted and usually lasts 3 to 4 months.

Feline pneumonitis

The onset is usually subacute with a small preauricular adenopathy and mild follicular conjunctivitis. A mild discharge is present. No pannus is noted, but one may see some subepithelial and epithelial infiltrates. No sequelae occur; the transmission is usually from cat to human.

DIAGNOSTIC AIDS

Ophthalmologists have at their disposal several laboratory and diagnostic aids to help in diagnosing the trachoma and inclusion conjunctivitis.[14] In the office, one may employ the Giemsa stain to look for the typical cystoplasmic inclusion bodies in the epithelial cells. The inclusions are numerous in smears from newborns with inclusion blennorrhea; however, they are present in small numbers in adult inclusion disease. Inclusion bodies are rarely seen in American Indians or others with chronic active trachoma.[2]

On a more sophisticated level, isolation of this agent can take place in the yolk sac of embryonated eggs. Immunofluorescent (FA) staining methods are available to aid in making a diagnosis. At the moment, this method is apparently the most sensitive of all the tests available; 40% of chronic trachoma cases are positive by the FA test.

The complement-fixation (CF) test measures antibody to chlamydial group antigen, so it is not specific for the trachoma inclusion conjunctivitis infection. An elevated CF titer of 1 to 16 or greater is seen in 50% of oculogenital cases. At least 4% of the general population have elevated titers. However, a fourfold increase in titers during the course of the illness suggests a chlamydial infection. Indirect immunofluorescent tests to measure serum or tear antibodies are being performed in some laboratories. The tests can be used to classify strains of trachoma inclusion conjunctivitis agent: types A, B, BA, and C are usually found in trachoma cases from endemic areas, whereas types D to I are found in oculogenital cases. Serum antibodies of the patient usually have a high titer against the infecting strain.

Table 7-3 compiles a correlation of features of chlamydial infections of the eye.

REFERENCES

1. Armstrong, J.H., Zacarias, F., and Rein, M.F.: Ophthalmia neonatorum: a chart review, Pediatrics **57**:884, 1976.
2. Bettman, J.W., Jr., Carreno, O.B., Szuter, C.F., and Yoneda, C.: Inclusion conjunctivitis in American Indians of the Southwest, Am. J. Ophthalmol. **70**:363, 1970.
3. Burdin, J.C., Weber, M., and Martin, F.: Epidemiological study of human listeriosis in France: considerations of about 62 cases observed in Lor-

raine, Rev. Epidemiol. Med. Soc. Sante Publique **22:**279, 1974.

4. Burns, R.P., and Florey, M.J.: Conjunctivitis caused by Mimeae, Am. J. Ophthalmol. **56:**386, 1963.

5. Cobbold, R.J.D., and MacDonald, A.: Molluscum contagiosum as a sexually transmitted disease, Practitioner **204:**416, 1970.

6. DeBord, G.G.: Species of the tribes Mimeae, Neisseriaceae, and Streptococceae which confuse the diagnosis of gonorrhea by smears, J. Lab. Clin. Med. **28:**710, 1943.

7. Endicott, J.N., Kirconnell, W.S., and Beam, D.: Granuloma inguinale of the orbit with bony involvement, Arch. Otolaryngol. **96:**457, 1972.

8. Engleman, E.P., and Weber, A.M.: Reiter's syndrome, Clin. Orthoped. Res. **57:**19, 1968.

9. Forster, R.K., Dawson, C.R., and Schachter, J.: Late follow-up of patients with neonatal inclusion conjunctivitis, Am. J. Ophthalmol. **69:**467, 1970.

10. Gow, J.A., Ostler, H.B., and Schachter, J.: Inclusion conjunctivitis with hearing loss, JAMA **229:**519, 1974.

11. Hansman, D.: Inclusion conjunctivitis, Med. J. Aust. **1:**151, 1969.

12. Harkness, A.H.: Reiter's disease, Br. J. Vener. Dis. **25:**185, 1949.

13. Holmes, K.K., Handsfield, H.H., Wang, S.P., Wentworth, B.B., Turck, M., Anderson, J.B., and Alexander, E.R.: Etiology of nongonococcal urethritis, N. Engl. J. Med. **292:**1199, 1975.

14. Jones, B.R.: Laboratory tests for chlamydial infection, Br. J. Ophthalmol. **58:**438, 1974.

15. Mathew, M., D'Souza, P., and Mehta, D.K.: A new treatment of phthiriasis palpebrarum, Ann. Ophthalmol. **14:**439, 1982.

16. Morax, V.: Les conjonctivites folliculaires, Paris, 1933, Masson et Cie.

17. Mordhorst, C.H., and Dawson, C.: Sequelae of inclusion conjunctivitis and associated disease in parents, Am. J. Ophthalmol. **71:**861, 1971.

18. Ostler, H.B.: Oculogenital disease, Surv. Ophthalmol. **20:**233, 1976.

19. Ostler, H.B., Dawson, C.R., Schachter, J., and Engleman, E.P.: Reiter's syndrome, Am. J. Ophthalmol. **71:**986, 1971.

20. Paronia, I.: Reiter's disease, Acta Med. Scand. Suppl. 212, 1948.

21. Poirier, R.H.: Chlamydial infection: diagnosis and management, Trans. Am. Acad. Ophthalmol. Otolaryngol. **79:**109, 1975.

22. Rhodes, A.J., and Van Rooyen, C.E.: Textbook of virology, ed. 5, Baltimore, 1968, The Williams & Wilkins Co.

23. Saari, K.M., and Kaurenen, O.: Ocular inflammation in Reiter's syndrome associated with *Campylobacter jejuni* enteritis, Am. J. Ophthalmol. **90:**572, 1980.

24. Saari, K.M., Vippula, A., Lassus, M., et al.: Ocular inflammation in Reiter's disease after *Salmonella enteritis*, Am. J. Ophthalmol. **90:**63, 1980.

25. Schachter, J.: Reply to letter to editor, JAMA **234:**592, 1975.

26. Schachter, J., Hanna, L., Hill, E.C., Massad, S., Sheppard, C.W., Conte, J.E., Jr., Cohen, S.N., and Meyer, K.F.: Are chlamydia infections the most prevalent venereal disease? JAMA **231:**1252, 1975.

27. Schachter, J., Lum, L., Gooding, C.A., and Ostler, B.: Pneumonitis following inclusion blennorrhea, J. Pediatr. **87:**779, 1975.

28. Scheie, H.G., Crandall, A.S., and Henle, W.: Keratitis associated with lymphogranuloma venereum, JAMA **135:**333, 1947.

29. Tabbara, K.F., Babb, A.A. Lacrimal system complications in trachoma, Ophthalmology **87:**298, 1980.

30. Thygeson, P.: Historical review of oculogenital disease, Am. J. Ophthalmol. **71:**975, 1971.

31. Thygeson, P., and Stone, W., Jr.: Epidemiology of inclusion conjunctivitis, Arch. Ophthalmol. **27:**91, 1942.

32. Wang, S., and Grayston, J.T.: Immunologic relationship between genital TRIC, lymphogranuloma venereum, and related organisms in a new microtiter indirect immunofluorescence test, Am. J. Ophthalmol. **70:**367, 1970.

33. Week, L.A., Smith, T.F., Pettersen, G.R., and Segura, J.W.: Urethritis associated with *Chlamydia:* clinical and laboratory diagnosis, Minn. Med. **59:**288, 1976.

34. Wile, V.J., and Kingery, L.B.: The etiology of common warts: preliminary report of an experimental study, JAMA **73:**970, 1919.

35. Yoneda, C., Dawson, C.R., Daghfous, T., Hoshiwara, I., Jones, P., Messadi, M., and Schachter, J.: Cytology as a guide to the presence of chlamydial inclusions in Giemsa-stained conjunctival smears in severe endemic trachoma, Br. J. Ophthalmol. **59:**116, 1975.

8 Viral diseases

Herpes simplex
THE VIRUS (Table 8-1)

The human herpesviruses—herpesvirus hominis, types 1 and 2 (HSV 1 and 2); cyto-megalovirus; varicella-zoster virus; and Epstein-Barr (EB) virus—are members of a large group of enveloped viruses that affect humans, animals, and birds. They have often been called "opportunistic viruses" because infection is often not apparent, and the clinical lesions commonly develop only after fever, shock, immunosuppression, ultra-violet light burns, or other trigger mechanisms.

After primary infection, these viruses can survive in a latent state, often in the spinal and cranial ganglia.[1] All members of the group appear morphologically identical by electron microscopy. They are composed of a central DNA core with a protein capsid of nucleoprotein and with 162 hollow, cylindric capsomeres. The capsid is surrounded by lipoprotein and glucoprotein; the completely enveloped virus has a diameter of 130 to

Table 8-1. Virus properties of herpes simplex and varicella-zoster viruses

Properties	Herpesvirus	
	Herpes simplex virus	Varicella-zoster virus
Morphologic characteristics		
Core	DNA	DNA
Capsid	Icosahedron; 162 hollow, cylindric capsomeres	Same
Envelope	Lipoprotein; glycoprotein	Same
Size	Core $75 \mu m$ Capsid 90 to $100 \mu m$ Enveloped 130 to $180 \mu m$ particle	Same
Inclusion body	Intranuclear, acidophilic Cowdry's type A	Same
Ether sensitivity	Positive	Positive
Antigenic types	Type 1: labial herpes Type 2: genital herpes	One immunologic type
Tissue tropism	Pantropic but prefers epithelium and nerve tissue	Pantropic but prefers epidermis, dermis, and nerve tissue
Animal hosts	Most animals susceptible, but particularly rabbit and mouse	Humans only
Lesions of chorioallantoic membrane	Type 1: small pocks Type 2: large pocks	None
Tissue culture	Growth on variety of cells	More fastidious and difficult to grow
Ganglion localization	Cranial and spinal ganglia, principally gasserian and sacral	Cranial and spinal ganglia
Primary attack	Herpetic stomatitis or acute herpetic keratoconjunctivitis; often inapparent	Varicella; rarely inapparent
Trigger mechanisms	Varied: for example, fever, stress, ultraviolet light, trauma, menstruation, immunosuppressive drugs	Any mechanism that depresses cellular immunity, such as tumors (especially Hodgkin's disease), old age, and immunosuppressive drugs
Importance of age	Primary attack in childhood; recurrence at any age	Primary attack (varicella) in childhood; recurrence (zoster) typically late in adult life
Characteristics of virus	Slow spread of viral cytopathogenic effect in contiguous linear fashion Cell-bound and not released into overlying medium Sensitive to freeze thaw	Simplex is not cell bound but is released throughout medium; therefore, produces diffuse CPE Hardy Produces classical dendrite in rabbit corneas

180 μm. Replication takes place in the nucleus of the cell, and Cowdry's type A eosinophilic intranuclear inclusion body is the remnant left after the virus has passed into the cytoplasm.

Several viruses cause central nervous system infection concomitantly with intraocular involvement in humans. These include cytomegalic inclusion disease, rubella, herpes simplex, measles, and maculopathy associated with subacute sclerosing panencephalitis.

Cytomegalic disease is seen in adults with hematologic malfunctions and in immunosuppressed patients.[2] The virus for cytomegalic inclusion disease can be found in the birth canal of pregnant women.

Herpesvirus hominis can cause neuroretinitis and encephalitis in an adult[29]; however, intraocular herpetic infection in adults is mostly limited to the anterior segment of the eye. Herpesvirus and herpes antigen have been isolated from the anterior chamber in cases of recurrent iritis without keratitis.[35]

Posterior intraocular herpetic involvement in the form of retinitis has been limited mostly to the neonatal period. The newborn usually acquires the virus (usually herpesvirus hominis type 2) from the mother's infected genital tract at delivery. The risk is 50%.[57] Ocular involvement occurs in 20% of cases of neonatal herpes and ranges from mild conjunctivitis to severe retinitis and encephalitis.

In the United States 60% of the population has been infected by 5 years of age, and 90% has been infected by 15 years of age, as demonstrated by serum–neutralizing antibody titers.[6] The virus can be recovered from the oral and nasal secretions and stools in 20% of patients less than 2 years of age and from 2.5% of older patients. The initial infection may remain subclinical in 85% to 99% of the cases,[48] but these patients all become carriers. Approximately 1% of primary infections will lead to a severe acute systemic illness.[5]

Herpes simplex virus produces many precipitating antigens, complement-fixing antibodies (IgM), and neutralizing antibodies (IgG) with a primary infection; however, a reinfection will not stimulate the production of these antibodies. The herpesvirus is a budding virus and can induce changes in infected cell surface antigens.[23]

TYPES

There are two types of herpes simplex virus (HSV): types 1 and 2. The antigens of types 1 and 2 can cross-react, but the two types are differentiated by the use of high serum antibody titers, by their preferential growth in differential cell species, by their plaque-forming ability on rabbit kidney-cell monolayers, and by pock size on the chorioallantoic membrane of embryonated hens' eggs.[50] Type 2 is more resistant to idoxuridine (IDU) and adenine arabinoside (Ara-A).[61] In rabbit keratitis, type 2 causes a more severe disease.[63] Type 2 herpesvirus is recovered principally from the genital sites,[8] from which it spreads either venereally from the mother to the newborn, by way of infected birth canal, or by ascending infection after premature rupture of the membranes.[39] Type 2 may cause genital herpes, neonatal systemic infections,[86,93] localized skin lesions, aseptic meningitis, and chronic neurologic disease and has been recovered from cervical cells from female patients with cervical cancer.[97] Bilateral conjunctivitis, dendritic keratitis,[25] and stromal keratitis can be seen but are not frequent findings. Chorioretinitis, retinitis, and cataracts have also been seen. In neonatal infection[21] and disseminated disease, about 10% of neonates may demonstrate ocular involvement.

Even though 80% of neonatal herpes simplex infections are caused by the type 2 virus, one may find that HSV type 1 can cause neonatal keratitis.[79] It is much less well appreciated that intrauterine infections can occur with associated congenital malformations and findings such as microcephaly,[20,54] chorioretinitis,[20,55] mental retardation, aseptic meningitis,[28] cutaneous vesicles, microphthalmia,[54] and cloudy posterior lens.[56] In these cases serum IgM may be elevated, suggesting an intrauterine infection. The congenital anomalies from this type of herpes infection are less specific than that seen with rubella.[39] The anomalies listed are probably not caused by primary disturbance of organogenesis but teratogenic sequelae resulting from disturbances of normally formed organs that may occur anytime from the ninth week to the late third trimester.[54] Rubella virus infects the embryo during embryogenesis in the critical first 8 weeks of pregnancy, with resulting nuclear cataracts, hearing loss, and cardiac anomalies.[90]

In adults, herpes infections of the eye are most often considered to be caused by HSV type 1. Although the genital type 2 virus may occasionally be recovered from herpetic lesions at extragenital sites, HSV isolates from eyes with herpetic keratitis or conjunctivitis have rarely been shown to be type 2. An exception to this is that in neonates genito-ocular spread of HSV type 2 occurs at the time of birth.[55,56,58,93] Several cases of HSV type 2 ocular infections in adults have been observed after genital herpetic disease.[62,63,64] Cases of ocular herpes attributed to HSV type 2 have demonstrated dendritic keratitis, ulcerative keratitis, interstitial keratitis, and corneal perforation.[59] Other cases that revealed HSV type 2 showed follicular conjunctivitis, preauricular gland enlargement, and the zoster form of distribution of vesicular lesions but with sparing of the medial parts of the face and almost all of the nose.[59] It can be stated that in adults only a small percentage of cases of HSV infection is caused by type 2; the vast majority of HSV ocular infections result from type 1.

PRIMARY INFECTION

Systemic infection with HSV 1 usually occurs within the first few years of life, but rare cases develop later. An increasing resistance comes with age, so that after early adult life primary infection is exceedingly rare. The young child is infected characteristically by salivary contamination from an adult with labial herpes; the characteristic clinical disease is an aphthous stomatitis, sometimes severe. This primary infection is often unrecognized or entirely subclinical. Primary infection outside the oral cavity is rare, but there are well-documented ocular cases, with or without associated oral lesions. The incubation period is 3 to 12 days and may be accompanied by fever, gastroenteritis, and diffuse adenopathy. Severe vesicular eruption associated with herpes, often referred to as Kaposi's varicelliform eruption, can occur and often is seen in patients who have an accompanying immune disease (atopy). Generalized infection and encephalitis may be seen in extremely serious cases.

The most characteristic lesion of primary HSV ocular infection is an acute conjunctivitis with lymphadenopathy and malaise, the mild cases of which are follicular in

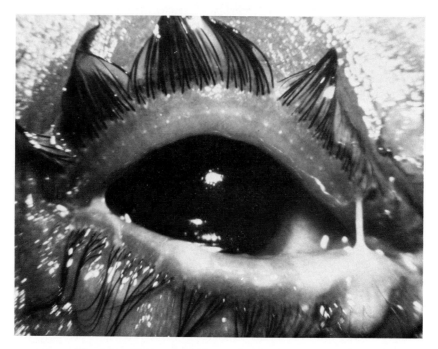

Fig. 8-1. Blepharoconjunctivitis of primary herpes simplex.

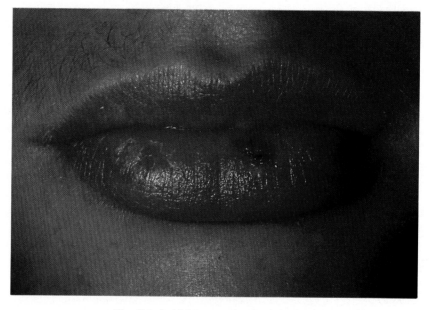

Fig. 8-2. Labial herpes simplex infection.

type; the more severe, pseudomembranous (50%) (Fig. 8-1); and some cases of which exhibit conjunctival dendrites. Dendritic keratitis accompanies the conjunctivitis in about half of the cases, and there also may be a unilateral ulcerative blepharitis (75%). The conjunctivitis may persist for 2 weeks, but the keratitis may last longer. Primary herpes can exhibit preauricular adenopathy, acute follicular conjunctivitis, and subepithelial dendritic opacities. Subepithelial dendritic keratitis has not been previously described. It is obvious that such a picture of herpes simplex infection would be difficult to differentiate from epidemic keratoconjunctivitis.[85] It seems probable that the common practice among parents of kissing their offspring on the eyes accounts for most of the primary ocular cases. Herpes simplex virus can sometimes be found in the mouths of labial herpes sufferers (Fig. 8-2), even during the intervals between attacks. Primary herpetic simplex infection may involve the lining of the lacrimal canaliculi and result in permanent strictures and epiphora.[22]

Diagnosis

A diagnosis is based on (1) history, (2) clinical appearance, (3) cytologic characteristics, (4) virus isolation, and (5) serologic findings. The history is important. A young child who develops acute follicular conjunctivitis 2 or 3 days after exposure to a parent or relative with labial herpes is almost certain to be suffering from a primary herpetic lesion.

The clinical appearance is highly suggestive. A young child with acute follicular or

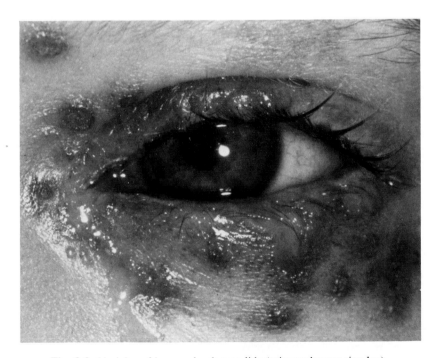

Fig. 8-3. Vesicles of herpes simplex on lids (primary herpes simplex).

pseudomembranous conjunctivitis probably has primary herpetic disease. If vesicles appear on the lids (Fig. 8-3) or a linear or dendritic corneal lesion is present, the diagnosis is certain.

Cytology is often helpful. If conjunctival scrapings, stained with Giemsa's stain, show a mononuclear exudate containing multinucleated giant epithelial cells, the diagnosis is almost definite.[80] If isolation of HSV 1 is successful, the question is settled. FA staining of herpes antigen in scrapings is most important and easy to do, and the response from the laboratory is quick.[34] Serologically, if an acute-phase blood specimen shows no HSV-neutralizing antibody, but a convalescent-phase specimen shows a significant titer, the diagnosis is definitive.

Primary infection results in the production of serum antiherpes antibodies, which rise to a peak in 2 to 3 weeks and then fall to a lower titer with spontaneous resolution of the disease. The virus becomes latent in the trigeminal or spinal ganglia and can be reactivated at any later time.[27] The pathogenesis of these recurrences is not understood. Serum antibodies rise only with primary infection and are of no diagnostic value for recurrent disease.

Treatment

Primary blepharoconjunctivitis may be treated with the application of prophylactic IDU ointment to eye and skin two to four times a day; IDU treatment should be stopped soon enough to avoid toxicity. Trifluorothymidine may also be used in lieu of IDU since it may be somewhat less toxic. A placebo and observation are probably of equal value, but treatment of keratitis is the same as for epithelial keratitis: that is, débridement and/or trifluorothymidine. The child may have to be restrained or anesthetized for débridement. This should be done gently with no injury to Bowman's layer.

RECURRENT HERPES

A general classification of recurrent herpes simplex infection with ocular involvement follows:

A. Vesicular eruption of the lids
B. Follicular conjunctivitis: may be accompanied by atypical punctate epithelial keratitis; can occur without skin lesions (cutaneous disease)
C. Cornea
    1. Epithelial keratitis: active viral replication
       a. Dendritic
       b. Geographic (ameboid)
       c. Marginal (limbal)
    2. Indolent and trophic ulceration (postinfectious herpes): epithelial and stromal ulceration with or without active stromal inflammation
    3. Stromal keratitis
       a. Sequential to epithelial keratitis
          (1) Confined to region of epithelial keratitis
          (2) Diffuse, central (disciform), or off the visual axis
          (3) Ulcerative keratitis
       b. Without epithelial involvement
          (1) Segmental

(2) Diffuse, central, interstitial keratitis
(3) Sclerokeratitis
4. Stromal scarring and edema secondary to permanent endothelial dysfunction
D. Uveitis
1. Iritis
2. Multifocal choroiditis
E. Trabeculopathy and ocular hypertension

Recurrent lesions generally are localized, superficial, and self-limited (labial "fever blister" or "cold sore," corneal dendrite) (Table 8-2), perhaps because of the protection provided by serum antibodies. Serum antibody titers do not change with these recurrent, localized infections. Healing of recurrent infections is presumably mediated by cellular immunity (sensitized lymphocytes)[52] rather than by humoral antibodies; such infections can become deep, extensive, and chronic in patients with deficient cellular immunity. Corneal lesions, although usually superficial and self-limited, can become deep and chronic even in healthy patients, perhaps because of the avascularity of the cornea; however, these problem cases may be the result of the unwise use of topical corticosteroids.

Table 8-2. Recurrent herpes simplex type 1

Characteristics	Dendritic keratitis	Herpes labialis
Latency	Gasserian ganglion	Gasserian ganglion
Trigger mechanisms	Fever most important; also sunburn, stress, menstruation, trauma, depression of cellular immunity by drugs, etc.	Fever most important; also sunburn, stress, menstruation, depression of cellular immunity by drugs, etc.
Premonitory symptoms	Foreign body sensation	Tingling and itching
Number of lesions	Varies from 1 to 10	Varies; often only 1
Intervals between recurrences	Vary with trigger mechanisms, especially with frequency of upper respiratory disease	Vary with trigger mechanisms, especially with frequency of upper respiratory disease
Subepithelial involvement	Varies from none to scar formation	No scarring
Secondary infection	Not seen in immunocompetent individuals	Not seen in immunocompetent individuals Note: Skin vesicles on face may be superinfected with S. aureus
Duration (untreated)	50% or more heal within a week; remainder in 2 to 3 weeks	2 days to 3 weeks; average, 9 to 10 days
Disease in patients (immunosuppressed by kidney transplantation, Wiskott-Aldrich syndrome, etc.)	May have severe, chronic stromal disease, keratouveitis, secondary fungal or bacterial infection, perforation	May have deep cutaneous ulceration, dissemination to skin and viscera
Sensitivity	Corneal sensitivity is reduced	Skin area may be sensitive

In an unsuspicious herpetic infection of the conjunctiva, which one may simply shrug off as a "conjunctivitis," applying topical steroids may "bring out" a dendrite. Doing so establishes the virus in the corneal nerve and allows it to travel from here to the cell body. The "trigger" mechanisms may then cause the virus to travel down the neuron and set up clinical disease. Once the virus enters the cornea, one may see live virus or antigen in the cells and dead virus particles, all of which may lead to the serious corneal stromal herpetic disease. One must remember that all type 1 is not identical to any other isolate of type 1 herpes. They may behave differently and respond to drugs differently. Apparently their DNA is not identical.

The HLA-B5 antigen appears to be more common in individuals with recurrent corneal herpes infection. This finding suggests a relationship between recurrences of herpes simplex and a genetically linked immunoreactivity.[98]

Recurrent eyelid herpes may appear as isolated vesicles or a group of vesicles and may be designated as *pseudozoster* (extensive cutaneous involvement in distribution of fifth cranial nerve on one side); one must think of herpes simplex in any "recurrent zoster." Erosive and ulcerative blepharitis can occur and should be considered in the differential diagnosis of this condition.[14]

Recurrent conjunctival herpes is exceedingly rare; however, one may see conjunctival dendrites and papillary, follicular, and ulcerative conjunctivitis. For practical purposes, conjunctival herpes occurs only with primary infections. Nevertheless, the clinical features of acute herpetic conjunctivitis—moderate to severe papillary and follicular reactions with epithelial and subepithelial corneal lesions—are, in the absence of typical corneal lesions of herpesvirus, closely similar to adenovirus infections, including types 8 and 9 keratoconjunctivitis. It is therefore important in cases of acute follicular conjunctivitis to consider herpes simplex as a possible cause of the disease. This is important if corticosteroids are considered to be administered.[10]

The best evidence suggests that the trigeminal ganglion is probably one source of the latent virus in human ocular disease. It has been shown that stereotaxic stimulation of the trigeminal ganglion of experimentally infected animals is a means of precipitating peripheral ocular shedding of HSV on command into the tears; in chronically infected animals this stimulation results in positive cultures within 2 days. Interruption of the ganglion before HSV infection reduces the incidence of recurrence of HSV.[60] Newer theories invoke prostaglandins in the mediation of recurrent herpes simplex.[24] The virus can be isolated from 75% of untreated patients with active dendritic keratitis[9]; tear film cultures are periodically positive, regardless of whether clinical disease is evident.

Trigger mechanisms must be considered in recurrent herpes so that they may be avoided or coped with more adequately. Recurrences are associated with febrile illnesses, overwork, psychologic disturbances, cold blowing wind, menstruation, or minor trauma. In addition, ocular recurrences may be seen when acute fever blisters appear on the lips and eyelids. These trigger mechanisms may be compatible with the theory that latent virus resides in the trigeminal ganglion.[1] Antibody is of no help in the prevention of recurrences.

Superficial punctate keratitis and stellate keratitis are variations of the epithelial infection that begin as fine punctate lesions that increase in size and later form white

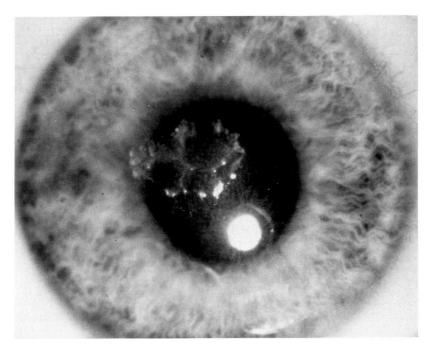

Fig. 8-4. Typical dendritic keratitis of herpes simplex.

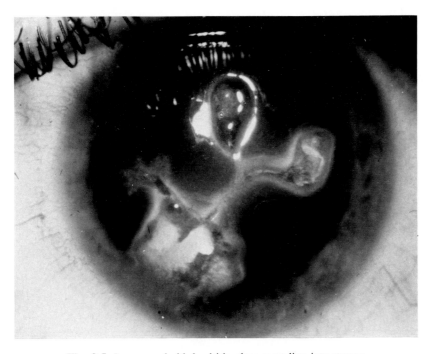

Fig. 8-5. Large ameboid dendritic ulcer spreading into stroma.

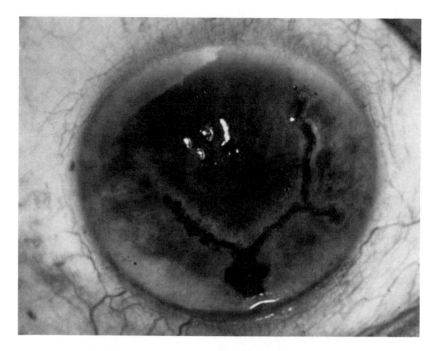

Fig. 8-6. Dendritic ulcer staining with rose bengal red.

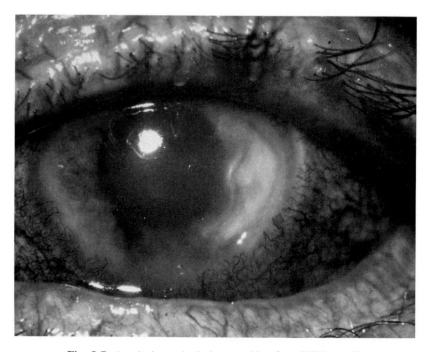

Fig. 8-7. Atypical marginal ulcer resulting from HSV type II.

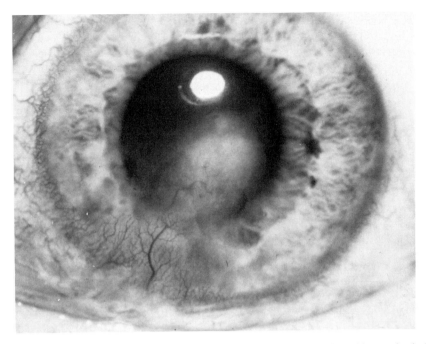

Fig. 8-8. Fascicular type of ulcer caused by herpes simplex and resembling phlyctenular lesion.

plaques of opaque epithelial cells 1 to 2 mm in diameter.[31] There can be a tendency toward palisading of epithelial cells at the periphery of each plaque. These plaques enlarge and develop into an easily recognized dendrite. The dendritic keratitis (Fig. 8-4) may occur at any location or at the site of the original (primary) lesion, even though the cornea completely heals before the recurrence.[33,36] After one attack of dendritic keratitis, the recurrence rate may be as high as 43% in 2 years.[7] The recurrent lesions may heal after 2 to 3 weeks, or they may progress. The dendrites can develop into geographic and ameboid ulcers and, spreading to the stroma, can occur in about 29% of these cases[13] (Fig. 8-5). Recovering the virus from a geographic ulcer may be more difficult, particularly if there is little epithelial lesion. Decreased corneal sensation and the presence of keratitic precipitates behind the lesion instead of on the lower part of the cornea as in iritis aid in the diagnosis of herpes. Clinically, the infected cells can be outlined with fluorescein, and the dead or desquamated cells can simultaneously be demonstrated by counterstaining with methylene blue or rose bengal (Fig. 8-6). A nondendritic marginal lesion caused by herpesvirus (Fig. 8-7) that involves the paralimbal region (marginal keratitis)[45] is clinically more resistant to treatment than a central keratitis and is predisposed to chronic trophic ulceration.[70] These lesions may also be prone to lipid deposits and may appear to be somewhat ''different'' in their total picture from the other herpes lesions.

The dendrite resembles the branches of a tree and is the characteristic corneal lesion of herpes simplex infection. The keratitis may occur as a fine epithelial or filamentary epithelial disease.

Bilateral corneal herpetic ulcers have been reported in children with measles. This is related to the lowered immune response during infection with measles.[84]

Fascicular ulcers resembling the fascicular phlyctenule may occur and should always be kept in mind (Fig. 8-8).

A pannus caused by herpetic keratitis is usually fascicular and associated with dendritic scars and decreased corneal sensitivity. One should remember that live virus may remain for a long time. It may be difficult in some cases to distinguish between a recurring erosion or active viral disease in recurring viral keratitis. In these doubtful instances it is advisable to take a viral culture or scraping of the lesion for fluorescent-antibody studies.

It has been postulated clinically that the greater the diminution of corneal sensitivity, the longer the ulcer will take to heal, and the greater will be the tendency for recurrence.[13] The corneal sensitivity should be tested carefully in all instances of epithelial corneal ulceration.

STROMAL HERPES (DISCIFORM KERATITIS)

This is a stromal edema with some cellular infiltration in a circular or oval pattern beneath a dendritic lesion[41] or under intact epithelium. It may appear as early as 5 to 10 days after the onset of a dendrite. Disciform keratitis may occur as a diffuse edematous keratitis (Figs. 8-9 and 8-10) or as an off–visual axis patch of disease. It can heal without complications or progress to an interstitial keratitis or corneal necrosis with deep scarring.[13,35,68] Similar lesions can be seen with herpes zoster ophthalmicus, vaccinia, mumps, varicella, infectious mononucleosis, and corneal trauma.[13] The edema can involve the full thickness of the cornea or may just involve the area beneath the epithelium.[41] Some degree of uveitis is usually concomitant, especially with more severe degrees of corneal involvement; complications of the uveitis, including secondary glaucoma, can occur.[38,48,69] Benign cases run a course of several months and heal with minimal scarring. In complicated cases late corneal thinning, scar formation, and neovascularization may occur.

It has been proposed that the disciform lesion represents an antigen-antibody reaction or a delayed hypersensitivity reaction[7,23] in which the epithelial viral antigen may soak into the stroma, where it could become fixed to react with antibody.[30] Furthermore, there has been substantiating evidence that virus does exist in these disciform lesions.[11,30,53,74] The endothelial cells under the disciform area are edematous and give the appearance of guttae. Virus has been cultured from or located morphologically in these infected corneal cells and from the anterior chamber[69] and iris.[13,95]

POSTINFECTIOUS HERPETIC EROSIONS (TROPHIC ULCERS)

The lesions usually follow viral epithelial and subepithelial disease. The virus cannot be cultured from the lesion. Small round or oval ulcers with sinuous or scalloped borders occur.[13] The corneal epithelium fails to cover the defect because of severe damage to its basement membrane[49] or to an associated neurotrophic element. The edges of the defect consist of piled-up epithelial cells that have failed to cover the ulcer base. The base of this lesion stains with rose bengal red (Fig. 8-11), in contrast to the fluorescein stain of the epithelium as noted in the typical dendritic lesion.

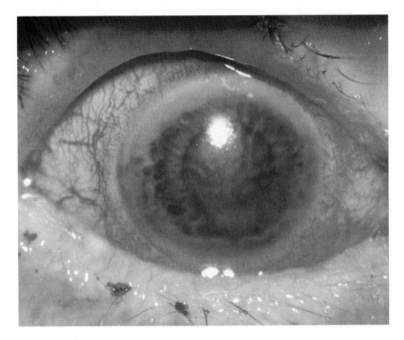

Fig. 8-9. Disciform keratitis.

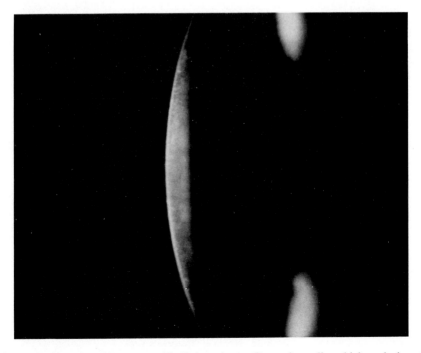

Fig. 8-10. Disciform keratitis as seen with slit-lamp beam. Cornea is swollen, thick, and edematous, as noted in section.

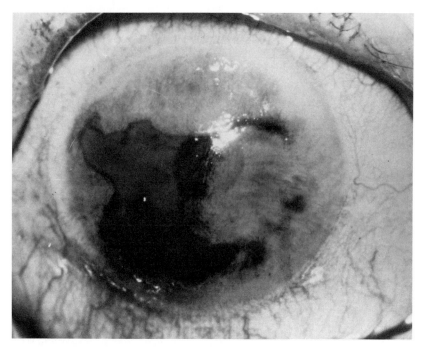

Fig. 8-11. Postinfectious herpes. Large base stains with rose bengal red. Edges are rolled and heaped up.

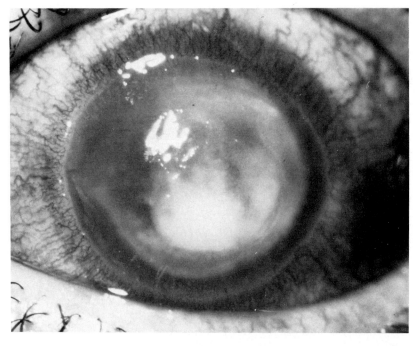

Fig. 8-12. Necrotic stromal herpes.

STROMAL KERATITIS (NECROTIZING HERPES)

These complicated cases of viral keratitis may follow chronic epithelial disease, disciform keratitis, superficial stromal disease, or recurrent disease of any type. Stromal keratitis may appear as a stromal abscess consisting of necrotic cheesy-white infiltrates with or without associated dendritic lesions[70] (Fig. 8-12). These infections may even resemble a bacterial or fungal abscess. In fact, cultures on the appropriate media should be used to rule out secondary bacterial invasion. Similar lesions may occur in the corneal periphery (marginal keratitis).

Necrotizing stromal keratitis is caused by viral invasion of stroma and subsequent humoral immune response (antigen-antibody complement-mediated reaction). A Wessely immune ring can be seen as a subepithelial ring surrounding the area of stromal disease (Fig. 8-13). This ring consists of polymorphonuclear leukocytes brought forth by an interaction of viral antigen—circulating antibody and the fixating of complement.

Keratitis may result from exposure to amoebas. Acanthamoeba keratitis has recently been reported. This may at first be mistaken for herpetic keratouveitis. Infections of this type presumably occur from a direct invasion.[37]

Interstitial (herpetic) keratitis

Also apparent is interstitial herpetic keratitis with dense vessels that represents an antibody-antigen complement-mediated reaction. Visual acuity may be involved if the visual axis is encroached on.

Additional comments

The sclera can become involved in a sclerokeratitis when one sees an interstitial keratitis caused by herpes simplex. There is much pain, and the corneal vascularization and uveitis are difficult to treat.

Other opacities in the superficial stroma are the ghost figures and small punctate granular lesions. The ghost opacities may be seen as areas of mild subepithelial edema and scarring underlying the site of an epithelial dendrite. Peculiar subepithelial flecks that appear greasy or granular are frequently seen after herpetic keratitis; the pathogenesis of these whitish-yellow particles is uncertain.

Severe complications may occur in stromal herpetic keratitis. The stroma may perforate as a result of the disease or because of improper treatment (Fig. 8-14). The cornea is compromised and may become infected with fungi or bacteria. Fig. 8-15 demonstrates a case of *Paecilomyces* organism superinfection of a herpetic stromal keratitis as a result of overzealous treatment with steroid drops. Severe keratitis may occur in atopic individuals (Fig. 8-16).

Herpetic uveitis may be a mild, nonviral iridocyclitis of immune or irritative origin, secondary to keratitis, or a severe iridocyclitis from viral invasion of anterior chamber and uvea. It is often hemorrhagic and may even result in a hypopyon (Fig. 8-17).[95] In addition, the virus may travel to the superior cervical ganglion of the sympathetic chain, in a way similar to that in which it travels to the trigeminal ganglion, and result in the keratouveitis. Chorioretinitis may occur in disseminated infections.

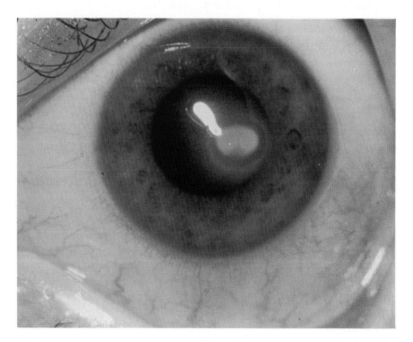

Fig. 8-13. Wessely immune ring of cornea.

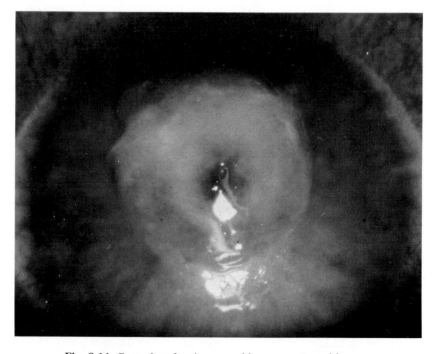

Fig. 8-14. Corneal perforation caused by severe stromal herpes.

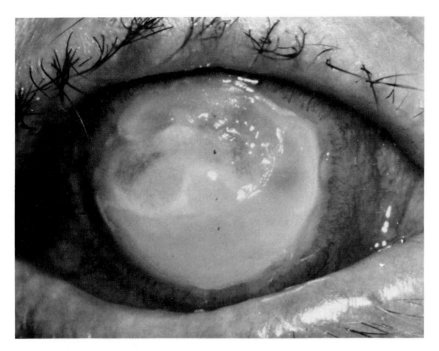

Fig. 8-15. Secondary *Paecilomyces* organism superinfection after prolonged treatment of herpes simplex keratitis with steroid drops.

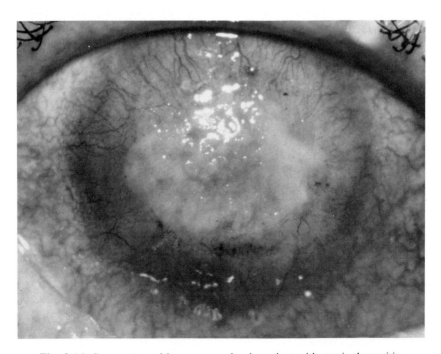

Fig. 8-16. Severe stromal herpes occurring in patient with atopic dermatitis.

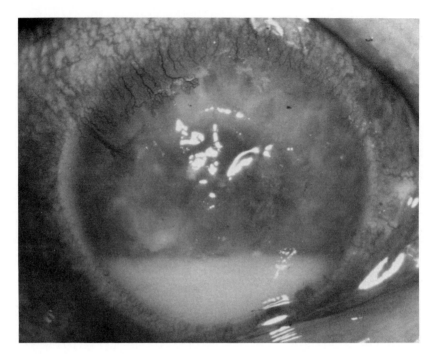

Fig. 8-17. Severe uveal reaction in herpes keratitis and uveitis. Hypopyon resulted from severe inflammatory reaction.

It must be remembered that in some cases the virus will be unresponsive to treatment, and, in spite of everything done, the corneal condition may steadily go downhill. Lysis of the cornea may result from a severe immunologic reaction with many polymorphonuclear cells being brought into the reaction. These will degranulate and release lytic enzymes, resulting in dissolution of collagen and lysis of the cornea.

LABORATORY AIDS

Multinucleated epithelial giant cells containing from 2 to 10 or more nuclei may be seen in the epithelial cell (Fig. 8-18) when scrapings are performed on the dendritic lesion. Although intranuclear eosinophilic inclusion bodies are seen with Giemsa's stains, they are infrequently found. Serum-neutralizing antibody is a test that one may consider. These titer levels are helpful in diagnosing primary types of infection, but they are not diagnostic in recurrent disease because the population already has a high circulating titer.[47] Very little change occurs in the level of circulating antibodies in recurrent infection.[12,47,48] Implantation of the corneal scrapings on rabbit kidney cells, HeLa cells, or chorioallantoic membranes of a developing chick embryo[49] may be done, but identification takes from 2 to 14 days.[40]

One of the most useful tests is the fluorescent-antibody test, which is a relatively simple and rapid test.[34] The results can be reported within 4 or 5 hours to the examining physician.[17,34]

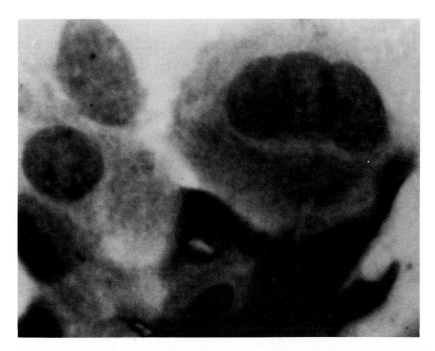

Fig. 8-18. Multinucleated epithelial cells seen in scraping of herpes simplex keratitis.

TREATMENT
Drugs for herpes simplex keratitis

Idoxuridine (IDU). IDU acts by competitively inhibiting the uptake of thymidine into the DNA molecule, thus producing a faulty DNA chain that cannot function in infection-producing viruses. IDU also affects the metabolism of the corneal epithelial cells, which take up the drug as well as the virus.[19,44,82]

IDU can cause a resolution of keratitis within 10 days in about 55% to 70% of the cases.[32,40,42] IDU is prescribed for the superficial, epithelial keratitis of herpes simplex. The treatment of herpetic uveitis and stromal disease is usually not helped by IDU. Some of the poor results in the treatment of deep stromal disease are explained by the instability and poor corneal penetration of the drug.[68] Resistance to IDU may be encountered. It also has been found that, when metabolized, IDU becomes inactive; certainly under these circumstances it is not effective and may even have detrimental effects on the treatment of deep stromal disease.[35] IDU can be toxic in repeated and long topical application and is even more toxic in the "dry eye" patients. In addition, it is topically sensitizing, producing drug-allergy contact dermatitis (Fig. 8-19). IDU may be responsible for narrowing and obliteration of the lacrimal punctum, follicular conjunctivitis[23,27] (Fig. 8-20), cicatricial conjunctivitis, inhibition of keratocyte mitosis, inhibition of corneal stromal repair, and decrease in the strength of healing corneal wounds[77,82] and, in addition, may affect epithelial regeneration.[19] One also can see severe changes in the

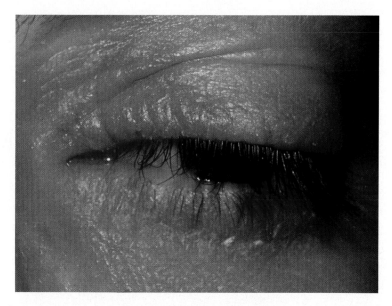

Fig. 8-19. Contact dermatitis caused by prolonged use of IDU in treatment of herpes simplex keratitis. (From Wilson, F.M., II: Surv. Ophthalmol. **24**:57, 1979).

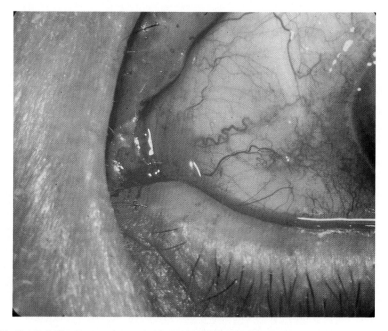

Fig. 8-20. Toxic follicular reaction secondary to IDU. Punctal occlusion is also seen and is part of toxic reaction. (From Wilson, F.M., II: Surv. Ophthalmol. **24**:57, 1979.)

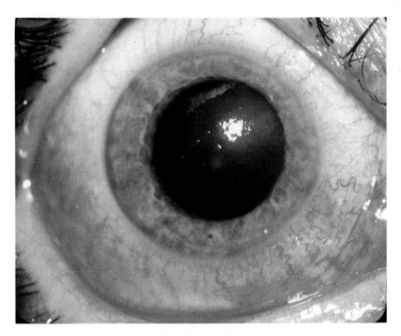

Fig. 8-21. Epithelial keratopathy and injection of inferior conjunctiva as manifestation of toxic reaction to IDU in treatment of herpes simplex keratitis. (From Wilson, F. M., II: Surv. Ophthalmol. **24:**57, 1979.)

cornea such as corneal pannus, punctate keratitis, epithelial opacification and irregularity (Fig. 8-21), subepithelial infiltration, corneal opacities, corneal ulceration, and patient discomfort. Overtreatment with IDU, especially in cases treated week after week for a number of months, destroys the epithelium and leads to stromal disease and even in some cases to lysis of the stroma.

Although IDU is insoluble and unstable and can cause toxicity and allergy on repeated therapy, it remains an effective drug for treatment of herpes simplex. Teratogenic properties of IDU medications have been reported in pregnant rabbits.[27]

Vidarabine (adenine arabinoside, Ara-A). Adenine arabinoside prevents the lengthening of the DNA chain and acts as an inhibitor of DNA polymerase. Ara-A is metabolized to arabinoside hypoxanthine (Ara-Hx), which, although it is more soluble and enters the stroma and aqueous, has only 2% of the antiviral activity of Ara-A or IDU. Ara-A is effective against IDU-resistant virus.[3,66,72,75] It may also be used in treatment of cases of IDU toxicity or IDU-resistant epithelial herpes.[26] Ara-A is as toxic as IDU but is without cross allergenicity to IDU. As the drug is used more often, the toxicity of Ara-A will unfold to a greater degree. Ara-A is equal to or may be slightly better than IDU for epithelial herpes.[67] It is equal to IDU for stromal disease and ineffective topically for herpes uveitis. It is usually equal to IDU for counteracting the adverse effects of steroids.[67] Ara-A is equal to IDU for impairment of stromal healing. It was not found to be teratogenic to rabbits.[18] There is no cross allergenicity with trifluorothymidine.

Adenine arabinoside is a beneficial drug; it is as effective as IDU in treating epithelial disease and can be used as an alternative in IDU failure and IDU toxicity for allergies. It is not immunosuppressive. Adenine arabinoside monophosphate (Ara-AMP) is an experimental drug that is more soluble and more slowly metabolized than Ara-A and may be more effective for stromal disease and keratouveitis.[87]

Since a definite variability exists in the herpesvirus hominis, one should not expect the patient to respond identically to treatment with these drugs. It is also important to keep in mind the fact that patients can and do develop resistance to drugs, so that switching of drugs may be of benefit.

Trifluorothymidine (TFT, F$_3$T). Trifluorothymidine is twice as potent and 10 times more soluble than IDU in a 1% solution.[50,51,77] TFT appears to be effective in treating the dendritic keratitis somewhat faster than IDU[17,91]; it has no cross toxicity to IDU or Ara-A; and it may produce epithelial keratopathy, topical allergy, and punctal narrowing only rarely.[43,92] TFT is effective for IDU-resistant epithelial herpes, and although it remains uncertain, it may be of value for stromal herpes uveitis since therapeutic levels of the drug can be obtained at intraocular sites such as the iris and anterior chamber.[73] It is useful in herpetic ulcers previously treated with topical steroids. TFT has a tendency to decrease central wound healing.

TFT seems to be more effective than IDU and Ara-A in treatment of superficial herpes.[32,50,71,91] Since it is more soluble, it may be effective in the treatment of stromal disease; its high activity also contributes to this action. Although toxicity in allergy states is rare, epithelial keratopathy and contact dermatitis can occur. TFT also has a tendency to impair stromal healing somewhat more than does IDU.

TFT also is significantly more effective and safer than IDU in treatment of herpetic ulcerations.[49] However, it must be noted that toxicity with the use of 1% TFT drops alone, especially if administered more than five times daily for more than a few days, can occur. The early signs are appearance of punctate epithelial erosions and epithelial microcysts. If this treatment continues, frank epithelial edema without stromal swelling will be noted. Punctal narrowing, microfilaments, and contact dermatitis can occur. Recent works certainly indicate that TFT is significantly more effective than IDU, not perhaps in the rate of healing but in chances of obtaining a successful healing at all. TFT is superior to IDU in the presence of concomitant corticosteroids.[51] Studies on wound healing have indicated similar but mild epithelial toxicity with either IDU or TFT. However, TFT is significantly less toxic to stromal wounding and healing, and suggestions of higher overall toxicity of IDU make TFT preferable.[51]

Steroids. Steroids may judicially be employed in treating certain types of herpetic involvement of the cornea. In stromal herpes, steroids will exhibit an anti-inflammatory effect and thus can affect the antigen-antibody complement reaction. They have a vasoconstrictor effect and may interfere with the afferent and efferent immune arcs. Steroids will slow neovascularization, which can be a threatening problem to the stroma and sight. It is well understood that steroids are of potential danger in cellular and humoral deficiency states and that they slow epithelial and stromal healing by interfering with collagen synthesis.

Steroids should be avoided in dendritic and geographic epithelial keratitis, in epithelial and stromal erosion, in stromal keratitis out of the visual axis, and in mild disciform keratitis. One may consider steroids in necrotizing and vascularizing central stromal keratitis in patients already receiving them for stromal keratitis or severe iridocyclitis. These steroid drops are to be used in gradually reduced frequency to the lowest level that prevents recurrent inflammation. They are to be used with topical antiviral therapy.[89]

Acyclovir. Acyclovir is an acyclic purine nucleoside analogue with highly potent and specific activity against HSV types 1 and 2. Although in vitro studies have shown acyclovir is a more potent antiherpetic drug than those currently in use, the present study indicates both acyclovir and vidarabine are equally effective in topical treatment of epithelial herpetic keratitis.[96] Significant side effects were not encountered with either drug over the 14-day therapy.

Acyclovir is efficacious in treating superficial herpetic keratitis. Neither topical acyclovir nor topical vidarabine is able to prevent the development of deeper secondary stromal changes in herpetic keratitis.[96] Systemic acyclovir results in a significant reduction in recovery of latent HSV from the trigeminal ganglia in mice following ocular infection.[76]

Rabbit ocular model experiments have shown that topical acyclovir treatment does not prevent the establishment of latent HSV infection.[88] Intravenous acyclovir therapy in rabbits with latent herpes infection reduces recoverable HSV in the central nervous system but does not eradicate existing latent herpetic infection. Further studies of recurrent herpes simplex keratitis, one of the leading causes of corneal blindness, are needed.

Acyclovir is active in vitro against varicella-zoster virus. Preliminary trials with intravenous acyclovir in herpes zoster suggest that the compound reduces the time of development of new lesions and the time for crustation of lesions. Unfortunately, intravenous acyclovir did not reduce the incidence or severity of ophthalmic complications. The drug also did not significantly alter the incidence of postherpetic neuralgia in this group. Acyclovir 3% has no significant detrimental effect on the quality of regenerating epithelium or the reepithelialization of epithelial wounds. In addition, it has no significant effect on the collagen content of stromal wounds.[46] Acyclovir in association with débridement appears to be more effective than using acyclovir alone.[94]

Specific treatment for the various types of herpes simplex infection

Recurrent dendritic keratitis without stromal involvement. Epithelial débridement may be equal or superior to IDU for epithelial herpes. Reepithelialization may take place faster; in addition, a lower incidence of "ghost images" is seen. One must be very careful about the delicacy with which epithelial débridement is performed, since existing stromal keratitis can be made worse. Patching the eye in conjunction with epithelial débridement is perhaps even superior to IDU therapy. Epithelial dendritic or geographic keratitis may also be treated by the use of (1) 0.5% IDU ointments five times a day for a week (this therapy may be more effective than the use of IDU drops every 2 hours); (2) 0.1% IDU drops every 1 or 2 hours for about 3 days, at which time staining of the lesion should disappear; then the dosage is decreased to five times a day for about 7 days[32]; (3) combined mechanical epithelial débridement with IDU ointment five times a day.

If no improvement occurs in 5 to 6 days and the patient is known to be carrying out the proper instructions, débridement of the epithelium and patching may be employed again. Antiviral ointment is instilled in the eye together with cycloplegic agents, and a pressure patch is applied for 24 hours until the patient is reexamined. If the epithelial defect persists, then pressure patching is still advocated. IDU is to be continued in lower doses for 10 days after the defect has healed, since a virus "rebound phenomenon" may occur if the drug is discontinued too early. One should always be on guard for toxic effects of the drug if it is continued for longer than 2 weeks. In a very young child, one may restrain the infant and debride the dendritic lesion. A general anesthetic may be required if the child is older.

Limbitis. Limbitis or limbal ulcers caused by herpes simplex appear to be extremely recalcitrant to treatment. Artificial tears are probably as effective as any therapy.

The lesions at the limbus are not typically dendritic and may be difficult to differentiate from other hypersensitivity reactions at the limbus. Scrapings of the area with the finding of multinucleated giant cells will help make a diagnosis, and in addition, a Papanicolaou stain may reveal eosinophilic intranuclear inclusions.

Disciform keratitis and uveitis. Opinion varies somewhat regarding the treatment of disciform keratitis. Some prefer to treat only with cycloplegia and watchful waiting, especially in off–visual axis cases. Others believe that treatment with steroids, such as 1% prednisolone acetate, as often as every hour for 2 or 3 days[40,68] and then tapering the use of them to a minimally effective dose is the best course to follow in cases in which the lesion is on the visual axis. It may be necessary to use a weak steroid every other day or perhaps every day to prevent a recurrence of the disciform keratitis.[36] Once the uveitis has been treated with steroids, it is difficult to control the recurrent inflammation without again using steroids.[40] One must be certain that steroids are essential to treat the disease, since the patient may become committed to steroids. Cycloplegics are used in all cases; in some instances the rational use of topical antibiotics is recommended to resist infection, since steroids are well known to lower the resistance of the cornea to infections. In addition, the herpes-infected cornea is a compromised area and predisposed to superinfection[40] (Fig. 8-15).

Postinfectious herpetic erosions. Trauma and inflammation from repeated attacks of herpes may result in injury to the basement membrane of the corneal epithelium. This will, in essence, result in the failure of the epithelium to cover the eroded area of the cornea. Virus is not cultured from these lesions. The erosion base stains with rose bengal red. One must be alert for a secondary infection. In addition, recurrent erosions and melting of the cornea may occur. If such a problem arises, soft contact lenses are used to promote reepithelialization, especially in postherpetic erosion problems. If the patient has been receiving a massive amount of antiviral drops, it is necessary to stop the antivirals and other medications such as gentamicin. These, it should be remembered, are toxic to the epithelium and the stroma. If the surrounding epithelium is hypertrophic, the loose and hypertrophic epithelium should be removed. Lubricating agents, including ointments, at night and patching are also in order; when the problems are moderately controlled, a bandage lens will aid in reepithelialization.

If severe and persistent corneal ulceration erosion occurs with no signs of healing in spite of the ointment or soft lens, one will have to take into consideration the possibility of performing a conjunctival flap[13] or a tarsorrhaphy. Collagenase inhibitors should be used if melting occurs; hypertonic saline drops may be employed if edema of the stroma is present under the erosion areas.

Recurrent epithelial disease with stromal involvement and iritis. One should investigate for a secondary infection by taking the appropriate cultures and scrapings. If there is a substantial amount of superficial necrotic tissue, it should be carefully debrided. Antivirals, cycloplegics, and soft lens application are employed if epithelial defects of any degree are present. Collagenase inhibitors such as L-cysteine or 10% acetylcysteine (Mucomyst) may be employed if stromal melting has occurred. They may be used as drops four to six times a day, but some question their effectiveness. The basic aim of therapy is to heal the epithelial defect. Once the epithelium has healed, the deep stromal disease vascularization and anterior chamber inflammation can be treated with judicious use of corticosteroids three times a day.[13,40,68] As improvement occurs, the steroids will have to be tapered, and only one drop a week may be necessary to keep the severe inflammation controlled.

It is necessary to weigh the secondary complications from a severe uveitis against the possibility of epithelial recurrence, stromal necrosis, perforation (Fig. 8-14), and bacterial and fungal infection (Fig. 8-15), all of which may occur with use of steroids. It follows, therefore, that if there is a minimal iritis with no hypopyon and no sign of endothelial decompensation, it is best to use a strong cycloplegic agent and antivirals without steroids.[40,68] If a severe iritis with corneal hypopyon ulceration has occurred, one may use systemic steroids; as the ulcer epithelializes and stromal inflammation and uveitis improve, the systemic steroids should be stopped and topical steroids started, gradually tapering their application. Topical antivirals are given when topical steroids are being used because the use of topical steroids may increase the penetration of the virus through the stroma.[68] Therefore an "umbrella" of IDU, Ara-A, or TFT is essential.

For a severe type of uveitis, Ara-A has been suggested to treat the herpetic kerato-uveitis by intravenous therapy in humans[75]; however, this is not advised.

If secondary glaucoma is a problem, it must be treated.

In chronic stromal herpes, if a descemetocele or perforation (Fig. 8-14) has occurred, a penetrating keratoplasty[65] may be necessary; recurrence of viral disease in a graft is not uncommon.*

Success following penetrating keratoplasty is greater if the operation is performed when the disease is inactive rather than when the disease is active.[15,16] Recurrence of herpetic disease in the graft can occur[78] in a high percentage of cases; in addition, there is a greater tendency for graft rejection and epithelial erosions. The success rate for regrafts is about half that for the primary graft. The failure rates are always high if a transplant is performed on an inflamed eye.[43] If the disease has been inactive for 6

---

*References 41, 43, 78, 81, 83.

months, there is a much better chance for a clear graft. Topical steroids are used in the postoperative management of eyes that have received corneal transplantation for viral scarring.[43] This is given regardless of whether topical steroids stimulate the recurrence of the disease. Topical IDU and Ara-A, even though they are known to be toxic to the epithelium, are used concurrently with the steroids in postoperative management.

Aggravation of a herpetic infection may occur in certain physical states and conditions: advanced age, pregnancy, alcoholism, malnutrition, malignancy, burns, use of immunosuppressive drugs, and immunodeficiency syndromes and in the newborn. In most of these conditions, the individual is in a compromised status.

From what has been suggested, it appears that herpes simplex hominis infection can lead to many complications, of which decreased visual acuity resulting from corneal scarring and destruction of the globe are but a few. Postinfectious disease with ulceration and poor healing of the epithelium over underlying diseased stroma can result in severe corneal scarring. Neurotrophic problems and loss of sensation can result in compromising states. Stromal necrosis, vascularization, and thinning and perforation of the cornea certainly are all possible complications. Secondary infection is an extremely serious problem in view of the fact that the actual site of the ulcer area and condition in which the herpes is seen is a compromised one. Endothelial decompensation in some instances is seen with resulting persistent corneal edema. Uveitis, glaucoma, and cataract formation are also problems that may occur.

Overtreatment of a simple epithelial keratitis may result in a severe problem caused by toxic effects of the medication. This appears to be a great fault of modern therapeutic attempts.

Dissemination of the herpes simplex infection can occur in patients with atopic eczema with the development of Kaposi's varicelliform eruption.[12]

Fingerprint striae of the cornea can be seen after herpes simplex[4] as well as in herpes zoster, trauma, and bullous keratopathy.

Cytologic study of herpetic keratitis and preparation of corneal scrapings are important. Intranuclear inclusions can be demonstrated by fixing the scrapings with Bouin's solution for an hour, storing them in 70% ethanol, and staining them with Papanicolaou's technique. Giemsa's staining may obscure nuclear details but remains an excellent technique for demonstrating cytoplasmic inclusions, giant cells, inflammatory cells, and microorganisms.[80]

Herpes zoster
VARICELLA-ZOSTER VIRUS[137]

The varicella-zoster (V-Z) virus is physically similar to the other herpesviruses. The major herpesviruses that infect humans are herpesvirus hominis, V-Z virus, and cytomegalovirus (inclusion or salivary gland virus of humans). Another virus, the B virus, causes a herpes simplex–like picture in monkeys and rarely infects humans; however, when it does, the outcome is usually fatal. The herpesviruses are DNA viruses and replicate in the cell nucleus.

The identity of the agents in these diseases was suggested in 1888 when it was noted that children developed varicella after contact with zoster patients.

The virus causing varicella (chickenpox) is believed to be identical to the virus causing herpes zoster[143] (Table 8-1). The varicella-zoster virus causes in the nonimmune host an acute exanthem, chickenpox. Varicella is a mild but highly contagious disease of childhood, characterized by successive crops of vesicular eruptions on the skin and mucous membranes. The peak incidence is from 2 to 6 years of age, and transmission is believed to be by respiratory droplets. The incubation period is 14 to 17 days.

In the partially immune host (usually an adult) the V-Z virus causes the herpes zoster syndrome. Immunologic evidence exists for this hypothesis, since antibodies in varicella are only present in convalescent serum, whereas in zoster there may be high antibody titers in the acute phase and even higher levels in the convalescent serum.

Immunity to exogenous reinfection with V-Z virus is long lasting. However, the neutralizing antibody produced does not protect against reactivation of latent virus. There is some evidence to indicate that varicella convalescent antibody may differ qualitatively from zoster antibody. Two subclasses of IgG have been separated from sera of patients with V-Z virus infection: slow IgG (varicella) and fast IgG. These differ in their neutralizing activity, which in varicella has been demonstrated to be slow IgG and in zoster, fast IgG. Thus the slow IgG fraction after varicella may not prevent subsequent development of zoster. A second exposure to V-Z virus in the form of zoster results in high levels of neutralizing antibody; thus few second attacks of zoster occur.

Isolates from cases of varicella and zoster are serologically indistinguishable. It seems that human and nonhuman primates are the only natural hosts of V-Z virus. The virus does not grow in embryonated eggs and can be carried in human or monkey cell cultures. Cytopathogenic effects are focal and slow to develop. Extension of individual lesions occurs by direct passage of virus by contiguous cells. Multinucleated giant cells form, and acidophilic inclusions are observed in the nucleus and occasionally in the cytoplasm of stained cells.

The V-Z virus may share minor antigenic determinants with HSV. Virus properties of the two are listed in Table 8-1.

The clinical picture of zoster occurs after activation of latent herpes zoster that has persisted after primary infection manifested as chickenpox. Herpes zoster clinical disease is caused by a viral inflammation of a dorsal root ganglion or a comparable cranial nerve ganglion. When the disease involves the first division of the fifth nerve, it is known as herpes zoster ophthalmicus and is of special importance because of the danger to the eye.

The differentiation of zoster from varicella is difficult before the appearance of unilaterally distributed lesions. If the eruption is atypical, it is indistinguishable from recurrent herpes simplex, which may occasionally also follow radicular lines. However, since secondary attacks of zoster are rare, most reported cases of recurrent zoster are probably herpes simplex infection.

In contrast to varicella, zoster is a sporadic disease and occurs more frequently in adults than in children. If a zoster patient transmits the virus to a susceptible child, the child develops varicella and may initiate an epidemic. The increased use of immunosuppressive drugs has increased the incidence of zoster, especially in life-threatening disseminated forms of the disease.

An increase in the incidence in severity of varicella-zoster infection is common in patients with Hodgkin's disease.[115] Zoster infections appear most frequently at a time when cellular immune response is maximally depressed, as indicated by the presence of cutaneous anergy or abnormalities in lymphocyte transformation in vitro. However, viral dissemination can occur if impairment of mechanisms such as a reduced level of interferon in vesicle fluid is present and if a failure to produce humoral varicella specific complement-fixing antibody occurs.[141] An increase in the incidence and severity of varicella-zoster, herpes simplex, and cytomegalovirus infections has been observed in patients with lymphomas. In chronic lymphocytic leukemia varicella-zoster infection may be severe.[104]

In extreme old age, cell-mediated and humoral antibody production is depressed. The incidence of V-Z infection is five times greater in individuals over 80 years of age than in adults between 20 and 40. Severe malnutrition, burns, eczema, and atopic dermatitis affect immune responses; patients who thus exhibit these compromising conditions are prone to zoster infection.

The pathologic changes are those that may give a clue to the pathogenesis of zoster. Zoster may be the result of reactivation of latent virus in the dorsal root ganglion. Lesions with typical intranuclear inclusions are found in the dorsal root ganglion of the sensory nerve supplying the affected area of skin. Pain may be caused by degeneration of small cutaneous nerve bundles and scarring of the segmental nerve and ganglion.

Virus is abundant in the vesicle fluid and occasionally may also be recovered from the spinal fluid. Varicella zoster is detected in trigeminal nerves and ganglia by immunofluorescence and electron-microscopic studies.

The pathogenesis of herpes zoster seems to be caused by a reactivation of the latent varicella-zoster virus in the posterior sensory root ganglion from a previous attack of varicella. After reactivation, the virus spreads peripherally from the dorsal root ganglion or extramedullary cranial nerve ganglion along the sensory nerve to the skin; hence pain may occur before the appearance of meningitis, myelitis, and encephalitis.[112] The skin eruption is limited to the dermatomes corresponding to the involved sensory ganglion.

CLINICAL PICTURE

The average age of the onset of herpes zoster is about 44 years. The disease may occur at any age but is more commonly seen among elderly patients. The greatest incidence occurs in the age groups of under 14 and over 40 years. There are numerous reports of herpes zoster ophthalmicus occurring in children as early as 18 months.[123] A 7-year-old boy who had had chickenpox at 2½ years old had absent IgA and deficiency of delayed hypersensitivity.[123]

The cutaneous lesions of zoster are histopathologically identical to varicella. Virus replicates in the strata germinativum and spinosum. The inflammatory reaction in the stratum corneum can be so severe as to be followed by scarring. This is rarely seen in varicella or herpes simplex infection.

The gasserian ganglion in its first division is often involved, although skin areas innervated by thoracic ganglia and cervical ganglia are on occasion involved, also.

Following are important facts concerning clinical zoster:

1. The first division of the fifth cranial nerve is affected 20 times more than the second and third divisions.

2. Second attacks of zoster are rare but can occur; frequent recurrences of zoster should raise the suspicion of malignancy.
3. The inflammatory reactions may involve the posterior and the anterior horns of the spinal cord; motor zoster occurs when the anterior horns are involved.
4. Diaphragmatic paralysis has been reported, as well as isolated facial nerve palsy with auricular eruption. The chorda tympani may be involved, and thus taste is affected.
5. Horner's syndrome with geniculate zoster can be seen occurring in association with trigeminal herpes in which the ophthalmic division is spared.[120]

SYMPTOMS AND SIGNS

The first symptom of herpes zoster is pain, which is accompanied by hyperesthesia of the skin within the distribution of one or more dermatomes. At the onset, a slight elevation of temperature might occur with some evidence of meningeal irritation. Sometimes simultaneously with the pain, but usually 3 to 4 days later, a blushing of the skin occurs, followed by the appearance of papules that quickly become vesicles. After a few days the clear fluid within the vesicles becomes turbid and yellow. In a short time, these burst, and crusts form. If secondary infection does not develop, the crusts disappear rapidly, leaving white scars in the area. The entire cycle usually takes 3 to 6 weeks. The most distressing symptom is the pain; occasionally it is mild, with a feeling of tingling and numbness, but usually the pain is throbbing and burning. The pain generally subsides with the eruption, but it may persist for years. The affected area is usually left with

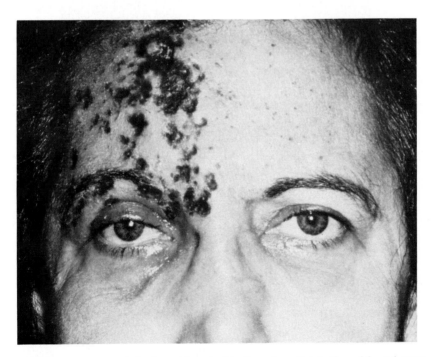

Fig. 8-22. Herpes zoster infection with typical lesions along distribution of frontal nerve.

decreased sensation and perhaps a slight feeling of numbness and tightness. Rarely the typical vesicles are absent.

The virus infection is invariably more severe and prolonged in older patients. Postherpetic neuralgia, absent in patients under 20 years, is frequent in patients over 50 years.

In herpes zoster ophthalmicus the frontal nerve is involved most often (Fig. 8-22), especially its medial branches (supratrochlear and supraorbital). The lacrimal and naso-ciliary branches are frequently not involved. The pain, scarring, and rash are usually more severe over the area of the skin supplied by the branches affected first. Hutchinson's rule that involvement of the eye is frequent if the side of the tip of the nose is involved is essentially true, but exceptions exist[139] (Fig. 8-23). Rarely does zoster pass the midline. Occasionally involvement of the ophthalmic and maxillary nerves may occur. Involvement of the maxillary and mandibular (second and third) divisions of the trigeminal nerve with sparing of the ophthalmic (first) division has rarely been reported.[120] The disease is rarely bilateral.[111]

Dissemination of the rash occurs most frequently in debilitated patients suffering

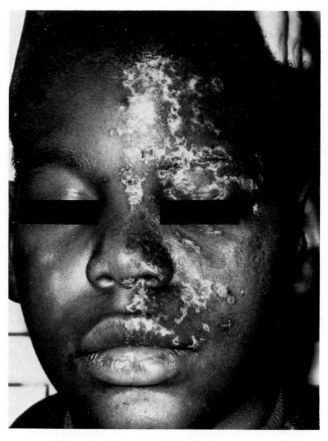

Fig. 8-23. Herpes zoster infection with hemifacial involvement and involvement of nasociliary nerve.

from other diseases.[133] Generalized encephalitis and pneumonia (primary varicella pneumonia) are two of the more serious complications that may prove fatal in debilitated patients.

OCULAR COMPLICATIONS

Ocular complications occur in about 50% of cases of ophthalmic zoster, appearing at any time during the eruptive phase or weeks to months after the rash has subsided.[110]

Upper lid

The upper lid generally participates because of the involvement of the frontal nerve branches. Marked edema of the upper lids with vesicle formation usually occurs. Lesions on the lid skin most often disappear with little or no scarring. Early in the disease ptosis is often present possibly because of mechanical edema or paresis of the sympathetic fibers to the levator muscle. Ptosis may also accompany third cranial nerve palsy. If marked scarring occurs, entropion or ectropion of the upper lid may occur. Canaliculitis has been seen in a patient with keratitis.[105] Necrosis of the lid and forehead can be seen, particularly in patients with malignant reticuloses.[115] Necrotizing zoster should alert the physician to the possibility of underlying malignancy.[104]

Conjunctiva

The conjunctiva is injected, edematous, and may exhibit petechial hemorrhages (Fig. 8-24). A follicular conjunctivitis with regional adenopathy may occur. Occasionally

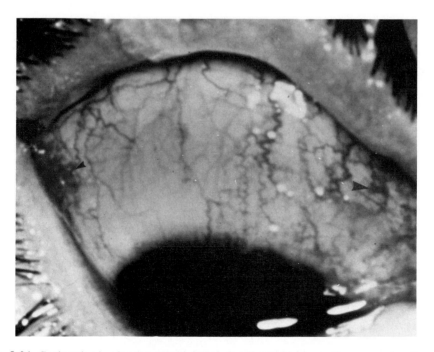

Fig. 8-24. Conjunctiva is edematous and injected. Small petechial hemorrhages occasionally may be seen in ophthalmic herpes zoster *(arrows)*.

vesicular lesions occur on the palpebral or bulbar conjunctiva and can cause scarring. Ulcers of the lids may also occur, possibly as a result of ischemic vasculitis.[124]

Cornea

Corneal complications may occur in 40% of zoster cases.[111]

Dendriform figures have been described by many authors.* Dendritic keratitis in herpes zoster ophthalmicus with confirmed reported isolations of herpes zoster virus from corneal tissue is now realized. Antibody titers also have demonstrated the zoster etiologic factors. The dendriform figures (Fig. 8-25) stain with fluorescein and are not excavated but are made up of swollen, heaped-up cells (Table 8-3). The often delicate pattern of herpes simplex dendrites is contrasted with the more coarse, ropy appearance of the zoster dendrite.[135] The terminal bulbs seen in simplex dendrites are not present in zoster dendrites. The dendrites of zoster stain with fluorescein irregularly and appear more linear with a gray, plaquelike appearance.

Punctate staining may occur and progress to small corneal infiltrates in the level of Bowman's layer. Superficial stromal opacities are also seen in the cornea.[126] These subepithelial opacities are nummular or coin shaped and may occur at any level of the cornea. They may be round and irregular and measure several millimeters. They usually occur 10 days after the onset of the rash and rarely may relapse as late as 2 years after the onset of the disease. Disciform keratitis and interstitial keratitis also occur.

---

*References 100, 101, 128, 135, 142.

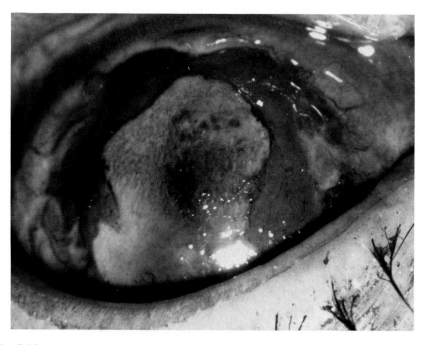

Fig. 8-25. Large gross dendritic figure stained with fluorescein (herpes zoster ophthalmicus).

Table 8-3. Differential points of dendritic lesions

Properties	Herpes zoster dendrite	Herpes simplex dendrite
Appearance	Medusoid "Painted-on" appearance Like plaque heaped on cornea Coarse, swollen epithelial cells reaching in different directions, either from a central focal point or in an elongated branching figure	Delicate, fine, lacy Denuded ulcer
Terminal bulbs	None	May or may not be seen
Staining	Stains poorly with fluorescein	Edges stain with rose bengal red dye; ulcer base stains well with fluorescein, which diffuses into surrounding diseased epithelium
Response to steroid drops	Good	Made worse
Dermatologic findings and distribution	Group vesicles with erythematous base; may occur in crops	Group vesicles with erythematous base; may occur in crops May be very similar to zoster; therefore what appears to be typical shingles caused by herpes zoster may be caused by simplex virus; dendrite on cornea may also be caused by herpes simplex
	Always in dermatomal distribution	May be in dermatomal distribution but usually is not
Healing	Heals usually in 2 to 3 weeks and lasts 5 to 6 weeks	May heal in 7 to 10 days, but may persist for 3 weeks
Symptoms	Prodrome of pain and tingling paresthesias or pruritis in two thirds of cases	May have pain and paresthesias
Age incidence	Peak: over 60 years; may occur in children also	1 to 15 years and 35 to 50 years
Inflammation	Less in histologic examination	More in skin lesions in pathologic examination
Recurrence	Rare; never in same distribution	Common

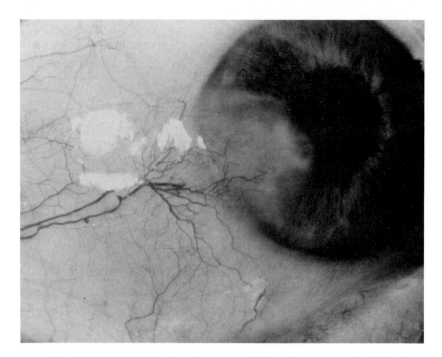

Fig. 8-26. Residual scarring that may result from herpes zoster keratitis.

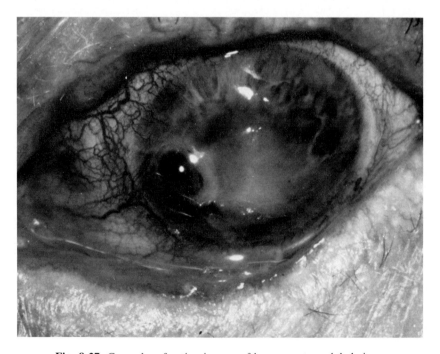

Fig. 8-27. Corneal perforation in case of herpes zoster ophthalmicus.

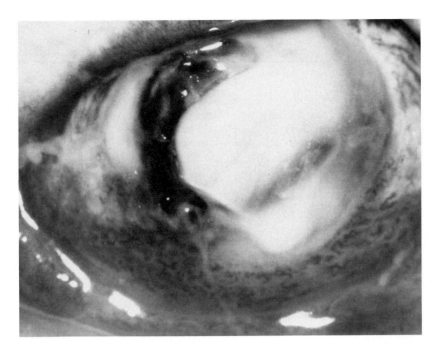

Fig. 8-28. Secondary infection by *Staphylococcus aureus* in compromised state of herpes zoster keratitis.

In addition to the listed causes of peripheral corneal ulcers, one has to consider herpes zoster as an etiologic factor. Replicating virus, vasculitis, or neurogenic disturbances may be factors in the development of the peripheral ulcers.[130]

Decreased corneal sensation usually occurs and may become permanent. In severe cases of decreased sensation a corneal picture similar to neurotrophic keratitis may occur. Corneal vascularization, edema, and scarring are not infrequent findings (Fig. 8-26). When the vascularization is substantial, secondary lipid keratopathy may develop. Perforation (Fig. 8-27) and granulomatous reaction of Descemet's membrane are rarer findings.[131] Secondary infection by *Staphylococcus aureus* can be seen in this compromised cornea (Fig. 8-28). Scleritis and scleromalacia are also complications of ophthalmic zoster.[109, 134] Scleritis may be seen immediately after the skin lesions have waned or a month or two later. The pain is relieved by cycloplegics. Steroids are not helpful.

Single or multiple patches of sectorial iris pigment epithelial loss and atrophy are seen.[127] Iris angiographic features reveal no vascular filling in the areas of atrophy. This supports the evidence that both nerves and arteries are involved in herpes zoster ophthalmicus and that many of the ocular findings may result from ischemia. In the extreme case, anterior-segment ischemia and necrosis may develop.[108]

A uveitis usually occurs when the cornea is involved. This is perhaps a mild and transient uveitis; however, in a considerable number of cases a severe anterior irido-

Table 8-4. Ophthalmic involvement in herpes zoster

External	Internal	External	Internal
Lid	Uvea	Cornea—cont'd	Nerve
Edema	Iritis	Subepithelial opacities	Intraneural lym-
Necrotic lesions	Sectorial atrophy	Nummular-like lesions	photic infiltration
Vesicles	Sectorial necrosis	Interstitial keratitis	of long posterior
Scar	of iris	Disciform keratitis	ciliary nerve
Entropion	Necrosis of	Decreased sensation	Optic atrophy
Ectroption	anterior ciliary	Neuroparalytic keratitis	Retrobulbar neuritis
Ptosis	body	Corneal ulcer	Optic neuritis
Canaliculitis	Iridocyclitis,	Vascularization	Chamber angle
Conjunctiva	exudative	Scarring	Trabeculitis
Edema	Choroiditis	Edema	glaucoma
Petechiae	Lens	Secondary lipid kera-	Pupil
Follicular reaction	Cataract	topathy	Horner's syn-
Edema	Vitreous	Sclera	drome
Vesicles	Cells may be	Scleritis	Adie's syndrome
Keratotic ulcer	present	Sclerokeratitis	
Scar	Retina	Scleromalacia	
Cornea	Vasculitis	Extraocular muscles	
Dendriform figures	Perivasculitis	Paralysis	
Plaquelike lesions	Bullous detach-		
Punctate lesions	ment		
	Thrombophlebitis		

cyclitis may develop, which tends to recur. Secondary glaucoma is a common complication resulting from trabeculitis. Focal areas of choroiditis may occur. Highly exudative types of iridocyclitis may occur and result in posterior synechiae, hypopyon, or hyphema.

Retina

Herpes zoster rarely affects the retina, but bilateral hemorrhagic retinopathy,[103] retinal arteritis,[106] retinal thrombophlebitis,[119] and bullous detachments are seen.[125]

Optic neuritis may appear as a retrobulbar neuritis with central scotoma and the appearance later of a pale disc[101,116,133] or as optic neuritis and neuroretinitis with swelling and blurring of the disc and retinal hemorrhages and exudates.[103] Pupillary, extraocular muscle paresis[114]; hemiplegias[99,113]; and Guillain-Barré[140] complications may occur.

Table 8-4 lists the external and internal ophthalmic involvement caused by herpes zoster virus.

LABORATORY DIAGNOSIS

Herpes zoster can usually be diagnosed readily on clinical grounds; however, laboratory confirmation can be made. Scrapings from vesicular fluid examined with Giemsa's stain show multinucleated giant epithelial cells and cells with intranuclear eosinophilic inclusion bodies. Cultures from cutaneous lesions can be inoculated in human embryonic kidney or human fibroblasts. The cultures become positive in 8 to 12 days in human embryonic kidney and as early as the fourth day when grown in human fibroblasts. The virus is recoverable only in the early cutaneous lesion, usually the first 72 hours. Cultures from corneal involvement have been grown in tissue culture.[132] The positive cultures were all taken within 48 hours of the zoster prodromata and did not become positive for an additional 10 to 16 days after the cutaneous cultures became positive.[132]

The antigen–varicella-zoster virus grown in tissue culture is used to detect complement–fixing antibody titers. Studies have also shown a usual rise of IgM followed by a rise of IgG in primary infections. In secondary infections only IgG rises as a rule; however, if preexisting antibody is low, a primary response with an increase of IgM followed by an increase of IgG may occur.[143]

Fluorescent-antibody stain is an effective adjunct in diagnosis.[117] High vesicle interferon titers are followed within 48 hours by cessation of dissemination.[132]

TREATMENT

The most commonly used therapy today in herpes zoster is topical and systemic corticosteroids. Lower incidences of postherpetic neuralgia and faster relief of pain in the acute phase are claimed[138] when systemic steroids are administered, but possible dissemination of the disease is the argument used against steroid treatment.[129] However, in some of these instances the patients may have serious underlying diseases.

Treatment with cytarabine and adenine arabinoside has been reported with reasonable results.[121,136] When used topically, the steroids may help the zoster dendrite,[102] but one must be absolutely sure of the diagnosis, since such treatment could be disastrous if the dendrite in truth were caused by herpes simplex virus. Passive immunization with zoster immune globulin has been found to be of some benefit in preventing the disease.[107]

Herpes zoster pain can be a serious problem to those afflicted. Administration of levodopa has been suggested for relief of pain of herpes zoster. Intensity of pain may be significantly reduced with 100 mg of levodopa three times a day for 10 days. Postherpetic neuralgia is also less frequent.[122]

Other virus infections

Virus infection of the external eye in mumps, varicella, rubeola, rubella, variola, and vaccinia occurs and should be recognized. The diseases are listed in Table 8-5 with differential diagnostic points and characteristics of each entity.

The characteristics of the virus inclusions in the preceding diseases and in the chlamydial diseases are listed in Table 8-6.

In addition, Table 8-7 summarizes the anterior segment ophthalmic changes and other virus-caused involvements of the eye.

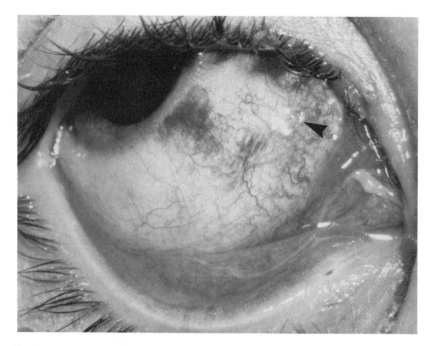

Fig. 8-29. Varicella vesicle of conjunctiva *(arrow)*. Also note conjunctival hemorrhage.

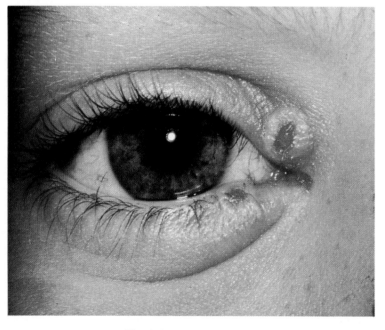

Fig. 8-30. Vaccinia of lid.

Table 8-5. Other viral diseases

Disease	General ophthalmic involvement	Characteristics	Conjunctiva	Cornea
Mumps* (paramyxovirus)	Episcleritis Scleritis[148]: usually bilateral and subsides quickly without vascularization Uveitis Optic neuritis Retinitis Dacryoadenitis Extraocular muscle paresis	Lifelong immunity Parotid and salivary glands affected	Catarrhal Follicular[144] (one case)	Fine epithelial keratitis Avascular interstitial keratitis of rapid onset and rapid resolution Usually unilateral Disciform keratitis may occur 5 to 7 days after onset of parotitis; clears in 1 to 4 weeks
Varicella† (varicella zoster)	Ocular palsies Internal ophthalmoplegia Uveitis (rare) Gangrene of lids Microphthalmia,[151] chorioretinitis, and cataracts in congenital varicella syndrome	Dendritic lesion is gray, intra-epithelial, plaquelike lesion staining only moderately with fluorescein. The figure is composed of sick and dying cells in the middle layer of the epithelium, which give it the gray appearance. The healthy basal cells lead to less rapid and less intense staining of the stroma with fluorescein Microcephaly, deafness, and heart disease in congenital varicella syndrome[151]	Catarrhal Conjunctival vesicles (Fig. 8-29) Conjunctival ulcer Phlyctenular-like lesions at limbus several months later	Corneal or limbal vesicle Fine punctate epithelial keratitis Disciform keratitis may occur late in the disease, even several months after onset Ulcerative keratitis Dendriform keratitis (raised and plaquelike) Interstitial keratitis (rare) Decreased sensation

Continued.

*References 147, 150, 153, 154, 156.
†References 144, 151, 152, 158.

Table 8-5. Other viral diseases—cont'd

Disease	General ophthalmic involvement	Characteristics	Conjunctiva	Cornea
Rubeola (measles) [146, 148]	Chorioretinitis (rare) Central vein occlusion (rare) Optic atrophy (rare) [153] Isolated extraocular muscle palsy (rare) [152]	Orbital pain, photophobia May have severe systemic disease: myocarditis, encephalitis, and pneumonia Malnutrition predisposes these patients to severe ocular complications	Acute catarrhal Swelling of plica Koplik spots‡ on caruncle (subepithelial mononuclear cells with overlying necrosis) and on conjunctival membranes (rare)	Fine, punctate, central epithelial keratitis and at times erosions Interstitial keratitis in severe cases (rare) Corneal ulcers (rare) with secondary bacterial involvement Corneal perforation in malnourished infants [154]
Rubella [145, 155, 157]		Rubella syndrome [158] may show cataracts, glaucoma, purpura, retinopathy, cardiac anomalies, microphthalmia, iris hypoplasia, subretinal neovascularization, [157] and microcornea	Mild catarrhal conjunctivitis	Fine epithelial keratitis [156]
Variola (smallpox)		Serious cause of blindness in India and North Africa	Catarrhal, hemorrhagic, or purulent Pustules	Pustules Disciform keratitis Ulcers Interstitial keratitis Perforation
Vaccinia [149] (Fig. 8-30)	Lid swelling	May respond to vidarabine [155]	Catarrhal or purulent	Fine epithelial keratitis Interstitial keratitis Disciform keratitis

‡Blue-white spots on an irregular bright red base appear with the rash on buccal mucosa, inner lip, and vagina.

Table 8-6. Virus inclusions

Viral disease	Characteristics				Iodine stain
	Cytoplasmic	Nuclear	Eosinophilic	Basophilic	
Herpes simplex	0	+	+	0	
Herpes zoster	0	+	+	0	
Varicella	0	+	+	0	
Variola	+	+	+	0	
Varccinia (Guarnieri's bodies)	+	0	+	0	
Trachoma	+	0	0	+	+
Inclusion conjunctivitis	+	0	0	+	+
Molluscum	+	0	+	0	
Lymphogranuloma venereum	+	0	0	+	0
Psittacosis	+	0	0	+	0

Table 8-7. Ocular DNA and RNA virus disease

Virus	Primary or systemic site	Ocular manifestations
DNA		
Pox virus family		
Variola	Smallpox	Conjunctivitis, keratitis, secondary hypopyon, ulcers, iritis, choroiditis
Vaccinia	Vaccinated area	Blepharoconjunctivitis keratitis, disciform edema
Molluscum contagiosum	Small epithelial tumors	Molluscum contagiosum lid tumors conjunctivitis, keratitis
Herpes virus family		
Herpes simplex	Local or systemic primary infection encephalitis, chronic recurrent infections	Keratitis, uveitis retinitis
Varicella-zoster	Chickenpox, herpes zoster	Conjunctival involvement keratitis, scarring, scleritis, iridocyclitis palsies, optic neuritis
Cytomegalovirus	Cytomegalic inclusion, disease of newborns	Uveitis, retinitis cataract
Epstein-Barr virus	Infectious mononucleosis syndrome	Rare conjunctivitis, uveitis optic neuritis
Adenovirus family		
Types 8 and 19	Upper respiratory infection	EKC, follicular or membranous conjunctivitis, keratitis, corneal opacities
Types 3, 4, 7, and others	Pharyngoconjunctival fever or upper respiratory infection	Follicular conjunctivitis, mild keratitis

From Nesburn, A.N.: Ophthalmology **87:**1204, 1980.   *Continued.*

Table 8-7. Ocular DNA and RNA virus disease—cont'd

Virus	Primary or systemic site	Ocular manifestations
Papova virus family		
Papilloma virus	Warts	Warts of lids, conjunctiva, rarely conjunctivitis, keratitis
RNA		
Paramyxovirus family		
Rubeola	Measles	Conjunctivitis, discharge Koplik's spot, punctate keratopathy, interstitial keratitis, uveitis, optic neuritis
	Slow virus manifestations-SSPE	Maculopathy
Mumps	Mumps	Conjunctivitis, dacryosystitis, keratitis, rarely scleritis, uveitis, optic neuritis, extraocular muscle palsies
Newcastle disease virus	Fowl pathogen	Follicular conjunctivitis, punctate keratopathy
Myxovirus family		
Influenza virus	Flu syndrome	Conjunctivitis
Togavirus family		
Rubella virus	Postnatal rubella	Conjunctivitis, rarely keratitis
	Congenital rubella syndrome	Cataracts, microophthalmos, corneal edema, glaucoma, iris atrophy, retinopathy, optic atrophy
Dengue virus	Dengue virus	Conjunctivitis, keratitis, iritis, retrobulbar pain
Yellow fever virus	Yellow fever	Lid and conjunctival hemorrhage, scleral jaundice
Sandfly fever virus	Sandfly fever	Conjunctival injection
Picornavirus family		
Enterovirus 70	Acute hemorrhage conjunctivitis syndrome, upper respiratory infection	Hemorrhage conjunctivitis, punctate keratopathy
Cattle foot and mouth disease virus	Virus transmitted to man	Conjunctivitis, keratitis

REFERENCES
Herpes simplex

1. Baringer, J.R., and Swoveland, P.: Recovery of herpes simplex virus from human trigeminal ganglions, N. Engl. J. Med. **288:**648, 1973.
2. Boniuk, I.: The cytomegaloviruses and the eye, Int. Ophthalmol. Clin. **12:**169, 1972.
3. Brightbill, F.S., and Kaufman, H.E.: Adenine arabinoside therapy in corneal stromal disease and iritis due to herpes simplex, Ann. Ophthalmol. **6:**25, 1974.
4. Brodrick, J.D., Dark, A.J., and Peace, G.W.: Fingerprint striae of the cornea following herpes simplex keratitis, Ann. Ophthalmol. **8:**481, 1976.
5. Brown, D.C.: Ocular herpes simplex, Invest. Ophthalmol. **10:**210, 1971.
6. Burns, R.P.: A double-blind study of IDU in human herpes simplex keratitis, Arch. Ophthalmol. **70:**381, 1963.
7. Carroll, J.M., Martola, E.L., Laibson, P.R., and Dohlman, C.H.: The recurrence of herpetic keratitis following idoxuridine therapy, Am. J. Ophthalmol. **63:**103, 1967.
8. Change, R., Fiumara, N.J., and Weinstein, L.: Genital herpes, JAMA **229:**544, 1974.
9. Coleman, V.R., Thygeson, P., Dawson, C.R., and Jawetz, E.: Isolation of virus from herpetic keratitis, Arch. Ophthalmol. **81:**22, 1969.
10. Darouger, S., Hunter, P.A., Viswalingam, J.A., et al.: Acute follicular conjunctivitis and and keratoconjunctivitis due to herpes simplex virus in London, Br. J. Ophthalmol. **62:**843, 1978.
11. Dawson, C.R., Togni, B., and Moore, T.E., Jr.: Structural changes in chronic herpetic keratitis, Arch. Ophthalmol. **79:**740, 1968.
12. Douglas, R.G., Jr., and Couch, R.B.: A prospective study of chronic herpes simplex infection and recurrent herpes labialis in humans, J. Immunol. **104:**289, 1970.
13. Duke-Elder, W.S., editor: System of ophthalmology, vol. 8. Diseases of the outer eye, pt. 1. Conjunctiva, London, 1965, Henry Kimpton.
14. Egerer, U., and Stary, A.: Erosive-ulcerative herpes simplex blepharitis, Arch. Ophthalmol. **98:**1760, 1980.
15. Fine, M.: Treatment of herpetic keratitis by corneal transplantation, Am. J. Ophthalmol. **46:**671, 1958.
16. Foster, C.S., and Duncan, J.: Penetrating keratoplasty for herpes simplex keratitis, Am. J. Ophthalmol. **92:**336, 1981.
17. Freyler, H., Hofmann, H., and Schwab, F.: Diagnosis of herpetic keratitis by immunofluorescence, Albrecht von Graefes Arch. Klin. Ophthalmol. **198:**155, 1976.
18. Gasset, A.R., and Akaboshi, T.: Teratogenicity of adenine arabinoside (Ara-A), Invest. Ophthalmol. **15:**556, 1976.
19. Gasset, A.R., and Katzin, D.: Antiviral drugs and corneal wound healing, Invest. Ophthalmol. **14:**628, 1975.
20. Hagler, W.S., Walter, P.V., and Nahmias, A.J.: Ocular involvement in neonatal herpes simplex virus infection, Arch. Ophthalmol. **82:**169, 1969.
21. Hanshaw, J.B.: Herpesvirus hominis infection in the fetus and newborn, Am. J. Dis. Child **126:**546, 1973.
22. Harris, G.J., Hyndiuk, R.A., Fox, M.J., and Taugher, P.J.: Herpetic canalicular obstruction, Arch. Ophthalmol. **99:**282, 1981.
23. Henson, D., Helmsen, R., Becker, K.E., et al.: Ultrastructural localization of herpes simplex virus antigens on rabbit corneal cells using sheep antihuman IgG anti-horse ferritin hybrid antibodies, Invest. Ophthalmol. **13:**819, 1974.
24. Hill, T.J., Blyth, W.A.: An alternative theory of herpes simplex recurrence and a possible role for prostaglandins, Lancet **1:**397, 1976.
25. Hutchison, D.S., Smith, R.E., Haughton, P.B.: Congenital herpetic keratitis, Arch. Ophthalmol. **93:**70, 1975.
26. Hyndiuk, R.A., Hull, D.S., Schultz, R.O., et al.: Adenine arabinoside in idoxuridine unresponsive and intolerant herpetic keratitis, Am. J. Ophthalmol. **79:**655, 1975.
27. Itoi, M., et al.: Teratogenicities of ophthalmic drugs. I. Antiviral ophthalmic drugs, Arch. Ophthalmol. **93:**46, 1975.
28. Jarratt, M., and Hubler, W.R., Jr.: Herpes genitales and aseptic meningitis, Arch. Dermatol. **110:**771, 1974.
29. Johnson, B.L., and Wisotzkey, H.M.: Neuroretinitis associated with herpes simplex encephalitis in an adult, Am. J. Ophthalmol. **83:**481, 1977.
30. Jones, B.R.: The management of ocular herpes, Trans. Ophthalmol. Soc. U.K. **79:**425, 1959.
31. Jones, B.R.: Differential diagnosis of punctate keratitis, Int. Ophthalmol. Clin. **2:**291, 1962.
32. Jones, B.R.: Rational regimen of administration of antivirals, Trans. Am. Acad. Ophthalmol. Otolaryngol. **79:**104, 1975.
33. Juel-Jensen, B.E., and MacCallum, F.O.: Herpes simplex, varicella, and zoster: clinical manifestations and treatment, Philadelphia, 1972, J.B. Lippincott Co.
34. Kaufman, H.E.: The diagnosis of corneal herpes simplex infection by fluorescent antibody staining, Arch. Ophthalmol. **64:**382, 1960.

35. Kaufman, H. E., Konai, A., and Ellison, E. D.: Herpetic iritis: demonstration of virus in the anterior chamber by fluorescent antibody techniques and electronmicroscopy, Am. J. Ophthalmol. **71:**465, 1971.

36. Kaufman, H. E., Nesburn, A. B., and Maloney, E. D.: IDU therapy of herpes simplex, Arch. Ophthalmol. **64:**382, 1960.

37. Key, N. S., Green, R., Willaert, E., et al.: Keratitis due to *Acanthamoeba castellani*, Arch. Ophthalmol. **98:**475, 1981.

38. Kimura, S. J.: Herpes simplex keratitis. In Infectious diseases of the conjunctiva and cornea: Symposium of the New Orleans Academy of Ophthalmology, St. Louis, 1963, The C. V. Mosby Co.

39. Komorous, J. M., Wheeler, C. E., Briggamen, R. A., and Caro, I.: Intrauterine herpes simplex infections, Arch. Dermatol. **113:**918, 1977.

40. Laibson, P. R.: Current therapy of herpes simplex virus infection of the cornea, Int. Ophthalmol. Clin. **13:**39, 1973.

41. Laibson, P. R.: Surgical approaches to the treatment of active keratitis, Int. Ophthalmol. Clin. **13:**65, 1973.

42. Laibson, P. R., Hyndiuk, R., Krachmer, J. H., and Schultz, R. O.: ARA-A and IDU therapy of human superficial herpetic keratitis, Invest. Ophthalmol. **14:**762, 1975.

43. Langston, R. H. S., and Pavan-Langston, D.: Penetrating keratoplasty for herpetic keratitis: decision making and management, Int. Ophthalmol. Clin. **15:**125, 1975.

44. Langston, R. H. S., Pavan-Langston, D., and Dohlman, C. H.: Antiviral medication and corneal wound healing, Arch. Ophthalmol. **92:**490, 1974.

45. Lanier, J. D.: Marginal herpes simplex keratitis (original article), Ophthalmol. Digest, p. 15, March 1976.

46. Lass, J. H., Pavan-Langston, D., and Park, N.: Acyclovir and corneal wound healing, Am. J. Ophthalmol. **88:**102, 1979.

47. Leopold, I. H., and Sery, T. W.: Epidemiology of herpes simplex keratitis, Invest. Ophthalmol. **2:**498, 1963.

48. Locatcher-Khorazo, D., and Seegal, B. C.: Microbiology of the eye, St. Louis, 1972, The C. V. Mosby Co.

49. Lowry, S. F., Melnick, J. L., and Rawls, W. E.: Investigation of plaque formation in chick embryo cells as a biological marker for distinguishing herpes virus type 2 from type 1, J. Gen. Virol. **10:**1, 1971.

50. McGill, J., Fraunfelder, F. T., and Jones, B. R.: Current and proposed management of ocular herpes simplex, Surv. Ophthalmol. **20:**358, 1976.

51. McGill, J., Holt-Wilson, A., McKennon, J., et al.: Some aspects of the clinical use of trifluorothymidine in the treatment of herpetic ulceration of the cornea, Trans. Ophthalmol. Soc. U. K. **94:**342, 1974.

52. Metcalf, J. F., and Kaufman, H. E.: Herpetic stromal keratitis: evidence for cell-mediated immunopathogenesis, Am. J. Ophthalmol. **82:**827, 1976.

53. Meyers, R. L., and Pettit, T. H.: Corneal immune response to herpes simplex virus antigens, J. Immunol. **110:**1575, 1973.

54. Montgomery, J. R., Flanders, R. W., and Yow, M. D.: Congenital anomalies and herpesvirus infection, Am. J. Dis. Child **126:**364, 1973.

55. Nahmias, A. J., Alford, C. A., and Korones, S. B.: Infection of the newborn with herpesvirus hominis, Adv. Pediatr. **17:**185, 1970.

56. Nahmias, A. J., and Hagler, W. S.: Ocular manifestations of herpes simplex in newborn (neonatal ocular herpes), Int. Ophthalmol. Clin. **12:**191, 1972.

57. Nahmias, A. J., Josey, W. E., Naib, Z. M., et al.: Perinatal risk associated with maternal genital herpes simplex virus infection, Am. J. Obstet. Gynecol. **11:**825, 1971.

58. Nahmias, A. J., and Rotzman, B.: Infection with herpes simplex virus 1 and 2, N. Engl. J. Med. **289:**781, 1973.

59. Neumann-Haefelin, D., Sundmacher, R., Wochnick, G., et al.: Herpes simplex virus types I and II in ocular disease, Arch. Ophthalmol. **96:**64, 1978.

60. Newburn, B. A., Dickinson, R., and Radnoti, M.: The effect of trigeminal nerve and ganglion manipulation on recurrence of ocular herpes in rabbits, Invest. Ophthalmol. **15:**726, 1976.

61. North, R. D., Pavan-Langston, D., and Geary, P.: Herpes simplex virus types 1 and 2: therapeutic response to antiviral drugs, Arch. Ophthalmol. **94:**1019, 1976.

62. Oh, J. O., Kimura, S. J., and Ostler, H. B.: Acute ocular infection by type 2 herpes simplex virus in adults, Arch. Ophthalmol. **93:**1127, 1975.

63. Oh, J. O., and Stevens, T. R.: Comparison of types 1 and 2 herpesvirus hominis infection of rabbit eyes, Arch. Ophthalmol. **90:**473, 1973.

64. Oh, J. O., Kimura, S. J., and Ostler, H. B.: Acute ocular infection in type 2 herpes simplex virus in adults. Report of 2 cases, Arch. Ophthalmol. **93:**1127, 1975.

65. Patten, J. T., Cavanagh, H. D., Pavan-Langston, D.: Penetrating keratoplasty in acute herpetic corneal perforations, Ann. Ophthalmol. **8:**287, 1976.

66. Pavan-Langston, D.: New developments in the therapy of ocular herpes simplex, Int. Ophthalmol. Clin. **13:**53, 1973.

67. Pavan-Langston, D.: Clinical evaluation of adenine arabinoside and idoxuridine in the treatment of ocular herpes simplex, Am. J. Ophthalmol. **80:**495, 1975.

68. Pavan-Langston, D.: Diagnosis and management of herpes simplex ocular infection, Int. Ophthalmol. Clin. **15:**19, 1975.

69. Pavan-Langston, D., and Brockhurst, R.J.: Herpes simplex panuveitis, Arch. Ophthalmol. **81:** 783, 1969.

70. Pavan-Langston, D., Dohlman, C.H., Geary, P., and Sulzewski, D.: Intraocular penetration of ARA-A and IDU: therapeutic implications in clinical herpetic uveitis, Trans. Am. Acad. Ophthalmol. Otolaryngol. **77:**455, 1973.

71. Pavan-Langston, D., and Foster, C.S.: Trifluorothymidine and idoxuridine therapy of ocular herpes, Am. J. Ophthalmol. **84:**818, 1977.

72. Pavan-Langston, D., Langston, R.H.S., and Geary, P.A.: Prophylaxis and therapy of experimental ocular herpes simplex. Comparison of idoxuridine adenine arabinoside and hypoxanthine arabinoside, Arch. Ophthalmol. **92:**417, 1974.

73. Pavan-Langston, D., and Nelson, D.J.: Intraocular penetration of trifluridine, Am. J. Ophthalmol. **87:**814, 1979.

74. Pavan-Langston, D., and Nesburn, A.B.: The chronology of primary herpes simplex infection of the eye and adnexal glands, Arch. Ophthalmol. **80:**258, 1969.

75. Pavan-Langston, D., North, R.D., Geary, P.A., and Kenkel, A.: Intravenous and possibly subconjunctival injection of soluble antiviral ARA AMP may be useful in treatment of deep ocular herpetic disease, Arch. Ophthalmol. **94:**1585, 1976.

76. Pavan-Langston, D., Park, N.H., and Lass, J.H.: Herpetic ganglionic latency: acyclovir and vidarabine therapy, Arch. Ophthalmol. **97:**1508, 1979.

77. Payrau, P., and Dohlman, C.H.: IDU in corneal wound healing, Am. J. Ophthalmol. **57:**999, 1964.

78. Pfister, R.R., Richards, J.S., and Dohlman, C.H.: Recurrence of herpetic keratitis in corneal grafts, Am. J. Ophthalmol. **73:**192, 1972.

79. Pierson, R.B., and Kirkham, T.H.: Neonatal keratitis due to herpesvirus: hominis type 1 infection, Can. J. Ophthalmol. **9:**429, 1974.

80. Plotkin, J., Reynaud, A., and Okumoto, M.: Cytologic study of herpetic keratitis, Arch. Ophthalmol. **85:**597, 1971.

81. Polack, F.M., and Kaufman, H.E.: Penetrating keratoplasty in herpetic keratitis, Am. J. Ophthalmol. **73:**908, 1972.

82. Polack, F.M., and Rose, J.: The effect of 5-iodo-2-deoxyuridine (IDU) in corneal healing, Arch. Ophthalmol. **71:**520, 1964.

83. Polack, F.M., Siverio, C., Bigar, F., and Centifanto, Y.: Immune host response to corneal grafts sensitized to herpes simplex virus, Invest. Ophthalmol. **15:**188, 1976.

84. Sachs, V., and Marcus, M.: Bilateral herpetic keratitis during measles, Am. J. Ophthalmol. **91:**796, 1981.

85. Stern, G.A., Zarn, S.Z., and Gutgesell, V.J.: Primary herpes simplex subepithelial dendritic keratitis, Am. J. Ophthalmol. **91:**496, 1981.

86. Tarkkanen, A., and Laatkainen, L.: Late ocular manifestations in neonatal herpes simplex infection, Br. J. Ophthalmol. **61:**608, 1977.

87. Trobe, J.D., Centifanto, Y., Zam, S., et al.: Antiherpes activity of adenine arabinoside monophosphate, Invest. Ophthalmol. **15:**196, 1976.

88. Trousdale, M.D., Dunkel, E.C., and Nesburn, A.B.: Effect of acyclovir on acute and latent herpes simplex virus infections in the rabbit, Invest. Ophthalmol. Vis. Sci. **19:**1336, 1980.

89. Waring, G.: Glucocorticosteroid therapy in ocular herpes simplex, Surv. Ophthalmol. **23:**35, 1978.

90. Warkany, J.: Congenital malformations, Chicago, 1971, Year Book Medical Publishers, Inc.

91. Wellings, P.C., Awdry, P.N., Bers, F.H., et al.: Clinical evaluation of trifluorothymidine in the treatment of herpes simplex corneal ulcers, Am. J. Ophthalmol. **73:**932, 1972.

92. Wellings, P.C., Awdry, P.N., Bers, F.H., Jones, B.R., Brown, D.C., and Kaufman, H.E.: Clinical evaluation of trifluorothymidine in the treatment of herpes simplex corneal ulcers, Am. J. Ophthalmol. **73:**932, 1972.

93. Wheeler, C.E., Jr., and Huffines, W.D.: Primary disseminated herpes simplex of the newborn, JAMA **191:**111, 1965.

94. Wilhelmus, K.R., Coster, D.J., and Jones, B.R.: Acyclovir and debridement in the treatment of ulcerative herpetic keratitis, Am. J. Ophthalmol. **91:**323, 1981.

95. Witmer, R., and Iwamoto, T.: Electron microscopic observations of herpes-like particles in the iris, Arch. Ophthalmol. **79:**331, 1968.

96. Yeakley, W.R., Laibson, P.R., Michelson, M.A., and Arentsen, J.J.: A double-controlled evaluation of acyclovir and vidarabine for the treatment of herpes simplex epithelial keratitis, Trans. Am. Ophth. Soc. **79:**168, 1981.

97. Zaib, Z.M., Nahmias, A.J., and Josey, W.E.: Genital herpes infections associated with cervical dysplasia and carcinoma, Cancer **23:**940, 1969.

98. Zimmerman, T. J., McNeill, J. I., Richman, A., Kaufman, H. E., and Wolfman, S. R.: HLA types and recurrent corneal herpes simplex infection, Invest. Ophthalmol. **16:**756, 1977.

Herpes zoster

99. Acers, T. E.: Herpes zoster ophthalmicus with contralateral hemiplegia, Arch. Ophthalmol. **71:**371, 1964.
100. Acers, T. E., and Vaille, V.: Co-existent herpes zoster and herpes simplex, Am. J. Ophthalmol. **63:**992, 1967.
101. Ahmad, M., Bowen, S. F., Jr., and Burke, R.: Optic atrophy following herpes zoster ophthalmicus in a child, Can. J. Ophthalmol. **4:**387, 1969.
102. Aronson, S. B., and Moore, T. E.: Corticosteroid therapy in cental stromal keratitis, Am. J. Ophthalmol. **67:**873, 1969.
103. Bartlett, R. E., Mumma, C. S., and Irvine, A. R.: Herpes zoster ophthalmicus with bilateral hemorrhagic retinopathy, Am. J. Ophthalmol. **34:**45, 1951.
104. Blodi, F.: Ophthalmic zoster in malignant disease, Am. J. Ophthalmol. **65:**686, 1968.
105. Bouzas, A.: Canalicular inflammation in ophthalmic cases of herpes zoster and herpes simplex, Am. J. Ophthalmol. **60:**713, 1965.
106. Brown, R. M., and Mendis, U.: Retinal arteritis complicating herpes zoster ophthalmicus, Br. J. Ophthalmol. **57:**344, 1973.
107. Brunell, P. A., Gershon, A. A.: Passive immunization against varicella-zoster infections and other modes of therapy, J. Infect. Dis. **127:**415, 1973.
108. Crock, G.: Clinical syndromes of anterior segment ischemia, Trans. Ophthalmol. Soc. U. K. **87:**513, 1967.
109. Dugmore, W.: Intercalary staphyloma in a case of herpes zoster ophthalmicus, Br. J. Ophthalmol. **51:**350, 1967.
110. Duke-Elder, W. S., editor: System of ophthalmology, vol. 8. Diseases of the outer eye, pt 1. Conjunctiva, London, 1965, Henry Kimpton.
111. Edgarton, A. E.: Herpes zoster ophthalmicus: report of cases and review of literature, Arch. Ophthalmol. **34:**40, 114, 1945.
112. Fierer, J., Bazeley, P., and Braude, A. I.: Herpes B virus encephalomyelitis presenting as ophthalmic zoster, Ann. Intern. Med. **79:**225, 1973.
113. Gilbert, G. J.: Herpes zoster ophthalmicus and delayed contralateral hemiparesis: relationships of the syndrome to central nervous system granulomatous angitis, JAMA **229:**302, 1974.
114. Goldsmith, M. O.: Herpes zoster ophthalmicus with sixth nerve palsy, Can. J. Ophthalmol. **3:**279, 1968.
115. Goodman, M. L., and Maher, E.: Four uncommon infections in Hodgkin's disease, JAMA **198:**1129, 1966.
116. Harrison, E. Q.: Complications of herpes zoster ophthalmicus, Am. J. Ophthalmol. **60:**1111, 1965.
117. Hayashi, K., Uchida, Y., and Oshima, M.: Fluorescent antibody study of herpes zoster keratitis, Am. J. Ophthalmol. **75:**795, 1973.
118. Hedges, T. R., III, and Albert, D. M.: The progression of the ocular abnormalities of herpes zoster, Ophthalmology **89:**165, 1982.
119. Hesse, R. J.: Herpes zoster ophthalmicus associated with delayed retinal thrombophlebitis, Am. J. Ophthalmol. **84:**329, 1977.
120. Jarrett, W. H.: Horner's syndrome with geniculate zoster, occurring in association with trigeminal herpes in which the ophthalmic division was spared, Am. J. Ophthalmol. **63:**326, 1967.
121. Johnson, M. T., Luby, J. P., Buchanan, R. A., and Mikulec, D.: Treatment of varicella-zoster infections with adenine arabinoside, J. Infect. Dis. **131:**225, 1975.
122. Kernbaum, S., and Hauchecome, J.: Administration of levodopa for relief of herpes zoster pain, JAMA **246:**132, 1981.
123. Kielar, R. A., Cunningham, G. C., and Gerson, K. C.: Occurrence of herpes zoster ophthalmicus in a child with absent immunoglobulin A and deficiency of delayed hypersensitivity, Am. J. Ophthalmol. **72:**555, 1971.
124. Kline, L. B., and Jackson, B. W.: Herpes zoster conjunctiva ulceration, Can. J. Ophthalmol. **12:**66, 1977.
125. Lincoff, H. A., Wise, G. N., and Romaine, H. H.: Total detachment and reattachment of the retina in herpes zoster ophthalmicus, Am. J. Ophthalmol. **41:**253, 1956.
126. Marsh, R. J.: Herpes zoster keratitis, Trans. Ophthalmol. Soc. U. K. **93:**181, 1973.
127. Marsh, R. J., Easty, D. L., and Jones, B. R.: Iritis and iris atrophy in herpes zoster ophthalmicus, Am. J. Ophthalmol. **78:**2, 1974.
128. Marsh, R. J., Fraunfelder, J. T., McGill, J. I., and Phil, D.: Herpetic epithelial disease, Arch. Ophthalmol. **94:**1899, 1976.
129. Merselis, J. G., Jr., Kaye, D., and Hook, E. W.: Disseminated herpes zoster: a report of 17 cases, Arch. Intern. Med. **113:**679, 1964.
130. Mondent, B. J., Brown, S. I., and Mondzelewski, J. P.: Peripheral corneal ulcers with herpes zoster ophthalmicus, Am. J. Ophthalmol. **86:**611, 1978.
131. Naumann, G., Gass, J. D. M., and Font, R. L.: Histopathology of herpes zoster ophthalmicus, Am. J. Ophthalmol. **65:**533, 1968.

132. Pavan-Langston, D., and McCulley, J. P.: Herpes zoster dendritic keratitis, Arch. Ophthalmol. **89:**25, 1973.

133. Pemberton, J. W.: Optic atrophy in herpes zoster ophthalmicus, Am. J. Ophthalmol. **58:**852, 1964.

134. Penman, G. G.: Scleritis as a sequel of herpes ophthalmicus, Br. J. Ophthalmol. **15:**585, 1931.

135. Piebenga, L. W., and Laibson, P. R.: Dendritic lesions in herpes zoster ophthalmicus, Arch. Ophthalmol. **90:**268, 1973.

136. Pierce, L. E., and Jenkins, R. B.: Herpes zoster ophthalmicus treated with cytarabine, Arch. Ophthalmol. **89:**21, 1973.

137. Scheie, H. G.: Herpes zoster ophthalmicus, Trans. Ophthalmol. Soc. U. K. **90:**899, 1970.

138. Scheie, H. G., and McLellan, T. G., Jr.: Treatment of herpes zoster ophthalmicus with corticotropin and corticosteroids, Arch. Ophthalmol. **62:**579, 1959.

139. Schwartz, D. E.: Herpes zoster ophthalmicus with nasociliary nerve involvement, Am. J. Ophthalmol. **74:**142, 1972.

140. Singh, S., Malhotra, V., and Malhotra, R. P.: Guillain-Barré syndrome in herpes zoster, N. Y. State J. Med. **72:**2094, 1972.

141. Stevens, D. A., and Merigan, T. C.: Interferon, antibody, and other host factors in herpes zoster, J. Clin. Invest. **51:**1170, 1972.

142. Sugar, H. S.: Herpetic keratouveitis: clinical experiences, Ann. Ophthalmol. **3:**355, 1971.

143. Weller, T. H., and Whitton, H. M.: The etiologic agents of varicella and herpes zoster: isolation, propagation, and cultural characterization in vitro, J. Exp. Med. **108:**843, 1958.

Other virus infections

144. Charles, N. C., Bennett, T. W., and Margolis, S.: Ocular pathology of the congenital varicella syndrome, Arch. Ophthalmol. **95:**2034, 1977.

145. Deutman, A. F., and Grizzard, W. S.: Rubella retinopathy and subretinal neovascularization, Am. J. Ophthalmol. **85:**82, 1978.

146. Ernest, J. T., and Costenbader, F. D.: Lateral rectus muscle palsy, Am. J. Ophthalmol. **65:**721, 1968.

147. Fields, J.: Ocular manifestations of mumps, Am. J. Ophthalmol. **30:**591, 1947.

148. Frederique, G., Howard, R. O., and Boniuk, I.: Corneal ulcers in rubeola, Am. J. Ophthalmol. **68:**996, 1969.

149. Hyndiuk, R. A., Okumoto, M., Domiano, R. A., Valenton, M., and Smolin, G.: Treatment of vaccineal keratitis with vidarabine, Arch. Ophthalmol. **94:**1363, 1976.

150. Meyer, R. F., Sullivan, J. H., and Oh, J. O.: Mumps conjunctivitis, Am. J. Ophthalmol. **78:**1022, 1974.

151. Nesburn, A. B., Borit, A., Pentelei-Molnar, J. C., and Lazaro, R.: Varicella dendritic keratitis, Invest. Ophthalmol. **13:**764, 1974.

152. Noel, L. P., and Watson, G. A.: Internal ophthalmoplegia following chicken-pox, Can. J. Ophthalmol. **11:**267, 1976.

153. North, D. P.: Ocular manifestations of mumps, Br. J. Ophthalmol. **37:**99, 1953.

154. Riggenburgh, R. S.: Ocular manifestation of mumps, Arch. Ophthalmol. **66:**739, 1961.

155. Roy, R. H., Hiatt, R. L., Korones, S. B., and Roane, J.: Ocular manifestations of congenital rubella syndrome, Arch. Ophthalmol. **75:**601, 1966.

156. Sivan, J. W., and Penn, R. F.: Scleritis following mumps, Am. J. Ophthalmol. **53:**366, 1962.

157. Smolin, G.: Report of a case of rubella keratitis, Am. J. Ophthalmol. **74:**436, 1972.

158. Thygeson, P.: Ocular viral diseases, Med. Clin. North Am. **43:**1419, 1959.

159. Uchida, Y., Kaneko, M., and Hayashi, K.: Varicella dendritic keratitis, Am. J. Ophthalmol. **89:**259, 1980.

ADDITIONAL READING
Herpes simplex

Abel, R., Jr., Kaufman, H. E., and Sugar, J.: The effect of intravenous adenine arabinoside against herpes simplex keratouveitis in humans, presented at the Fourteenth Interscience Conference on Antimicrobial Agents and Chemotherapy, San Francisco, Sept. 11-14, 1974.

Abel, R., Kaufman, H. E., and Sugar J.: Intravenous adenine arabinoside against herpes simplex keratouveitis in humans, Am. J. Ophthalmol. **79:**659, 1975.

Bloom, J. N., Katz, J., and Kaufman, H. E.: Herpes simplex retinitis and encephalitis in an adult, Arch. Ophthalmol. **95:**1798, 1977.

Cogan, D. G., et al.: Herpes simplex retinopathy in an infant, Arch. Ophthalmol. **72:**641, 1964.

Coleman, V. R., Thygeson, P., Dawson, C. R., and Jawetz, E.: Isolation of virus from herpetic keratitis, Arch. Ophthalmol. **81:**22, 1969.

Hyndiuk, R. A., Charlin, R. E., Alpren, T. V. P., and Schultz, R. O.: Trifluridine in resistant human herpetic keratitis, Arch. Ophthalmol. **96:**1839, 1978.

Hyndiuk, R. A., Hull, D. S., Schultz, R. O., Chin, G. N., Laibson, P. R., and Krachmer, J. H.: Adenine arabinoside in idoxuridine unresponsive and intolerant herpetic keratitis, Am. J. Ophthalmol. **79:**655, 1975.

Kaufman, H. E.: Disease of the corneal stroma after herpes simplex infection, Am. J. Ophthalmol. **63:**878, 1967.

Kaufman, H. E.: Herpes virus keratitis: management of herpetic keratitis with IDU, Ann. Ophthalmol. **1:**199, 1968.

Kaufman, H. E.: Herpetic stromal disease, Am. J. Ophthalmol. **80:**1092, 1975.

Kaufman, H. E.: Antimetabolite drug therapy in herpes simplex, Ophthalmology **87:**1980.

Kaufman, H. E., Ellison, E. D., and Townsend, W. M.: The chemotherapy of herpes iritis with adenine arabinoside and cytarabine, Arch. Ophthalmol. **84:**783, 1970.

Kaufman, H. E., Martola, E. L., and Dohlman, C. H.: Herpes simplex treatment with IDU and corticosteroids, Arch. Ophthalmol. **69:**468, 1963.

Meyers-Elliott, R. H., Pettit, T., and Maxwell, A.: Viral antigens in the immune ring of herpes simplex stromal keratitis, Arch. Ophthalmol. **98:**897, 1980.

Patterson, A., and Jones, B. R.: The management of ocular herpes, Trans. Ophthalmol. Soc. U. K. **87:**59, 1967.

Pavan-Langston, D., and Brockhurst, R. J.: Herpes simplex panuveitis: a clinical report, Arch. Ophthalmol. **81:**783, 1969.

Pavan-Langston, D., Campbell, R., and Lass, J.: Acyclic antimetabolite therapy of experimental herpes simplex keratitis, Am. J. Ophthalmol. **86:**618, 1978.

Pavan-Langston, D., and Dohlman, C. H.: A double-blind clinical study of adenine arabinoside therapy of viral keratoconjunctivitis, Am. J. Ophthalmol. **74:**81, 1972.

Pavan-Langston, D., Dohlman, C. H., Geary, P., and Sulzewski, D.: Intraocular penetration of ARA-A and IDU: therapeutic implications in clinical herpetic uveitis, Trans. Am. Acad. Ophthalmol. Otolaryngol. **77:**455, 1973.

Pavan-Langston, D., and Nesburn, A. B.: The chronology of primary herpes simplex infection of the eye and adnexal glands, Arch. Ophthalmol. **80:**258, 1968.

Smolin, G., Okumoto, M., and Friedlaender, M.: Treatment of herpes simplex keratitis with levamisole, Arch. Ophthalmol. **96:**1078, 1978.

Smith, J. P., and Lavine, D. M.: Cicatricial ectropion of the upper lid secondary to herpes zoster ophthalmicus, Ann. Ophthalmol. **13:**579, 1981.

Sugar, J., Stark, W., Bender, P. S., et al.: Triflurothymidine treatment of herpes simplex epithelial keratitis and comparison with idoxuridine, Ann. Ophthalmol. **12:**611, 1980.

Waring, G. O.: Viewpoints: glucocorticoid therapy in ocular herpes simplex, Surv. Ophthalmol. **23:**35, 1978.

9 Blepharitis

Conditions that affect the anterior lid margins are (1) staphylococcal blepharitis, (2) seborrheic blepharitis, (3) rosacea blepharitis, and (4) parasitic blepharitis. The posterior lid margins are affected by meibomian gland dysfunction.

ANTERIOR LID MARGIN

Marginal blepharitis often affects the eye.[18] The most common causes are staphylococcal infection[2,16,19] and seborrhea. The staphylococcus organism is present throughout life in the nasopharyngeal tissues and can be a cause of a number of infections. The staphylococcus organism can remain viable for an interval of time and can produce chronic and smoldering infections of long duration,[14] such as is seen in chronic staphylococcal blepharitis. The delayed type of hypersensitivity to staphylococcal antigens is common in human beings. In addition to the infections of the lid margins, external ocular signs of staphylococcal origin are (1) catarrhal corneal ulceration or infiltrations, which are antigen-antibody reactions, and (2) phlyctenulosis, which is a delayed hypersensitivity to staphylococcal antigen. In 1937 Thygeson[17] and Allen demonstrated that the topical application of a filtrate prepared from a culture of S. aureus produced a toxic type of conjunctivitis and keratitis in a human volunteer. The secretion of this necrotizing type of toxin is a mechanism by which S. aureus can attack the external eye.[3,16] It also has been noted that a significant and possibly less severe toxigenic conjunctivitis is produced by S. epidermidis filtrates.[20] A definite relationship exists among the exotoxin, the conjunctivitis, and the inferior punctate epithelial keratitis seen in chronic staphylococcal blepharoconjunctivitis. Also interesting is that the phage group II staphylococci are etiologic agents in exfoliative dermatitis in newborns (Ritter's disease), in toxic epidermal necrolysis in older patients, in scarlatiniform rash, and in bullous impetigo.[10,21]

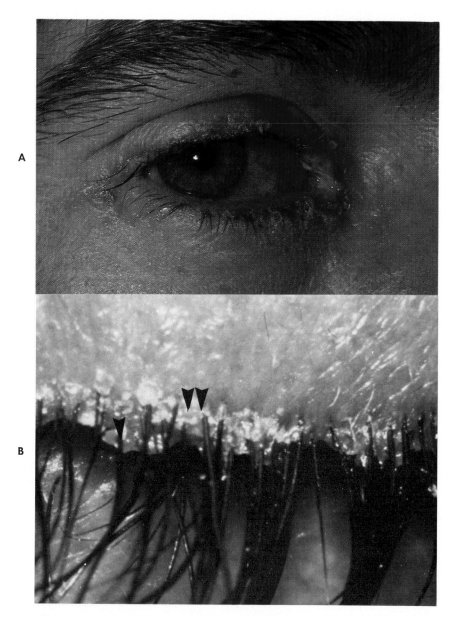

Fig. 9-1. A, Ulcerative blepharitis with intensive crusting of lid margin. **B,** When this was removed, bleeding area was visible *(double arrow)*. Collarette formation *(single arrow)* is noted around cilium.

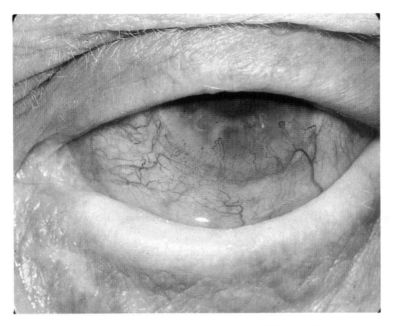

Fig. 9-2. Loss of cilia after staphylococcal blepharitis.

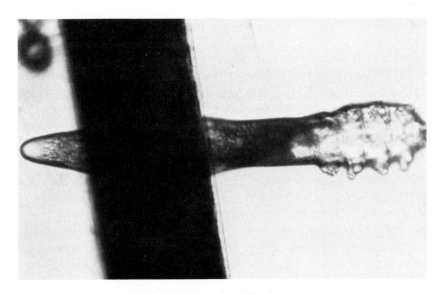

Fig. 9-3. *Demodex folliculorum.*

These diseases are caused by the extracellular protein produced by the phage group II staphylococcus[9] and manifest external disease signs.

Clinical signs

Staphylococcal blepharitis. The two types of staphylococcal blepharitis are squamous and ulcerative. The more commonly occurring squamous type exhibits brittle, fibrinous scales; the less common ulcerative type is characterized by matted, hard crusts surrounding the individual cilium (Fig. 9-1). When crusts are removed, small ulcers of the hair follicles can be seen, and bleeding may occur. Both types of staphylococcal blepharitis may exhibit dilated blood vessels on the lid margins, madarosis, white lashes (poliosis), misdirected lashes (trichiasis), broken lashes, irregularity of the lid margins (tylosis), and loss of lashes (Fig. 9-2). The scales that encircle the lash are known as collarettes. These collarettes are formed from fibrin from the ulcerated blepharitic base. The fibrin is carried from the skin-lid margin by the growing cilium; the cilium appears to pierce the scale. The lids may, in addition, exhibit hordeola, both internal and external, as well as angular blepharitis.

Blepharoconjunctivitis can develop as a side effect of basal cell carcinoma treatment, keratinizing dermatoses, and cystic acne with oral 13-*cis*-retinoic acid.[4] The *Moraxella* organism also causes angular blepharitis. The conjunctiva is often affected in staphylococcal blepharitis so that one may see a chronic papillary conjunctivitis and a reasonable amount of mucopurulent exudate containing polymorphonuclear (PMN) leukocytes. The conjunctivitis is worse, as are the symptoms, on awakening.

Since *Staphylococcus aureus* is a facultative intracellular parasite (unlike other pyogenic cocci such as pneumococci), it is resistant to the usual sulfonamide and antibiotic therapy, particularly when *S. aureus* infects the lid margin and produces chronic squamous or ulcerative blepharitis. Infection of the meibomian, sweat, and sebaceous glands of the cilia follicles probably also accounts for much of the resistance to therapy since it is difficult or impossible to obtain a therapeutic concentration of any drug in these structures.

The conjunctivitis and epithelial keratitis in staphylococcal blepharitis are in part the result of dermatonecrotoxin released from staphylococci proliferating on the lid margin. Eradication of a lid margin infection is one of the most difficult problems in infectious disease. Often the disease persists throughout the patient's lifetime. Blepharitis itself is relatively symptomless or at least well tolerated, but when it is accompanied by conjunctivitis or especially keratitis, it is a curse to its victims.

Microbiologic cure of the lid margin infection can rarely be achieved by chemotherapeutic means. Supplementary immunotherapy is therefore highly desirable, particularly to prevent the recurrence of staphylococcal marginal ulceration and staphylococcal phlyctenular keratoconjunctivitis and to relieve the staphylococcal epithelial keratitis that usually accompanies blepharitis. Graduated doses of *Staphylococcus* toxin have been useful, often dramatically so, both in neutralizing toxicity and in desensitizing the patient to the organism. Recent experience with Staphage Lysate has been encouraging in both marginal ulceration and phlyctenulosis. Immunotherapy in persistent epithelial keratitis, recurrent marginal ulceration, and staphylococcal phlyctenulosis seems to be a worthy alternative.

Corneal complications are frequently seen in staphylococcal blepharitis and include toxic epithelial keratitis (punctate erosions, PEE), catarrhal infiltration, ulceration, phlyctenules, and pannus formation.

The epithelial keratitis is seen in the inferior quadrants of the cornea predominantly and consists of fine, small, flat, punctate lesions that are regular and may stain with fluorescein, as well as with rose bengal red. The dermatonecrotoxin is concentrated in the tears and is responsible for the keratitis. Lid closure concentrates this toxin and enhances the formation of keratitis. This fine epithelial keratitis should be differentiated from the blotchy corneal lesions that are seen in keratoconjunctivitis sicca.

The catarrhal ulcer or infiltrate of the cornea that may accompany the blepharitis usually occurs at the 10, 2, 4, and 8 o'clock positions. A lucid interval exists between the lesion and the limbus. The infiltrate appears first, and ulceration may follow. After the ulcer heals, there may be a peripheral wedge of pannus at the ulcer site.

The phlyctenular disease of staphylococcal origin may also accompany this type of blepharitis.

The roles of *Pityrosporum ovale* and *Demodex folliculorum* in staphylococcal blepharitis are in question. *D. folliculorum* is a microscopic, eight-legged, transparent mite (Fig. 9-3) that probably infests about 40% of humans. The parasite lives in sebaceous follicles. It covers the base of the lash with a tubular sleeve (Fig. 9-4). Waxy debris forms cuffs around the lashes. Since bacteria are found on *D. folliculorum* bodies, it is possible that the mite serves as a vector for staphylococcal infection, with the bacteria probably acting as mechanical transmitters of the organism.[5,7] The epithelial keratitis seen in infestation by the *Demodex* organism can easily be associated with a staphylococcal infection. *D. folliculorum* should not be confused with *Phthirus pubis* (pediculosis). Pubic lice have a predilection for cilia as well as pubic hairs because of the appropriate spacing of the cilia (Fig. 9-5). Nits are usually seen stuck to the lashes as small oval bodies (Fig. 9-6). The feces of the organism are toxic and cause a follicular conjunctivitis and mild epithelial keratitis.

Phthiriasis palpebrarum is an uncommon cause of blepharitis and conjunctivitis and may easily be overlooked.[6] A high index of suspicion and careful examination of the patient's lid margins and eyelashes will lead to the proper diagnosis. Treatment of Phthiriasis palpebrarum is best accomplished by careful removal of the lice and nits (louse eggs) from the patient's lashes. Local application of a pediculicide such as yellow mercuric oxide 1% ophthalmic ointment applied twice daily for 1 week or 0.25% physostigmine (Eserine) ointment applied twice daily to the lid margins for a minimum of 10 days should be considered when the total removal of *Phthirus pubis* and nits is not possible mechanically. Body hair should be examined for infestation with lice and treated with gamma benzene hexachloride shampoo. This medication should be used with caution in infants, children, and pregnant women. Family members, sexual contacts, and close companions should be examined and treated appropriately; clothing, linen, and personal items should be disinfected at 50° C for 30 minutes.

The diagnosis of the *D. folliculorum* infection may be made by extracting the lash and suspending it in viscous fluid; examination of the base will reveal the mite clinging to the lash. When treating the *Demodex* parasite, lid hygiene scrubs of soap and water or lid treatment with polysulfide ointment are effective. When dealing with pediculosis,

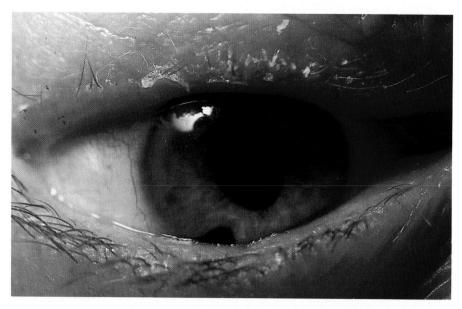

Fig. 9-4. Cuffing of base of cilium as seen in *Demodex folliculorum* infection of lid margin.

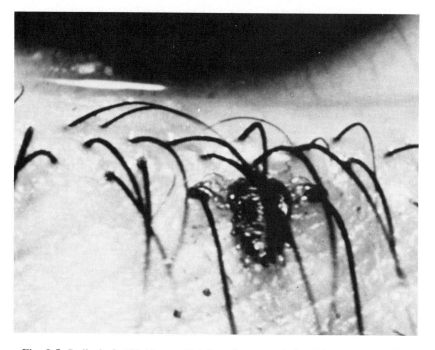

Fig. 9-5. Pediculosis *(Phthirus pubis)*. Parasite suspends itself between two cilia.

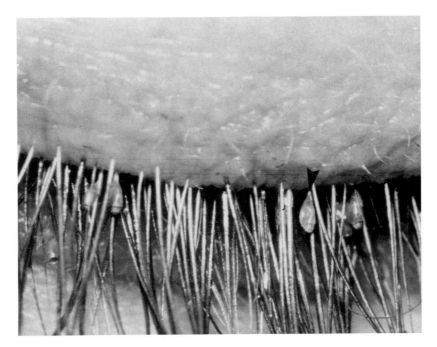

Fig. 9-6. Nits *(arrow)*.

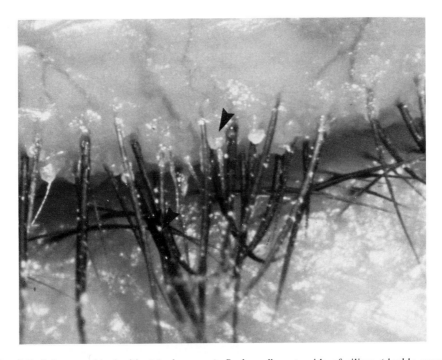

Fig. 9-7. Sebaceous blepharitis *(single arrow)*. Scales adhere to side of cilium *(double arrow)*.

the nits should be removed manually, and the adult organism dealt with by application of petroleum jelly, which smothers the organism.

Seborrheic blepharitis. This common type of marginal blepharitis (Fig. 9-7) often has a superimposed staphylococcal infection.

Seborrheic blepharitis is seen as an excessive sebaceous gland secretion from glands of Zeis, with the clinical appearance of redness of the lid margins without ulceration and large, yellow, gray, greasy scales (oily form) that are loosely attached to the side of the cilia (scurf) (Fig. 9-7). The condition may be associated with seborrheic dermatitis of the scalp, nose, or chest; oily skin is also seen. Accumulation of scales such as dandruff is seen on the scalp, eyebrows, and lashes (dry form) in other cases. The role of dandruff itself in the disease is questionable.

The cultures usually yield no organisms, but *P. ovale,* a yeastlike organism that buds on axis, is frequently seen on scrapings, the significance of which is not particularly known. It has been postulated that *P. ovale* produces disease by splitting lipids into irritating fatty acids.

Lid hygiene and removal of excess lipid by expression of glands may help alleviate the symptoms of burning, watering, and discharge.

Other rarer forms of marginal inflammation

Patients with rosacea have a greater than normal predisposition to staphylococcal infection and are frequently afflicted with staphylococcal blepharoconjunctivitis. In this condition, one can see a paralytic dilation of the superficial blood vessels leading to telangiectasia and erythema of the lid margins. In addition, one may find papules, pustules, and pustular acneiform lesions that heal without scarring.

Patients with atopic disease also have a predilection for herpetic and staphylococcal infections. Atopic patients have a defect with cellular immunity and possibly a defect in the IgA antibody response.[11] The high prevalence of staphylococcal blepharitis in the atopic population may be a result of these factors.

POSTERIOR LID MARGIN

The meibomian gland may show dysfunction with hypersecretion of the glands associated with lid inflammation. A liquid residue may occur on the mucocutaneous strip of the lid with foamy tears accumulating in the canthi, or a thick greasy film may be noted. Hyperemia, thickening, irregularity, and a loss of contour of the posterior lid margin may occur together with a normal-appearing anterior lid margin. This condition may be associated with inspissated meibomian material, which may be semisolid or yellow and oily in consistency. One may see chalazia, tarsitis, or nodules on the posterior lid; occasionally, the Zeis glands may become inflamed.

Conjunctivitis and superficial epithelial keratitis may also occur in meibomian gland dysfunction.[13]

The cause of this condition and that of "conjunctivitis meibomiana" is not clear. In the chronic stage, in which there are minimal external eyelid signs, cultures are frequently negative. *Staphylococcus epidermidis* and *S. aureus* are the most commonly isolated aerobes.

The symptoms include tearing, burning, itching, dryness, irritation, and photophobia.

The more prominent ocular signs are occasional scarring from chronic infection, occasional decreased corneal sensation, papillary conjunctival hypertrophy, staining with rose bengal red, and rapid breakup of the precorneal tear film.

The lid margins exhibit pouting meibomian orifices, inspissated meibomian plugs, and little or no inflammation anterior to the gray line.

The clinical signs in the chronic stage of meibomian keratoconjunctivitis represent a nonspecific inflammatory response by the eye and its adnexa, with the exception of the superficial punctate keratopathy and the stagnation of the meibomian glands. The superficial punctate keratopathy looks like that seen in conditions with an unstable tear film, not like that described as secondary to staphylococcus toxin,[17] which is more typically seen with blepharitis involving the anterior eyelid and cilia line.[3] An unstable tear film in patients with meibomian keratoconjunctivitis accounts for the keratopathy without suggesting the presence of a bacterial exotoxin; however, this may be only one of several pathways producing a superficial punctate keratopathy in patients with blepharitis. Abelson and Holly[1] recently described a blink abnormality that would contribute to the superficial punctate keratopathy to be produced by an unstable tear film.

The stagnation of the meibomian glands, which produces the lipid layer of the tear film, may account for the tear film instability. This is in accordance with the stabilization of the tear film when fresh secretions from deep within the glands are added by expressing these directly into the tear film.[13] The observed instability is not caused by a quantitative decrease in the tear lipid layer, since the presence of normal or increased interference patterns in the tear film can be used as a measure of the amount of lipid present.[13]

Consistent finding of a generalized sebaceous gland dysfunction suggests diffuse abnormality of the sebaceous glands (the meibomian gland is a specialized sebaceous gland), which predisposes patients to dermatitis or blepharitis centered around these glands.[13]

DIFFERENTIAL DIAGNOSIS

A number of entities should be considered in a differential diagnosis of marginal lid ulcers. Lid marginal ulcers may be caused by vaccinia virus and other pox viruses as well as the herpesvirus. Definite attempts should be made to rule out these entities, which often are associated with characteristic skin lesions or with follicular conjunctivitis. Scrapings may show giant cells and a mononuclear cell response.

Angular blepharitis is often associated with *Moraxella* organism infections; the organism, of course, can be identified by scrapings. It should be remembered that children with *Moraxella* species blepharitis often exhibit follicular conjunctivitis.

One of the complications of chronic blepharitis is poliosis, a sign also seen in Waardenburg's and Behçet's syndromes. Loss of lashes is also seen in *Candida albicans* lid infections and trichotillomania.

Staphylococcal blepharitis is frequently noted in dry eyes. The two conditions, of course, may occur separately. However, the corneal staining in staphylococcal blepharitis usually involves the lower one third of the cornea, but the dry eye is associated with diffuse stain in the interpalpebral zone. Filaments are usually not seen in staphylococcal blepharitis, but they may be seen in dry eye.

TREATMENT

If seborrhea is present, the scalp should be shampooed with antiseborrheic products such as regular selenium sulfide. The meibomian secretion should be investigated and, if found excessive, should be expressed from the glands at home daily. The lids should be cleansed daily with a cotton-tipped applicator and shampooed with a mild baby shampoo.

In long-standing cases of staphylococcal blepharitis, the antibacterial therapy of the lids is most important. The order of preference of antibiotic ointments to be applied with a cotton-tipped applicator is (1) bacitracin, (2) erythromycin, and (3) chloramphenicol. The severity of the blepharitis will determine the frequency of the application. Severe cases may require three to four applications daily. It should be noted that *S. aureus* can survive in an intraleukocytic environment after being phagocytized by PMN neutrophils.[14] The bacterial survival within the phagocytes is seen and protected from the action of high concentrations of most antibiotics. Rifampin, however, is able to kill intraleukocytic staphylococci and should be considered in recalcitrant cases of staphylococcal blepharitis.[12, 16]

If after a while one reaches a plateau with staphylococcal blepharitis, the condition does not seem to improve, redness and keratitis persist, and the bacterial cultures are negative, it may be necessary to apply steroid ointment to the lid margins twice daily for several weeks. This may result in improvement and final amelioration of the problem.

If one sees recurrent styles or chalazia in addition to the blepharitis, one might consider the use of topical antibiotics plus the use of systemic antibiotics.

If catarrhal ulceration occurs, prednisolone drops should be added to the usual blepharitis treatment, ranging from very dilute steroid such as 0.12% prednisolone to a more formidable concentration of 1% two or three times a day. One should always be aware of the complications of corticosteroid therapy.

Complicating staphylococcal phlyctenulosis may be treated with the antibiotics mentioned. The corticosteroids are less effective in the staphylococcal type of phlyctenular disease than in the tuberculosis type.[15]

In cases in which the blepharitis is largely associated with meibomitis and seborrhea, systemic antibiotics may be useful; 1 g tetracycline initially and then 250 mg daily are advocated. It should be cautioned that they never be used in children or expectant mothers. Evidence supports the role of *Propionibacterium acnes* in acne vulgaris and similar conditions such as seborrhea. The principal hypothesis proposes that free fatty acids initiate comedogenesis and inflammation of sebaceous follicles.[8] These free fatty acids are probably derived from sebum triglycerides through the lipolytic action of microbial lipases contained within the glands. *P. acnes* appears to be a major source of these lipases.[8] The similarity of the meibomian glands to sebaceous glands, the frequency of *P. acnes* in lid cultures, and preliminary experience with oral tetracycline has led to speculation that *P. acnes* may have a comparable role in seborrheic blepharitis.[8]

Erythromycin in the same dose as tetracycline is also effective.

If *Demodex* organism infection is present, lid hygiene with lid scrubs of soap and water and application of polysulfide ointment are effective. When dealing with pediculi, the nits should be removed manually, and the adult organism dealt with by application of petroleum jelly.

It is important to realize that difficulties exist in treating staphylococcal blepharo-keratoconjunctivitis. Treatment may have to be continued for a long period; the patient's understanding of the chronicity of the disease should be established. One must recognize the atypical forms of the disease, different types of corneal involvement, and the influence on the disease of tear dysfunction and allergic complications.

REFERENCES

1. Abelson, M.B., and Holly, F.J.: Inferior punctate keratopathy: a tentative mechanism, Am. J. Ophthalmol. **83**:866, 1977.
2. Allen, H.F.: *Staphylococcus aureus* and *Pseudomonas* in conjunctivitis and keratitis. In Infectious diseases of the conjunctiva and cornea: Symposium of the New Orleans Academy of Ophthalmology, St. Louis, 1963, The C.V. Mosby Co.
3. Allen, J.H.: Staphylococcic conjunctivitis, Am. J. Ophthalmol. **20**:1025, 1937.
4. Blackman, H.J., Peck, G.L., Olsen, T.G., et al.: Blepharoconjunctivitis: a side effect of 13-*cis*-retinoic acid therapy for dermatologic diseases, Ophthalmology **86**:753, 1980.
5. Couch, J.M., Green, W.R., Hirst, L.W., and De La Cruz, Z.C.: Diagnosing and treating *Phthirus pubis* palpebrarum. In Friedman, A.H., and Boniuk, M.M.: Clinical pathological review, Surv. Ophthalmol. **26**:219, 1982.
6. English, F.P., Iwamoto, T., Darrell, R.W., et al.: The vector potential of *Demodex folliculorum*, Arch. Ophthalmol. **84**:83, 1970.
7. Jeffery, M.P.: Ocular diseases caused by nematodes, Am. J. Ophthalmol. **40**:411, 1955.
8. Jones, D.B., and Robinson, N.M.: Anaerobic ocular infections, Trans. Am. Acad. Ophthalmol. Otolaryngol. **83**:309, 1977.
9. Kapral, F.A., and Miller, M.M.: Product of *S. aureus* responsible for scaled-skin syndrome, Infect. Immun. **4**:541, 1971.
10. Lillibridge, C.B., Melish, M.E., and Glasgow, L.A.: Site of action of exfoliative toxin in staphylococcal scalded skin syndrome, Pediatrics **50**:728, 1972.
11. Luckansen, J.R., Sabad, A., Goltz, R.W., et al.: T and B lymphocytes in atopic eczema, Arch. Dermatol. **110**:375, 1974.
12. Mandell, G.L., and Vest, T.K.: Killing of intraleukocytic *S. aureus* by rifampin, J. infect. Dis. **125**:486, 1972.
13. McCulley, J.P., and Sciallis, G.F.: Meibomian keratoconjunctivitis, Am. J. Ophthalmol. **84**:788, 1977.
14. Mudd, S., and Shayegani, M.: Delayed type hypersensitivity to *S. aureus* and its uses, Ann. N.Y. Acad. Sci. **236**:244, 1974.
15. Ostler, H.B., and Lanier, J.D.: Phlyctenular keratoconjunctivitis with special reference to the staphylococcal type, Trans. Pac. Coast Otoophthalmol. Soc. **55**:237, 1974.
16. Smolin, G., and Okumoto, M.: Staphylococcal blepharitis, Arch. Ophthalmol. **95**:812, 1977.
17. Thygeson, P.: Bacterial factors in chronic catarrhal conjunctivitis; rôle of toxin-forming staphylococci, Arch. Ophthalmol. **18**:373, 1937.
18. Thygeson, P.: The etiology and treatment of blepharitis; study in military personnel, Milit. Surg. **98**:191, 1946.
19. Thygeson, P.: Complications of *Staphylococcus* blepharitis, Am. J. Ophthalmol. **68**:446, 1969.
20. Valenton, M., and Okumoto, M.: Toxin producing strains of *Staphylococcus epidermidis*, Arch. Ophthalmol. **89**:186, 1973.
21. Warren, R., Rogolsky, M., Wiley, B.B., et al.: Effect of ethidium bromide on elimination of exfoliative toxin and bacteriocin production in *Staphylococcus aureus*, J. Bacteriol. **118**:980, 1974.

ADDITIONAL READING

Burton, J.L., and Shuster, S.: The relation between seborrhea and acne vulgaris, Br. J. Dermatol. **85**:197, 1971.

Coston, T.O.: Demodex folliculorum blepharitis, Trans. Am. Ophthalmol. Soc. **65**:361, 1967.

English, F.P., Iwamato, T., Darrell, R.W., et al.: The vector potential of *Demodex folliculorum*, Arch. Ophthalmol. **84**:83, 1970.

Frankel, R.K., Strauss, J.S., Yim Yip, S., et al.: Effect of tetracycline on the composition of sebum in acne vulgaris, N. Engl. J. Med. **273**:850, 1965.

Jones, D.B., and Robinson, N.M.: Anaerobic ocular infections, Trans. Am. Acad. Ophthalmol. Otolaryngol. **83**:309, 1977.

Keith, C.G.: Seborrheic blepharo-kerato-conjunctivitis, Trans. Ophthalmol. Soc. U.K. **87**:85, 1967.

Kligman, A.M.: An overview of acne, J. Invest. Dermatol. **62**:268, 1974.

Marples, R.R., Downing, D.T., and Kligman, A.M.: Control of free fatty acids in human surface lipids by *Corynebacterium acnes*, J. Invest. Dermatol. **59**:127, 1971.

10 Involutional changes and degenerations

Involutional changes

MORPHOLOGIC CHANGES

Advancing age frequently brings about minor alterations in the gross morphologic characteristics of the cornea, including flattening of the vertical meridian, generalized thinning that is most prominent peripherally, increased stromal relucency, and decreased transparency and luster. Histopathologically there is irregular thickening of the epithelial basement membrane and Descemet's membrane and nonspecific degeneration of stromal ground substance and collagen. Increased visibility of the corneal nerves occurs idiopathically in some elderly people.

There is little or no clinical importance to these changes, except that the vertical flattening of the cornea may require the prescription of relatively more plus cylinder at the 180-degree axis.

The aging conjunctiva undergoes changes similar to those of the cornea in that the tissue becomes thinner, less transparent, and more relucent, mainly because of atrophy in the subepithelial tissues. Looseness occurs as a result of the loss of elastic tissue, occasionally producing frank redundancy known as conjunctivochalasis. The conjunctival vessels become more prominent, particularly in the interpalpebral area, and tortuosities, varicosities, and small telangiectases may appear.

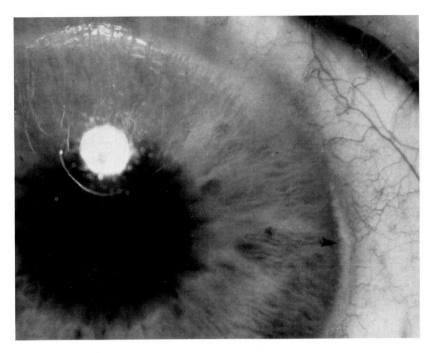

Fig. 10-1. Vogt's limbal girdle, type II. No lucid interval is seen; chalklike flecks are noted in opacity *(arrow)*.

Table 10-1. Differentiation of types I and II limbal girdles of Vogt

Type I (early calcific band keratopathy)	Type II (true Vogt's girdle)
Lucid interval	No lucid interval
Fine crystals	Chalklike flects
"Swiss-cheese holes"	No "holes"
Slightly more superficial	Slightly deeper
Rather smooth central edge	Thornlike extensions from central edge
Calcium	Elastosis
Calcium adjacent conjunctiva	Pinguecula adjacent conjunctiva

LIMBAL GIRDLE (WHITE LIMBAL GIRDLE OF VOGT) (Fig. 10-1)

Vogt's girdle is a narrow, crescentic, yellow-white line running along the nasal and temporal limbal areas of the cornea in the interpalpebral zone. It is composed of small, irregular, chalklike flecks and opacities lying immediately beneath the epithelium and is usually more prominent nasally. As described by Vogt (Table 10-1), type I is separated from the limbus by a narrow lucid interval, and type II extends to the limbus without an intervening clear zone. Other differentiating features are that type I contains tiny, round "holes" (areas of relative lucency), has a relatively sharp central edge, and is slightly more superficial in the subepithelial tissues than is type II. Along its central edge, type II has small, linear extensions that point toward the central cornea.

Type II appears to consist of elastotic degeneration of subepithelial collagen[14] such as that found in pinguecula and is considered to be the characteristic and true Vogt's girdle, whereas type I actually is thought to represent early calcific band keratopathy. The lucid interval of type I can be explained by the fact that calcium deposition ends at the termination of Bowman's membrane, still some distance from the opaque sclerolimbal junction. The elastosis of type II occurs between the end of Bowman's membrane and the sclerolimbal junction so that no lucid interval occurs.

Vogt's girdle (type II) can be found in about 60% of patients over age 40 if searched for carefully by indirect lateral illumination.[14] Its occurrence probably depends to a large extent on exposure to sunlight, as is true of pinguecula.

Vogt's girdle has no clinical significance except that it needs to be differentiated from minimal calcific band keratopathy. Perhaps the severity of the girdle can provide some insight into the degree of actinic exposure to which a patient has been subjected.

SPHEROID DEGENERATION[10] (Fig. 10-2)

This is one of many names* (Table 10-2) applied to spherical, golden-brown, translucent, droplike deposits that may be seen in the subepithelial layers of the cornea and conjunctiva.

The histopathologic composition of spheroid degeneration has long been unclear

---

*References 1, 3, 9, 11, 12.

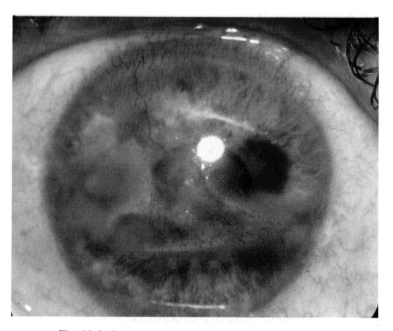

Fig. 10-2. Spheroid degeneration in bandlike distribution.

and, to some extent, controversial. Different workers[1,4,9,12] have described the material variously as being hyaline, colloid, high-tyrosine protein, lipid, keratin-like, a secretory product of abnormal fibrocytes, and elastotic degeneration of collagen. It seems clear, however, that the material is acidophilic and amorphous by light microscopy (Fig. 10-3), finely granular by electron microscopy, extracellular, and proteinaceous.

Histopathologic investigations led Garner, Morgan, and Tripathi[8] to conclude that the material represents an incomplete form of keratin and thus that it originates from the epithelium; however, Hanna and Fraunfelder[9] were of the opinion that the substance is of stromal origin, consisting of a fibrocyte-derived granular protein deposited on adjacent collagen fibrils. Both groups of workers agreed that the composition is not lipid, despite the "oil-droplet" clinical appearance. Most workers now think that the process is basically a stromal one and that epithelial involvement occurs only secondarily after destruction of Bowman's membrane.[1,9,11,12] The present weight of evidence seems to support the contention that spheroid degeneration is a type of elastotic degeneration of collagen.[1,11,12]

The clinically descriptive term of spheroid degeneration will be employed until the histopathologic nature of the disorder is finally determined. Fraunfelder, Hanna, and Parker[3,4,9] refer to three types:

Primary corneal
  Age
  Possibly heredity

Table 10-2. Various names applied to spheroid degeneration of the cornea and conjunctiva

Name	Year
Hyaline degeneration	1892
Colloid degeneration	1898
Degeneratio sphaerularis elaiodes	1935
Blindness of Dahlak	1937
Degeneratio hyaloidea granuliformis	1953
Degeneratio primaria oleoguttata centrale et superficiale	1953
Tropical dystrophy	1954
Bietti nodular dystrophy of tropical, barren lands	1955
Fisherman's keratopathy	1961
Nodular band-shaped dystrophy of tropical countries of arid soil	1962
Band-shaped nodular dystrophy	1964
Gelatinous dystrophy	1964
Labrador keratopathy	1965
Keratinoid degeneration	1970
Chronic actinic keratopathy	1972
Spheroid degeneration	1972
Bietti's degeneration	1973
Nama keratopathy	1973
Proteinaceous degeneration	1973
Climatic droplet keratopathy	1973
Elastoid degeneration	1973
Corneal elastosis	1975

Modified from Freedman, A.: Arch. Ophthalmol. **89:**193, 1973.

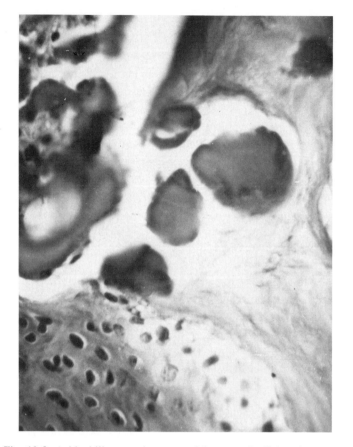

Fig. 10-3. Acidophilic amorphous material as seen by light microscopy.

Secondary corneal
  Chronic ocular diseases (glaucoma, herpes, dystrophies)
  Chronic climatic insults (possibly with hereditary influence)
Conjunctival
  Age
  Possibly actinic exposure
  With primary or secondary corneal types

The *primary corneal* type is unrelated to the coexistence of any other ocular disease but is related to advancing age and is usually bilateral. The *secondary corneal* type is a degenerative change that can occur after various long-standing ocular diseases, including glaucoma, herpetic infection, and dystrophies (especially Fuchs' endothelial dystrophy and lattice dystrophy). This type can be unilateral or bilateral depending on the location of the predisposing disease. The secondary corneal form may be caused also by chronic climatic insults. These cases are usually bilateral, can occur in young people, and are often referred to as tropical or climatic corneal degenerations. The *conjunctival* form can occur alone or with either of the corneal types. It is more common in older age groups and may be associated with pinguecula or pterygium.

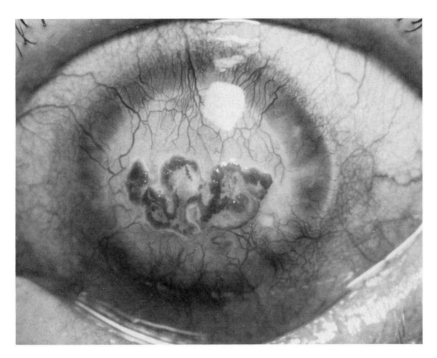

Fig. 10-4. Spheroid degeneration occurring secondarily in failed corneal graft.

Spheroid degeneration occurs almost exclusively in the interpalpebral zones of the cornea and conjunctiva, suggesting that actinic exposure plays a role in its development. The spheroids tend to be most prominent in the paralimbal areas, although the secondary corneal form is not infrequently central when that is the location of the underlying corneal disease (Fig. 10-4). Extensive spheroid degeneration, like that seen in the tropical and climatic degenerations, can extend in plaquelike fashion across the corneal center, causing serious impairment of vision (noncalcific, spheroid band keratopathy).

The spheroids are located mainly in the superficial stroma, but they may occasionally be seen in the deep stroma or within the epithelium. Clinically and histopathologically they show bright autofluorescence in the presence of ultraviolet light.

CORNEAL ARCUS (ARCUS CORNEAE, GERONTOXON, ARCUS SENILIS)

Corneal arcus is a yellow-white, hazy ring of cholesterol, cholesterol esters, phospholipids, and triglycerides in the peripheral cornea (Fig. 10-5). The deposits appear first in the inferior, and then the superior, aspect of the cornea but eventually advance to encircle the entire cornea. The lipids are found extracellularly in the corneal stroma, typically in an anvil-shaped distribution. A lucid interval occurs between the peripheral border of the arcus and the limbus. This area is free of lipid, however, only in the superficial and middle layers of the cornea, whereas the deposits extend across the limbus into the adjacent sclera at the level of Descemet's membrane. The lucid interval is attributed to the tendency for the superficial lipid deposits to end abruptly at the point of

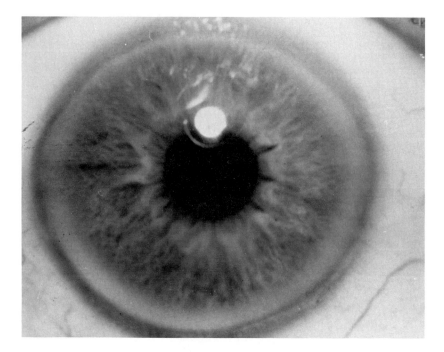

Fig. 10-5. Corneal arcus.

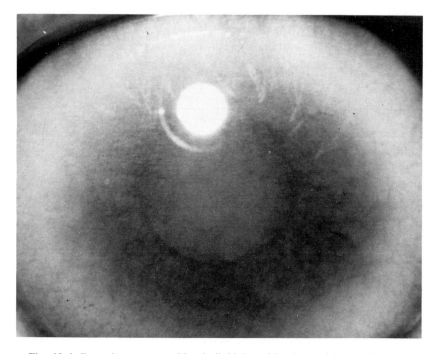

Fig. 10-6. Extensive arcus resulting in lipid deposition into axial area of cornea.

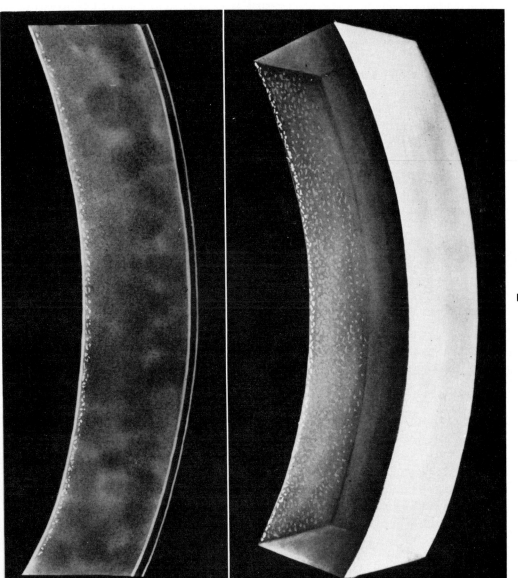

B

Fig. 10-7. A, Cornea farinata consists of punctate opacities in deep stroma as seen in parallele-piped section. These are best seen by retroillumination. **B,** Same lesion and location in optical section.

termination of Bowman's layer, but it apparently relates, in some poorly understood way, also to the presence of the limbal vasculature, since the arcus and its lucid interval can be seen to be displaced centrally in an area of abnormal corneal vascularization. On slit-lamp examination one can see numerous crisscrossing lines of relative clarity throughout the arcus, and in very early arcus these lines may be more apparent than the arcus itself. Occasionally, these lines are misdiagnosed as some obscure corneal dystrophy.

Corneal arcus generally carries no implication of systemic abnormality, although some cases are related to hypercholesterolemia (Chapter 17). Arcus as a congenital finding is discussed in Chapter 3. Most cases seem to develop simply on the basis of a genetic predisposition in combination with the effects of aging, but no specific hereditary pattern has been established. At times the arcus can be rather extensive and extend axially, at which time it probably should be classified as a lipid keratopathy (Fig. 10-6).

The term *corneal arcus* would seem to be preferable to the older *arcus senilis*, in keeping with the current trend toward avoiding the use of the word *senile* in medical terminology.

CORNEA FARINATA (Fig. 10-7)

This age-related corneal change consists of innumerable, tiny, dustlike, gray dots and flecks in the deep corneal stroma. The name *farinata* refers to the farinaceous, or flourlike, appearance of the deposits. They are classically more prominent centrally and are best seen with indirect retroillumination. The condition is usually bilateral, but unilateral cases have been reported. The deposits do not interfere with vision. Cornea farinata sometimes occurs as a familial trait.

The histopathologic characteristics of cornea farinata are unknown, but it is likely that the deposits are composed of lipofuscin,[2] a degenerative pigment that accumulates in aged cells. Lipofuscin has been found in pre-Descemet dystrophy, a condition that bears a close clinical resemblance to cornea farinata (Chapter 11). Degenerative changes that occur with age in the deep stromal collagen are decreased interfibrillar distances, breakdown of fibers, and multiple, small, collagen-free spaces. The relationship of these changes to cornea farinata is uncertain.

Cornea farinata sometimes is mistaken for cornea guttata. Careful examination of the posterior surface of the cornea by specular reflection reveals the normal endothelial mosaic pattern underlying the opacities of cornea farinata, which are smaller and more gray-white than those of cornea guttata.

DESCEMET'S STRIAE (GLASS STRIAE)

Small, linear striations in Descemet's membrane are often seen in otherwise normal corneas, perhaps more commonly in older patients.[13] The striae are finer and more subtle than those of striate keratopathy and are not large enough to cause gross irregularities of Descemet's membrane or of the posterior corneal surface. Descemet's striae are generally oriented vertically, but they may tilt slightly away from the vertical in either the nasal or the temporal direction. They have a double-walled (pipestem) configuration. They are

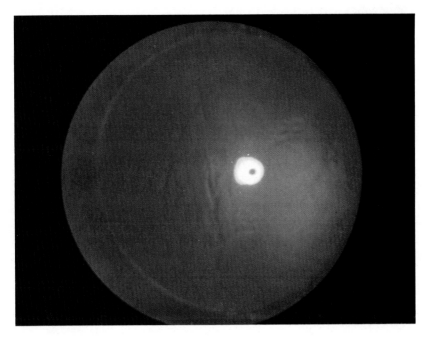

Fig. 10-8. Glassy striae or Descemet's striae are vertically oriented.

of no clinical significance except that they have been thought by some workers to be slightly more common in diabetic patients (Fig. 10-8).

HASSALL-HENLE BODIES

The basement membrane (Descemet's membrane) of the corneal endothelium is normally of rather uniform thickness except in the corneal periphery, where localized areas of overproduction are common, particularly with advancing age. These nodular thickenings are called Hassall-Henle bodies or Descemet's ''warts.'' They project toward the endothelium and are visible in the area of specular reflection as small, circular, dark areas within the normal endothelial mosaic.

Hassall-Henle bodies are histopathologically the same as the excrescences that occur in cornea guttata but are peripheral, are considered to be physiologic age changes, and are clinically harmless, whereas the excrescences are central and may be associated with endothelial decompensation and corneal edema (Chapter 11).

DELLEN (FUCHS' DIMPLES)

Dellen are localized thin spots of the cornea or sclera that occur in areas of tear film instability and dryness. The thinning is caused by water loss from the corneal stroma or sclera. Dellen are discussed more fully in Chapter 13 but are mentioned here because they may occur idiopathically in elderly people.

MOSAIC (CROCODILE) SHAGREEN

Following are types of mosaic (crocodile) shagreen:

Anterior
   Involutional
   Traumatic
   Juvenile
   Nontraumatic atrophy bulbi
Posterior
   Involutional

Anterior mosaic shagreen

In this entity the central, anterior area of each cornea develops a pattern of gray-white, polygonal opacities separated by relatively clear spaces, creating an appearance that has been likened to that of crocodile leather. Vascularization does not occur, but there may be some decrease of corneal sensation. Only rarely are the opacities dense enough to cause slightly decreased visual acuity.

Most cases of anterior mosaic shagreen are of involutional (senile) origin, although posttraumatic and juvenile forms have been described, as has a case in an eye with atrophy bulbi. The juvenile form has been reported in association with megalocornea, peripheral calcific band keratopathy, and iris malformations. The exact cause of all forms is unknown.

The polygonal areas are composed of plaques of fibrous tissue that form in areas of interruption of Bowman's layer. The deep epithelium is disrupted by the fibrous plaques, but the epithelial surface remains normal.

Anterior mosaic shagreen is not to be confused with the anterior corneal mosaic, a pattern that is demonstrable after pressure is applied to the normal, fluorescein-stained cornea.

Posterior mosaic shagreen (Fig. 10-9)

This bilateral involutional corneal change closely resembles anterior mosaic shagreen, except that it affects the deep stroma and Descemet's membrane. Gray polygonal patches, separated by dark, clear lines, are found in the deep layers of the cornea; the opacities frequently are dense enough to obscure examination by specular reflection of the underlying endothelium.

At times a subepithelial opacity is present, suggesting associated involvement of Bowman's layer. The epithelium is normal.

PINGUECULA

A pinguecula is a triangular to polygonal, gray-white to yellowish, slightly elevated nodule of degenerated conjunctiva adjacent to the limbus in the horizontal meridian. It is particularly common on the nasal side.

Histopathologically the lesion consists of a mass of subepithelial collagen that has undergone elastotic degeneration (elastosis), so named because the degenerated collagen fibrils take on the staining characteristics of elastic tissue; that the material is not elastin

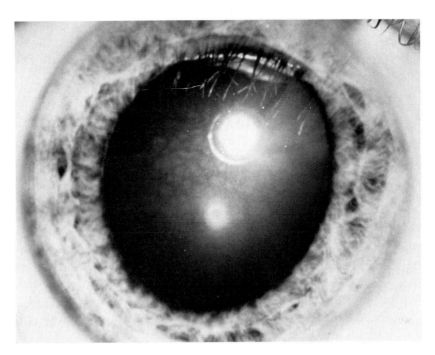

Fig. 10-9. Posterior mosaic shagreen. Gray polygonal patches are noted in deep stroma and Descemet's membrane area.

is evident from the fact that it is resistant to digestion by elastase. Microscopically the elastotic collagen fibrils are basophilic and are arranged in clumps of irregular curlicues on a background of hyaline degeneration. The overlying epithelium is usually normal or slightly thinned, but it may be thickened or even mildly dysplastic.

Elastotic degeneration of collagen is thought to be caused by the combined effects of age and exposure to sunlight, perhaps with some influence being exerted also by exposure to dust and wind. The predilection of pinguecula for the nasal aspect of the interpalpebral conjunctiva is probably related to the fact that this area of the conjunctiva is known to receive the greatest amount of ultraviolet exposure from sunlight because of reflection from the side of the nose.

Pingueculae have little clinical significance, although they have been mistaken for epithelial tumors; the two should be differentiated easily by the subepithelial location of pingueculae, their lack of staining with topical rose bengal, and their fluorescence in ultraviolet light. Conjunctival scrapings from pingueculas show essentially normal epithelial cells, whereas scrapings from epithelial tumors usually show neoplastic characteristics and some degree of keratinization. A patient sometimes first notices a pinguecula when it is rendered more conspicuous by the hyperemia of coincidental conjunctivitis or episcleritis, which makes the relatively avascular pinguecula more apparent by contrast. Rarely a pinguecula itself becomes inflamed (pingueculitis). It is not clear whether this represents an immunologic response to antigenically altered collagen or merely an incidental episcleritis in the area of the pinguecula.

Treatment other than reassurance is generally not required for pingueculae, although they can be excised easily should they become troublesome. Pingueculitis can be treated with observation only, topical steroids, or excision.

The relationship of pinguecula to pterygium is discussed later in the chapter.

OTHER INVOLUTIONAL CHANGES

On occasion one may find increased visibility of the corneal nerves in an aging cornea. The Hudson-Stähli line can be seen as an involutional change; however, this finding can be observed also as a pigmentary change in old traumatized corneas.

Degenerations

The term *degeneration* represents changes in tissue or tissue reactions related to a specific disease process. The various types of degenerations may be listed as hyaline, amyloid, lipid, and calcific degeneration. The condition can be found unilaterally or bilaterally. A family history is not associated with the problem.

In contrast the term *dystrophy* refers to bilateral disease with specific pathologic changes associated with a genetic pattern. Vascularization of the cornea does not occur in most of the dystrophies; however, in the degenerations the specific underlying disease process may be associated with vascularization of the cornea.

AMYLOID DEGENERATION (Figs. 10-10 and 10-11)

Amyloid may appear as a small, salmon-pink to yellow-white, fleshy, waxy, sometimes nodular mass or masses on the cornea or conjunctiva.

Secondary localized amyloidosis is seen on the cornea and the conjunctiva or lid after chronic ocular diseases (Figs. 10-10 and 10-11). Some of the problems causing amyloidosis of a secondary localized nature are trachoma, interstitial keratitis, uveitis, glaucoma, retrolental fibroplasia, sarcoidosis, leprosy, and keratoconus. When one sees amyloid associated with severe chronic disease of the eye, the cornea may exhibit vascularization. Amyloid exists in the eye in conditions other than degenerations. It is seen as a dystrophic element in primary localized disease such as lattice dystrophy of the cornea and gelatinous dystrophy of the cornea (Chapter 11). Systemic disease such as primary systemic amyloidosis with eye involvement is discussed in Chapter 15.

BAND-SHAPED KERATOPATHY[21] (Fig. 10-12)

Band keratopathy of calcific origin occurs from drugs, localized ocular inflammatory disease, or systemic disease causing hypercalcemia. The deposition of hydroxyapatite deposits of calcium carbamate in Bowman's layer and in the basement membrane of the epithelium and the superficial portions of the stroma is seen.[36,37] The deposits of this material will often coalesce and eventually destroy Bowman's layer. Calcific degeneration may involve all layers of the cornea as is seen in phthisis bulbi, necrotic intraocular neoplasm, and conditions in which "bone" is formed in other parts of the eye.[44]

Band keratopathy is most often seen in the interpalpebral area.[21] A lucid interval is

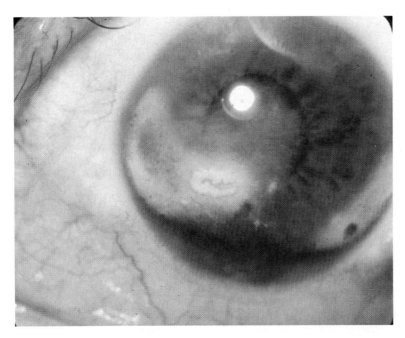

Fig. 10-10. Secondary localized amyloid in case with interstitial keratitis and band keratopathy. (Courtesy F. Wilson II, M.D., Indianapolis, Ind.)

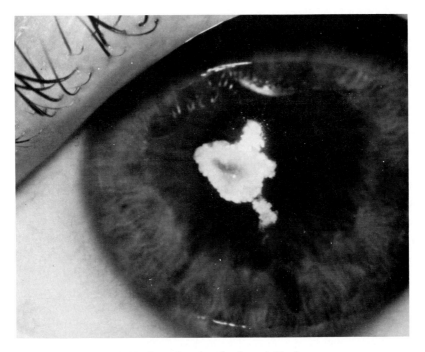

Fig. 10-11. Secondary localized amyloid of cornea.

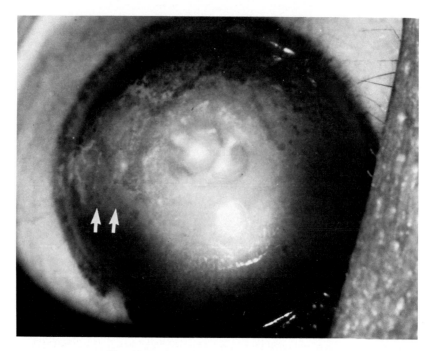

Fig. 10-12. Band keratopathy *(double arrow).*

seen between the calcific band and the limbus. The deposition of the calcium in Bowman's layer accounts for the lucid interval, since Bowman's layer does not extend to the absolute limbus. Small holes in the calcific opacity are noted throughout the band keratopathy and represent areas in which corneal nerves penetrate Bowman's layer. These small holes give a ''Swiss-cheese'' appearance to the layer on slit-lamp examination. Histologically, the earliest changes consist of a basophilic staining of the basement membrane of the epithelium, which is followed by involvement of Bowman's layer with calcium deposition and fragmentation of Bowman's layer. The calcium is deposited in extracellular fashion in local disease, whereas in systemic hypercalcemia the deposits are intercellular.

The true mechanism of calcium deposition has not been determined.[36,37] There is some laboratory evidence to associate local inflammatory reactions with hypercalcemia as a cause.[22] Uveitis may alter corneal metabolism, resulting in a rise in tissue pH and thus favoring precipitation of calcium salts.[19] The deposits of calcium salts usually take a long time, but cases of rapid deposition of calcium salts have been observed. In such instances all cases had in common aqueous tear deficiency, suggesting that with decreased tear production a higher concentration of calcium may be present, since tears contain calcium. The other factors common to all cases were exposed and inflamed corneal stroma and frequent application of artificial tears containing mercurial preservatives. It has been observed that band keratopathy can develop in individuals who use glaucoma medications containing phenylmercuric nitrate.[32] The use of the latter chemical probably results in the corneal disease, and the calcium deposits resolve on cessation of this substance. The depositions were identified histochemically as calcium. In addition, chronic exposure to mercury can result in the development of band keratopathy.[32,33]

Keratopathy, in a band form, may be seen as depositions of urate crystals in the cornea. In this instance, the band keratopathy takes on a brownish color instead of the gray-white opacity that one sees in calcific band keratopathy. Keratopathy in band form can also occur in extensive spheroid degeneration of the cornea.

Following are some of the other conditions that result in band keratopathy:

A. Hypercalcemia
    1. Sarcoidosis
    2. Fanconi's disease
    3. Still's disease (granulomatous uveitis)
    4. Hypercalcemia (uremia, parathyroid adenoma)
    5. Hypophosphatasia
    6. Multiple myeloma
    7. Discoid lupus
    8. Hyperphosphatemia
    9. Vitamin D toxicity
    10. Metastatic disease (lung and bone disease with increased calcium)
    11. Ichthyosis
B. Gout
C. Ocular disease
    1. Chronic nongranulomatous uveitis (juvenile rheumatoid arthritis)
    2. Prolonged glaucoma
    3. Long-standing corneal edema
    4. Degenerated globe
    5. Spheroid degeneration in band form
    6. Norrie's disease
D. Idiopathy
E. Toxic mercury vapors
F. Irritants, climatic or otherwise, and eyedrops containing mercurial drugs
G. Dry eye[35] with rapidly developing band keratopathy

Band keratopathy of calcific origin may be treated by the use of ethylenediamine tetraacetic acid (EDTA).* To apply EDTA, it is necessary first to instill 4% cocaine drops or other topical anesthetic into the cul-de-sac. The cocaine will facilitate the removal of the epithelium, which is necessary for the medication (EDTA) to be effective. The EDTA, a chelating agent, is dropped on a small strip of cellulose sponge that is resting on the cornea; the cellulose strip is kept moist by dropping the solution onto the sponge continuously. The surface of the cornea is scraped gently with a sterile scalpel blade; flecks of calcium come off as one continues the procedure. Patching, cycloplegics, and mild antibiotics are employed until reepithelialization has taken place.

If no EDTA is available, a simple method to employ is to scrape the cornea with a no. 15 scalpel after having instilled anesthetic drops.[43] Continue the scraping until all gritty-feeling material is removed.

---

*To prepare solution, use Endrate (Abbott Laboratories), 20 ml ampule containing 150 mg/ml. Dilute the ampule to 175 ml with water. (A 0.05 M, 1.7% solution of neutral disodium EDTA is obtained.)

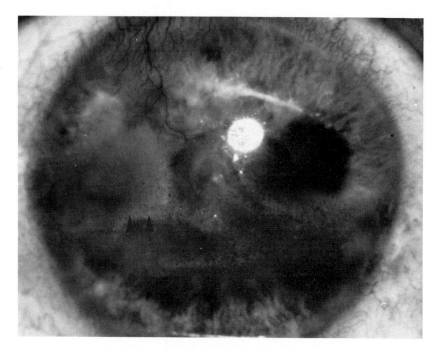

Fig. 10-13. Spheroid degeneration may occur in band-shaped form *(double arrow).*

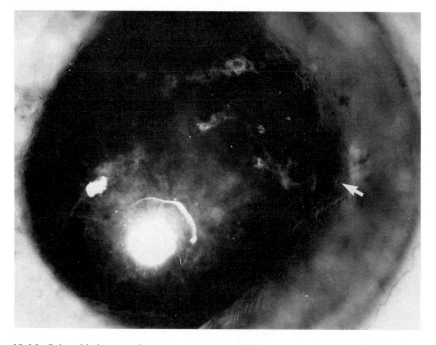

Fig. 10-14. Spheroid degeneration can occur secondarily, as seen in case of lattice dystrophy *(arrow).*

SPHEROID DEGENERATION

This degenerative condition of the cornea was discussed earlier in the chapter and has been described by many people.*

The "oil-droplet" hyaline-like deposits occur in the superficial corneal stroma, usually bilaterally, in a variety of chronic ocular or corneal disorders having in common a relationship to climate and outdoor exposure. The condition may result from the degenerative effects of chronic actinic irradiation, presumably ultraviolet radiation, or other diseases of the cornea. The degeneration is characterized by the appearance of yellow, oily droplets under the epithelium and in the anterior stroma most often seen in the 3 and 9 o'clock meridians. The droplets may replace Bowman's layer and, in very extensive conditions, form a band keratopathy (Fig. 10-13).

Spheroid degeneration may occur as a primary disease, at which time the described findings are bilateral and located in superficial corneal stroma. Secondary types can be seen unilaterally. There is usually some associated disease (Fig. 10-14) or chronic irritation in the secondary type. Spheroid degeneration has been seen in association with lattice dystrophy.

Histologically, the granules and concretions of variable size and shape are located in the superficial stroma and in and around Bowman's layer. The deposits resemble most the degenerative connective tissue of pingueculae and are considered a form of elastotic degeneration of collagen.

Electron-microscopic evidence reveals that the small, oily lesions are developed from extracellular material deposited on the collagen fiber. The extracellular material is secreted by abnormal fibrocytes and forms spheroids of collagen.[31] The deposits are periodic acid-Schiff (PAS) negative and have a fine granular structure. The degeneration is not considered keratinoid, as suggested by Garner.[29]

Both primary and secondary forms fluoresce with ultraviolet light.

A conjunctival form may be seen with primary and secondary forms and may be associated with pingueculae.

SALZMANN'S DEGENERATION

This noninflammatory condition consists of elevated bluish-white and sometimes yellow-white corneal nodules usually arranged in a circular fashion around the pupillary area (Fig. 10-15). However, these nodules may appear in any area of the cornea and at the edge of a long-standing pannus. The raised areas consist of hyaline plaques located between the epithelium and Bowman's layer, replacing Bowman's layer in most areas. The epithelium shows areas of hypertrophy and areas of atrophy with a marked increase of subepithelial basement membrane material.

Salzmann's degeneration is often associated with previous disease such as long-standing phlyctenular and trachomatous disease. It is seen in chronic luetic corneal disease as well as old viral disease. The finding of electron-dense hyaline bodies suggests a relationship between this disease and spheroidal degeneration.

---

*References 15, 16, 27-29, 31, 38, 43.

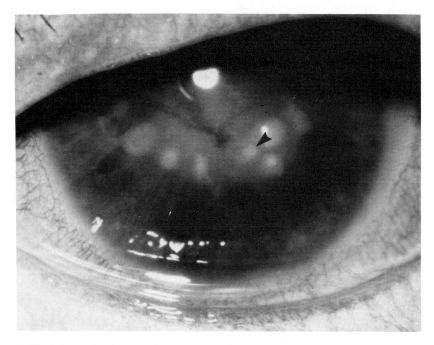

Fig. 10-15. Salzmann's degeneration is characterized by small, elevated, round, bluish-white lesions *(arrow)* in cornea.

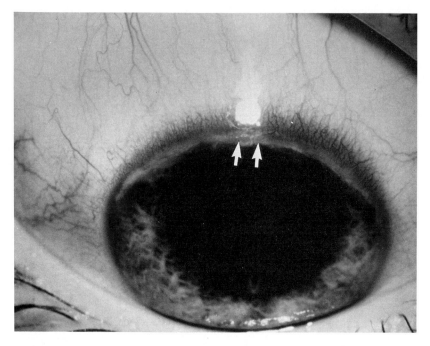

Fig. 10-16. Terrien's marginal thinning in superior aspect of cornea. Thin lipid line occurs axial to marginally thinned area *(double arrow)*.

Usually treatment is not necessary; however, if encroachment is on the pupillary area and the visual acuity is markedly decreased, a penetrating keratoplasty may be necessary.

TERRIEN'S MARGINAL DEGENERATION

This degeneration is an uncommon marginal thinning of the cornea. It is said to occur more often in older males and bilaterally. However, I have seen a number of cases that occurred in the early teens, at which time the condition was unilateral. Therefore one must expect a rather broad spectrum of findings in this degenerative condition of the peripheral cornea. The marginal opacification with superficial peripheral vascularization is a prominent feature. The peripheral cornea progresses to a marked thinning, and one can see a yellow-white line in the most axial portion of the thinned area that appears to be a lipid deposition at the advancing edge of the thin area[19,20] (Figs. 10-16 and 10-17). This is seen as a yellowish-white, small, spherical deposit in the deep layers of the in-

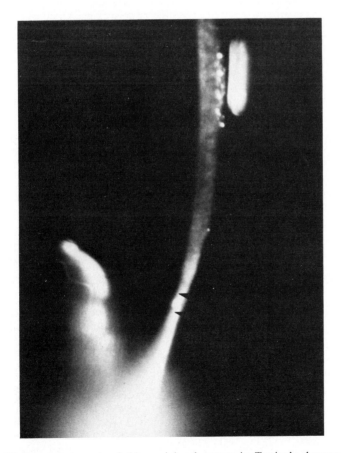

Fig. 10-17. Slit-lamp photograph of thin peripheral cornea in Terrien's degeneration *(double arrow).*

volved area. The epithelium remains intact, although slight irritation at intervals may occur. As the condition progresses, one can see a large amount of astigmatism develop because of the tilting forward of the entire cornea. Perforation, although it does not occur with any frequency, is a threat.

The cause of Terrien's marginal degeneration is unknown. An electron microscopic study of the pathologic conditions demonstrated that the collagen tissue was apparently phagocytized by histiocytic cells with a high degree of lysosomal activity. These cells penetrated the cornea along the blood vessels and caused the severe thinning.

If the thinning becomes so extreme that perforation is threatened, a reconstructive full-thickness or lamellar corneoscleral graft is necessary to alleviate the problem. These grafts must be hand-fashioned to fit the defect.

Terrien's marginal degeneration may be confused with Mooren's ulcer. The differences between these two conditions are listed in Table 10-3.[17]

Table 10-3. Comparative evaluation of Mooren's ulcer and Terrien's ulcer

Mooren's ulcer	Terrien's ulcer
Epithelial breakdown at central edge of ulcer with central progression; fluorescein stain at central edge	No fluorescein stain at central edge; no central progression; marginal and circumferential spread with thinning
Unilateral or bilateral	May be symmetrical and bilateral; may be unilateral
Mild or severe peripheral and central spread of ulcer	Peripheral, fine, yellow, white punctate stromal opacities frequently associated with corneal vascularization; deposits are lipid in nature
Severe corneal melting; destructive	Peripheral corneal gutter formation with vascularization of the base
Number of ulcers are probably on immune basis; plasma cells in conjunctival biopsies	Cause is in doubt; may be degenerative or inflammatory in origin and possible involvement of immune factors
Pain and inflammation	Recurrent and intermittent attacks of pain and inflammation
May be rapidly destructive; other mild cases may heal spontaneously	Extremely slow; starts in superior or inferior cornea; corneal ectasia and furrow formation
Perforation occurs in severe cases; severe cases treated with conjunctival resection, cryotherapy, and cytotoxic drugs	Perforation can occur; seen in 15% of cases
	Formation of pseudopterygial growth onto the cornea at oblique angles and Terrien's ulcer may occur early where thinning is not too evident; thinned areas may have to be structurally improved via grafting

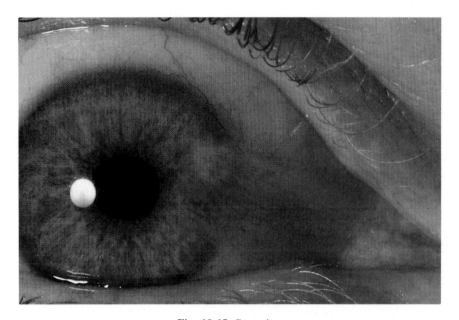

Fig. 10-18. Pterygium.

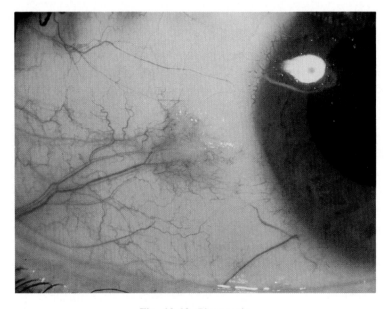

Fig. 10-19. Pinguecula.

PTERYGIUM

Pterygia are fibrovascular connective tissue overgrowths of the bulbar conjunctiva onto the cornea (Fig. 10-18). They are usually horizontally located in the palpebral fissure and on the nasal side of the cornea, but they may occur on the temporal side. An iron line called Stocker's line may be seen in advance of the pterygium head. It is believed that pterygia and pingueculae are the result of actinic degeneration from ultraviolet energy. The wearing of eyeglasses can decrease the incidence, since ultraviolet transmission is decreased. Histologically, pingueculae (Fig. 10-19) and pterygia appear to be identical except that there is no corneal involvement with pingueculae. In both instances one may see elastotic degeneration (basophilic degeneration) of the subepithelial tissue caused by breakdown of the collagen.[34,39] The subepithelial abnormal material stains for elastin but is not sensitive to elastase. In addition, one may see changes of mild dysplastic nature in the overlying epithelium as well as a dissolution of Bowman's layer in this area.

The rate of pterygium recurrence is rather high—up to 40%. The recurrence comes from the cut conjunctival edge and not from the corneal side. The most favorable type of treatment is the excision of the pterygium with recession of the conjunctiva and baring of the sclera. Attention should be paid to the area of the cornea and limbus, which should be carefully cleared of pathologic conditions so that the corneal epithelium can regenerate reasonably rapidly. The regrowth of corneal epithelium should take place before the conjunctival epithelium regrows to the area of the limbus; it will probably reduce the number of recurrences. Immediate postoperative application of strontium 90 beta radiation and another application 2 weeks later will have a tendency to reduce the number of recurrences as well. Approximately 1350 reps may be applied each time. More often than not, extensive regrowth can occur, resulting in cicatricial limitation of ocular mobility. One should adopt a conservative attitude toward minor pterygia, thereby eliminating treatment of the more bothersome recurrences. The principal reason for excising the pterygium is either the cosmetic defect that is produced by the lesion or the encroachment of the pterygium on the visual axis. Unless the pterygium is the cause of a severe cosmetic defect, there is no reason to excise a pterygium that has only reached the limbus.

Topical corticosteroids may be useful in reducing the postoperative inflammatory reaction but may have no influence on the prevention of recurrences. As has already been stated, the most popular treatment is the use of beta radiation provided by a strontium 90 applicator. Triethylenethiophosphoramide (Thiotepa) has been used topically to prevent recurrence. Allergy to the drug and permanent depigmentation of the skin of the lids are complications of this therapy. Because of this latter complication, triethylenethiophosphoramide should be used with particular caution in darkly pigmented individuals.

One must distinguish between a true pterygium and a pseudopterygium. Pseudopterygia occur with corneal ulcers or other inflammatory problems in which the conjunctiva is entrapped on the cornea. A probe can be passed beneath the conjunctiva and above the sclera, which is not possible in the case of a true pterygium.

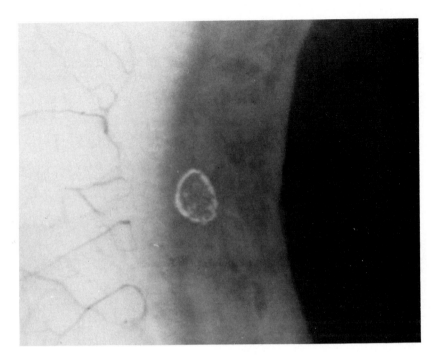

Fig. 10-20. Coats' white ring.

COATS' WHITE RING (Fig. 10-20)

This small corneal opacity is located where a previous foreign body was noted. It is a small, granular, white, oval ring noted on slit-lamp examination. The deposit contains iron.

LIPID DEGENERATION

Lipid degeneration of the cornea occurs as a primary[21,22] or secondary problem.[18,20] Secondary lipid deposition may occur in the cornea as a result of local or systemic disease. Secondary fatty degeneration in a diseased cornea or one with a history of previous trauma is not uncommon to find, especially if the cornea has become vascularized.

Lipid degeneration may occur after corneal ulceration, trauma, corneal hydrops[40] interstitial keratitis, or herpes zoster keratitis (Fig. 10-21) or late in the course of congenital aniridia.

A much less frequent occurrence is the presence of primary lipid material with no previous history of disease or vascularization in a cornea.[23] Corneal lipid infiltrates with neither a previous history of corneal disease before onset of the bilateral corneal opacification nor any evidence of trauma or other identifiable factors leading to the corneal lipid deposits can be seen.[26] Serum lipids usually are within normal limits except for a mildly elevated serum cholesterol.

In primary lipoidal degeneration of the cornea, as well as in corneal arcus,[41] phos-

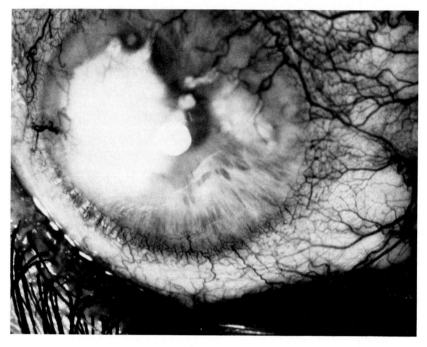

Fig. 10-21. Lipid degeneration following herpes zoster keratitis.

pholipids have been demonstrated in the presence of neutral fats and cholesterol. Fibrin can also be demonstrated in the corneal button excised at the time of keratoplasty.[41]

The opacity in lipid degeneration of the cornea usually is a dense, yellow-white opacity in the affected area of the cornea. The opacity may fan out with feathery edges from a prominent blood vessel that leads into it (Fig. 10-22). One may also see multi-colored crystals at the edge of the opacity where it is not so dense. Histologically, the material consists of cholesterol crystals, which may be present in the superficial layer or in the stroma of the cornea.

As a differential diagnosis one might consider some rare lipid changes in the cornea such as Tangier disease and lecithin cholesterol–acyltransferase deficiency. In Tangier disease the visual acuity is good, and hazy stromal infiltrates consisting of fine dots are distributed in the cornea. The plasma cholesterol is low, and the high-density lipoproteins are usually markedly deficient. In lecithin cholesterol–acyltransferase deficiency the vision is usually not affected, and a prominent corneal arcus is noted.[30] Lipoproteins of abnormal structure are seen in the plasma as well as in other tissues of the body, including the cornea.[30]

The phenomenon of the deposition of lipids in the cornea without any previous vascularization or history of trauma may occur from an excess production of lipids or the inability to metabolize them.[25] The corneoscleral limbal blood vessels may show abnormal permeability to the substances that are deposited in the cornea. This etiologic mechanism is suggested to explain the presence of corneal arcus and the sometimes poor

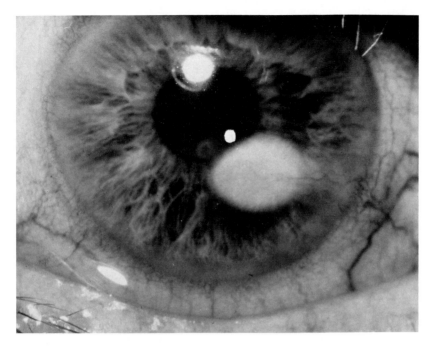

Fig. 10-22. Lipid deposit with feathery edges and central blood vessel.

correlation between corneal arcus and elevated serum lipids. It should also be remembered that the permeability of human corneoscleral limbal vessels to low-density lipoproteins, IgM, and fibrin increases with age.[41] In addition, local inflammatory processes associated with corneoscleral and limbal microvascular changes may account for the lipid deposits in some cases.[26,41]

REFERENCES
Involutional changes

1. Brownstein, S., Rodrigues, M.M., Fine, B.S., and Albert, E.N.: The elastotic nature of hyaline corneal deposits: a histochemical fluorescent, and electron microscopic examination, Am. J. Ophthalmol. **75:**799, 1973.
2. Curran, R.E., Kenyon, K.R., and Green, W.R.: Pre-Descemet's membrane corneal dystrophy, Am. J. Ophthalmol. **77:**711, 1974.
3. Fraunfelder, F.T., and Hanna, C.: Spheroid degeneration of the cornea and conjunctiva. III. Incidences, classification and etiology, Am. J. Ophthalmol. **76:**41, 1973.
4. Fraunfelder, F.T., Hanna, C., and Parker, J.M.: Spheroid degeneration of the cornea and conjunctiva. I. Clinical course and characteristics, Am. J. Ophthalmol. **74:**821, 1972.
5. Freedman, A.: Climatic droplet keratopathy. I.

Clinical aspects, Arch. Ophthalmol. **89:**193, 1973.
6. Freedman, J.: Nama keratopathy, Br. J. Ophthalmol. **57:**688, 1973.
7. Garner, A.: Keratinoid corneal degeneration, Br. J. Ophthalmol. **54:**769, 1970.
8. Garner, A., Morgan, G., and Tripathi, R.C.: Climatic droplet keratopathy. II. Pathologic findings, Arch. Ophthalmol. **89:**198, 1973.
9. Hanna, C., and Fraunfelder, F.T.: Spheroid degeneration of the cornea and conjunctiva. II. Pathology, Am. J. Ophthalmol. **74:**829, 1972.
10. Johnson, G.T.: Etiology of spheroidal degeneration of the cornea in Labrador, Br. J. Ophthalmol. **65:**270, 1981.
11. Klintworth, G.K.: Chronic actinic keratopathy: a condition associated with conjunctival elastosis (pingueculae) and typified by characteristic extracellular concretions, Am. J. Pathol. **67:**327, 1972.

12. Rodrigues, M.M., Laibson, P.R., and Weinreb, S.: Corneal elastosis: appearance of band-like keratopathy and spheroidal degeneration, Arch. Ophthalmol. **93**:111, 1975.
13. Sturrock G.: Glassy corneal striae, Albrecht von Graefes Arch. Klin. Ophthalmol. **188**:245, 1973.
14. Sugar, S.H., and Kobernick, S.: The white limbal girdle of Vogt, Am. J. Ophthalmol. **50**:101, 1960.

Degenerations

15. Ahmad, A., Hogan, M., Wood, I., and Ostler, H.B.: Climatic droplet keratopathy in a 16-year-old boy, Arch. Ophthalmol. **95**:149, 1977.
16. Anderson, J., and Fuglsang, H.: Droplet degeneration of the cornea in North Cameroor: prevalence and clinical appearance, Br. J. Ophthalmol. **60**:256, 1976.
17. Austin, P., and Brown, S.I.: Inflammatory Terrien's marginal corneal disease, Am. J. Ophthalmol. **92**:189, 1981.
18. Andrews, J.S.: The lipids of arcus senilis, Arch. Ophthalmol. **68**:264, 1962.
19. Doughman, D.J., Olson, G.A., Nolan, S., and Hajny, R.G.: Experimental band keratopathy, Arch. Ophthalmol. **81**:264, 1969.
20. Duke-Elder, S., and Leigh, A.G.: Cornea and sclera. In Duke-Elder, S., editor: System of ophthalmology, vol. 8. Diseases of the outer eye, pt. 2, St. Louis, 1965, The C.V. Mosby Co.
21. Duke-Elder, S., and Leigh, A.G.: Cornea and sclera. In Duke-Elder, W.S., editor: System of ophthalmology, vol. 8. Diseases of the outer eye, pt. 2, London, 1965, Henry Kimpton.
22. Economon, J.W., Silverstein, A.M., and Zimmerman, L.E.: Band keratopathy in a rabbit colony, Invest. Ophthal. **2**:361, 1963.
23. Fine, B.S., Townsend, W.M., and Zimmerman, L.E.: Primary lipoidal degeneration of the cornea, Am. J. Ophthalmol. **78**:12, 1974.
24. Forstat, S.L., and Gassett, A.R.: Transient traumatic posterior annular keratopathy of Payrau, Arch. Ophthalmol. **92**:527, 1974.
25. Fredrickson, D.S.: Hereditary systemic diseases of metabolism that affect the eye. In Mausolf, F.A., editor: The eye and systemic disease, ed. 2, St. Louis, 1980, The C.V. Mosby Co.
26. Freedlaender, M.H., Cavanaugh, H.D., Sullivan, W.R., et al.: Bilateral central lipid infiltrates of the cornea, Am. J. Ophthalmol. **84**:781, 1977.
27. Freedman, A.: Climatic droplet keratopathy. I. Clinical aspects, Arch. Ophthalmol. **89**:193, 1973.
28. Freedman, J.: Nama keratopathy, Br. J. Ophthalmol. **57**:688, 1973.
29. Garner, A., Morgan, G., and Tripathi, R.: Climatic droplet keratopathy. II. Pathologic findings, Arch. Ophthalmol. **89**:198, 1973.
30. Gjone, E., and Bergaust, B.: Corneal opacity in familial plasma cholesterol ester deficiency, Acta Ophthalmol. **47**:222, 1969.
31. Johnson, G.J., and Ghosh, M.: Labrador keratopathy: clinical and pathological findings, Can. J. Ophthalmol. **10**:119, 1975.
32. Kennedy, R.E., Roca, P.D., and Landers, P.H.: Atypical band keratopathy in glaucomatous patients, Am. J. Ophthalmol. **72**:917, 1971.
33. Kennedy, R.E., Roca, P.D., and Platt, D.S.: Further observations on atypical band keratopathy in glaucomatous patients, Trans. Am. Ophthalmol. Soc. **72**:107, 1974.
34. Klintworth, G.K.: Chronic actinic keratopathy—a condition associated with conjunctival elastosis (pingueculae) and typified by characteristic extracellular concretions, Am. J. Pathol. **67**:32, 1972.
35. Lemp, M.A., and Ralph, R.A.: Rapid development of band keratopathy in dry eyes, Am. J. Ophthalmol. **83**:657, 1977.
36. O'Connor, R.G.: Calcific band keratopathy, Trans. Am. Ophthalmol. Soc. **70**:58, 1972.
37. Pouliquen, Y.: Ultrastructure of band keratopathy, Arch. Ophthalmol. **27**:149, 1967.
38. Rodger, F.C.: Clinical findings, course, progress of Bietti's corneal degeneration in the Dahlak Islands, Br. J. Ophthalmol. **57**:657, 1973.
39. Rodrigues, M.M., Laibson, P.R., and Weinreb, S.: Corneal elastosis. Appearance of band-like keratopathy and spheroidal degeneration, Arch. Ophthalmol. **93**:111, 1975.
40. Shapiro, L.A., and Farkas, T.G.: Lipid keratopathy following corneal hydrops, Arch. Ophthalmol. **95**:456, 1977.
41. Walton, K.W.: Studies on the pathogenesis of corneal arcus formation, J. Pathol. **111**:263, 1973.
42. Wood, T.O., and Walker, G.G.: Treatment of band keratopathy, Am. J. Ophthalmol. **80**:553, 1975.
43. Young, J.D.H., and Finlay, R.D.: Primary spheroidal degenerations of the cornea in Labrador and Northern Newfoundland, Am. J. Ophthalmol. **79**:129, 1975.
44. Zeiter, H.J.: Calcification and ossification in ocular tissue, Am. J. Ophthalmol. **53**:265, 1962.

CHAPTER

11 Dystrophies

Although a dystrophy may manifest itself at birth, it is often seen initially in the first or second decade of life. Dystrophies exhibit a hereditary pattern, are bilateral, and may be progressive. Often the etiologic agent is unknown. Involvement of the cornea can affect the anterior limiting membrane, Bowman's layer, the corneal stroma, and the posterior limiting membrane area. The dystrophies can be identified clinically by the morphologic characteristics and distribution of the abnormal material; they may be identified individually by the specific histopathologic and histochemical characteristics of the deposited substances.

Dystrophies of the epithelium and Bowman's layer

The epithelium of the cornea consists of five to six layers of cells. The basal cells produce and also rest on the basement membrane, which is PAS positive. The basal cells of the epithelium and the basement membrane are connected by desmosomes. The surface of the epithelium exhibits fingerlike projections (microvilli and microplicae) that serve to increase the epithelial surface and to stabilize the adherence of the tear film (mucin layer). Bowman's layer is actually part of the corneal stroma and is made up of collagen fibers that are somewhat irregularly distributed. This layer is in intimate contact with the basement membrane anterior and with the remainder of the corneal stroma posteriorly.

Anterior corneal dystrophies affect the epithelium, the basement membrane, and Bowman's layer (Table 11-1). Primary involvement of any one of these layers frequently leads to, or is accompanied by, changes in the other two layers, so that exact classification as to level of involvement often is difficult and arbitrary.

EPITHELIUM AND BASEMENT MEMBRANE DYSTROPHIES

Dystrophies that affect primarily the epithelium and basement membrane include the following:
1. Meesmann's dystrophy
2. Cogan's dystrophy (map-dot-fingerprint dystrophy)
3. Dystrophic recurrent erosions

Meesmann's dystrophy (juvenile epithelial corneal dystrophy)

Meesmann's dystrophy is a rare, bilateral, symmetrical, familial corneal disease that begins early in life. Epithelial vesicles, which may be seen as early as 6 months of age, tend to increase with age. Meesmann's dystrophy is inherited as an autosomal dominant trait with incomplete penetrance.[32,35,36,40]

This epithelial dystrophy may be accompanied by symptoms of lacrimation, photophobia, and irritation of the eye in middle age. The discomfort is caused by rupture of microcysts onto the epithelial surface. Visual acuity, in most instances, remains good, but corneal surface irregularity and some opacification, which occurs in older patients, can produce some decrease in vision.

The small bleblike lesions in epithelium appear in direct focal illumination as small, white-gray, punctate opacities that are diffusely distributed over the corneal surface

Table 11-1. Epithelial and Bowman's layer dystrophies

Dystrophy	Vision	Inheritance	Manifestation	Pathologic features
Meesmann's	Not usually affected but may decrease	Dominant	Childhood	Intraepithelial cysts that contain cellular debris PAS-positive material within epithelial cells and in basement membrane zone
Recurrent erosions	Reduced if in pupillary area	May show dominant trait, but most are acquired	Seen in childhood and adult life	Defect in epithelial basement membrane and in hemidesmosome formation, resulting in epithelial loss, microcysts, and bullae
Map-dot-fingerprint	Reduced	None	Adulthood	Debris containing intraepithelial cysts Insinuation of basement membrane and collagen intraepithelially accounting for fingerprint and map appearance Recurring epithelial erosions
Bleblike	Usually not affected	Dominant	Adulthood	Fibrillogranular material between basement membrane and Bowman's layer No micropseudocysts visible
Reis-Bücklers'	Reduced	Dominant	Childhood	Abnormal Bowman's layer Replacement of Bowman's layer with abnormal collagen fibers Degenerative anterior stroma and keratocytes in anterior layers of the cornea Recurrent epithelial erosions
Grayson-Wilbrandt	Reduced	Dominant	Adolescence	PAS-positive material in abnormal amounts in basement membrane zone extend in undulating fashion into epithelium Erosions of epithelium
Honeycomb	Reduced	Dominant	Childhood	May be variant of Reis-Bücklers' dystrophy
Inherited band keratopathy	Can be reduced	Dominant	Adulthood	Calcific deposition in basement membrane and in Bowman's layer
Anterior crocodile shagreen	Not usually affected	None	Adulthood	Anterior polygonal opacities seen as involutional change
Local mucopolysaccharide accumulation	May be reduced	None	Infants	Bilateral diffuse clouding caused by acid mucopolysaccharide in Bowman's layer

to the limbus but are more pronounced in the interpalpebral zone (Fig. 11-1). On retro-illumination, the opacities appear as clear, spherical vesicles that are regular in size and shape. The intervening epithelium is clear. Rarely, unusual forms may be seen such as a whorllike pattern at the level of Bowman's layer and peripheral limbal lesions or focal, wedge-shaped lesions.[50] Some opacities may stain with fluorescein and rose bengal dyes.[7,50] The corneal sensation may be reduced.

Histopathologically, the epithelial layer may vary in thickness; in addition, the epithelial cells are disorganized with poor maturation from basal layer to surface. PAS-positive, debris-containing cysts appear primarily within the anterior epithelium, and autofluorescence is noted. The cysts, which are the vesicles seen with retroillumination on slit-lamp examination, occur throughout the epithelial layer, and some may open to the surface of the cornea. The amorphous material within the cysts, which stains positively with alcian blue and with colloidal iron, demonstrating the presence of glycosamino-glycans, may result from degenerating epithelial cells. In one study, the most anterior portion of a thick epithelial basement membrane, as well as the adjacent region of Bowman's layer, also stained for acid mucopolysaccharides.[17] Bowman's layer, stroma, endothelium, and Descemet's membrane otherwise appear normal. The basement membrane appears thick and may show small fingerlike projections extending into the basal epithelium, possibly representative of increased epithelial activity.[17]

A material called *peculiar substance* is apparent by electron microscopy and is de-

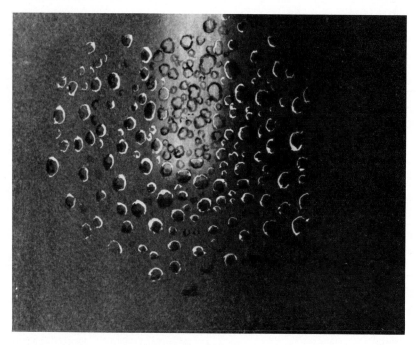

Fig. 11-1. Meesmann's dystrophy. Bleblike lesions are seen on retroillumination but appear as gray round opacities on direct illumination with slit lamp. (From Grayson, M., and Keates, R.H.: Manual of diseases of the cornea, Boston, 1969, Little, Brown & Co.)

scribed as a mass of fibrillogranular material intermixed with cytoplasmic filaments.[10, 17] This peculiar substance is considered a characteristic structural change within the cytoplasm of the basal epithelial cells in this dystrophy. A vacuolated, homogeneous substance also appears within the epithelial cysts.[17] In addition, as noted, production of the thick basement membrane is dependent on altered epithelial cells and so is not specific. Increased glycogen in the basal cells as is seen in some cases does not correlate with the presence of peculiar substance and may be caused by the rapid turnover of cells.[13] It appears to be a nonspecific change.[10, 13] In some instances electron-dense bodies occur in the basal epithelial cells and appear similar to lysosomes.[38] These bodies are engulfed by vacuoles in the more superficial layers of the cornea. The vacuoles increase in number until they result in destruction of cells.[38]

It is helpful in making a diagnosis of Meesman's dystrophy to establish the familial nature of the disease, since a similar corneal picture can be produced by other conditions, including vernal conjunctivitis, meibomian gland disease, insensitive cornea, reduced tear production and healing erosions,[4] mild epithelial edema, and bleb pattern of epithelial basement membrane dystrophy.

Treatment. Treatment is often unnecessary. Lamellar or penetrating keratoplasty develops the disease in the epithelium. Epithelial débridement is of little value, since recurrence of the epithelial pathologic condition occurs. It is claimed that superficial keratectomy results in reepithelialization without recurrence of epithelial disease.[13]

Recurrent erosions

Recurrent corneal erosions are associated with defects in adherence of the epithelial cells to the underlying basement membrane. The adherence of the basal cells to the basement membrane is enhanced by the presence of numerous hemidesmosomes[30] (Fig. 11-2).

When repeated instances of nonadherence occur, the patient experiences pain, photophobia, tearing, and foreign body sensation.[12]

By far the majority of cases of recurrent erosion are caused by corneal injury from fingernails and paper.[11]

Acquired recurrent erosions, in addition to the trauma from fingernails or paper, are observed also after photocoagulation or vitrectomy[34] and secondary to other corneal dystrophies (lattice, Fuchs', and anterior membrane dystrophies[8]), alkali burns, foreign bodies with concretion, postinfectious ulcer from herpes simplex, exposure, and Cockayne's syndrome.[2]

Familial erosions are usually seen as a bilateral problem, occurring primarily in women.[52] The epithelium may exhibit a "slipped-rug" appearance; often filaments are seen. The recurrent erosions may occur over multiple sites on the cornea, a situation different from traumatic erosions.

Attacks of pain and ocular irritation usually occur in the early morning hours or on awakening, which seems plausible, since corneal hydration from lid closure may be a factor affecting epithelial adhesion. An abnormal adherence between lid and cornea during sleep may be a factor in setting the stage for an attack of epithelial erosion. During an acute attack one may see epithelial loss, epithelial microcysts, bullae, lack of adherence of sheets of epithelium, and epithelial filament formation. In these instances the visual acuity may be severely impaired if the pathologic condition occurs in the pupillary area.

Recurrences affect the area of the cornea previously injured. In the interval between attacks one can, on slit-lamp examination, detect epithelial cysts, surface irregularity, and some subepithelial scarring.[49,52] The healed epithelial area may even resemble a dendritic figure, a pseudodendrite. This fact should be kept in mind to avoid prescribing unnecessary medication.

The epithelial basement membrane is a most important factor in the adhesion of regenerating epithelium. If the basement membrane and superficial stroma are intact, the regenerating epithelium will require only a few days to demonstrate its adhesion. If not, it may take the basement membrane and hemidesmosomes several months to regenerate. If the basal cells of the epithelium do not adhere because of lack of regenerating basement membrane or associated hemidesmosomes or because of the presence of abnormal basement membrane, the epithelial cells will "rub" off, and the clinical picture of erosion will occur.[20,29,30]

It has been suggested that corneal erosions may be associated with an immunologic etiologic agent in some cases.[37] Tissue-fixed antibodies to complement have been demonstrated by direct immunofluorescence in conjunctival epithelium. Circulating antibodies to normal corneal and conjunctival epithelium were demonstrated in the patient's serum by the indirect immunofluorescence technique; the titer of circulating antibodies was found to correlate with the disease activity.[37] This concept has yet to be verified.

It has also been suggested that catecholamines and prostaglandins, which increase the cyclic AMP intracellularly, reduce the mitotic activity, cell locomotion, and cell glycogen. An increase in the cyclic guanine monophosphate has the opposite effect. This interesting finding may influence healing of corneal erosions; however, the clinical application and significance in treatment of persistent epithelial defects must still be established.[11]

Treatment. The treatment of recurrent corneal erosion is directed toward reestablishment of a normal basement membrane and toward securing tight adhesion of the epithelium to the basement membrane through normal junction complexes. Pressure patching may be tried for several days to encourage epithelial regeneration; when this is established, 5% sodium chloride ointment may be used. This hyperosmotic agent will dehydrate the epithelium and also help reduce friction between the lids and the cornea. This should be continued for as long as 4 to 6 months three times a day after the last episode. In addition, therapy with topical colloidal dextran (Dehydrex) polysaccharide solution (pH 7.0, 280 to 310 mOsm) may be tried. It is given five times a day and before sleep. Treatment is continued for 3 months.[19] Cycloplegics may be used in an acute case to reduce ciliary spasm and pain; topical antibiotic drops may be used to minimize the possibility of infection. It may be necessary to remove loose epithelium. A big flap of loose epithelium must be removed, followed by patching. In resistant cases, a therapeutic soft lens will aid in alleviating the pain and will promote epithelial healing. The contact lens is kept in place for 1 to 2 months before cleansing it and is continued for a total of at least 6 months.

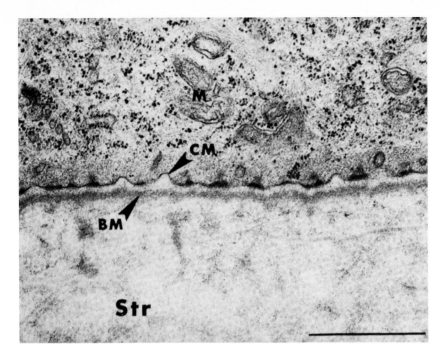

Fig. 11-2. Adherence of basal cells of epithelium *(CM)* to basement membrane *(BM)* is enhanced by presence of hemidesmosomes. *M*, Mitochondria; *Str*, stroma. (From Khodadoust, A.A., Silverstein, A.M., Kenyon, K.R., and Dowling, J.E.: Am. J. Ophthalmol. **65:**339, 1968.)

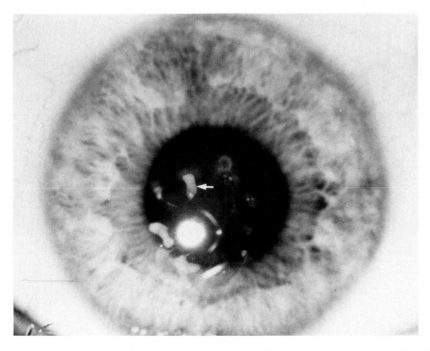

Fig. 11-3. Cogan's microcystic dystrophy. Typical puttylike lesions *(arrow)* and maplike lines are noted in epithelium.

Map-dot-fingerprint dystrophy

Map, dot, and fingerprint dystrophy (also called Cogan's microcystic epithelial dystrophy and anterior basement membrane dystrophy) is considered to be a nonhereditary, bilateral, epithelial dystrophy of the cornea.* However, an autosomal dominant pattern can, in some instances, be demonstrated.[33] It occurs in adults, perhaps slightly more frequently in women; the majority of patients are between the ages of 40 and 70 years.

Dots. Dotlike opacities appear as gray-white intraepithelial opacities that may be round, oblong, or comma shaped (Fig. 11-3). With focal illumination the dot opacities have the appearance of deposits of putty. They may occur in the pupillary zone, which may result in a decrease in vision, or in the periphery without any alteration in acuity. Fluorescein may stain the superficial pseudomicrocysts. The dots, in addition to being larger and puttylike, may also be small, fine, closely clustered, and clear. The latter are best seen on retroillumination. Another pattern in net form consists of rows of blebs. Blebs and nets, when seen with maps or fingerprints, are associated with erosions.

Usually there are no symptoms, but corneal erosions can occur; the patient may

---

*References 13, 14, 31, 51, 54.

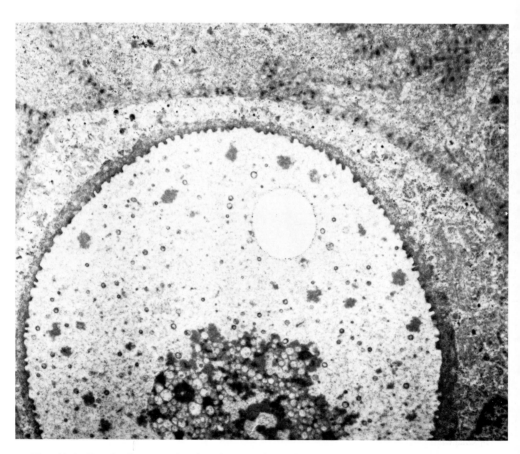

Fig. 11-4. Pseudomicrocyst showing degenerating cell. Pyknotic nucleus and cellular debris are seen. Cyst wall is created by normal border of neighboring cell.

then complain of foreign body sensation, pain, and photophobia. The areas of erosion stain with fluorescein.[7,13]

The gray-white opacities correspond to epithelial microcysts (pseudocysts). The epithelial cells posterior to an extension of aberrant intraepithelial basement membrane may become insinuated in the middle zone of the epithelium and then degenerate and contribute to the formation of microcysts. These microcysts (pseudocysts) (Fig. 11-4) contain pyknotic nuclei and cellular debris with no visible lining. The cyst wall is created by the normal border of the neighboring cell. The cysts may spontaneously discharge onto the corneal surface and thus disappear,[42] but when they open to the corneal surface, they produce an erosion. Epithelial cells adjacent to the normal basement membrane remain normal, whereas those adjacent to aberrant basement membrane become vacuolized and liquified. Epithelial cells superficial to the aberrant membrane have a normal appearance. Anomalous basement membrane deficient in hemidesmosomes, together with abnormal attachments of basal epithelium to Bowman's membrane, may result in corneal erosions.[12] Small epithelial dots are noted also on retroillumination in healing recurrent epithelial erosions.

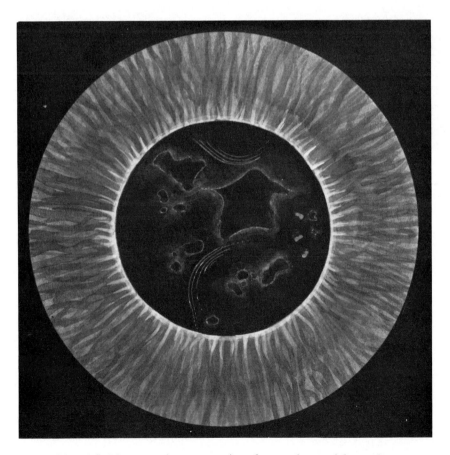

Fig. 11-5. Diagrammatic representation of maps, dots, and fingerprints.

245 of the cornea

Fingerprints. Fingerprint changes may occur in combination with dotlike or maplike changes* (Fig. 11-5). The "fingerprints" are concentric, contoured lines that may occur in any area of the cornea. The fingerprint lines are formed by subepithelial sheets of fibrillogranular material plus basement membrane.[3]

The finding of fingerprints was at one time thought to be a rare occurrence, but careful slit-lamp examination reveals that this is not so. Similar findings may be seen as a secondary problem in Fuchs' dystrophy. Fingerprint dystrophy is usually asymptomatic.[3] However, occasionally an eye may be irritated because of epithelial erosions of the

---

*References 3, 5, 13, 14, 27, 42, 46.

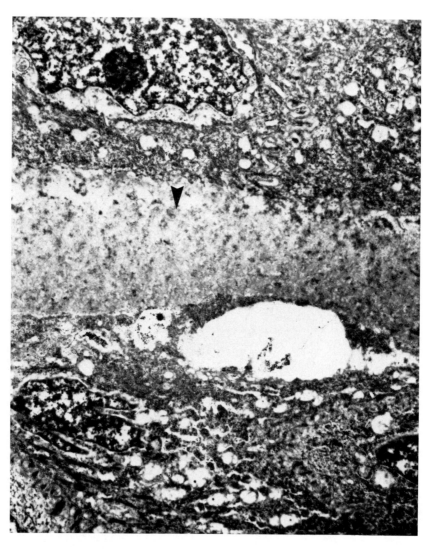

Fig. 11-6. Electron microscopic study showing insinuation of basement membrane substance *(arrow)* between epithelial cells in case of map-dot-fingerprint dystrophy.

cornea. Irregular astigmatic changes may occasionally result in decreased visual acuity.[4] The fingerprints, as with microcysts, are seen best against the red fundus reflex with a dilated pupil or on retroillumination with the slit-lamp beam reflected off the iris.

Map. In addition to the more orderly fingerprint designs, which are related to reduplication and thickening of the basement membrane, and deposits of fibrillogranular material extending below the epithelium, irregular geographic designs are distributed throughout the epithelium[4,14,46] (Fig. 11-5). These appear as gray-white, interlacing lines resembling the architecture of a map. These opacities may be diffuse gray patches containing clear areas and may be extensive or slight. The maplike changes are probably related to proliferation of collagen material into the corneal epithelium,[46] resulting in a thick basement membrane extending into the epithelium as multilaminar sheets, 2 to 6 μm in thickness (Fig. 11-6). Hemidesmosomes are not formed in epithelial cells that are adjacent to this abnormal intraepithelial basement membrane.

Treatment. Removal of the diseased corneal epithelium in patients who exhibit epithelial erosion, followed by tight patching, may in some cases be effective treatment. If these efforts do not help, a soft lens may be prescribed. Treatment of erosions was described previously.

Summary. The major problems in the foregoing group of anterior basement membrane dystrophies are (1) the formation of pseudomicrocysts; (2) the thick abnormal basement membrane, which is PAS positive and AMP negative; (3) the accumulation of fibrillogranular material between the epithelial basement membrane and Bowman's layer.* The erosions result from the presence of abnormal basement membrane and lack of hemidesmosomal attachments of the epithelium. There is insinuation of epithelial cells beneath the sheets of basement membrane and fibrillogranular material so that normal maturation is interfered with and results in the formation of the micropseudocysts.

In addition, it has been suggested[16] that fingerprint/bleb dystrophy and Cogan's dystrophy are separate entities entirely, based on histochemical and ultrastructural findings. However, they probably should be considered as a spectrum of the same disease entity.

Bleblike dystrophy

Other dotlike lesions that appear in the epithelium are fine, clear, round blebs seen on retroillumination. This bleb pattern may also be associated with another pattern called *nets,* which follows the anterior corneal mosaic and consists of rows of blebs.[6,7] These nets do not result in erosions per se, but when they occur with maps and fingerprints, one may see erosions. The blebs are formed by the accumulation of fibrillogranular material between the basement membrane and Bowman's layer,[15] which indents the basal epithelium, resulting in the slit-lamp appearance. The blebs do not represent pseudomicrocysts.

BOWMAN'S LAYER DYSTROPHIES

Dystrophies that affect Bowman's layer include the following:

1. Reis-Bücklers' dystrophy
2. Grayson-Wilbrandt dystrophy
3. Anterior crocodile shagreen (mosaic dystrophy)
4. Hereditary calcific band keratopathy

---

*References 3, 13, 18, 46, 49, 54.

Reis-Bücklers' corneal dystrophy

This dystrophy is transmitted as an autosomal dominant trait with strong penetrance.[9,25,43,44] It is bilateral and symmetrical. The corneal disease is discernible in early childhood; symptoms usually begin about 5 years of age, with recurring attacks of erosion resulting in photophobia, foreign body sensation, injection, and pain lasting for several weeks. The cornea becomes progressively more cloudy with superficial, reticu-

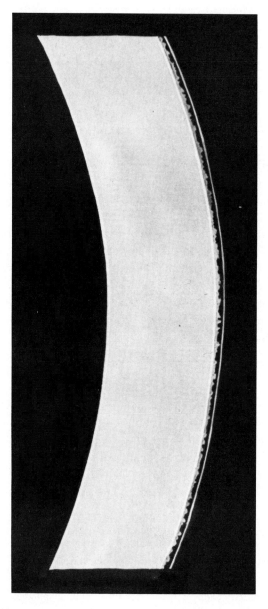

Fig. 11-7. Peaklike projections from area of Bowman's layer extend into epithelium.

lated, gray-white opacities and epithelial defects.[41] The opacities are diffuse and geographic in nature at the level of Bowman's layer, with peaklike projections into the epithelial layer (Fig. 11-7). The corneal surface is rough and irregular with a loss of transparency, producing an irregular astigmatism. The opacities may take on various sizes and shapes and be crescent or ringlike figures, all of which are interwoven into a geographic-like surface[25,43] (Fig. 11-8). The extreme periphery of the cornea remains transparent, whereas dense opacities occur more in the midperiphery. The epithelial breakdown seems to subside later in life since Bowman's layer is replaced by scar tissue. Vision deteriorates during the twenties. Corneal sensation is decreased, and no vascularization is noted.[23,24]

Degenerative changes occur in the basal epithelial cells, and the basement membrane may be irregularly present, but the main pathologic condition is found in Bowman's layer.[22,26,53] Bowman's layer is absent in many areas and is replaced by fibrocellular connective tissue[1,22,24,44] (Fig. 11-9). Similar material projects into the epithelium.[1] Such intraepithelial projections, together with variations in subepithelial scar tissue, account for the clinical appearance of the corneal opacity. When Bowman's layer is absent, there are no hemidesmosomes or basement membrane; thus the faulty epithelial adherence accounts for the recurrent erosions seen in this disease.[1] Numerous superficial keratocytes in varying stages of activity are found in the collagenous material.

It is likely that the primary and basic problems are in the superficial keratocytes that produce abnormal fibrils and replace Bowman's layer with secondary epithelial injury. It is possible, however, that the changes resulting from epithelial breakdown result in activation of stromal cells, and thus absorption of Bowman's layer ensues.[1] In addition, the fibrocellular material may involve the anterior stroma. This finding may correspond to the stromal opacity noted in most advanced cases.[1,53]

The posterior stroma, Descemet's membrane, and endothelium do not exhibit any disease.

Treatment. The management of the erosions is similar to that already described and includes hyperosmotic drops during the day, hyperosmotic ointment at bedtime, a pressure patch, and if necessary, a thin, loosely fitting, soft contact lens with a high degree of gas permeability.

Lamellar and penetrating keratoplasty can be done, but the superficial opacities may recur in the graft.[22,23,25,39] A superficial keratectomy may offer some help.[22,26] Removal of the subepithelial fibrous tissue by blunt dissection may be an effective technique and may eliminate the necessity for a penetrating graft.[55]

Anterior membrane dystrophy (Grayson-Wilbrandt)[21]

A clinical picture resembling Reis-Bücklers' dystrophy, but with some differences, has been reported.[21] The onset of the disease in these cases did not occur until 10 to 11 years of age, and the pathologic condition was mostly confined to the basement membrane. Episodes of injection and pain are infrequent. Irregular epithelial surfaces may account for some patients exhibiting a visual acuity of 20/200. Corneal sensation is normal.

Slit-lamp examination exhibits opacities with a gray-white, macular appearance in

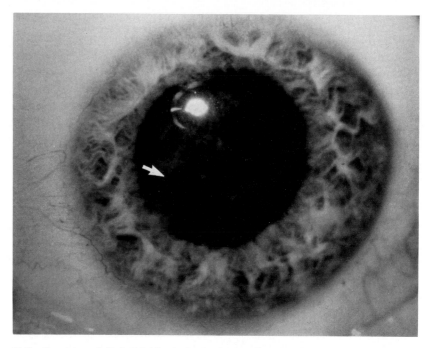

Fig. 11-8. Opacities of Reis-Bücklers' dystrophy are interwoven ringlike figures making up geographic pattern *(arrow)*.

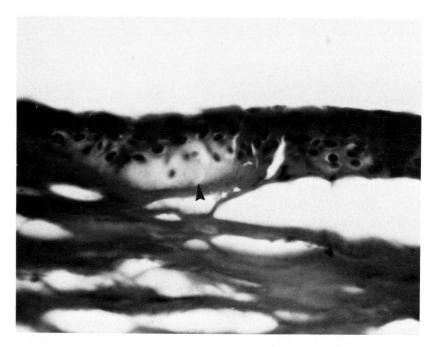

Fig. 11-9. Bowman's layer is absent in some areas and replaced by fibrocellular connective tissue *(arrow)*. (From Grayson, M.: Degenerations, dystrophies, and edema of the cornea. In Duane, T.D. [ed.]: Clinical Ophthalmology. Hagerstown, Md.: Harper & Row, 1978, vol. 4, chap. 16.)

Bowman's area extending into the epithelial layer. The lesions vary in size. The cornea between these lesions is clear.

With light microscopy, the epithelium varies in thickness and may be reduced to several layers; the epithelial cells are irregular in size and shape. PAS-staining material is apparent between Bowman's layer and the epithelium, which is irregular in thickness and corresponds to the opacity described with a fine-slit beam.

Griffith and Fine[22] have described a case that appears to belong in this group of anterior membrane dystrophies. It is possible that this disorder is an attenuated form of Reis-Bücklers' dystrophy, but the variable effect on the vision, the normal corneal sensation, and the partial affection of the cornea suggest that this is a separate but related disorder.

Penetrating keratoplasty can be performed[23]; however, there is a tendency for the superficial opacity to recur.

Honeycomb dystrophy[48] (Thiel and Behnke)

This bilateral subepithelial dystrophy is transmitted as an autosomal dominant trait. It begins in childhood, appearing as a progressive course of recurrent erosions and decreasing vision. The vision varies from 20/25 in younger patients to 20/100 in the age group of 40 to 60 years. Corneal erosions disappear by the thirties to fifties. The dystrophy exhibits a bilateral honeycomb-like opacity in the subepithelial region of the cornea with projections into the anterior region. The corneal sensation is not reduced.

The typical honeycomb appearance, smooth corneal surface, normal sensation, and less visual involvement make this slightly different from Reis-Bücklers' disease[48]; it may be a variant of Reis-Bücklers' dystrophy.

Inherited band keratopathy

Although band keratopathy is usually seen in local ocular diseases and in systemic diseases (Chapter 10), it can occur as an inherited trait.[47]

Anterior crocodile shagreen and mosaic pattern

This condition is discussed in detail in Chapter 10.

Table 11-1 summarizes some of the pathologic and hereditary features of the more frequently occurring primary anterior corneal dystrophies.

Local anterior mucopolysaccharide accumulation
(Fig. 11-10)

Bilateral diffuse corneal clouding with increased acid mucopolysaccharide accumulation in Bowman's layer occurred in two infants without evidence of systemic mucopolysaccharidosis.[45] There was no evidence of intracellular vacuoles containing fibrogranular inclusions or extracellular granular material.

The corneal epithelium is normal, but as noted, Bowman's layer shows diffuse thickening with abnormal acid mucopolysaccharide. There is normal stromal collagen and keratocytes. The endothelium and Descemet's membrane are normal.

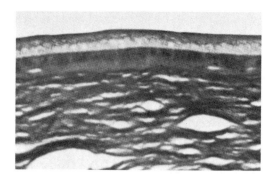

Fig. 11-10. Corneal clouding as result of accumulation of acid mucopolysaccharide in Bowman's layer. (From Rodrigues, M.M., Calhoun, J., and Harley, R.D.: Am. J. Ophthalmol. **79:**916, 1975.)

Stromal dystrophies

These disorders of the cornea are typified by the development of noninflammatory, nonvascularized opacifications of various sizes and shapes. The opacities are bilateral and hereditary and exhibit specific physical characteristics on examination with the slit lamp. Recent work has helped to identify the histochemical makeup of some of the opacities. In instances in which the vision is threatened, the problem can be treated surgically.

GRANULAR DYSTROPHY (Tables 11-2 and 11-3)

This dystrophy is transmitted as an autosomal dominant disease. It is bilateral and symmetrical.

The corneal opacities have an early onset, but the visual acuity at this stage of development is not impaired, and the patient experiences no discomfort. The early lesions, which are mostly located in the axial portion of the cornea, are small, discrete, sharply demarcated, grayish-white opacities occurring in the stroma of both eyes (Fig. 11-11). The lesions are usually grossly visible in adolescence. As the condition advances, the lesions become larger, coalesce, increase in number, and extend into the deeper layers of the stroma. The epithelium shows some irregularity; the stroma, in advanced cases, may become somewhat cloudy between the lesions.

The opacities may take on varying shapes; the grayish-white, well-demarcated lesion can be in the form of a "Christmas tree" (Fig. 11-12). The clearly defined opacities in this figure are mostly confined to the axial portion of the cornea. Clear corneal tissue exists between the discrete opacities until late in the disease when a haze is noted between the superficial stromal masses. The opacities may extend toward the periphery of the cornea but do not actually reach it.

Although epithelium involvement has not been verified histologically at the inception of this dystrophy, ultrastructural examination has revealed some epithelial and subepithelial granules. The characteristic rod-shaped crystalline structures of granular dys-

Table 11-2. Stromal corneal dystrophies: histopathologic features

Dystrophy	Sensitivity	Masson trichrome stain	PAS stain	Alcian blue	Congo red	Oil red O	Thioflavine "T"	Birefringence*	Dichroism†
Granular (Groenouw's type I)	Normal	+ (Red)	–	–	–	–	–	–	–
Macular (Groenouw's type II)	Decreased	–	+ (Pink)	+ (Blue)	–	–	–	–	–
Lattice (Biber-Haab-Dimmer)	Decreased	+ (Red)	+ (Pink)	–	+ (Orange)	–	+	Increased	+ (Red and green)
Schnyder's crystalline	Decreased or normal	–	–	–	–	+ (Red)	–	–	–
Fleck (speckled or mouchetée)	Normal: few cases decreased	–	–	+ (Keratocytes) Blue	–	–	–	–	–
Pre-Descemet	Normal	–	–	–	–	+ (Red)	–	–	–
Hemochromatosis	Normal	Violet to black	–	–	–	–	–	–	–

*Birefringence[106]:
1. Place a Polaroid filter in front of the eyepiece lens.
2. Place a Polaroid filter between the microscope light and slide.
3. When perpendicular to each other, no light is seen, but when the amyloid fibrils stained with Congo red lie in a parallel direction, polarization of the light results. Thus some of the light passing through the first Polaroid filter is rotated by the amyloid and passes through the second filter as yellow-green color against a black background.

†Dichroism[106] (the linear molecules of the Congo-red dye arrange themselves along the axis of the amyloid fibrils, and, because of this, dichroism and birefringence can be demonstrated):
1. Place a green filter in front of the microscope light.
2. Place a polarizing filter between the green light and the slide.
3. The parallel-stained Congo-red amyloid fibrils absorb green light.
4. If the polarizing plane is parallel to the fibril axis, the green light is absorbed.
5. If the polarizing plane is at right angles to the fibril, it is not absorbed.
6. Rotation of the polarizing filter will therefore result in red and green colors.

Table 11-3. Stromal corneal dystrophies

Dystrophy	Character of opacity	Clinical features
Granular (Groenouw's type I)	Discrete, gray-white opacities with sharp borders Clear cornea between opacities	Axial region; all depths of stroma No involvement of epithelium or Descemet's membrane
Lattice (Biber-Haab-Dimmer)	Gray lines resembling pipestem-like threads that are translucent by retroillumination; dot and stromal opacities between these give ground-glass appearance. Threadlike opacities may show bulbous areas and dichotomous branching	Scattered latticelike network with bifurcating pipestemlike threads, mainly limited to zone between center of cornea and periphery, usually extending to limbus; seen throughout the stroma and may involve epithelium but usually not endothelium
Macular (Groenouw's type II)	Poorly demarcated, gray-white opacities Diffusely cloudy cornea between large, irregular opaque areas	Entire cornea may be involved, but more dense in axial region; some spots extend to limbus; deep epithelium and endothelial layers are affected
Schnyder's crystalline	Crystalline deposits, usually	Mostly located on axial area of cornea
Fleck (speckled or mouchetée)	Well demarcated, small, round, doughnutlike opacities	Opacities are located in all levels of stroma
Pre-Descemet	Small opacities of varied shapes and sizes: round, comma, dots, dendritic, or linear	Best seen in retroillumination; all opacities are in deep stroma
Congenital hereditary stromal	Bilateral, inherited, present at birth; progressive with epithelial changes; deep stromal opacity	Deep stromal opacity, no edema, cornea normal thickness; flakey, feathery and central
Marginal crystalline (Bietti)[59]	Crystals in cornea	Superficial stromal deposition in paralimbal area

Vision	Transmission electron–microscopic studies	Inheritance	Erosion symptoms
Usually good until age 40	Electron-dense, rhomboid-shaped rods Endothelium not affected	Autosomal dominant Rarely sporadic	−
Reduced early in life (in late adolescence)	Nonbranching fibrils (8) characteristic of amyloid Endothelium not affected	Autosomal dominant Autosomal recessive	+ +
Affected in late teens	Membrane-bound vacuoles with fibrillogranular material Endothelium affected		
Usually not markedly disturbed; may be decreased to 20/40 level If extremely extensive pathologic condition is present, vision can be worse	Notched rectangular crystals	Autosomal dominant	−
Vision is usually not affected; however, photophobia may be marked	Cytoplasmic, membrane-bound vacuoles with fibrillogranular material	Autosomal dominant	−
Vision is not affected	Cytoplasmic membrane-bound vacuoles with fibrillogranular material	Autosomal dominant	−
Poor	Cornea normal thickness; no secondary changes in anterior stroma; uniform distribution of loose and compact lamellae composed of collagen filaments of small diameter; loose lamellae is always related to a keratocyte; normal Descemet's membrane	Autosomal dominant	−
Vision is not affected by crystals Fundus albipunctatus is noted	No studies available	Not definitely established	−

Continued.

Table 11-3. Stromal corneal dystrophies—cont'd

Dystrophy	Character of opacity	Clinical features
Central cloudy (François)	Diffuse posterior opacity in pupillary zone broken up into segmental areas seen best via sclerotic scatter; in direct illuminations, opacities are multiple, small, fuzzy-outlined gray areas, polygonal in shape and separated by clearer areas	Opacity extends to level of Bowman's layer; in this location, opacities are smaller and less numerous; segmentation of diffuse posterior opacity does not involve Descemet's membrane; at this level, opacity resembles Vogt's posterior crocodile shagreen
Parenchymatous (Pillat)	Central punctate opacities; peripheral ones are also seen but are finer; central opacities affect posterior, middle, and to a lesser extent, anterior stroma	Most opacities are larger than those seen in pre-Descemet dystrophy. Appears gray on focal illumination and clear on retroillumination
Posterior amorphous[126]	Gray sheets of indistinct corneal opacities	Opacities are at various levels of deep stroma and may involve endothelium, which is normal
Corneal hemochromatosis	Diffuse gray opacity of entire stroma; microincineration suggests lesions are of ferrous nature	Many refringent dots in anterior third of stroma. Descemet's membrane may be thick and irregular, and endothelium thin or absent in some areas

trophy have been seen within the epithelial cells. A number of morphologic findings in the cases presented support the contention of an epithelial origin of the dystrophic deposits.

The nature of the material in granular dystrophy is not known. It is described as hyaline, which says nothing about its chemical nature. Recently it has been suggested that the deposits may represent some kind of pathologic keratohyaline.[83]

There is neither vascularization of the stroma nor decreased corneal sensitivity except in the atypical forms. In the latter case, the lesions are snowflake-like opacities in the superficial stroma, which may extend to the periphery and develop a diffuse superficial haze by the teens. The eosinophilic-staining opacities, which stain intensely red with Masson trichrome stain[78] (Fig. 11-13) and negatively or weakly positively with PAS stain,[84] have been identified as extracellular hyaline deposits.[107] Recent histochemical studies demonstrated that the opacities may be noncollagenous protein with tyrosine, tryptophan, arginine, and sulfur-containing amino acids.[76]

The electron microscopic picture of this dystrophy has been extensively studied and found to be characteristic.* The opacities are in the form of electron-dense trapezoid-

---

*References 56, 91, 96, 99, 119, 124, 127.

Vision	Transmission electron–microscopic studies	Inheritance	Erosion symptoms
No decrease in vision	No studies available	Autosomal dominant	–
No decrease in vision	No studies available	Autosomal dominant	–
Vision may be reduced	No studies available	Autosomal dominant	–
Decrease in vision	No studies available	—	–

shaped or rod-shaped "crystals." They are 100 to 500 μm wide, are found in cross section, show several morphologic patterns (homogeneous, filamentous, moth eaten), and are considered to be typical of granular dystrophy[119] (Fig. 11-14). The stromal keratocytes in some instances exhibit degenerative changes and scattered vacuoles and may be the source of the abnormal product. The endothelial cells on electron microscopic examination are normal.

It has been suggested that granular dystrophy may have some relationship to lattice dystrophy[98] since some cases of granular dystrophy, like all cases of lattice dystrophy, have demonstrated finely filamentous, possibly amyloid, material around stromal lesions.[127]

Treatment

If the visual acuity is decreased enough so that the patient is incapacitated, the treatment of choice is a penetrating keratoplasty. It should be noted that granular dystrophy in corneal grafts has recurred in a number of cases* and may be seen as early as a year

*References 62, 108, 115, 123, 127.

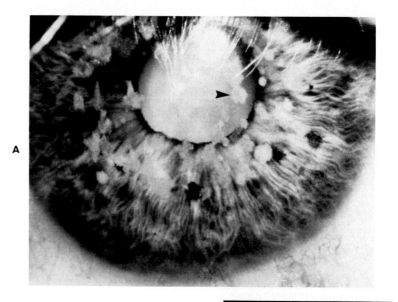

A

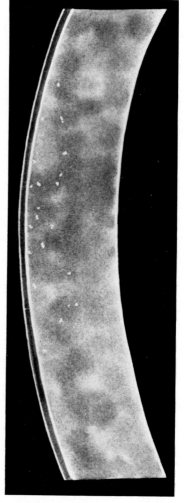

B

Fig. 11-11. A, Lesions in granular dystrophy
are discrete, gray-white opacities *(arrow)*
with clear corneal stroma between opacities. B,
Optical section showing destruction of lesions
throughout stroma.

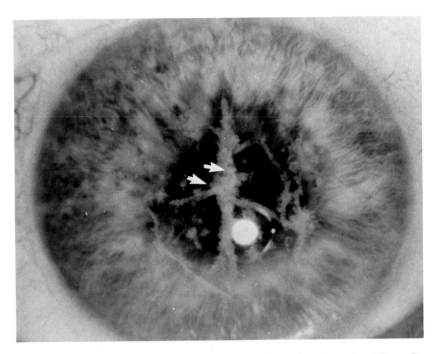

Fig. 11-12. Christmas tree opacity *(arrows)* in case of granular dystrophy. (From Grayson, M.: Degenerations, dystrophies, and edema of the cornea. In Duane, T.D. [ed.]: Clinical Ophthalmology. Hagerstown, Md.: Harper & Row, 1978, vol. 4, chap. 16.)

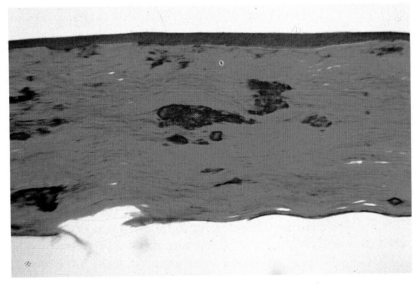

Fig. 11-13. Positive Masson trichrome stain seen in granular dystrophy.

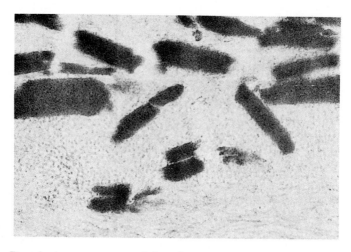

Fig. 11-14. Densely homogeneous, rod-shaped structures characteristic of granular dystrophy as noted with transmission electron microscopy. (×36,000.) (From Haddad, R., Font, R.L., and Fine, B.S.: Am. J. Ophthalmol. **83:**213, 1977.)

after the keratoplasty.[62,81,123,127] Deposits of the electron-dense, trapezoid-shaped and rod-shaped structures occur in the subepithelial area below Bowman's layer and in the stroma.[81] It is presumed that such occurrences are the result of either involvement of the donor material by genetically abnormal keratocytes from the stroma of the host cornea or some metabolic disturbance in the host's corneal tissue. Avascular fibrous tissue, which is also seen between the epithelium and Bowman's layer and accounts for the diffuse corneal haze in recurrences, is not considered a part of the dystrophic recurrence but a nonspecific reaction. This fibrous layer can be removed at the level of Bowman's layer; a clear cornea results after epithelialization of the keratectomized area.

LATTICE DYSTROPHY (Tables 11-2 and 11-3)

Lattice dystrophy is inherited as a dominant hereditary pattern.[89] Bilateral manifestations of corneal disease appear at an early age, usually 2 to 7 years. The majority of cases are bilateral, but unilateral cases have been reported.[111] Increasing visual difficulties result in marked visual handicap by the twenties or thirties. Patients often complain of photophobia and irritation, which are results of corneal erosions.

The early corneal lesions in individuals as young as 2 years appear to be located in the area of the anterior stroma and Bowman's layer.[120] They are primarily in the axial portions of the cornea and appear as fine, irregular lines and dots. As the pathologic condition increases, the corneal surface becomes irregular; this irregular astigmatism results in early decrease in vision. The characteristic lesions are dotlike nodules, threadlike spicules, and double-contoured branching filaments that advance to a point; the cornea exhibits a ground-glass appearance on biomicroscopic examination (Fig. 11-15). In late cases the opacities increase in severity, becoming more confluent. The threadlike spicules, which now resemble lattice striae and may branch dichotomously, are present

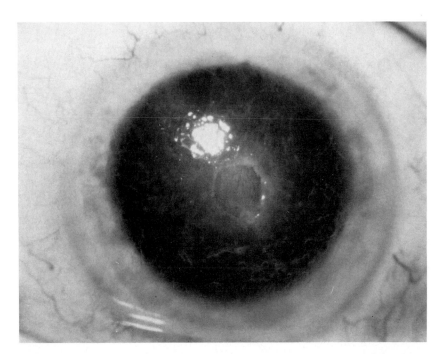

Fig. 11-15. Lattice dystrophy. Opacity on biomicroscopic examination exhibits ground-glass appearance.

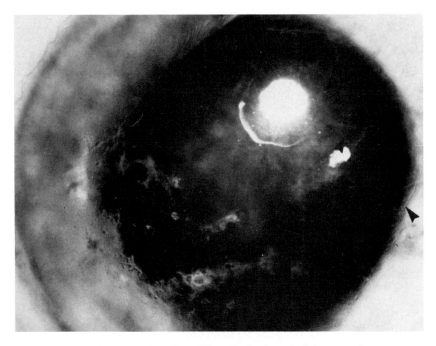

Fig. 11-16. Lattice dystrophy. Threadlike spicules branch dichotomously *(arrows)*.

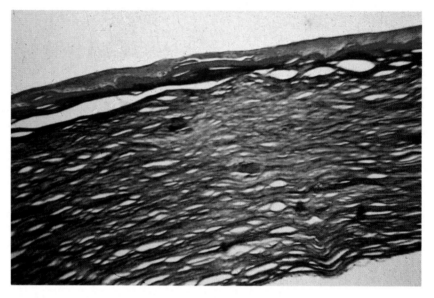

Fig. 11-17. Lattice dystrophy. Lesions may be seen subepithelially and in all levels of stroma.

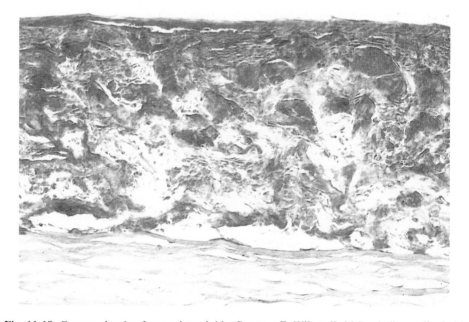

Fig. 11-18. Congo red stain of corneal amyloid. (Courtesy F. Wilson II, M.D., Indianapolis, Ind.)

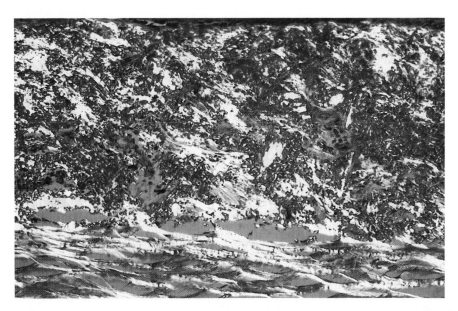

Fig. 11-19. Corneal amyloid as seen with polarized light. (Courtesy F. Wilson II, M.D., Indianapolis, Ind.)

in all layers of the stroma (Fig. 11-16). In addition, there is invasion of the epithelial and subepithelial areas (Fig. 11-17). A central subepithelial dense opacity is seen in this late stage. No endothelial involvement is seen. The lattice lines are not degenerated nerves in hereditary stromal lattice dystrophy.[129]

Histologically the epithelium may be irregularly thick or thin.[86] Degenerated epithelial cells occur, the basement membrane of the epithelium is not continuous,[130] and Bowman's layer is, on occasion, absent, thin, or thickened in various areas. The epithelial basement membrane is defective and without hemidesmosomes, resulting in erosions.[72] The deposit found between the epithelium and Bowman's layer is PAS positive, Masson stain positive, and alcian-blue negative. These deposits stain positively with Congo red and thioflavine "T." The amyloid nature of the deposits has been confirmed by electron microscopy and by immunofluorescent studies using antisera against human amyloid. The deposits are extracellular and are made up of fine, electron-dense, nonbranching fibrils of 8 to 10 nm diameter without periodicity,[99] as compared to the 30 nm diameter of the normal corneal collagen fibers. Most of the fibrils are highly aligned, which explains the phenomena of dichroism and birefringence. The 8 nm collagen fibers fluoresce when stained with thioflavine "T." Congo red stains the stromal deposits consistent with the findings of amyloid[117] (Fig. 11-18).

When these deposits are examined with a polarizing filter on the microscope, the property of dichroism of Congo red–stained amyloid is demonstrated[73,82] (Fig. 11-19). With the polarizing filter (Table 11-3) in place, one color is noted in transmitted light and another in reflected light; for example, yellow, orange, or red is seen in transmitted light, and, when the filter is turned, the deposits will take on a white-green effect in reflected light. This amyloid material, as noted, may collect between the epithelium and Bowman's layer, but it is also distributed throughout the lamellae of the stroma. The lesions may appear in the middle and deep stroma and correspond to the lattice lines and white dots seen with the slit lamp. Descemet's membrane and endothelium are essentially normal, although some amyloid deposit has been seen rarely in the former. This abnormal material may originate in the keratocytes,[90] or it may be a product of collagen degeneration.[99] The number of keratocytes is decreased; some of them appear quite active, but others appear degenerated.[73]

Amyloid is a noncollagenous, fibrous protein containing 2% to 5% carbohydrate. It may be similar in structure to the light chains of immunoglobulins, as is noted in primary systemic amyloidosis. The major component of amyloid deposits associated with secondary systemic amyloidosis and with familial Mediterranean fever is a protein (protein AA) that is unrelated to immunoglobulins. Both primary and secondary amyloid deposits are associated with a structural protein, the plasma (P) component, now known as AP.[102] Studies have shown protein AA and protein AP in the amyloid deposits of lattice dystrophy. In secondary localized and primary localized amyloid changes, the types of amyloid have not yet been fully established.

Differential diagnosis

Lattice dystrophy is considered to be or to represent a primary localized form of amyloidosis.[112,117] However, "latticelike dystrophy" may occur only rarely with systemic amyloidosis. In this instance the disease may manifest in 20- to 30-year-old patients in the form of "latticelike dystrophy"; in later decades one sees involvement of the skin, fifth cranial nerve palsies, peripheral neuropathies with muscle atrophy, and cachexia.[96,98,100,101] Biopsy of the peripheral nerves shows amyloid. The clinical difference between rarely occurring lattice corneal changes with generalized amyloidosis and lattice dystrophy without systemic involvement should be noted. The "dystrophy" in the former instance is milder and later in onset; the individual retains good visual acuity until age 50. In the systemic disease corneal nerve degeneration shows latticelike refractile lines that spare the central cornea. The lines are radially arranged and are not randomly placed. The white dots of typical lattice dystrophy are not seen.[96,98] Thus it appears that patients who develop systemic amyloidosis may show corneal disease that is clear out to the periphery, but in cases in which the periphery of the cornea is clear, no systemic findings are seen.

Amyloid deposits, which are transparent on retroillumination and punctate, filiform, and glasslike in indirect illumination, have been described.[97] The findings are at all levels, but mostly at the middle and deep stroma. The lesions, which stain positive for Congo red and display dichroism with polarized light, are found in middle- to older-aged groups. There is no progression, vision is not affected, and the cornea remains lustrous. No demonstrable hereditary disease is noted. This sporadic disorder appears to be bilateral and seen equally in both men and women.[97]

It may be associated with systemic disease. The corneal findings have been seen in Kaposi's sarcoma and in a case in which skin biopsies of nodular lesions proved to be amyloid.

Secondary deposits of amyloid are seen in the cornea after or associated with local

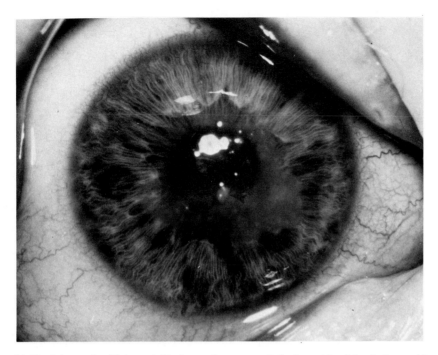

Fig. 11-20. Primary familial amyloid change in cornea. Raised, multinodular lesions with subepithelial formations of amyloid *(arrow)*.

ocular diseases of long duration such as trachoma, phlyctenular disease, interstitial keratitis, or chronic indolent corneal ulcers. These lesions are secondary deposits and are not considered dystrophic in nature.

Primary familial amyloidosis of the cornea is an extremely infrequent finding and, when seen, is characterized by central, raised, multinodular, subepithelial formation of amyloid[87,121] (Fig. 11-20). These lesions are similar to those described by Akiya, Ito, and Matsui,[57] who characterized the clinical appearance as a gelatinous, droplike corneal dystrophy.

It must be noted that lattice dystrophy may clinically appear as atypical granular dystrophy, and one should be aware of these unusual cases.[130]

Treatment

The treatment of lattice dystrophy, when the visual acuity has been impaired to a point that the patient is incapacitated, is penetrating keratoplasty (Fig. 11-21). Recurrence of the dystrophy can take place in the graft after 3 to 5 years.[81,92,94] Lattice dystrophy recurs more frequently than granular or macular dystrophy. Stromal lattice figures or white spots may not be found in the central graft; one may see peripheral stromal lattice and dots and diffuse subepithelial opacities, which may stain with Congo red and have a filamentous appearance.[81,92] In addition, nonamyloid material is seen in the superficial stroma.[92,94] When recurrent erosions are seen, one may employ the use of a soft contact lens to alleviate the annoying symptoms and to aid in the reepithelialization of the erosion.

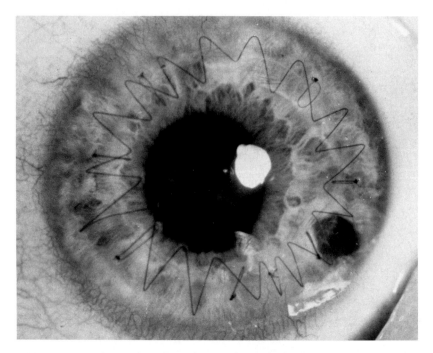

Fig. 11-21. Penetrating keratoplasty is used to obtain good visual results in patients with lattice dystrophy.

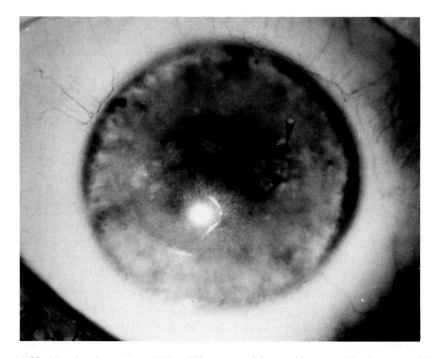

Fig. 11-22. Macular dystrophy exhibits diffuse corneal haze with gray-white dense opacities in this area of haze *(arrows)*.

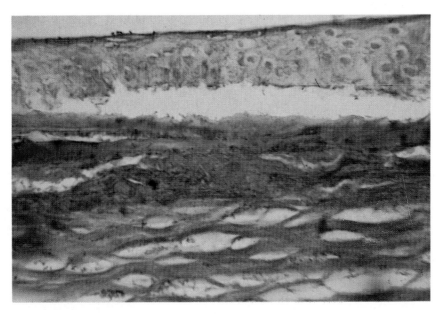

Fig. 11-23. Macular dystrophy. Colloidal iron stain in macular dystrophy with accumulation of acid mucopolysaccharide under epithelium.

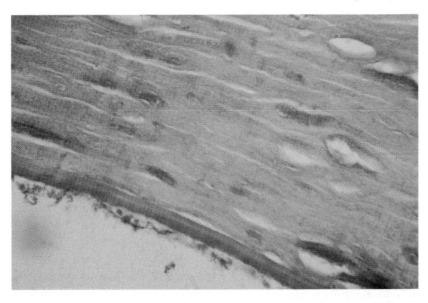

Fig. 11-24. Macular dystrophy. Colloidal iron stain exhibiting accumulation of acid mucopolysaccharide in endothelium.

MACULAR DYSTROPHY[90] (Tables 11-2 and 11-3)

This dystrophy may be detected as early as the first year of life and is transmitted as an autosomal recessive trait. The corneal changes are usually seen in the ages between 3 and 9 years. At this time, a diffuse clouding occurs in the more superficial portions of the cornea. However, the opacification that is seen at first in the axial portions of the cornea soon extends to the periphery; by the teens the opacification involves the entire thickness of the cornea and may extend out to the limbal area. As the condition progresses, the cornea becomes increasingly cloudy; within this sea of haziness are gray-white, denser opacities with indistinct borders (Fig. 11-22). These denser, macular opacities may be found in the anterior stroma, and their proximity to the corneal surface may result in irregularity of the epithelial surface (Fig. 11-23). Some of these denser, macular opacities are seen in the area of the posterior cornea and endothelium, which causes Descemet's membrane to appear gray and guttae to form (Fig. 11-24).

Of the three classic stromal dystrophies, macular dystrophy appears to be the most serious one. The patient experiences progressive loss of vision and attacks of irritation and photophobia. This dystrophy may result in blindness in the twenties or thirties.

Subepithelial tissue produces areas of epithelial thinning, and basement membrane–like and fibrillar material collects beneath the epithelium. Fibroblasts and histiocytes collect in this fibrillar material and may contribute to irregular corneal surface and opacity.[85]

Histologically, macular dystrophy is characterized by the accumulation of excess glycosaminoglycan deposits between the stromal lamellae, underneath the epithelium, within the stromal keratocyte, surrounding the stromal keratocyte, and within the endothelial cells.[84] A positive reaction for glycosaminoglycan (acid mucopolysaccharide) with the colloidal iron and alcian blue tests[93] is noted in the keratocyte; these deposits contain keratin sulfate and a hexose or a deoxyhexose acid mucosubstance.[75,77]

Electron-microscopic studies lead to the belief that the primary defect in metabolism rests with the keratocyte, which leads to abnormal storage of mucopolysaccharide.* The corneal keratocyte is distended by numerous intracytoplasmic vacuoles.[74] These vacuoles appear as dilated cisternae of the rough-surfaced endoplasmic reticulum and contain granular material as well as fine fibrillar material. Occasionally, one may see membranous lamellae material. Some vacuoles are clear, but many contain fibrils of 10 to 15 nm diameter, probably keratin sulfate,[74] and lamellar bodies that may contain glycolipid. Subepithelial histiocytes demonstrate similar intracellular material, but the epithelium is not affected. The endothelium, however, contains material similar to that found in the keratocyte. Descemet's membrane, especially the posterior portion, is infiltrated by vesicular and granular material deposited by the abnormal endothelium during the membrane's development. The banded anterior portion of the membrane is free of this material. The maternal factor correct for the enzyme defect, since the cornea is clear at birth, and deposits are absent from the fetal part of Descemet's membrane.[77,118] The basic defect therefore appears to be in the nuclear DNA, which produces defective enzymes involved in keratin sulfate metabolism. The vacuoles within the keratocytes possess a stronger affinity for colloidal iron, which identifies them as sites of acid mucopolysaccharide accumulation.[90]

*References 68, 77, 90, 103, 125.

It is interesting that a deficiency of lysosomal α-galactosidase in macular dystrophy of the cornea and in conjunctiva fibroblasts has been demonstrated; theoretically this fact would favor the inclusion of macular dystrophy among the inborn lysosomal disorders.[68] However, this is not substantiated.

It appears that, although macular dystrophy may be a disorder of acid mucopolysaccharide metabolism as seen from the present histochemical electron microscopic and biochemical studies, it would be necessary to establish basic biochemical defects from metabolic studies from cultured keratocytes. Systemic mucopolysaccharidosis and macular corneal dystrophy differ in that, in most cases of the former, one sees normal conjunctival and skin fibroblasts, sparing of the epithelium, and involvement of Descemet's membrane and endothelium.[110]

Rodrigues, Calhoun, and Harley[114] describe a case of bilateral, diffuse clouding of the cornea, which was associated with an accumulation of acid mucopolysaccharide in Bowman's layer. There was neither involvement of other corneal layers nor evidence of systemic mucopolysaccharidosis. This type of case must be kept in mind when making a diagnosis of macular dystrophy.

Treatment

Good results are obtained from penetrating keratoplasty for macular dystrophy (Fig. 11-25). After 10 years I have seen no recurrences of macular dystrophy in any of the grafts performed. However, this problem exists because host keratocytes that are

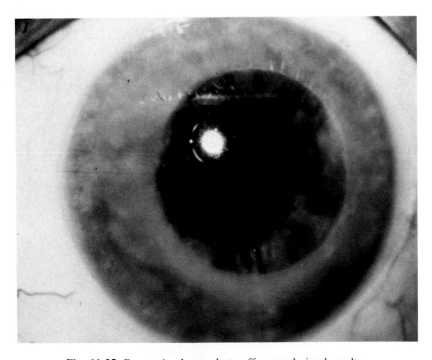

Fig. 11-25. Penetrating keratoplasty offers good visual results.

genetically involved in the disease perform their disease-oriented tasks in the donor stroma.[90, 113]

FLECK DYSTROPHY (SPECKLED OR MOUCHETÉE) (Tables 11-2 and 11-3)

This dystrophy is transmitted as an autosomal dominant trait.[80] The condition is stationary with no loss of visual acuity and may first be seen in early childhood.[58] The lesions are bilateral and are present in all layers of the corneal stroma, except Bowman's

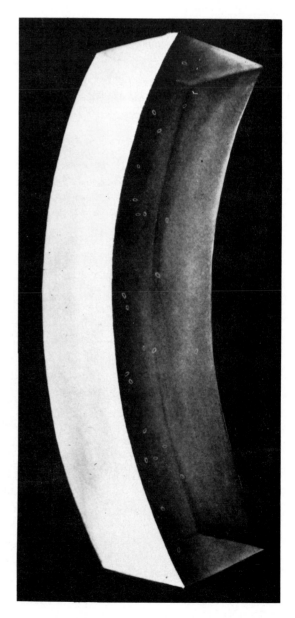

Fig. 11-26. Fleck dystrophy. Small, oval, doughnut-shaped, gray-white lesions are seen in stroma.

layer. They may involve the peripheral as well as the central stroma of the cornea. The lesions are semiopaque, flattened opacities that may be oval, round, doughnut-shaped, or gray-white, granular lesions[109] (Fig. 11-26). These small opacities are well outlined and demarcated, and the intervening cornea is clear.[60, 104] The best way to demonstrate them is on retroillumination. Although the vast number of cases have not incurred decreased corneal sensation, some cases may present this finding.[60, 104] Some degree of photophobia may be present, but this has not been a serious problem; the patient is often unaware of the corneal findings.[105] Corneal biopsies have been performed on patients who have both fleck dystrophy and keratoconus. Occasionally cases have been seen in pseudoxanthoma elasticum and in instances with limbal dermoids.[109] Collier[67] demonstrated the occurrence of central cloudy dystrophy and speckled dystrophy of the cornea in the same patient and in different members of the family.

The histopathologic studies reveal abnormal keratocytes with variable numbers of membrane-limited intracytoplasmic vacuoles containing a fibrillogranular material that stains positively for mucopolysaccharide. In addition, lipid material seen with oil red O stain as small, membrane-bound vesicles containing electron-dense lamellar bodies has been demonstrated.[88, 104]

CENTRAL CRYSTALLINE DYSTROPHY (SCHNYDER)
(Tables 11-2 and 11-3)

This entity is transmitted as an autosomal dominant trait; it is absent at birth but may be seen occurring as early as 18 months of age.[69, 95] The chief characteristic of the dystrophy is the presence of bilateral, round or oval, ring-shaped, discoid, or annular

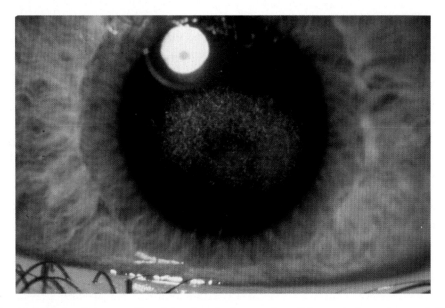

Fig. 11-27. Schnyder's crystalline dystrophy. Lesion consists of fine, polychromatic, needlelike crystals in area of Bowman's layer and anterior stroma.

opacities located in the centers of the corneas that consist of fine, polychromatic, needle-shaped crystals (Fig. 11-27). In addition, a diffuse, noncrystalline haze may be seen. The changes are not always visible grossly, but on slit-lamp examination the crystals can be seen as a meshwork of yellow, needlelike crystals with a polychromatic luster.[61] The yellowish-white opacity is located in the anterior part of the corneal stroma, including Bowman's layer, in a disc or ring form.[69,78,79,109] The epithelium is not involved, and the surrounding stroma is not involved with crystals. The cornea is not vascularized; the sensation is disturbed in some cases. Some cases have been reported of the occurrence of small, white, punctate opacities scattered in the stroma in Schnyder's crystalline dystrophy, but in most cases, as mentioned before, the stroma may be clear except where the crystals are deposited.[95] In some instances the stroma exhibits a milky opalescence.[61] Small clumps of electron-dense material adjacent to the crystals in the superficial stroma correspond to the diffuse noncrystalline haze.[70] Although the crystals are cholesterol, the more rounded globules of diffuse haze contain neutral fats, triglycerides, and noncrystalline cholesterol.[78]

Corneal arcus, in both children or adults, and the presence of Vogt's limbal girdle have been seen with sufficient frequency that they can be included as parts of the crystalline dystrophy picture.

The crystals have been identified as cholesterol,[116] and, although hyperlipidemia may exist with the corneal dystrophy, one can find normal values in the serum.[61] Xanthelasma has been reported, together with elevated serum cholesterol. Primary genu valgum has been seen in more than one pedigree.[69] However, these later changes are regarded as separately inherited manifestations.

This entity rarely affects the visual acuity, but on occasion it may be reduced. Usually the dystrophy does not progress. In any event, the disease may be considered a localized corneal defect of lipid metabolism, but in some cases a systemic defect also occurs. The keratocyte may be the stromal cell involved in the abnormal lipid metabolism. Burns,[63] working with radiolabeled cholesterol administered intravenously to a patient with crystalline dystrophy, showed that radioactivity in the blood decayed at a normal rate, but the keratoplasty button obtained from the patient showed a higher level of radioactivity and cholesterol than did the serum, suggesting an active uptake and storage of cholesterol in the cornea.

The histopathologic features of Schnyder's dystrophy include the presence of cholesterol crystals in the superficial stroma and in cases associated with hyperlipoproteinemia, as described by Bron, Williams, and Carruthers[61]; neutral fat and noncrystalline cholesterol were also demonstrated in the stroma, which may correlate with the diffuse stromal clouding seen in the cases of Bron et al. Destruction of Bowman's zone and superficial stroma with disorganization of collagen has been observed, although these changes may be secondary.

Usually treatment is not necessary for the corneal dystrophy; however, in cases in which visual acuity is reduced to a point that the patient is visually incapacitated, a penetrating corneal graft may be necessary. If the dystrophy is associated with certain systemic hyperlipidemia, treatment is directed toward this condition.

If material is taken from a graft, a frozen section should be made; the crystals will dissolve if regular methods of preparation are used. Oil red O stains neutral fats red; the Schultz method stains cholesterol blue-green for half an hour and then turns it brown.

The corneal crystals seen in Schnyder's dystrophy must be differentiated from other conditions causing corneal crystals, such as the following:

A. Multiple myeloma
B. Diseases of amino acid metabolism
   1. Infantile (nephropathic) form of cystinosis
   2. Adolescent cystinosis
   3. Adult cystinosis
C. Lipid keratopathy
   1. Associated with systemic disease: familial lecithin cholesterol–acyltransferase deficiency
   2. Associated secondarily with local corneal disease and corneal vascularization
D. Marginal crystalline dystrophy of Bietti
E. Cornea urica
F. Schnyder's crystalline dystrophy
G. Tyrosinosis
H. Calcium deposition
   1. Primary band keratopathy
   2. Secondary to systemic disease: kidney failure with uremia
I. Sap from dieffenbachia plant[71]
J. Hyperbilirubinemia

MARGINAL CRYSTALLINE DYSTROPHY (BIETTI) (Table 11-3)

This dystrophy was described in a case in which two brothers manifested the presence of crystalline material in the superficial corneal stroma in the region of the paralimbal cornea (Fig. 11-28). Both brothers showed fundus albipunctatus.[59] The corneal changes do not affect the vision at all.

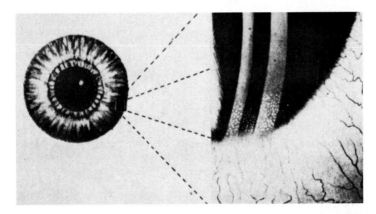

Fig. 11-28. Marginal crystalline changes in cornea. (From Bagolini, B., and Ioli-Spada, G.: Am. J. Ophthalmol. **65:**53, 1968.)

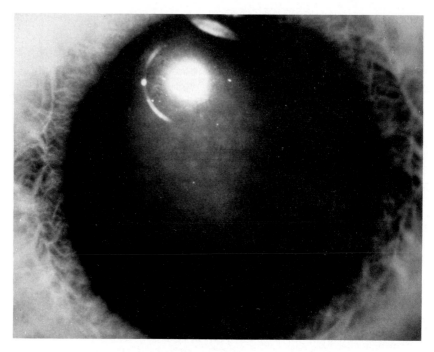

Fig. 11-29. Central cloudy dystrophy of François. General clouding of cornea is broken up into segmental areas of opacity by intervening clear tissue.

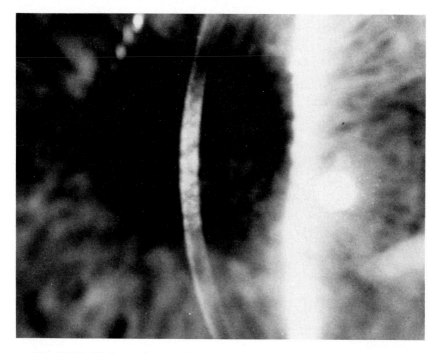

Fig. 11-30. Slit-lamp photograph showing distribution of opacity of François.

CENTRAL CLOUDY DYSTROPHY (FRANÇOIS) (Table 11-3)

This dystrophy is transmitted as an autosomal dominant trait appearing in persons from 8 to 70 years of age. There is neither decrease in visual acuity nor any symptoms. The condition is nonprogressive.

The opacity that occupies the pupillary zone is more dense posteriorly and appears to fade anteriorly and peripherally (Figs. 11-29 and 11-30). It is a diffuse clouding that is broken into segmental areas of opacity by intervening clear tissue. Sometimes the opacification extends to or, very rarely, involves Bowman's layer; in this location the opacities are smaller and less numerous.[122]

No involvement of the epithelium or Descemet's membrane occurs, but pre-Descemet involvement is seen. At this level the dystrophy exhibits similarities to Vogt's posterior crocodile shagreen in which a mosaic pattern is seen in the deep cornea. There is no vascularization and no inflammation. The stromal opacities can be seen well by scleral scatter.

Central cloudy dystrophy has been reported to have occurred in patients with fleck dystrophy and pseudoxanthoma elasticum,[66] fleck dystrophy,[65] and pre-Descemet dystrophy.[67]

PARENCHYMATOUS DYSTROPHY (PILLAT) (Table 11-3)

Parenchymatous dystrophy of the cornea is quite rare, and few cases have been reported. In one of two studies, the central portion of the cornea was involved; in the other the periphery was afflicted. The central opacities affect the posterior, middle, and, to a lesser degree, anterior stroma. Most of the opacities are larger than those seen in pre-Descemet dystrophy, appearing gray on focal illumination and clear on retroillumination. The peripheral opacities are finer than the central ones and are separated from them by clear stroma. The opacities are of a punctate nature.

The corneal changes have little effect on vision and do not depress the corneal sensitivity. There are no symptoms of discomfort in parenchymatous dystrophy.

POSTERIOR AMORPHOUS DYSTROPHY[64] (Table 11-3)

In some instances of this autosomal, dominant bilateral dystrophy the visual acuity is reduced to the 6/12 level.

Gray sheets form indistinct patches at various levels of the deep stroma across the entire stroma. The opacity may extend to the level of Descemet's membrane; the endothelium may be involved, also.

Posterior amorphous dystrophy appears in the first decade of life, remains asymptomatic, and progresses to a thinner cornea than is seen normally. The epithelium remains normal.

CORNEAL HEMOCHROMATOSIS[128] (Tables 11-2 and 11-3)

This entity is an unusual type of corneal dystrophy involving the anterior stroma and both limiting membranes. A decrease in vision is noted, but no pain, congestion, or photophobia occurs.

A fine, diffuse, gray cloudiness of the entire cornea appears. Sensitivity is undisturbed. The stromal opacity is confined to the anterior third of the cornea and appears to consist of many minute, refringent dots resembling lipid droplets. No change is noted in the posterior two thirds of the stroma. Descemet's membrane may be thick and irregular. The endothelium may be thin or absent in some areas.

The results of the Masson and Mallory stains in hemochromatosis indicate the presence of nucleic acid. Perls' test gives a green color to the corneal accumulations, which are found between the stromal fibers, in contrast to the usual stromal dystrophies in which the accumulations appear to originate from the destruction of the fibers themselves. The positive Perls' test and positive findings by way of microincineration of the stromal lesions and anterior layer of Descemet's membrane indicate the presence of a ferrous compound.

No primary or secondary evidence exists of systemic hemochromatosis. No enlargement of the liver, diabetes, pigmentation of the skin, or excess iron in the serum occurs. Nevertheless, the cornea in the localized form is laden with iron attached to nucleoprotein.

This local corneal disease with accumulation in the tissues of an abnormal iron protein should be considered as a purely local disturbance akin to that which leads to the appearance of a nonsystemic amyloidosis in the case of lattice dystrophy.

Pre-Descemet dystrophies

CORNEA FARINATA (Fig. 10-7)

This prototype of the so-called pre-Descemet dystrophies is sometimes classified with them, although cornea farinata is generally considered to be an age-related degeneration. Cornea farinata consists of tiny, punctate, gray opacities in the deep stroma immediately anterior to Descemet's membrane and is discussed in Chapter 10.

PRIMARY PRE-DESCEMET DYSTROPHY (Tables 11-2 and 11-3)

This corneal abnormality resembles cornea farinata but has larger and more polymorphous pre-Descemet opacities. It may be primary (of unknown or hereditary origin) or secondary (associated with ocular or systemic diseases). Vision is unaffected.

Grayson and Wilbrandt[137] described pre-Descemet dystrophies that consisted of admixtures of six types of tiny, deep, stromal opacities: (1) dendritic or stellate, (2) boomerang, (3) circular or dot, (4) comma, (5) linear, and (6) filiform (Fig. 11-31). The deposits were axial, peripheral, or diffuse in various cases. The type and location of the opacities showed no correlation with age or with the presence or absence of coexisting ocular or systemic disease.

Curran, Kenyon, and Green[134] used light and electron microscopy to study a case of primary pre-Descemet dystrophy that demonstrated dot, linear, semicircular, and filamentary opacities. The pathologic condition was limited to the keratocytes of the posterior stroma with sparing of collagen, Descemet's membrane, and endothelium. Within the keratocytes were cytoplasmic vacuoles (secondary lysosomes) that appeared to con-

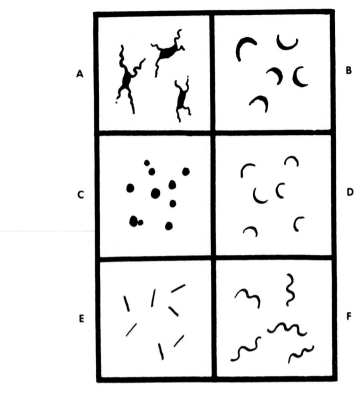

Fig. 11-31. Patterns of opacities in the pre-Descemet dystrophies. **A,** Dendritic. **B,** Boomerang. **C,** Circular. **D,** Comma. **E,** Linear. **F,** Filiform.

tain lipofuscin, which is a degenerative, "wear-and-tear," lipoprotein pigment that accumulates in aging cells.

These findings raise the questions of whether the pre-Descemet dystrophies are merely variants of cornea farinata and whether they might be better regarded as degenerations rather than as dystrophies. Cornea farinata is regularly classified as an involutional degeneration, even though its histopathologic picture remains uncertain. Pre-Descemet dystrophies, however, can occur in patients who are in their thirties,[137] suggesting that aging may not be the only cause. Heredity apparently can play a part, and both cornea farinata and pre-Descemet dystrophy can be familial.[131-133] In one of the families reported by Grayson and Wilbrandt,[137] the mother had typical cornea farinata, whereas her daughter had pre-Descemet dystrophy. The secondary pre-Descemet dystrophies, discussed next, could easily be classified as degenerations because of their clinical associations with other abnormalities; however, despite the evidence that pre-Descemet opacities may be more degenerative than dystrophic, I prefer to adhere to the tradition of referring to them (except for cornea farinata) as dystrophies until they are better understood.

Table 11-4. Abnormal substance of stromal dystrophies

Dystrophy	Abnormal substance
Granular	Hyaline
Lattice	Amyloid
Macular	Glycosaminoglycan
Central crystalline	Cholesterol
Fleck	Intracellular glycosaminoglycan
Congenital hereditary stromal	None identified
Pre-Descemet	Intracellular lipids

SECONDARY PRE-DESCEMET DYSTROPHY

Pre-Descemet opacities in association with other ocular or systemic abnormalities are often called secondary pre-Descemet dystrophies, although the cause-and-effect relationships are unclear. Pre-Descemet dystrophy has occurred several times in association with keratoconus and has been referred to in this situation as deep filiform dystrophy of Maeder and Danis.[138] It has occurred also with anterior membrane dystrophies,[137] with posterior polymorphous dystrophy,[137] with ichthyosis (deep punctate dystrophy of Franceschetti and Maeder),[135, 136] and in female carriers of sex-linked ichthyosis.[139]

A summary of abnormal substances of stromal dystrophies is listed in Table 11-4.

Endothelial dystrophies and corneal edema

CORNEAL STATUS

To appreciate the dystrophies of the posterior layer of the cornea, the electron microscopic appearance of the endothelium and Descemet's membrane must be considered.

The transmission electron microscopic (TEM) appearance of the normal endothelial cell demonstrates pinocytotic vesicles on the anterior and posterior borders. Microvilli can be seen protruding into the anterior chamber, but these are sparse in number (Fig. 11-32). The endothelial cells are joined together by zonular occludens; however, no true desmosomes are found (Fig. 11-33). Interdigitation of the cell borders is seen, as well as a rich supply of organelles (Fig. 11-33). A well-developed Golgi system, abundant mitochondria, and smooth and rough endoplasmic reticulum are seen (Fig. 11-34). Intracytoplasmic filaments are not normally present.

The scanning electron microscopic (SEM) features of the normal endothelium reveal orderly and well-demarcated cell borders, which take on a zigzag configuration (Fig. 11-35). One may find occasional microvilli and blunt ciliary processes. Pinocytotic vacuoles are seen on the surface; the nucleus of the endothelial cell may make a surface feature as well (Fig. 11-35).

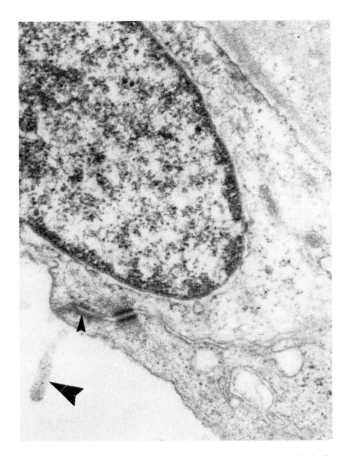

Fig. 11-32. Microvilli *(large arrow)* are sparce in number in normal endothelium. Endothelial cells are joined by zonula occludens *(small arrow)*.

The morphologic status of the endothelium can be studied with the specular microscope. With this instrument the status of the endothelium from the standpoint of size, number, and cell shape can be studied. The degree of "cell spread," which is an attempt of the endothelium to cover defects induced by trauma or disease, may be evaluated. One cannot, however, determine the metabolic status of the endothelial cells with the use of the specular microscope.

Deep incisions into the cornea as in radial keratotomy procedure may cause endothelial damage. It is believed that cuts in Bowman's membrane and in the stromal tissue may cause corneal stretching, resulting in a continuing process of injury to the endothelial cell layer.[214]

Another instrument that is helpful in studying the clinical status of the cornea is the pachymeter. The degree of corneal thickness is examined with this instrument, and thus stromal edema can be evaluated and followed.

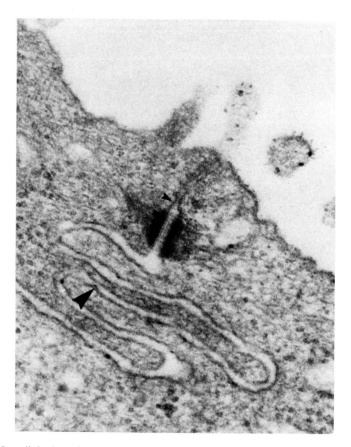

Fig. 11-33. Interdigitation of cell borders is prominent *(large arrow)*. Endothelial cells are joined by zonula occludens *(small arrows)*.

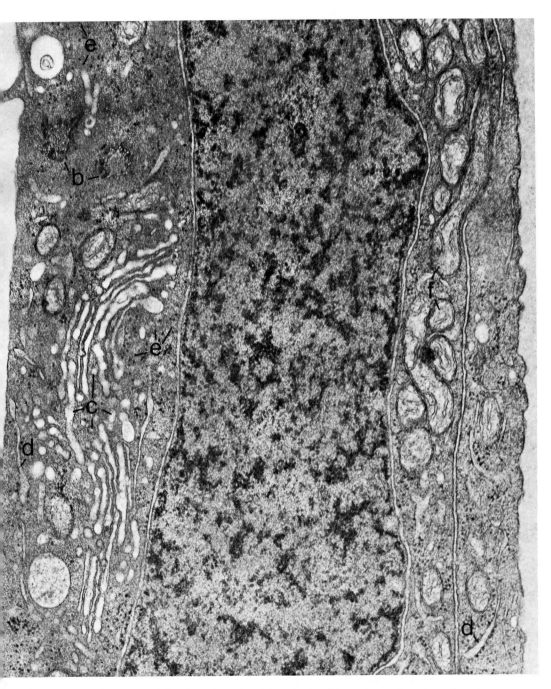

Fig. 11-34. Well-developed Golgi system, abundant mitochondria, and smooth and rough endo-plasmic reticulum. *a,* Microvillus; *b,* cisternae; *c,* Golgi system; *d,* endoplasmic reticulum; *e,* ribosomes; *f,* mitochondria. (From Hogan, M.J., Alvarado, J.A., and Weddell, J.E.: Histology of the human eye, Philadelphia, 1971, W.B. Saunders Co.)

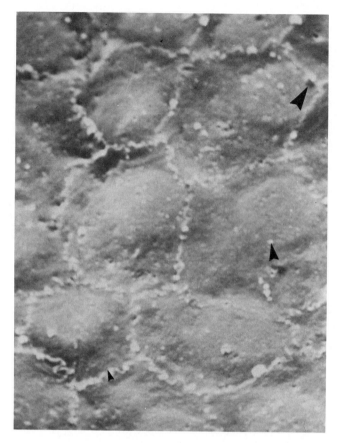

Fig. 11-35. Scanning electron microscopy exhibits well-demarcated and outlined endothelial cells in normal subject *(small arrow)*. Microvilli *(medium arrow)* and pinocytotic vacuoles are occasionally seen *(large arrow)*.

DESCEMET'S MEMBRANE

Descemet's membrane is the distensible and elastic basement membrane produced by the corneal endothelium. A typical basement membrane, it is a compact connective tissue consisting of small-diameter collagen fibrils and filaments bonded to a matrix of glycoproteins. It provides support for the posterior cornea and functions as a semipermeable barrier to molecules entering and leaving the cornea from the anterior chamber. Descemet's membrane is located between the corneal stroma and endothelium and terminates at Schwalbe's ring. It is poorly adherent to both stroma and endothelium, allowing for easy separation.

Two distinct regions are apparent. The anterior third is 1 to 4 μm thick and displays a banded pattern.[147] The posterior two thirds is 5 to 15 μm thick and appears amorphous and granular (Fig. 11-36). The posterior granular-appearing two thirds of Descemet's membrane contains smaller, less regularly arranged fibrils (Fig. 11-36).

Descemet's membrane increases in thickness throughout life, measuring 10 to 40 μm in the adult. The endothelium forms new basement membrane on the posterior sur-

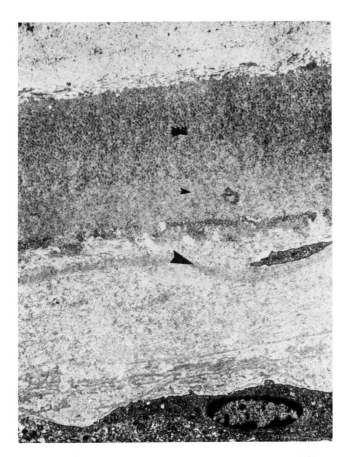

Fig. 11-36. Descemet's membrane consists of anterior banded layer *(medium arrow)* and non-banded area *(small arrow)*. Multilaminar basement membrane is laid down by altered endothelial cells *(large arrow)*.

face of the banded, embryonic Descemet's membrane in a discontinuous pattern, resulting in a lamellar appearance of the adult Descemet membrane. In addition, the endothelium produces more basement membrane in some areas. These peripherally located focal thickenings are called *Hassall-Henle warts*.

As with other basement membranes, Descemet's membrane is best seen by light microscopy after staining with PAS. Endothelial cell proliferation and Descemet membrane production may be excessive, resulting in specific clinical problems as noted in the following paragraphs.

Postinflammatory Descemet's ridges and membranes can be seen and may be confused with a prominent Schwalbe ring, anterior chamber tubes from proliferation of endothelial cells, Descemet's membrane proliferating around vitreous strands, pieces of Descemet's membrane stripped during surgery that hang into the anterior chamber, and folds in Descemet's membrane after trauma.

The corneal endothelium may also proliferate over free surfaces; spread around the chamber angle and across the iris, vitreous surface, zonules, ciliary body, and retina; and may even line the entire anterior chamber. In so doing, it produces ectopic Descemet's membrane, which has been referred to as glassy, cuticular, or hyaline membrane. In chronic interstitial keratitis the regenerating endothelium produces diffuse multilaminar thickening, secondary cornea guttata, retrocorneal ridges, and anterior chamber strands and networks.[208] The proliferative response occurs most commonly after trauma in children because of the greater regenerative potential of young endothelium[179] and after blunt trauma with angle recession.[167] It is also seen following penetrating injury and in chronic iridocyclitis, essential iris atrophy, congenital glaucoma, and the anterior chamber cleavage syndrome. Descemet's membrane lining the trabecular meshwork[153] may produce intractable glaucoma, as seen in late glaucoma of interstitial keratitis. In addition, it may extend over an iris nevus and resemble an iris melanoma.[213]

Breaks in Descemet's membrane from birth trauma usually occur from compression of the globe by forceps. They are usually unilateral, although bilateral cases occur. The breaks are fusiform and almost always centrally located, with a vertical or oblique orientation. In contrast, the breaks in congenital glaucoma are irregular, bilateral, and randomly oriented. If the break occurs in an infant or child, the regenerating endothelium will cover the posterior cornea and clear the overlying edema within about a month. Breaks in Descemet's membrane occur in keratoconus, resulting in the clinical picture of acute hydrops. The regenerated Descemet membrane within the break often contains guttatelike lesions.

The interposition of fluid such as blood, edema,[185] or leukocytes may separate Descemet's membrane from the overlying stroma. In bacterial keratitis, posterior abscesses may develop; this also may be seen in interstitial keratitis and metastatic spread of tubercle bacilli.[177] The abscess may displace Descemet's membrane posteriorly, may perforate, resulting in a central posterior ulcer; or may split Descemet's membrane between the banded and non-banded portions.

Deposits in and on Descemet's membrane and endothelium occur in corneal arcus,[141] keratoconus (Fleischer's ring), cornea guttata, macular corneal dystrophy, corneal hemochromatosis,[205] argyrosis, drug deposition (phenothiazine), hypercupremia, and multiple myeloma.

The formation of a retrocorneal membrane[160] may be prompted by injury or inflammation caused by chemical burns, vitrectomy,[175] vitreous touch,[202] herpes keratitis, and interstitial keratitis.[157]

Acquired autosensitivity to degenerating Descemet's membrane, resulting in granulomatous inflammation in both eyes, an effect similar to that seen in sympathetic ophthalmia or phacoanophylactic uveitis, although rare, can occur.[211]

ENDOTHELIUM

The endothelium is a single layer of cells, loosely attached to Descemet's membrane. No desmosomes attach the endothelial cell to Descemet's membrane. The endothelium continues to produce Descemet's membrane throughout life. As with Bowman's layer, the fibrils do not run parallel to bundles as they do in the stroma.

The endothelial cells can be photographed. Difference in size and enlarged cells are seen (Fig. 11-37). They should be studied and counted before insertion of intra-ocular lenses. In addition, donor endothelial cells can be counted and studied before keratoplasty. Polymegathism is demonstrated in Fig. 11-37. Some cells are quite large and irregular.

The endothelial cell is the main barrier regulating the flow of fluid and molecules in and out of the cornea and is much less permeable than Descemet's membrane.

At birth, the endothelium is a compact, cellular monolayer with a high nucleus: cytoplasm ratio. In humans the regenerative function of the endothelium declines with age. The endothelial cells become larger and flatter with age and continue, by spreading, to cover the posterior corneas as a continuous sheet. Cell division may play a minor role.

Stimuli to endothelial regeneration in childhood may provoke marked proliferation of the endothelial cells and Descemet's membrane, whereas an identical stimulus in the adult may produce barely enough response to maintain corneal integrity.

Degenerating and regenerating endothelial cells may undergo metaplasia (or dedifferentiation) to form fibroblast-like cells. The term *fibroblast-like* indicates that these cells possess features of both endothelial cells and fibroblasts. More severe insults result in fibroblast-like transformation. The fibroblastic characteristics include (1) an increased amount of rough endoplasmic reticulum containing electron-dense substance, (2) intracytoplasmic filaments, which are probably collagen precursors, (3) increased cortical densities adjacent to the cell surface, (4) intracytoplasmic vacuoles, and (5) lack of apical tight junctions.

The fibroblast-like cells may, in addition, redifferentiate into endothelial cells, which resume the production of Descemet-like basement membrane, or regenerating endothelial cells may migrate from undamaged areas to produce a layer of basement membrane. Thus the cells covering the posterior cornea in disease and dystrophic

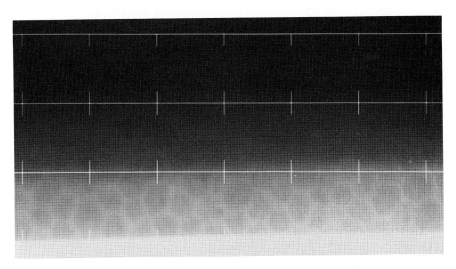

Fig. 11-37. Polymegathism. Endothelial cell photography makes it possible to count cells and study their size and shape.

states may alternate between the fibroblast-like and endothelial types, each producing its own characteristic contribution to Descemet's membrane. The result is a multi-laminar Descemet membrane consisting of the original membrane anteriorly and the newly produced material posteriorly (Fig. 11-36).

The other course that may be taken is metaplasia into an epithelial-like cell with desmosomal structures, sparse organelle system, and many tonofibrils (Fig. 11-38).

It has been suggested that the corneal endothelium is a mesothelial structure. A mesothelium is the surface lining of a serous cavity. It is mesodermally derived (as are fibroblasts) and can undergo fibroblastic metaplasia, in contrast to a true endo-thelium, which in fact is the lining of a vascular channel and does not convert to a fibroblast. In essence, the anterior chamber is truly a serous cavity lined anteriorly by mesothelium. As noted before, the fibroblast-like cells, resulting from metaplasia, produce a ''fibrous layer'' on the posterior surface of the original Descemet membrane. This layer consists of basement membrane–like substance of collagen and may occur in a variety of clinical situations, such as congenital hereditary corneal dystrophy (CHCD), Fuchs' endothelial dystrophy, posterior polymorphous de-

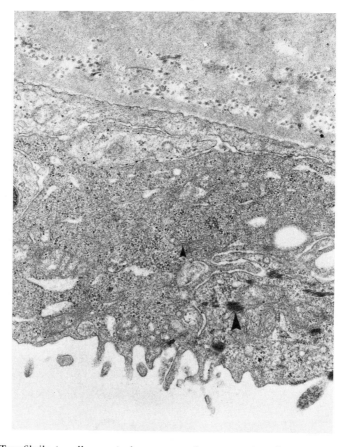

Fig. 11-38. Tonofibrils *(small arrow)*, desmosomes *(large arrow)*, and sparcity of organelles are seen in this epithelial-like cell.

generation, macular corneal dystrophy, or irritative stimuli, including penetrating wounds, keratoplasty, homograft reaction, interstitial keratitis,[157] uveitis, vitreous touch, freezing, dichloroethane poisoning, alkali burn,[179] and contusion angle–deformity injuries. In each instance, the reactive endothelial cells respond by producing excesses of basement membrane–like material, collagen fibrils, and fine filaments to form the abnormal posterior layer of Descemet's membrane and retrocorneal membranes (Fig. 11-36).

The ultrastructural similarity of the endothelial reaction to CHCD and a variety of other dystrophic diseases and irritative influences seems to reflect a common pattern in the pathogenesis of these familial and acquired disorders of the corneal endothelium. Understanding this concept will aid in the study of both the clinical and pathologic conditions and responses of the foregoing posterior membrane entities.

Mesodermal growth factor (MGF) is isolated from mouse submaxillary glands. It is a powerful mitogenic substance for corneal fibroblasts in tissue culture. In rabbits with injured corneas MGF accelerated the healing response by rapidly repopulating the zone of killed endothelium and by increasing the width of the zone of activated cells peripheral to the dead zone. In patients 59 years of age or younger, MGF stimulated an increase in the number of mitotic figures.[203]

EDEMA OF THE CORNEA

With the use of the pachymeter, one may observe the status of corneal thickness as well as edematous tendencies. The status of endothelial cell morphologic characteristics can be studied with the specular microscope.

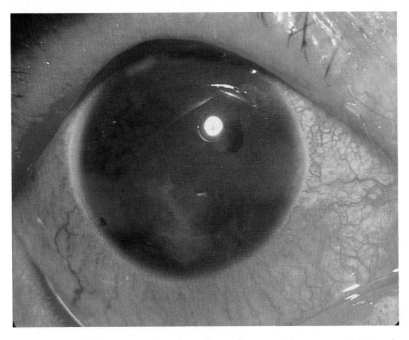

Fig. 11-39. Cogan-Reese syndrome showing edema of cornea, iris nevus, and heterochromia.

Several factors can cause decompensation that eventually leads to corneal edema. The endothelium of the cornea heals by cellular spreading; cell loss may result in decompensation sooner or later.[182] The number of endothelial cells decreases with age; this decrease may be sufficient enough so that decompensation ensues and edema results. If the cornea is traumatized and endothelial cells are lost, the ongoing decrease in cells with age may lead to decompensation.

Corneal edema can occur a number of years after initial trauma or surgery. A donor graft that initially had a sufficient number of endothelial cells to maintain metabolic integrity may, as additional cells die, become edematous.

Study of donor endothelium with the specular microscope before corneal transplant surgery will aid in evaluating the donor endothelium. This certainly would be most important in studying the endothelium of individuals who are anticipating intraocular lens insertion. Loss of endothelial cells occurs with this procedure; thus it is important to be certain that the number and appearance of the endothelial cells is adequate before this type of surgery is performed. Apparently, the contact of the methylmethacrylate lens with the endothelium is a factor in the loss of endothelial cells. The lens can adhere to the endothelial surface, and the cells "rip-off" in manipulation. Dipping the lens in 40% polyvinylpyrrolidone (PVD K29-31) may minimize this tendency.

Commercially prepared dilutions (1:10,000) of epinephrine can cause increased corneal thickness and loss of endothelial cells when injected into the anterior chamber. Endothelial toxicity is caused by the buffer capacity of the epinephrine solution, which is controlled by the concentration of antioxidant (sodium bisulfite) as well as by vehicle formulation and a low pH.[156]

Thimerosal, which is generally used as a preservative agent in topical ophthalmic solutions, even in low concentrations of 0.0001% and 0.005% can cause both structural and functional damage to the endothelium on prolonged exposure and thus should not be used during intraocular surgery since corneal edema may result. Other solutions that are irrigated into the anterior chamber have undesirable effects on the endothelium.[154, 155] For example, sterile physiologic saline and lactated Ringer's solution may result in progressive degeneration of the endothelium. Balanced salt solution will cause some degeneration but only after prolonged irrigation. Anterior chambers irrigated with Ringer's solution containing bicarbonate, reduced glutathione, and adenosine do not exhibit any increase in the thickness of the cornea. This solution is more physiologic and is a better infusion solution for intraocular surgery. It is controversial as to whether air has a detrimental effect on the endothelium.

It has been claimed that the elimination of vitreous contact may result in clinical reversal of corneal edema despite a prolonged period of vitreous contact and seemingly irreversible endothelial changes.[184]

Following are conditions that may be etiologic factors in producing corneal edema:

A. Trauma and insult
    1. Foreign body in the anterior chamber, especially in the inferior chamber angle

   2. Birth trauma
   3. Penetrating and contusion wounds to the eye
   4. Air blast injury[180, 181]
   5. Continuous wear of a contact lens[145]
   6. Freezing of endothelium with cryoprobe during cataract extraction
   7. Acid burns
   8. Alkali burns[187]
B. Congenital
   1. Congenital hereditary corneal dystrophy
   2. Congenital glaucoma
C. Dystrophies — adult onset
   1. Fuchs' epithelial-endothelial dystrophy
   2. Macular corneal dystrophy
   3. Lattice corneal dystrophy
   4. Deep posterior polymorphous dystrophy
D. Surgical
   1. Trauma of the surgical procedure
   2. Vitreous endothelial touch[184]
   3. Epithelial downgrowth
   4. Hemorrhage into the anterior chamber
   5. Infection (postoperative)
   6. Stripping of Descemet's membrane
   7. Graft failure
   8. Retrocorneal membrane and synechiae formation
   9. Intraocular lens insertion[148, 171]
  10. Pars plana vitrectomy
  11. Phacoemulsification[146, 191]
  12. Anterior segment necrosis[194, 207]
  13. Irrigating solutions[154, 155] and drugs[206]
E. Inflammatory
   1. Herpes simplex keratitis
   2. Herpes zoster keratouveitis
   3. Severe uveitis and iritis
   4. Graft rejection reaction
   5. Corneal ulcers
F. Drugs[206] — epinephrine and pilocarpine instilled into the anterior chamber
G. Glaucoma
   1. Acute narrow angle
   2. Sustained increase in intraocular pressure (IOP) in chronic simple glaucoma with poor endothelium
H. Acute hydrops caused by keratoconus
I. Others (rare causes)
   1. Cerebrohepatorenal syndrome of Zellweger
   2. Ectodermal dysplasia
   3. Cogan-Reese syndrome[200, 213]* (Fig. 11-39)
   4. Chandler's syndrome[161]

---

*Cogan-Reese syndrome involves unilateral glaucoma, corneal edema, iris whorls or nodules, iris stromal atrophy, heterochromia (darker eye is involved), ectropion uvea, peripheral anterior synechiae, non-malignant diffuse nevus, and overgrowth of endothelium and Descemet's membrane onto the iris surface.

ENDOTHELIAL DYSTROPHIES
Cornea guttata

Cornea guttata is a condition usually seen in the middle- to older-aged group. An inheritance pattern is not always determined but the condition can occur as an auto-somal dominant trait.

Slit-lamp examination of this condition reveals dewdroplike, wartlike endothelial prominences that are mushroomlike excrescences on Descemet's membrane (Fig. 11-40). Seen at first in the posterior central surface of the cornea, these wartlike excrescences are abnormal products of the endothelial cells.[166] The endothelial cells bordering these excrescences may degenerate or may lay down excessive basement membrane.

The guttate lesions are often located in the axial areas of the cornea. A golden-brown pigmentation may be seen at the level of the guttae; if the guttate spots are concentrated in the axial areas of the cornea with heavy pigmentation, the visual acuity may be reduced. A typical beaten-metal appearance to the endothelial layer with scattered pigment is seen on slit-lamp examination. On specular reflection the endothelial warts are seen as dark guttate spots, and the normal hexagonal appearance of the endothelium is disturbed. The cells are irregular in size and shape.

If the "warts" are numerous and the endothelial cells are compromised or de-stroyed to a point at which metabolism becomes inefficient, then stromal edema occurs, followed by epithelial edema and bullous keratopathy (Fig. 11-41). The average case of mild-to-moderate cornea guttata remains stationary for years.

Guttate lesions are located in the periphery of the cornea in young individuals. In this instance, they are called Hassall-Henle bodies and are innocuous. Hassall-Henle bodies are more dome shaped than are the guttate of cornea guttata, which are shaped like mushrooms, and the endothelial cells are not as thinned over their surface, as is seen in true cornea guttata.

In some instances the endothelial change is not in guttate form but is seen as a diffusely increased relucency of the endothelium, giving the appearance of a grayish membrane.[140, 150] In these cases the warts may be buried in a thickened Descemet layer and thus are without the appearance of guttate formation.

Secondary cornea guttata may be associated with degenerative corneal disease, trauma, or inflammations. The corneal endothelium is adversely affected in iritis, deep stromal inflammation, corneal ulcers, corneal abscesses, injury, keratoconus, and interstitial keratitis.[212] In severe inflammation endothelial cells may become edematous and, in this instance, may resemble a guttate appearance.[178] The guttata sub-sides when the causative agent is removed, but with true cornea guttata, of course, the lesion is permanent. Secondary linear guttate lesions may fuse together to form hyaline ridges on the posterior cornea, as is seen in chronic keratouveitis, luetic interstitial keratitis, recurrent corneal ulcers,[215] neuroparalytic keratitis,[199] herpes simplex disciform keratitis,[159] endothelial dystrophy,[172] and mesodermal dysgenesis of the iris.[176]

It has been shown that air has an effect on human corneal endothelium. There is a loss of endothelial cells, as well as a peau d'orange effect or pseudoguttate formation. These effects are transient and disappear with the reabsorption of the air from the anterior chamber.[158]

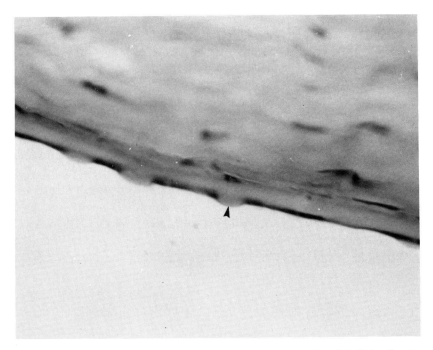

Fig. 11-40. Cornea guttata. Descemet's warts are noted with loss of endothelial cells *(arrow)*.

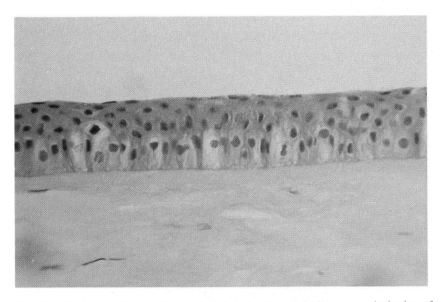

Fig. 11-41. Early bullous keratopathy in Fuchs' dystrophy, clinically seen as bedewing of epithelium. (From Grayson, M., and Keates, R.H.: Manual of diseases of the cornea, Boston, 1969, Little, Brown & Co.)

On occasion, one may see fine networklike structures extending from the posterior surface of the cornea into the anterior chamber. These hyaline strands vary in size from fine threads to larger netlike structures.

Fuchs' endothelial dystrophy[186] (Fig. 11-42)

This condition is a bilateral dystrophy of the endothelium seen in the thirties to fifties.[148] It is probably dominantly transmitted[196] and occurs more often in women. Fuchs' dystrophy is a progressive corneal disease with resulting corneal edema caused by metabolic incompetency of the endothelial cells and their failure to act as an effective "pump." The end result is gradual opacification of the stroma with epithelial and stromal edema; the course of the disease extends over several decades.

The Descemet membrane–endothelial area is characterized by wartlike excrescences (Fig. 11-43), fine pigment dusting, moderate graying, and thickening of Descemet's membrane with progressive endothelial degeneration. However, one may see only irregular endothelial disturbance and no prominent "warts." The process begins in the axial portion of the cornea and spreads to the periphery. Phagocytized brown pigment may appear in the endothelial cells.[165]

The epithelium at first may exhibit bedewing. Epithelial edema appears first in the basal layers and later in the more superficial layers. On retroillumination the bedewing appears as a fine patina. However, as the condition progresses, the bedewing gives way to the formation of the epithelial bullae (Fig. 11-44). These bullae may rupture, and

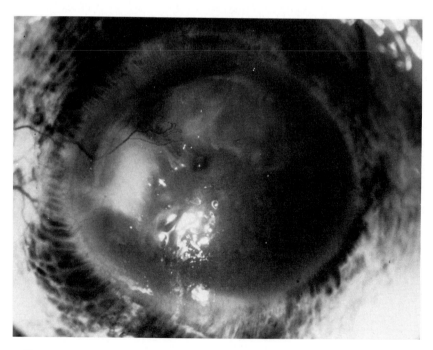

Fig. 11-42. Fuchs' dystrophy with epithelial bullae, scarring, and vascularization.

the patient will experience pain and foreign body sensation, with the eye becoming red and irritated. At this point the cornea in its compromised state may be susceptible to microbial invasion. The epithelial edema is more intense in the morning hours and in humid weather. Subepithelial fibrosis (Fig. 11-45) and vascularization may occur in more advanced cases. Corneas with long-standing edema may show increase in base-

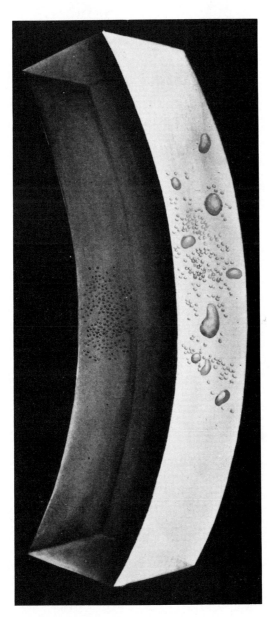

Fig. 11-43. Diagrammatic representation of wartlike excresences on Descemet's membrane and epithelial bullae seen in advanced Fuchs' dystrophy.

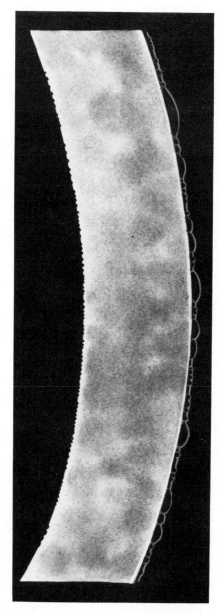

Fig. 11-44. Optical section diagrammatically depicts guttate and epithelial bullae of advanced Fuchs' dystrophy.

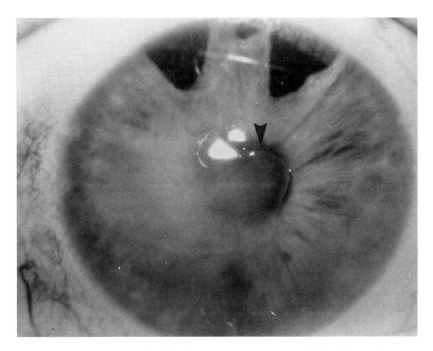

Fig. 11-45. Subepithelial fibrosis *(arrow)* may occur in Fuchs' dystrophy.

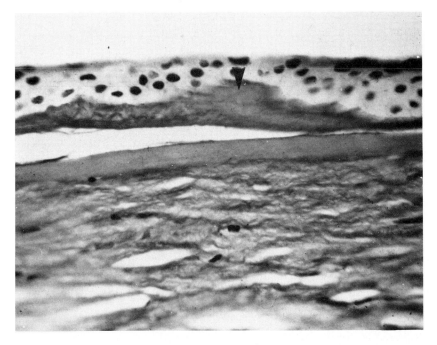

Fig. 11-46. In long-standing Fuchs' dystrophy, increase in basement membrane substance *(arrow)* and alterations in Bowman's layer may be seen.

ment membrane substance (Fig. 11-46), patchy loss of basement membrane and fewer hemidesmosomes. These all can result in recurring erosions.

Other signs of epithelial edema and involvement of the epithelial basement membrane are secondary fingerprint patterns and other linear opacities in the deep corneal epithelium. As the edema progresses, the stroma becomes more involved and may become opaque because of fibrosis and edema. An increase in relucency of the posterior stroma and the appearance of fluid clefts is also noted. In addition, Descemet's membrane may demonstrate an undulating appearance and thus can be thrown into folds (Fig. 11-47).

The irregularity of epithelium and light scatter at the surface of the cornea cause the decreased visual acuity in most of these patients. In addition, the subepithelial fibrosis may contribute to decreased vision. When the stroma becomes opacified, the visual acuity will suffer. In the early stages of epithelial edema, visual symptoms are worse on waking, before evaporation of the tears can clear the epithelium.

As noted, the main pathologic condition lies in the endothelium. The cells show changes in cell size and density, with thinning over Descemet's warts. The collagen tissue shows an increase posterior to Descemet's membrane. The new membrane consists of a basement membrane–like material, together with collagen material. The source of the new material is the diseased endothelial cells,[166] that is, both abnormal basement membrane with long-spaced collagen and layers of looser fibrillar collagen. Some cells take on morphologic features of fibroblasts that produce the collagen. In addition, some

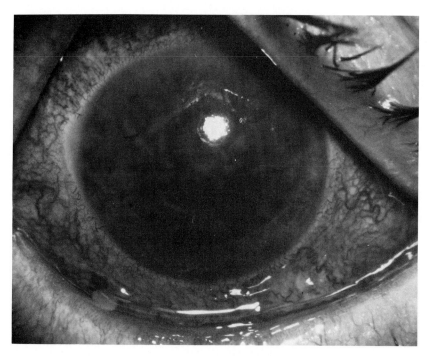

Fig. 11-47. Edema of stroma and large folds in Descemet's membrane occur in Fuchs' dystrophy.

cells show tonofilaments, surface microvilli, and desmosomes similar to epithelial cells.[162] As was noted, connective tissue is seen subepithelially and may arise from the epithelium itself or from fibroblasts from adjacent areas.

As the apical junctions of the epithelium deteriorate, and as the endothelium further undergoes deterioration, excess aqueous humor penetrates the stroma and fluid. The diseased endothelium can no longer act as an effective metabolic pumping agent; thus corneal edema results. As more scarring occurs, fewer bullae are seen, and the patient's complaints, which are caused by rupture of the bullae, become fewer and fewer.

Although no systemic problems are noted with Fuchs' endothelial dystrophy, one may observe that ocular hypertension and open-angle glaucoma may occur with more frequency than in the general population.[149] Narrow-angle glaucoma may also be seen, since the thick cornea may involve the angle even more.

Treatment. Patients with early epithelial edema may be treated conservatively at first with 5% sodium chloride drops six to eight times daily and 5% sodium chloride ointment at night before sleep if the edema is mild. This medication decreases the epithelial edema and affords better visual acuity for a short while during the day. The hyperosmotic agents act primarily on the epithelial edema and have no influence on the stromal edema. A hair dryer held at arm's length from the surface of the cornea may help "dry out" the corneal surfaces and may be repeated two or three times a day.

A therapeutic soft lens (bandage lens) is beneficial in alleviating any discomfort

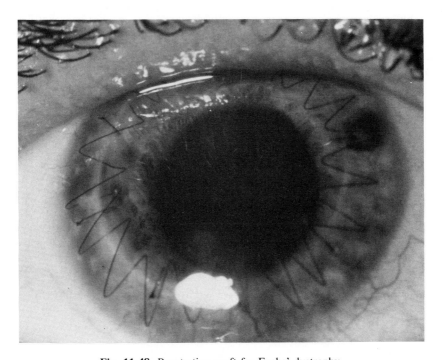

Fig. 11-48. Penetrating graft for Fuchs' dystrophy.

Table 11-5. Suggested method of treatment of endothelial dystrophy with or without cataract

Condition of cornea	Vision	Measurement of intraocular pressure	Suggested treatment
Cornea guttata with no gross epithelial edema in presence of cataract or without cataract	Usually good if no cataract is present or if corneal pigmentation is not great in axial area of cornea	May be measured with applanation tonometer when edema of epithelium not present	If no cataract present, watch May use hyperosmotic agents (drops), if there is decreased visual acuity in morning Hair dryer to be used at arm's length. Allow warm air to flow on surface of cornea for 1 to 2 minutes If cataract is present, may use regular technique of intracapsular cataract extraction
No *gross* epithelial edema Cataract	Cloudy in morning and clear in evening	May be measured with applanation tonometer when no epithelial edema is present; otherwise use MacKay-Marg tonometer	May perform cataract extraction with care not to touch endothelium; avoid bleeding in and excessive irrigation of anterior chamber Hyperosmotic agents when necessary Hair dryer when epithelial edema is noted
Epithelial edema with thick stroma but no cataract or posterior corneal folds Include aphakia	Cloudy Visual acuity is decreased, but *not* debilitating as yet	MacKay-Marg tonometer may show increased IOP Applanation tension is inaccurate under these circumstances	Hair dryer Hyperosmotic agents Control IOP Soft contact lens if corneal erosions and epithelial bullae are causes of symptoms
Epithelial edema with posterior corneal folds and stromal thickening and cataract Not controlled by usual medical methods	Poor vision	MacKay-Marg tonometer may demonstrate increase in IOP	Combined corneal graft and cataract extraction Try contact lens to decrease irregular astigmatism caused by epithelial edema if patient is too ill to undergo surgery Corneal graft in aphakic patients Watch for cystoid macular edema in all aphakic patients; this is limiting factor for obtaining good vision postoperatively in presence of clear graft
Bullous keratopathy without cataract	Poor vision	MacKay-Marg tonometer may have increase in IOP	Corneal graft
Bullous keratopathy with cataract	Poor vision	MacKay-Marg tonometer Watch for increased IOP	Combined cataract extraction and graft

resulting from bullae formation and rupture. This lens has made life more pleasant particularly for older patients who do not desire or cannot undergo corneal transplantation.

However, if both eyes are involved with 20/80 vision or less, it is advisable to perform a penetrating keratoplasty on one eye. If the patient has only one remaining eye and has a severe bullous keratopathy with vision of 20/200 or less, a penetrating graft on the remaining eye may be attempted (Fig. 11-48). The success rate for aphakic keratoplasty has appreciably increased since the introduction of microsurgical techniques, microinstruments, 10-0 sutures, and anterior vitrectomy techniques. However, the recognition of cystoid macular edema as a cause of poor visual acuity in the face of a clear graft can be frustrating.

Fuchs' endothelial dystrophy in the presence of a cloudy lens should be treated with a combined procedure (Table 11-5). The fact that the duration of a clear graft, even when all parameters are in excellent order, may be limited[204] must also be considered. Keratoplasty in the presence of very narrow angles should be accompanied by lens extraction.

If the intraocular pressure is elevated, this should be treated because it will increase the fluid in the cornea. This may be done with carbonic anhydrase inhibitors, miotics, or epinephrine. The IOP must be taken with the electronic applanometer (MacKay-Marg) since there is a tendency for Goldmann applanation to give falsely low readings.

Congenital hereditary endothelial dystrophy (CHED)[174, 188]

This corneal dystrophy is hereditary, but various modes of inheritance have been reported, such as autosomal recessive or autosomal dominant.[189] The recessive form is more common, whereas the dominant form is rare and more associated with other ocular and systemic abnormalities.[169, 170] The recessive form is present in the neonatal period or at birth. Nystagmus often occurs; usually there are no other signs or symptoms. The dominant form generally exhibits clear corneas early in life, but opacification is slowly progressive.[168]

The essential feature of CHED is congenital, bilateral diffuse corneal edema unrelated to commonly known etiologic factors such as congenital glaucoma,[142, 143] intrauterine infections, or mucopolysaccharidosis.

The opacity is seen at or shortly after birth.[142-144]

The clinical picture may vary from a mild haziness to a moderately severe, diffuse, homogeneous, gray-white, ground-glass appearance of the central cornea that extends to the periphery. A thickening of the cornea by two to three times is also seen and is one way in which a cloudy cornea caused by CHED may be differentiated from one caused by posterior polymorphous dystrophy, in which instance the cornea is of normal thickness. Diffuse cloudiness with corneal thickening caused by edema usually prevents clinical evaluation of endothelium and Descemet's membrane. There is no vascularization, and corneal sensitivity and intraocular pressure are normal. The corneal opacity may be stationary but may show slow progression with epithelial disease. Discomfort rarely occurs since bullae are not usually seen; however, epithelial edema and bedewing can occur. If the problem occurs early in life, a fixation nystagmus and esotropia are seen.

The basic problem seems to be an endothelial degeneration, which may have its onset in utero or a few months to a year after birth. If the endothelial defect or absence occurred during fetal life, it is likely that Descemet's membrane will be poorly formed,[169, 170] and marked stromal edema and opacity will be present at birth.[144] In CHED the normal appearance of the 3 μm thickness of the banded anterior fetal portion of Descemet's membrane indicates that the endothelium is functionally normal throughout most of uterine life. However, with the onset of endothelial dysfunction, at the fifth month of gestation the affected endothelium secretes abnormal and excessive basement membrane, which accumulates as aberrant, nonbanded posterior portion of Descemet's membrane.[169, 172, 173, 195] As the condition progresses, secondary changes occur in the epithelium and Bowman's layer. Collagen fibers of the stroma are separated by fluid. The collagen fibers are of normal or larger diameter with no apparent relation to keratocytes. Descemet's membrane is thickened.

One may find asymptomatic relatives with CHED; this recognition is important because these persons run a high risk of producing offspring with severe visual loss.[183] The asymptomatic individuals have normal visual acuity and corneal thickness.[183] However, clear, vacuole-like lesions with surrounding white haze, irregular endothelial mosaic, and beaded white lines may extend across the level of Descemet's membrane. The lesions in this group are similar in appearance to those described with posterior polymorphous dystrophy.[189] On occasion one may find patients with progressive sensorineural deafness in association with CHED.[163, 190]

Differential diagnosis. The preceding discussion of CHED raises the question of opacification of the cornea at birth. In addition to CHED, the following conditions must be taken into consideration:

1. Congenital glaucoma
2. Anterior segment malformation
3. Birth trauma
4. Congenital lues
5. Inborn errors of metabolism
6. Trisomy 13
7. Acid mucopolysaccharide accumulation in Bowman's layer
8. Peters' anomaly
9. Intrauterine infection—posterior corneal ulcers

Treatment. Poor results with penetrating keratoplasty are caused by the frequency of surgical complications and to the inability of technically satisfactory grafts to remain clear.[209] This latter development results from failure of the donor endothelial cells and their replacement by the defective cells of the host.[189] It is to be stressed that the donor endothelium must be of high quality so that a penetrating keratoplasty will have a chance for success. Recently long-term clear grafts have been reported.[208]

Congenital hereditary stromal dystrophy (CHSD)[210]

Congenital hereditary stromal dystrophy is seen as an autosomal dominant trait that is present at birth and is mostly stationary with no epithelial disease. The corneal stroma exhibits a flaky, feathery appearance. No secondary changes are noted in the anterior

Table 11-6. Comparative classification of diffuse congenital dystrophies appearing in the first year of life

Characteristic	Posterior polymorphous dystrophy (congenital corneal edema)	Congenital hereditary stromal dystrophy	Congenital hereditary endothelial dystrophy
Inheritance	Autosomal dominant	Autosomal dominant	Autosomal recessive
Laterality	Bilateral	Bilateral	Bilateral
Time of appearance of opacity	At birth or within first year	At birth	At birth
Progression	Slowly progressive	None	Minimal
Corneal thickness	Probably normal	Normal	Severely increased
Location of opacity	Diffuse	Central	Diffuse
Appearance of opacity	Ground glass	Ground glass, flaky, feathery	Ground glass, few white maculae
Histopathology			
Epithelium	Mild edema	Normal	Mild edema
Bowman's layer	Fragmented or intact	Normal	Intact or fragmented
Stroma	Edema, some large collagen fibrils (700 nm diameter)	Entire stroma; small diameter collagen fibrils (15 nm) form alternating loose and compact lamellae	Edema, some large collagen fibrils (700 nm diameter)
Descemet's membrane	Thin original Descemet's membrane covered by multilaminar collagen tissue	Normal anterior banding not prominent	Thin original Descemet's membrane covered by acellular feltwork of 30 nm diameter collagen fibrils
Endothelium	Epithelial-like: many microvillae, desmosomes, and tonofilaments	Normal	Often atrophic

layers of the cornea. The stroma shows loose and compact lamellae composed of collagen filaments of small diameter. The loose lamellae are related to a keratocyte. Descemet's membrane is normal, as is the endothelium.

It is seen therefore that CHSD essentially is a disorder of stromal fibrillogenesis and an underlying disturbance of the composition and distribution of acid mucopolysaccharide in the lamellae on which the sizes, shapes, and arrangements of collagen fibers depend. Table 11-6 lists the important differences among CHSD, PPD, and CHED.

Posterior polymorphous dystrophy (PPD)

Posterior polymorphous dystrophy is usually transmitted as a dominant trait but it also has been claimed to be transmitted as a recessive trait.[164] This most often bilateral dystrophy may be congenital or may develop early in life; in many instances it is asymmetrical. Occasionally it is unilateral or more advanced in one eye than the other.[147] Usually patients with PPD demonstrate normal vision and are asymptomatic, so that age of onset may be difficult to determine. However, if the lesions are severe and are concentrated in the visual axis with edema, the visual acuity may be reduced.[162] Ordinarily, since the epithelium is not edematous, the stroma is spared, and the vision is not reduced. Normal corneal sensitivity is noted, and vascularization is not ordinarily seen except in severe cases. PPD can be slowly progressive.

Nodular, grouped vesicular and blisterlike lesions on Descemet's membrane area occur[201] (Figs. 11-49 and 11-50). Gray-white halos surrounding the vesicles are seen as are flat, gray-white opacities resembling the hazy, white-gray zones that surround the vesicles. In addition, sinuous broad bands and gray thickened areas of Descemet's membrane are noted.[162] The lesions stand out on retroillumination from the iris. The vesicles were at one time thought to be caused by herpes. The broad bands consist of elevated ridges that are roughly parallel to each other and must be differentiated from traumatic breaks in Descemet's membrane. Although PPD is said to be nonprogressive, in fact it is slowly progressive; however, the condition may be severe enough to require keratoplasty.[162]

Posterior polymorphous corneal dystrophy may be associated with band kera topathy,[162] anterior segment mesodermal dysgenesis with prominent ring of Schwalbe,

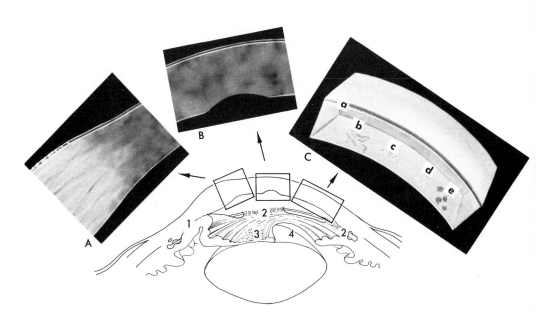

Fig. 11-49. A, Posterior polymorphous dystrophy. Diagrammatic representation of biomicroscopic findings: *(1)* iridocorneal adhesions obliterating trabeculum, *(2)* abnormal iris processes, and *(3)* patchy iris atrophy involving iris stroma. **B,** Area of circumscribed posterior keratoconus. **C,** Section en bloc showing *(a)* calcific deposition in Bowman's membrane layer, *(b)* "sinuous" opacities, *(c)* vesicular lesions, *(d)* flat gray-white macular lesions, and *(e)* aggregations of guttata. (From Grayson, M.: Trans. Am. Ophthalmol. Soc. **72:**517, 1974.)

iridocorneal adhesions, abnormal iris processes, iris atrophy, displaced pupil,[162] glaucoma,[147, 162, 193, 198] deposition of calcium apatite crystals in the deep stroma,[164] cornea guttata with edema, and posterior circumscribed keratoconus (Fig. 11-49 and Table 11-7).

Electron-microscopic study has revealed the main change to be in the endothelial cell.[147, 162] It is stated that the endothelial cell may undergo metaplasia into an epithelial-

Text continued on p. 308.

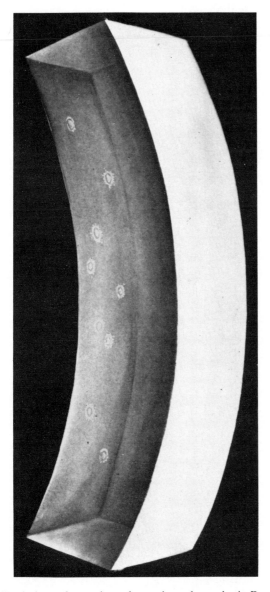

Fig. 11-50. Blisterlike lesions of posterior polymorphous dystrophy in Descemet's membrane.

Table 11-7. Disease spectrum noted in deep posterior polymorphous dystrophy and anterior mesodermal dysgenesis

Type A	Type B	Type C	Type D	Type E (Hogan and Bietti)	Congenital hereditary edema
Nonprogressive	Nonprogressive	Progressive	Iris processes and broad synechiae	No anterior segment anomaly	Cornea edema
Vesicular lesions projecting into anterior chamber from posterior corneal surface	Vesicular lesions on posterior surface of cornea project into anterior chamber	Iris processes in chamber angle	Iris atrophy	Calcium deposition deep in stroma	Descemet membrane alterations with electron microscope, which resemble those changes seen in types C and D
No anterior segment disease	Iris processes in angle of anterior chamber	Posterior embryotoxon	Corectopia	Posterior membrane lesions that are "sinuous" and elevated	
		No glaucoma	Glaucoma		
		Posterior membrane changes exhibit blisterlike droplets, flat macular-like and sinuous opacities	Band keratopathy		
		Corneal edema	Corneal edema		
		Cornea guttata	Posterior embryotoxon		
			Posterior keratoconus		
			Cornea guttata		
			Progressive posterior membrane changes: sinuous lesions, blisterlike and macular-like lesions in Descemet's area		
			Sclerocornea		

From Grayson, M.: Trans. Am. Ophthalmol. Soc. **72:**517, 1974.

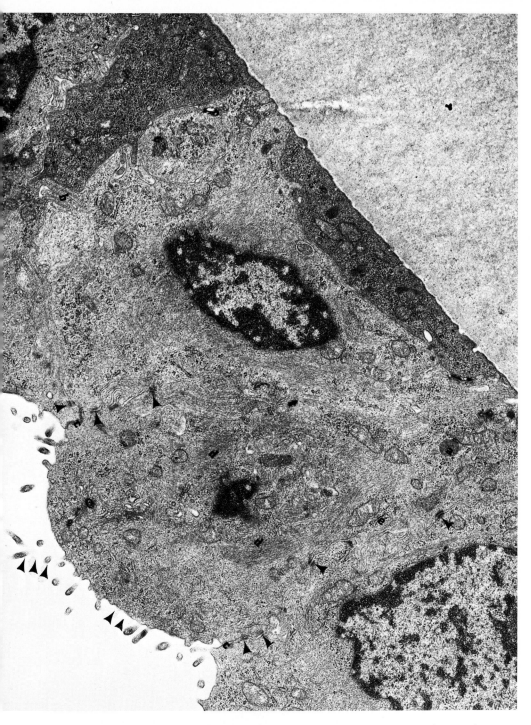

Fig. 11-51. Polymorphous dystrophy. Mitochondria are few, and those present are degenerating *(a)*. Desmosomes *(single arrows)* are abundant, and microvilli are numerous *(triple arrow)*. Extensive interdigitation between cells *(b)* and zonulae occludens are noted *(c)*. *d,* Extensive intracytoplasmic filaments; *e,* elongated endoplasmic reticulum. Double arrows indicate rounded edge or elevated apices of altered cells. (×8714.5.) (From Grayson, M.: Trans. Am. Ophthalmol. Soc. **72:**517, 1974.)

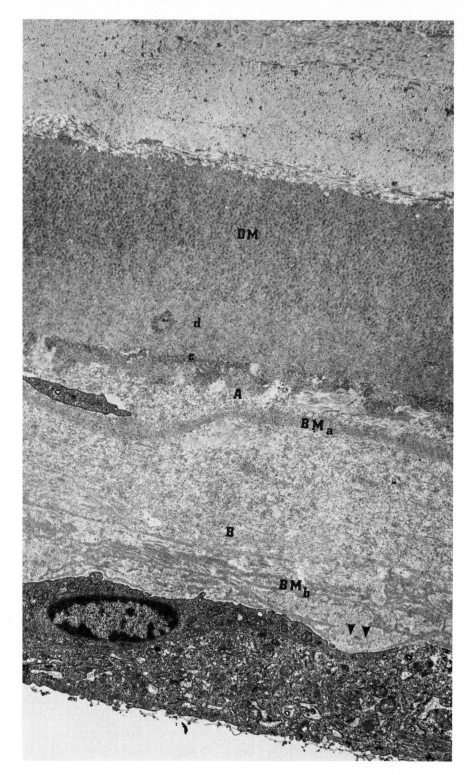

Fig. 11-52. Posterior polymorphous dystrophy. Abnormal membrane has been laid down in layers *A* and *B*. Abnormal membrane consists of collagen fibers and laminated areas of basement membrane (BM_a and BM_b). Demarcation line *(c)* is visible. BM_a separates collagen fiber layers *A* and *B*. Double arrow indicates area in which indentations are made into the posterior cellular layer, possibly representing early guttate lesions. Descemet's membrane *(DM)* shows narrow nonbanded zone *(d)*. (×6394.5.) (From Grayson, M.: Trans. Am. Ophthalmol. Soc. **72:**517, 1974.)

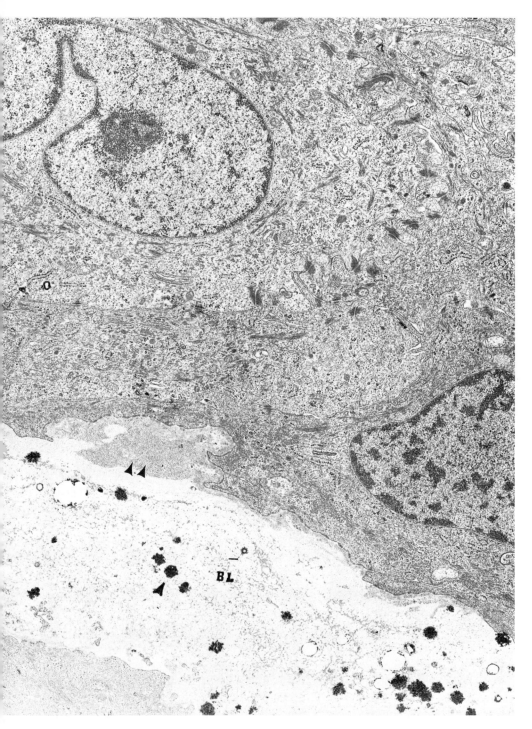

Fig. 11-53. Irregular thickening of basement membrane *(double arrow)* of epithelium is present. Calcium deposits *(single arrow)* are noted in Bowman's layer *(BL)*. Note normal presence of many desmosomes and cytoplasmic filaments in epithelial cells. (×8714.5.) (From Grayson, M.: Trans. Am. Ophthalmol. Soc. **72:**517, 1974.)

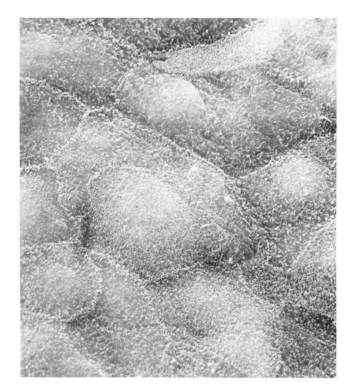

Fig. 11-54. Posterior polymorphous dystrophy. Myriads of microvilli may be seen on scanning electron microscopy.

like cell. The fact that the anterior banded layer of Descemet's membrane is of normal thickness suggests that the problem develops in the neonatal period. These cells exhibit mitochondrial changes, intracytoplasmic filaments, hemidesmosomes, a decreased number of organelles, and many microvilli[162] (Figs. 11-51 and 11-52). In addition to these changes, deposition of abnormal multilaminated basement membrane has been found[162, 165] (Fig. 11-52). The latter is deposited by these abnormal endothelial cells.[162, 195]

In advanced cases, intercellular and intracellular epithelial edema occurs, and the epithelial basement membrane is thick and fragmented. Bowman's layer is usually normal, although subepithelial fibrous tissue is seen in advanced cases,[162] and calcific deposits that form band keratopathy may be seen (Fig. 11-53).

Scanning electron microscopy shows myriads of microvilli and microplicae (Fig. 11-54).[192]

Treatment. In uncomplicated cases no treatment is essential, but keratoplasty is occasionally indicated. In rare instances the corneal edema in adults decreases spontaneously with improvement in visual acuity.[151] If edema is a direct problem, hypertonic solutions or a soft contact lens may be tried.[151, 162]

It is noted that glaucoma, iridocorneal adhesions, and corneal edema are seen in PPD and Chandler's syndrome.[197] However, there are differences, as listed in Table 11-8.

Table 11-8. Disease spectrum in PPD and Chandler's syndrome

PPD	Chandler's syndrome
Inherited dystrophy Usually dominant Ridges, vesicles, and plaques on posterior surface of the cornea Endothelial decompensation leads to epithelial and stromal edema Some patients have iridocorneal adhesions, ectropion of iris pigment, and glaucoma Bilateral Slowly progressive Endothelialization of the anterior chamber angle as is seen in Chandler's syndrome; ultrastructural characteristics of epithelial cells	Spectrum of iris atrophy syndromes, which includes essential iris atrophy and iris nevus syndrome Corneal edema secondary to endothelial dystrophy Iris atrophy confined to stroma is minimal; no through and through holes; normal pupil (classic essential iris atrophy shows true iris dissolution with holes and irregular pupil) Anterior chamber angle shows peripheral anterior synechia and glaucoma Nonfamilial Rapidly progressive Unilateral Ectopic endothelium and abnormal Descemet's membrane covering the trabecular meshwork and extending on to the iris (also seen in essential iris atrophy) Endothelial cells were degenerated but retained their endothelial ultrastructural characteristics

Traumatic corneal endothelial change

This has been noted after nonpenetrating "blast injuries" to the eye. Small, multiple, corneal foreign bodies of the superficial cornea are associated with ring-shaped opacities of the endothelium, which disappear in several days.[152]

Ectatic dystrophies

ANTERIOR KERATOCONUS (Fig. 11-55)

This condition is commonly called conical cornea; it may be congenital but usually appears at puberty or soon after. It has a tendency to progress for about 7 to 8 years and then remain stable. However, exacerbations of progression may occur at any time. The apex of the cone is usually displaced nasally and inferiorly with an oblique conical deformation of the cone. It is bilateral, but formes fruste can be found in family members or in the other eye of a seemingly unilateral case. The optical problem is one of high irregularity or high astigmatism, as demonstrated by keratometry. In the office a Klein keratoscope or Placido's disc may be used to demonstrate distortion of the corneal mires.

Two cone types are described. The first is the more common round, or nipple, cone. The cone center most often lies inferiorly and nasally often within a few millimeters of the visual axis. The other cone, the oval or sagging cone, is less common, is larger, and lies in the inferotemporal quadrant. It is more often associated with corneal hydrops and scarring. The oval cone optical center is further away from the visual axis. It is

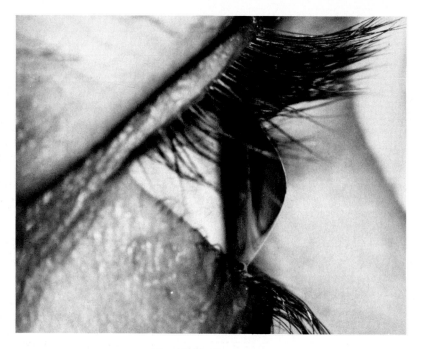

Fig. 11-55. Keratoconus.

closer to the limbus, which makes it more difficult to fit a contact lens and to surgically correct it.[237]

Apical thinning of the cornea occurs; however, the cornea seldom, if ever, perforates. The conical deformation of the cornea results in a convexity of the lower lid on downward gaze called Munson's sign. Vertical stress lines appear deep in the cornea stroma. Increased visibility of the corneal nerves and Fleischer's ring are diagnostic features of keratoconus. Fleischer's ring is an annular, brown-pigmented ring near the base of the cone. Hemosiderin is found in the basal epithelial cells; it is seen with the slit lamp in low magnification and with diffuse cobalt-blue light.[232] Ruptures of and scars in Bowman's layer, as well as increased visibility of the corneal nerves, are also seen. Occasionally one will see ruptures of Descemet's membrane and endothelial shagreen in the area of the cone and guttae. Speculation has been advanced that the wearing of contact lenses by patients with low scleral rigidity might occasionally cause the development of keratoconus or permanent with the rule of astigmatism.

Histopathologic examination reveals fragmentation and fibrillation of Bowman's layer and the basement membrane (Fig. 11-56). Islands of fibroblastic activity occur in the area of Bowman's layer, basement membrane, and anterior stroma. This fragmentation of Bowman's layer with islands of fibrolytic activity is seen consistently in the histopathologic findings of keratoconus. Electron microscopic studies suggest that the early changes may be in the basal epithelial cells, which degenerate and release proteolytic enzymes that lead to the destruction of Bowman's layer and basement membrane. The anterior stromal keratocytes undergo fibroblastic activity. It has been shown that in

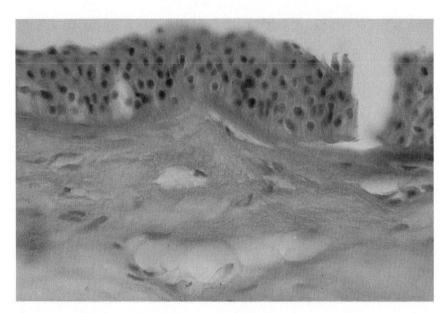

Fig. 11-56. Fragmentation and fibrillation of Bowman's layer and basement membrane in kerato-conus. (From Grayson, M.: Degenerations, dystrophies, and edema of the cornea. In Duane, T.D. [ed.]: Clinical Ophthalmology. Hagerstown, Md.: Harper & Row, 1978, vol. 4, chap. 16.)

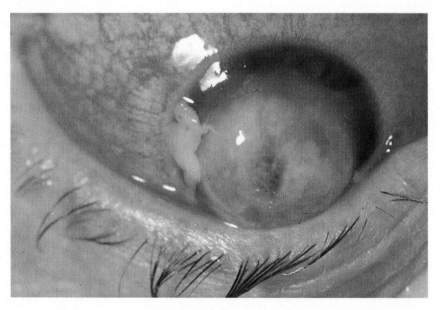

Fig. 11-57. Acute corneal hydrops.

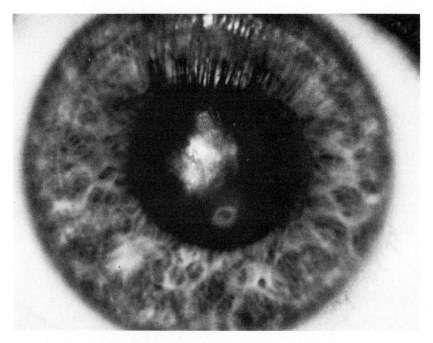

Fig. 11-58. Residual scarring from hydrops of cornea secondary to keratoconus.

cross sections of the normal cornea there are about 340 lamellae, but the collagen fibers themselves are of normal diameter.[238] Keratocytes near the cone demonstrate degenerative changes. Fleischer's ring, on electron-microscopic study, has been characterized by the accumulation of ferritin particles in intercellular spaces of the epithelium; 50% of the cases probably demonstrate this pigmented ring. Tears in Descemet's membrane occur, and degeneration of endothelium is seen with localized overproduction of Descemet's material. When Descemet's membrane ruptures, acute hydrops occurs; it may occur suddenly with an increase in corneal clouding as a result of ensuing edema (Fig. 11-57). The visual acuity becomes markedly decreased, and the eye becomes mildly irritable. The condition usually clears over an 8- to 10-week period, although some scarring (Fig. 11-58) or chronic edema may remain. Contraction of the scar may improve some of the optical aberrations by flattening the cone if there is no scarring in the pupillary area.

Keratoconus[223] may be associated with other ophthalmic findings such as[222] retinitis pigmentosa, ectopia lentis, congenital cataract, aniridia, microcornea, and blue sclera.

Systemic association with keratoconus consists of vernal catarrh[220]; atopy[220, 242]; hypothyroidism osteogenesis imperfecta[226]; and Down's,[241] Marfan's,[236] Apert's, Duane's,[230] Ehlers-Danlos,[236] Little's,[224] Noonan's,[240] and Crouzon's syndromes.[243] In Ehlers-Danlos[224] and Laurence-Moon-Biedl syndromes[224] keratoconus has been reported in association with microcornea, whereas it has been seen in association with megalocornea in van der Hoeve's syndrome,[231] Apert's syndrome, acrocephalo-syndactyl, and retrolental fibroplasia.[235]

Management

The keratoconus patient's vision should be corrected as long as is possible with spectacles. Refraction in these patients, especially of the subjective aspect, should be performed very carefully. If spectacles do not correct the vision, the patient may be fitted with contact lenses. Although keratoconus can develop in patients wearing contact lenses, I do not believe that contact lenses are responsible for the entity of clinical keratoconus. The patient may have started to wear contact lenses with undiagnosed keratoconus, or the keratoconus may have developed while the patient was wearing the lens.[228] It requires great patience on the part of the ophthalmologist and high motivation on the part of the patient to fit contact lenses in a moderate-to-severe case of keratoconus.[229]

Thermokeratoplasty has been used with limited success. At the present time patients indicated for a thermokeratoplasty are few. A good number of patients with keratoconus, including those with relatively steep cones, can be fitted with contact lenses. Only after exhaustive trial fittings with single-cut or multicurve lenses have been unsuccessful should thermokeratoplasty be considered. A cornea must be sufficiently clear to allow adequate visual acuity. The patient with dense stromal and Descemet membrane opacities in the visual axis is not a candidate for thermokeratoplasty. Unfortunately the patients who are difficult to fit with contact lenses are the patients with steep cones and corneal scarring. Some of the complications of thermokeratoplasty are stromal scarring or the recurrence of a steep cone. In a number of cases delayed reepithelialization or persistent epithelial defects have developed. Thermokeratoplasty can damage the basement membrane complexes at the interface between the basal epithelial cells and Bowman's layer and result in defects of the epithelial healing.

Association of keratoconus and mitral valve prolapse has been reported.[216]

Keratoplasty or penetrating keratoplasty should be considered if there is much scarring with poor visual acuity or if chronic edema persists after an acute attack of hydrops. It also must be considered when the contact lenses, either hard or soft, no longer suffice in providing adequate visual acuity. It is wise to follow carefully the degree of thinning in a patient so that the graft can be performed before too much thinning occurs in the periphery of the cornea. Occasionally a paretic pupil[221, 225] occurs after keratoplasty for keratoconus; the likely etiologic agent for this peculiarity will be found on the basis of ischemic atrophy of the sphincter pupillae muscle, secondary to iris "strangulation" and ischemia during surgery.[218, 221]

Epikeratophakia has been introduced as a surgical procedure that may be beneficial.[28]

Acute hydrops[225] should be treated conservatively, and assurance given to the patient that the condition nearly always improves; however, some residual scarring might persist. One may use a pressure patch during the day to put direct pressure on the cornea to counteract its swelling and thus decrease the edema. However, the patch should be removed at bedtime, since the pressure would be on the inferior sclera when the eyes roll up during sleep, which could actually result in an increase in the edema. If a mild anterior chamber reaction occurs, one may advise mild cycloplegia; if there is extensive epithelial edema, hyperosmotic agents may be of help; however, these treatments are usually of limited value. Anterior keratoconus usually heals in about 6 to 8 weeks, possibly with a residual scar. Topical steroid drops may be used to minimize scarring.

KERATOGLOBUS

In this bilateral, globular configuration of the cornea,[233] the cornea is thin, especially peripherally, and transparent, and the base diameter is either normal or slightly increased. Keratoglobus may be linked to keratoconus on a genetic basis: one family was reported to include a father with keratoglobus and a son with keratoconus.[219] A patient with thyroid ophthalmopathy developed keratoglobus in adulthood. In addition, keratoglobus has been associated with blue sclera,[217] hyperextensibility of the joints of the hand and ankles, sensorineural hearing defects, and mottling of the teeth. A prominent feature of this syndrome is corneal perforation after minimal trauma.

Pellucid marginal degeneration of the cornea has been described. It is considered a bilateral clear, inferior, corneal-thinning disorder. Protrusion of the cornea occurs above the band of thinning, which is located 1 to 2 mm from the limbus. It results in high astigmatic, against-the-rule errors. There are no cones, scars, or Fleischer rings, but there are stress lines, and hydrops can develop. I have called these cases keratoglobus when there was peripheral thinning and believe that keratoconus, keratoglobus, and pellucid marginal degeneration are variants of one and the same thing.   .

Differential diagnosis

It is important to differentiate among keratoglobus, keratectasia, and congenital anterior staphyloma. A keratectasia is a bulging, opaque cornea protruding through the palpebral aperture with variable thinning and scarring of the stroma. It usually occurs unilaterally and is probably caused by an intrauterine keratitis with perforation. The corneal tissue subsequently undergoes metaplasia to skinlike tissue. Keratectasia also may be caused by a failure of mesoderm to migrate into the cornea, with subsequent thinning and bulging. The condition of congenital anterior staphyloma is similar to keratectasia, but in this instance uveal tissue is incorporated in the cornea as a lining. Megalocornea may appear similar to keratoglobus, but the corneal diameter is normal in keratoglobus.

POSTERIOR KERATOCONUS[227, 234, 239]

Posterior keratoconus may be total or diffuse with a generalized increase in the curvature of the posterior corneal surface. Central thinning can result; but the anterior surface is normal. The condition is nonprogressive, with no evidence of hereditary transmission. Most cases have been found in women. The cornea remains clear or may show a mild stromal haze. The condition is probably a developmental arrest since the posterior curve is usually more marked in the embryonic cornea. The posterior surface is slightly more curved than the anterior surface, even in normal individuals.

This total or diffuse posterior keratoconus should not be confused with the more circumscribed keratoconus. In posterior keratoconus, a localized crater defect occurs on the posterior corneal surface with the concavity toward the anterior chamber. Descemet's membrane and epithelium are absent, and the stroma is thin. Stromal opacities overlie this lesion. The etiologic agent of posterior keratoconus is unknown but presumed to represent a local overabsorption of a defect in the mesodermal development, probably as a result of some problem with lens vesicle separation. The term von Hippel's posterior corneal ulcer is used as a synonym by some; others limit the use of this term to cases in which there is evidence of intrauterine inflammation.

The heredity of circumscribed posterior keratoconus is unclear; however, some cases may be familial. There have been instances in which various ocular abnormalities have been found, such as Fleischer's ring, cleavage anomalies, anterior lenticonus, aniridia, iris atrophy, and ectropion uvea. In addition systemic abnormalities may occur, such as hypertelorism, poorly developed nasal bridge, bull neck, mental retardation, stunted growth, and brachydactyly.

REFERENCES
Epithelium and Bowman's layer

1. Akiya, S., and Brown, S.E.: The ultrastructure of Reis-Bücklers dystrophy, Am. J. Ophthalmol. **72**:549, 1971.
2. Broderick, J.D., and Dark, A.J.: Corneal dystrophy in Cockayne's syndrome, Br. J. Ophthalmol. **57**:391, 1973.
3. Broderick, J.D., Dark, A.J., and Peace, G.W.: Fingerprint dystrophy of the cornea, Arch. Ophthalmol. **92**:483, 1974.
4. Bron, A.J., and Brown, N.A.: Some superficial corneal disorders, Trans. Ophthalmol. Soc. U.K. **91**:13, 1971.
5. Bron, A.J., and Jones, D.B.: Net-like degeneration of Bowman's membrane, Br. J. Ophthalmol. **53**:490, 1969.
6. Bron, A.J., and Tripathi, R.C.: Anterior corneal mosaic: further observations, Br. J. Ophthalmol. **53**:760, 1969.
7. Bron, A.J., and Tripathi, R.C.: Cystic disorders of the corneal epithelium. I. Clinical aspects, Br. J. Ophthalmol. **57**:361, 1973.
8. Brown, N.A., and Bron, A.J.: Recurrent erosion of the cornea, Br. J. Ophthalmol. **60**:84, 1976.
9. Bücklers, M.: Ueber eine weitere familiäre Hornhautdystrophie (Reis), Klin. Monatsbl. Augenheilkd. **114**:386, 1949.
10. Burns, R.D.: Meesmann's corneal dystrophy, Trans. Am. Ophthalmol. Soc. **66**:531, 1968.
11. Cavanaugh, D.W., Pihlaja, D., Thoft, R., and Dohlman, C.H.: Pathogenesis and treatment of persistent epithelial defects, Trans. Am. Acad. Ophthalmol. Otolaryngol. **81**:754, 1976.
12. Chandler, P.A.: Recurrent erosions of the cornea, Am. J. Ophthalmol. **28**:355, 1945.
13. Cogan, D.G., Donaldson, D.D., Kuwabara, R., and Marshall, D.: Microcystic dystrophy of the corneal epithelium, Trans. Am. Ophthalmol. Soc. **62**:213, 1964.
14. Cogan, D.G., Kuwabara, T., Donaldson, D.D., and Collins, E.: Microcystic dystrophy of the cornea, Arch. Ophthalmol. **92**:470, 1974.
15. Dark, A.J.: Bleb dystrophy of the cornea: histochemistry and ultrastructure, Br. J. Ophthalmol. **61**:65, 1977.
16. Dark, A.J.: Cogan's microcystic dystrophy of the cornea: ultrastructure and photomicroscopy, Br. J. Ophthalmol. **62**:821, 1979.
17. Fine, B.S., Yanoff, M., Pitts, E., and Slaughter, F.D.: Meesmann's epithelial dystrophy of the cornea, Am. J. Ophthalmol. **83**:633, 1977.
18. Fogle, J.A., Kenyon, K.R., Stack, W.J., and Green, W.R.: Defective epithelial adhesion in anterior corneal dystrophies, Am. J. Ophthalmol. **79**:925, 1975.
19. Foulks, G.N.: Treatment of recurrent corneal erosion and corneal edema with topical osmotic colloidal solution, Ophthalmology **88**:801, 1981.
20. Goldman, J.M., Dohlman, C.H., and Kravitt, B.A.: The basement membrane of the human cornea in recurrent epithelial erosion syndrome, Trans. Am. Acad. Ophthalmol. Otolaryngol. **73**:471, 1969.
21. Grayson, M., and Wilbrandt, H.: Dystrophy of the anterior limiting membrane of the cornea (Reis-Bücklers type), Am. J. Ophthalmol. **63**:345, 1966.
22. Griffith, D.G., and Fine, B.S.: Light and electron microscopic observations in a superficial corneal dystrophy, Am. J. Ophthalmol. **63**:1659, 1967.

23. Hall, P.: Reis-Bücklers dystrophy, Arch. Ophthalmol. **91**:170, 1974.
24. Hogan, M., and Wood, I.: Reis-Bücklers corneal dystrophy, Trans. Ophthalmol. Soc. U.K. **91**:41, 1971.
25. Jones, S.T., and Stauffer, L.H.: Reis-Bücklers corneal dystrophy, Trans. Am. Acad. Ophthalmol. Otolaryngol. **74**:417, 1970.
26. Kanai, A., Kaufman, H.E., and Polack, F.M.: Electron microscopic study of Reis-Bücklers dystrophy, Ann. Ophthalmol. **5**:953, 1973.
27. Kaufman, H.G., and Clowe, F.W.: Irregularities of Bowman's membrane, Am. J. Ophthalmol. **62**:227, 1966.
28. Kaufman, H.E., and Werblin, T.P.: Epikeratophakia for the treatment of keratoconus, Am. J. Ophthalmol. **93**:342, 1982.
29. Kenyon, K.: The synthesis of basement membrane by epithelium in bullous keratopathy, Invest. Ophthalmol. **8**:156, 1969.
30. Khodadoust, A.A., Silverstein, A.M., Kenyon, R.K., and Dowling, J.E.: Adhesion of regenerating corneal epithelium. The role of the basement membrane, Am. J. Ophthalmol. **65**:339, 1968.
31. King, R.G., Jr., and Geeraets, R.: Cogan-Guerry microcystic corneal epithelial dystrophy, Med. Coll. Va. Q. **8**:241, 1972.
32. Kuwabara, R., and Ciccarelli, E.C.: Meesmann's corneal dystrophy, Arch. Ophthalmol. **71**:676, 1964.
33. Laibson, P.R., and Krachmer, J.H.: Familial occurrence of dot, map and fingerprint dystrophy of the cornea, Invest. Ophthalmol. **14**:397, 1975.
34. Mandelcorn, M.S., Blankenship, G., and Machemer, R.: Pars plana vitrectomy for management of severe diabetic retinopathy, Am. J. Ophthalmol. **81**:561, 1976.
35. Meesmann, A.: Ueber eine bisher nicht beschriebene dominant vererbte Dystrophia epithelialis corneae, Ber. Dtsch. Ophthalmol. Ges. **52**:154, 1938.
36. Meesmann, A., and Wilke, F.: Klinische und anatomische Untersuchungen über eine bisher unbekannte, dominant vererbte Epitheldystrophie der Hornhaut, Klin. Monatsbl. Augenheilkd. **103**:361, 1939.
37. Mondeno, B.J., Brown, S.I., Robin, B.S., and Temp, M.A.: Autoimmune phenomena of the conjunctiva and cornea, Arch. Ophthalmol. **95**:468, 1977.
38. Nakaniski, I., and Brown, S.I.: Ultrastructure of epithelial dystrophy of Meesmann, Arch. Ophthalmol. **93**:259, 1975.
39. Olson, R.J., Kaufman, H.E.: Recurrence of Reis-Bücklers corneal dystrophy in a graft, Am. J. Ophthalmol. **85**:349, 1978.
40. Pameijer, J.K.: Ueber eine fremdartige familiäre oberflächliche Hornhautveränderung, Klin. Monatsbl. Augenheilkd. **95**:516, 1935.
41. Paufique, L., and Bonnet, M.: La dystrophie cornéenne hérédo-familiale de Reis-Bücklers, Ann. Oculist **199**:14, 1966.
42. Polack, F.M.: Contributions of electron microscopy to the study of corneal pathology, Surv. Ophthalmol. **20**:375, 1976.
43. Reis, W.: Familiäre, fleckige Hornhautentartung, Dtsch. Med. Wochenschr. **43**:575, 1917.
44. Rice, N.S.C., Ashton, N., Jay, B., and Black, R.K.: Reis-Bücklers dystrophy, Br. J. Ophthalmol. **52**:577, 1968.
45. Rodrigues, M.M., Calhoun, J., and Harley, R.D.: Corneal clouding with increased acid mucopolysaccharide accumulation in Bowman's membrane, Am. J. Ophthalmol. **79**:916, 1975.
46. Rodrigues, M.M., Fine, B.S., Laibson, P.R., and Zimmerman, L.E.: Disorders of the corneal epithelium, Arch. Ophthalmol. **92**:475, 1974.
47. Streiff, E.B., and Zwahlen, P.: Une famille avec dégénérescence en bandelette de la cornée, Ophthalmologica (Paris) **111**:129, 1947.
48. Thiel, H.J., and Behnke, H.: Eine bisher unbekannte subepitheliale hereditäre Hornhautdystrophie, Klin. Monatsbl. Augenheilkd. **150**:862, 1967.
49. Tripathi, R.C., and Bron, A.J.: Ultrastructural study of nontraumatic recurrent erosion, Br. J. Ophthalmol. **56**:73, 1972.
50. Tripathi, R.G., and Bron, A.J.: Cystic disorders of the corneal epithelium. II. Pathogenesis, Br. J. Ophthalmol. **57**:375, 1973.
51. Trobe, J.D., and Laibson, P.R.: Dystrophic changes in the anterior cornea, Arch. Ophthalmol. **87**:378, 1972.
52. Wales, H.J.: A family history of corneal erosions, Trans. Ophthalmol. Soc. N.Z. **8**:77, 1955.
53. Winkelman, J.E., and Delleman, J.W.: Reis-Bücklers Hornhautdystrophie und die Rolle der Bowmanschen Membran, Klin. Monatsbl. Augenheilkd. **155**:380, 1969.
54. Wolter, J.R., and Fralick, F.B.: Microcystic dystrophy of the corneal epithelium, Arch. Ophthalmol. **75**:380, 1966.
55. Wood, T.O., Fleming, J.C., Dotson, R.S., and Cotton, M.S.: Treatment of Reis-Bücklers corneal dystrophy by removal of subepithelial fibrous tissue, Am. J. Ophthalmol. **85**:360, 1978.

Stromal dystrophies

56. Akiya, S., and Brown, S.I.: Granular dystrophy of the cornea: characteristic electron microscopic lesions, Arch. Ophthalmol. **84**:179, 1970.

57. Akiya, S., Ito, I., and Matsui, M.: Gelatinous drop-like dystrophy of the cornea, Jpn. J. Clin. Ophthalmol. **26:**815, 1972.

58. Aracena, T.: Hereditary fleck dystrophy of the cornea: report of a family, J. Pediatr. Ophthalmol. **12:**223, 1975.

59. Bagolini, B., and Ioli-Spada, G.: Bietti's tapetoretinal degeneration with marginal corneal dystrophy, Am. J. Ophthalmol. **65:**53, 1968.

60. Birndoft, L.A., and Ginsberg, S.P.: Hereditary fleck dystrophy associated with decreased corneal sensitivity, Am. J. Ophthalmol. **73:**670, 1972.

61. Bron, A.J., Williams, H.P., and Carruthers, M.E.: Hereditary crystalline stromal dystrophy of Schnyder: clinical features of a family with hyperhypoproteinemia, Br. J. Ophthalmol. **56:**383, 1972.

62. Brownstein, S., Fine, B., Sherman, M., and Zimmerman, L.: Granular dystrophy of the cornea: electron microscopic confirmation of recurrence in a graft, Am. J. Ophthalmol. **77:**701, 1974.

63. Burns, R.: Personal communication, 1976.

64. Carpel, E.F., Sigelman, R.J., and Doughman, D.J.: Posterior amorphous corneal dystrophy, Am. J. Ophthalmol. **83:**629, 1977.

65. Collier, Mt: Dystrophie mouchetée du parenchyme cornéen avec dystrophie nuageuse centrale, Bull. Soc. Ophtalmol. Fr. **64:**608, 1964.

66. Collier, M.: Elastorrhexie systématisée et dystrophies cornéennes chez deux soeurs, Bull. Soc. Ophtalmol. Fr. **65:**301, 1965.

67. Collier, M.: Dystrophie nuageuse centrale et dystrophie ponctiforme prédescemétique dans une même famille, Bull. Soc. Ophtalmol. Fr. **66:**575, 1966.

68. Cotlier, F., and Hughes, W.F.: Enzymatic deficiency in macular dystrophy (Groenouw II), presented at the Spring Meeting of the Association for Research in Vision and Ophthalmology, Sarasota, Fla., 1972.

69. Delleman, J.W., and Winkelman, J.E.: Degeneratio corneae cristallinea hereditaria: a clinical, genetical and histological study, Ophthalmologica (Basel) **155:**409, 1968.

70. Ehlers, N., and Matthiessen, M.: Hereditary crystalline dystrophy of Schnyder, Acta Ophthalmol. **51:**1, 1967.

71. Ellis, W., Barfort, P., and Mastman, G.J.: Keratoconjunctivitis with corneal crystals caused by the dieffenbachia plant, Am. J. Ophthalmol. **76:**143, 1973.

72. Fogle, J.A., Kenyon, K.R., Stark, W.J., and Green, W.R.: Defective epithelial adhesion in anterior corneal dystrophies, Am. J. Ophthalmol. **79:**925, 1975.

73. François, J., and Fehér, J.: Light microscopical and polarisation optical study of lattice dystrophy of the cornea, Ophthalmologica **164:**1, 1972.

74. François, J., Hanssens, M., Teuchy, H., et al.: Ultrastructural findings in macular dystrophy (Groenouw type II), Ophthalmol. Res. **7:**80, 1975.

75. François, J., Victoria-Troncoso, V., Mandgla, P.C., and Victoria-Ihler, A.: Study of the lysosomes by vital stain in normal keratocytes and in keratocytes from macular dystrophy of the cornea, Invest. Ophthalmol. **15:**599, 1976.

76. Garner, A.: Histochemistry of corneal granular dystrophy, Br. J. Ophthalmol. **53:**799, 1969.

77. Garner, A.: Histochemistry of corneal macular dystrophy, Invest. Ophthalmol. **8:**473, 1969.

78. Garner, A., and Tripathi, R.D.: Hereditary crystalline stromal dystrophy of Schnyder. II. Histopathology and ultrastructure, Br. J. Ophthalmol. **56:**400, 1972.

79. Gillespie, F.D., and Covelli, B.: Crystalline corneal dystrophy, Am. J. Ophthalmol. **56:**465, 1963.

80. Goldberg, M.F., Krimmer, B., Sugar, J., Sewell, J., and Wong, E.: Variable expression in flecked (speckled) dystrophy of the cornea, Ann. Ophthalmol. **9:**889, 1977.

81. Herman, S.J., and Hughes, W.F.: Recurrence of hereditary corneal dystrophy following keratoplasty, Am. J. Ophthalmol. **75:**689, 1973.

82. Hogan, M., and Alvarado, S.: Ultrastructure of lattice dystrophy of the cornea: a case report, Am. J. Ophthalmol. **64:**656, 1967.

83. Johnson, B.L., Brown, S.I., and Zaidman, G.W.: A light electronmicroscopic study of recurrent granular dystrophy of the cornea, Am. J. Ophthalmol. **92:**49, 1981.

84. Jones, S.T., and Zimmerman, L.E.: Histopathologic differentiation of granular, macular, and lattice dystrophies of the cornea, Am. J. Ophthalmol. **51:**394, 1961.

85. Jones, S.T., and Zimmerman, L.E.: Macular dystrophy of the cornea (Groenouw II), Am. J. Ophthalmol. **47:**1, 1959.

86. Kani, A., Tanaka, M., Kaneko, H., et al.: Clinical and histopathological studies of the lattice dystrophy of the cornea, Acta Soc. Ophthalmol. Jpn. **17:**357, 1973.

87. Kirk, H.Q., Rabb, M., Hahenhauer, J., and Smith, R.: Primary familial amyloidosis of the cornea, Trans. Am. Acad. Ophthalmol. Otolaryngol. **77:**411, 1973.

88. Kiskaddon, B.M., Campbell, R.J., Waller, R.R., and Bourne, W.: Fleck dystrophy of the cornea: case report, Ann. Ophthalmol. **12:**700, 1980.

89. Klintworth, G.K.: Lattice corneal dystrophy: an inherited variety of amyloidosis restricted to the cornea, Am. J. Pathol. **50:**371, 1967.

90. Klintworth, G.K., and Vogel, F.S.: Macular corneal dystrophy: an inherited acid mucopolysaccharide storage disease of corneal fibroblasts, Am. J. Pathol. **45:**565, 1964.

91. Kuwabara, U., Akiya, S., and Azawa, H.: Electron microscopic study on the stromal lesions in granular dystrophy of the cornea, Acta Soc. Ophthalmol. Jpn. **74:**1468, 1970.

92. Lanier, J.D., Fine, M., and Togni, B.: Lattice corneal dystrophy, Arch. Ophthalmol. **94:**921, 1976.

93. Livni, N., Abraham, F.A., and Zauberman, H.: Groenouw's macular dystrophy: histochemistry and ultrastructure of the cornea, Doc. Ophthalmol. **37:**327, 1974.

94. Lorenzetti, D.W.C., and Kaufman, H.E.: Macular lattice dystrophies and their recurrences after keratoplasty, Trans. Am. Acad. Ophthalmol. Otolaryngol. **71:**112, 1967.

95. Luxenburg, M.: Hereditary crystalline dystrophy of the cornea, Am. J. Ophthalmol. **63:**507, 1967.

96. Malbran, E.: Corneal dystrophies: a clinical, pathological, and surgical approach, Trans. Am. Acad. Ophthalmol. Otolaryngol. **76:**563, 1972.

97. Mannis, M.J., Krachmer, J.H., Rodriguez, M.M., et al.: Polymorphic amyloid degeneration of the cornea, Arch. Ophthalmol. **99:**1217, 1981.

98. Matsuo, N., Fujiwara, H., and Ofuchi, Y.: Electron and light microscopic observations of a case of Groenouw's granular dystrophy, Folia Ophthalmol. Jpn. **18:**436, 1967.

99. McTigue, J.: The human cornea: a light and electron microscopic study of the normal cornea and its alterations in various dystrophies, Trans. Am. Acad. Ophthalmol. Otolaryngol. **65:**591, 1968.

100. Meretoja, J.: Comparative histopathological and clinical findings in eyes with lattice corneal dystrophy of two types, Ophthalmologica **165:**115, 1972.

101. Meretoja, J.: Genetic aspects of familial amyloidosis with corneal lattice dystrophy and cranial neuropathy, Clin. Genet. **4:**173, 1973.

102. Mondino, B.J., and Sundar Raj, C.V.: Protein AA and lattice corneal dystrophy, Am. J. Ophthalmol. **89:**380, 1980.

103. Morgan, G.: Macular dystrophy of the cornea, Br. J. Ophthalmol. **50:**57, 1966.

104. Nicholson, D.H., Green, W.R., and Cross, H.E.: A clinical and histopathological study of François-Neetens speckled corneal dystrophy, Am. J. Ophthalmol. **83:**554, 1977.

105. Patten, J.T., Hyndiuk, R.A., Donaldson, D.D., Herman, S.J., and Ostler, H.B.: Fleck (Mouchetée) dystrophy of the cornea, Ann. Ophthalmol. **8:**25, 1976.

106. Pearse, A.C.: Histochemistry, theory and applied, Boston, 1968, Little, Brown & Co.

107. Polack, F.: Contributions of electron microscopy to the study of corneal pathology, Surv. Ophthalmol. **20:**375, 1976.

108. Pouliquen, Y., Frouin, M.A., Faure, J.P., and Offret, S.: Ophthalmol Clinic, Hotel-Dieu, Place de Parvis, Notre-Dame, Paris, Exp. Eye Res. **18:**163, 1974.

109. Purcell, J.J., Jr., Krachmer, J.H., and Weingeist, T.A.: Fleck corneal dystrophy, Arch. Ophthalmol. **95:**440, 1977.

110. Quigley, H.A., and Goldberg, M.F.: Scheie syndrome and macular dystrophy. An ultrastructural comparison of skin and conjunctiva, Arch. Ophthalmol. **85:**553, 1971.

111. Rabb, M.R., Blodi, F., and Boniuk, M.: Unilateral lattice dystrophy of the cornea, Trans. Am. Acad. Ophthalmol. Otolaryngol. **78:**440, 1974.

112. Ramsey, M.S., Fine, B.S., and Cohen, S.W.: Localized corneal amyloidosis, Am. J. Ophthalmol. **73:**360, 1973.

113. Robin, A.L., Green, W.R., Lapsa, T.P., Hoover, R.E., and Kelley, J.S.: Recurrence of macular corneal dystrophy after lamellar keratoplasty, Am. J. Ophthalmol. **84:**457, 1977.

114. Rodrigues, M.M., Calhoun, J., and Harley, R.D.: Corneal clouding with increased acid mucopolysaccharide accumulation in Bowman's membrane, Am. J. Ophthalmol. **79:**916, 1975.

115. Rodrigues, M.M., and McGavic, J.S.: Recurrent corneal granular dystrophy: a clinicopathologic study, Trans. Am. Ophthalmol. Soc. **73:**306, 1975.

116. Sedan, J., and Valles, A.: Cristaux de cholestral dans la cornée, Bull. Mem. Soc. Fr. Ophthalmol. **59:**127, 1946.

117. Smith, M., and Zimmerman, L.: Amyloid in corneal dystrophies, Arch. Ophthalmol. **79:**407, 1968.

118. Snip, R.C., Kenyon, K.R., and Green, R.D.: Macular corneal dystrophy: ultrastructural pathology of the corneal endothelium and Descemet's membrane, Invest. Ophthalmol. **12:**88, 1973.

119. Sornson, E.: Granular dystrophy of the cornea: an electron microscopic study, Am. J. Ophthalmol. **59:**1001, 1965.

120. Stansbury, F.C.: Lattice type of hereditary corneal degeneration: report of five cases, including one of a child of two years, Arch. Ophthalmol. **40:**189, 1974.

121. Stock, E.L., and Kielar, R.A.: Primary familial amyloidosis of the cornea, Am. J. Ophthalmol. **82:**266, 1976.

122. Strachan, I.M.: Central cloudy corneal dystrophy of François: five cases in the same family, Br. J. Ophthalmol. **53:**192, 1969.

123. Stuart, J.C., and Mund, M.L.: Recurrent granular corneal dystrophy, Am. J. Ophthalmol. **79:**18, 1975.

124. Teng, C.C.: Granular dystrophy of the cornea. A histochemical and electron microscopic study, Am. J. Ophthalmol. **63:**772, 1967.

125. Teng, C.C.: Macular dystrophy of the cornea. A histochemical and electron microscopic study, Am. J. Ophthalmol. **62:**436, 1966.

126. Thomsett, J., and Bron, A.J.: Polymorphic stromal dystrophy, Br. J. Ophthalmol. **59:**125, 1975.

127. Tripathi, R., and Garner, A.: Corneal granular dystrophy: a light and electron microscope study of its recurrence in a graft. Br. J. Ophthalmol. **54:**361, 1970.

128. Urrets-Zavalia, A., Jr., and Katz, C.: Corneal hemochromatosis: a unique type of corneal dystrophy involving the anterior stroma and both limiting membranes, Am. J. Ophthalmol. **72:**88, 1971.

129. Wolter, J.R., and Henderson, J.W.: Neurohistology of lattice dystrophy of the cornea, Am. J. Ophthalmol. **55:**475, 1963.

130. Yanoff, M., Fine, B.S., Colosi, N.J., and Katowitz, J.A.: Lattice corneal dystrophy: report of an unusual case, Arch. Ophthalmol. **95:**651, 1977.

Pre-Descemet dystrophies

131. Collier, M.: Caractère hérédo-familial de la dystrophie ponctiforme prédescemétique, Bull. Soc. Ophtalmol. Fr. **64:**731, 1964.

132. Collier, M.: Dystrophie filiforme profonde de la cornée, Bull. Soc. Ophtalmol. Fr. **64:**1034, 1964.

133. Collier, M.: Dystrophie nuageuse centrale et dystrophie ponctiforme prédescemétique dans une même famille, Bull. Soc. Ophtalmol. Fr. **66:**575, 1966.

134. Curran, R.E., Kenyon, K.R., and Green, W.R.: Pre-Descemet's membrane corneal dystrophy, Am. J. Ophthalmol. **77:**711, 1974.

135. Franceschetti, A., and Maeder, G.: Dystrophie profonde de la cornée dans un cas d'ichthyose congénitale, Bull. Mem. Soc. Fr. Ophtalmol. **67:**146, 1954.

136. Franceschetti, A., and Schlaeppi, V.: Dégénérescence en bandelettes et dystrophie prédescemétique de la cornée dans un cas d'ichthyose congénitale, Dermatologica **115:**217, 1957.

137. Grayson, M., and Wilbrandt, H.: Pre-Descemet dystrophy, Am. J. Ophthalmol. **64:**276, 1967.

138. Maeder, G., and Danis, P.: Sur une nouvelle forme de dystrophie cornéenne (dystrophia filiformis profunda corneae) associée à un kératocône, Ophthalmologica **114:**246, 1947.

139. Sever, R.J., Frost, P., and Weinstein, G.: Eye changes in ichthyosis, JAMA **206:**2283, 1968.

Endothelial dystrophies

140. Abbott, R.L., Fine, B.S., Webster, R.E., et al.: Specular microscopic and histologic observations in non-guttate corneal endothelial degeneration, Ophthalmology **88:**788, 1981.

141. Andrews, J.S.: The lipid of arcus senilis, Arch. Ophthalmol. **68:**264, 1972.

142. Antine, B.E.: Congenital corneal dystrophy, Am. J. Ophthalmol. **70:**656, 1970.

143. Antine, B.E.: Congenital hereditary corneal dystrophy (CHCD), South. Med. J. **63:**946, 1970.

144. Antine, B.E.: Histology of congenital hereditary corneal dystrophy, Am. J. Ophthalmol. **69:**964, 1970.

145. Aquavella, J.V.: Chronic corneal edema, Am. J. Ophthalmol. **76:**201, 1973.

146. Arentsen, J.J., Rodriguez, M.M., and Laibson, P.R.: Corneal opacification occurring after phacoemulsification and phacofragmentation, Am. J. Ophthalmol. **83:**794, 1977.

147. Boruchoff, S.A., and Kuwabara, T.: Electron microscopy of posterior polymorphous degeneration, Am. J. Ophthalmol. **72:**879, 1971.

148. Bourne, W.M., and Kaufman, H.E.: Endothelial damage associated with intraocular lenses, Am. J. Ophthalmol. **81:**482, 1976.

149. Buxton, J.N., Preston, R.W., Reechers, R., et al.: Tonography in cornea guttata: a preliminary study, Arch. Ophthalmol. **77:**602, 1967.

150. Chi, H.H., Teng, C.C., and Katzin, H.M.: Histopathology of primary endothelial-epithelial dystrophy of the cornea, Am. J. Ophthalmol. **45:**518, 1958.

151. Cibis, G.W., Krachmer, J.A., Phelps, C.D., and Weingist, T.A.: The clinical spectrum of posterior polymorphous dystrophy, Arch. Ophthalmol. **95:**1529, 1977.

152. Cibis, G.W., Weingeist, T.A., and Krachmer, J.H.: Traumatic corneal rings, Arch. Ophthalmol. **96:**485, 1978.

153. Colosi, N.J., and Yanoff, M.: Reactive corneal endothelialization, Am. J. Ophthalmol. **83:**219, 1977.

154. Edelhauser, H.F., Van Horn, D.L., Hyndiuk, R.A., and Schultz, R.D.: Intraocular irrigating solutions, Arch. Ophthalmol. **93:**648, 1975.

155. Edelhauser, H.F., Van Horn, D.L., Schultz, R.O., and Hyndiuk, R.A.: Comparative toxicity

of intraocular irrigating solutions on the corneal endothelium, Am. J. Ophthalmol. **81:**473, 1976.

156. Edelhauser, H.F., Hyndiuk, R.A., Zeeb, A., and Schultz, R.O.: Corneal edema and the intraocular use of epinephrine, Am. J. Ophthalmol. **93:**327, 1982.

157. Edmonds, C., and Iwamoto, T.: Electron microscopy of late interstitial keratitis, Ann. Ophthalmol. **4:**693, 1972.

158. Eiferman, R.A., Wilkins, E.L.: The effect of air on human corneal endothelium, Am. J. Ophthalmol. **92:**328, 1981.

159. Forgács, J.: Stries hyalines rétrocornéennes postinflammatoires en toiles araignées, Ophthalmologica **145:**301, 1963.

160. Friedman, A.H., and Henkind, P.: Corneal stromal overgrowth after cataract extraction, Br. J. Ophthalmol. **54:**528, 1970.

161. Gassett, A.R., and Worthen, D.M.: Keratoconus and Chandler's syndrome, Ann. Ophthalmol. **6:**819, 1974.

162. Grayson, M.: The nature of hereditary deep polymorphous dystrophy of the cornea: its association with iris and anterior chamber dysgenesis, Trans. Am. Ophthalmol. Soc. **72:**516, 1974.

163. Harboyan, G., Mamo, J., der Kaloustian, V., and Karam, F.: Congenital corneal hereditary dystrophy: progressive sensorineural deafness in a family, Arch. Ophthalmol. **85:**27, 1971.

164. Hogan, M.J., and Bietti, G.: Hereditary deep dystrophy of the cornea (polymorphous), Am. J. Ophthalmol. **65:**777, 1968.

165. Hogan, M.J., Wood, I., and Fine, M.: Fuchs' endothelial dystrophy of the cornea, Am. J. Ophthalmol. **78:**363, 1974.

166. Iwamoto, T., and DeVoe, A.G.: Electron microscopic studies on Fuchs' combined dystrophy. I. Posterior portion of the cornea, Invest. Ophthalmol. **10:**9, 1971.

167. Iwamoto, T., and DeVoe, A.G.: Light and electron microscopy in absolute glaucoma with pigment dispersion phenomena and contusion angle deformity, Am. J. Ophthalmol. **72:**420, 1971.

168. Judisch, G.F., and Maumanee, I.H.: Clinical differentiation of recessive congenital hereditary endothelial dystrophy and dominant hereditary endothelial dystrophy, Am. J. Ophthalmol. **85:**606, 1978.

169. Kanai, A.: Further electron microscopic study of hereditary corneal edema, Invest. Ophthalmol. **10:**545, 1971.

170. Kanai, A., Waltman, S., Polack, F., et al.: Electron microscopic study of hereditary corneal edema, Invest. Ophthalmol. **2:**197, 1971.

171. Kaufman, H.E., and Katz, J.I.: Endothelial damage from intraocular lens insertion, Invest. Ophthalmol. **15:**996, 1976.

172. Kaufman, H.E., Robbins, J.E., and Capella, J.A.: The endothelium in normal and abnormal corneas, Trans. Am. Acad. Ophthalmol. Otolaryngol. **69:**931, 1965.

173. Kenyon, K.R., and Antine, B.: The pathogenesis of congenital hereditary endothelial dystrophy of the cornea, Am. J. Ophthalmol. **72:**787, 1971.

174. Kenyon, K.R., and Maumenee, A.E.: The histological and ultrastructural pathology of congenital hereditary corneal dystrophy: a case report, Invest. Ophthalmol. **7:**475, 1968.

175. Kenyon, K.R., Stark, W.J., and Stone, D.L.: Corneal endothelial degeneration and fibrous proliferation after pars plana vitrectomy, Am. J. Ophthalmol. **81:**486, 1976.

176. Kirkham, T.H.: Hyaline corneal opacities in a case of Rieger's anomaly, Br. J. Ophthalmol. **53:**354, 1969.

177. Klien, B.A.: Acute metastatic syphilitic corneal abscess: a clinical and histopathologic study, Arch. Ophthalmol. **14:**612, 1935.

178. Krachmer, J.H., Schnitzer, J.I., and Fratkin, J.: Cornea pseudoguttata: a clinical and histopathologic description of endothelial cell edema, Arch. Ophthalmol. **99:**1377, 1981.

179. Lauring, L.: Anterior chamber glass membranes, Am. J. Ophthalmol. **68:**308, 1969.

180. Leibowitz, H.N., Laing, R.A., and Sandstrom, M.: Continuous wear of hydrophilic contact lens, Arch. Ophthalmol. **89:**575, 1973.

181. Lemp, M.A.: Air blast keratopathy, Arch. Ophthalmol. **88:**575, 1972.

182. Levenson, J.E.: Corneal edema: cause and treatment, Surv. Ophthalmol. **20:**190, 1975.

183. Levenson, J.E., Chandler, J.W., and Kaufman, H.E.: Affected asymptomatic relatives in congenital hereditary endothelial dystrophy, Am. J. Ophthalmol. **76:**967, 1973.

184. Leibowitz, H.M., Laing, R.A., Chang., P.R., et al.: Corneal edema secondary to vitreocorneal contact, Arch. Ophthalmol. **99:**417, 1981.

185. Mackool, R.J., and Holtz, J.: Descemet membrane detachment, Arch. Ophthalmol. **95:**459, 1977.

186. Marbran, E.S.: Corneal dystrophies: a clinical pathological and surgical approach. Am. J. Ophthalmol. **74:**771, 1972.

187. Matsuda, H., and Smelser, G.K.: Endothelial cells in alkali burned cornea: ultrastructural alterations, Arch. Ophthalmol. **89:**402, 1973.

188. Maumenee, A.E.: Congenital hereditary corneal dystrophy, Am. J. Ophthalmol. **50:**1114, 1960.

189. Pearce, W.G., Tripathi, R.C., and Morgan, G.: Congenital endothelial corneal dystrophy: clinical, pathological and genetic study, Br. J. Ophthalmol. **53:**477, 1969.

190. Pietruschka, G.: Ueber eine familiäre Endothel-dystrophie der Hornhaut (in Kombination met Glaukom, Vitiligo, und Otosklerose), Klin. Monatsbl. Augenheilkd. **136:**794, 1960.

191. Polack, F.M., and Sugar, A.: The phacoemulsi-fication procedure. III. Corneal complications, Invest. Ophthalmol. **16:**39, 1977.

192. Polack, F.M., Bourne, W.M., Forstot, S.L., and Yamaguchi, T.: Scanning electron micros-copy of posterior polymorphous corneal dys-trophy, Am. J. Ophthalmol. **89:**575, 1980.

193. Pratt, A.W., Saheb, M.E., and Leblanc, R.: Posterior polymorphous corneal dystrophy in juvenile glaucoma, Can. J. Ophthalmol. **11:**180, 1976.

194. Robertson, D.M.: Anterior segment ischemia after segmental episclera buckling and cryopexy, Am. J. Ophthalmol. **79:**871, 1975.

195. Rodrigues, M.M., Waring, G.O., Laibson, P.R., and Weinreb, S.: Endothelial alterations in con-genital corneal dystrophy, Am. J. Ophthalmol. **80:**678, 1975.

196. Rosenblum, P., Stark, W.J., Maumenee, I.H., et al.: Hereditary Fuch's dystrophy, Am. J. Ophthalmol. **90:**455, 1980.

197. Rodriques, M.M., Phelps, C.D., Krachmer, J.H., et al.: Glaucoma due to endothelialization of the anterior chamber angle: a comparison of posterior polymorphous dystrophy of the cornea and Chandler's syndrome, Arch. Ophthalmol. **98:**688, 1980.

198. Rubenstein, R.A., and Silverman, J.J.: Heredi-tary deep dystrophy of the cornea associated with glaucoma and ruptures in Descemet's membrane, Arch. Ophthalmol. **79:**123, 1968.

199. Rushton, R.H.: Hyaline membrane in the an-terior chamber, Proc. R. Soc. Med. **31:**1098, 1938.

200. Scheie, H.G., and Yanoff, M.: Iris nevus (Cogan-Reese) syndrome, Arch. Ophthalmol. **93:**963, 1975.

201. Snell, A.C., Jr., and Irwin, E.S.: Hereditary deep dystrophy of the cornea, Am. J. Ophthal-mol. **45:**636, 1958.

202. Snip, R.C., Kenyon, K.R., and Green, W.R.: Retrocorneal fibrous membrane in the vitreous touch syndrome, Am. J. Ophthalmol. **79:**233, 1975.

203. Squires, E.L., and Weiman, V.L.: Stimulation of repairs of human corneal endothelium in organ culture by mesodermal growth factor, Arch. Ophthalmol. **98:**1462, 1980.

204. Stocker, F.W., and Irish, A.: Fate of successful corneal graft in Fuchs' endothelial dystrophy, Am. J. Ophthalmol. **68:**820, 1969.

205. Urrets-Zavalia, A., Jr., and Katz, C.: Corneal hemochromatosis: a unique type of corneal dys-trophy involving the anterior stroma and both limiting membranes, Am. J. Ophthalmol. **72:**88, 1971.

206. Van Horn, D.L., Edelhauser, H.F., Prodano-vich, G., Eiferman, R., and Pederson, H.J.: Effect of ophthalmic preservative thimbusol on rabbit and human endothelium, Invest. Ophthal-mol. **16:**273, 1977.

207. Von Noorden, G.K.: Anterior segment ischemia following the Jensen procedure, Arch. Ophthal-mol. **94:**845, 1976.

208. Waring, G.O., Font, R.L., Rodrigues, M., and Mulenberger, R.D.: Alterations of Descemet's membrane in intersititial keratitis, Am. J. Oph-thalmol. **81:**773, 1976.

209. Waring, G.O., and Laibson, P.R.: Keratoplasty in infants and children, Trans. Am. Acad. Oph-thalmol. Otolaryngol. **83:**283, 1977.

210. Witschel, H., Fine, B.S., Grutzner, P., and McTigue, J.W.: Congenital hereditary stromal dystrophy, Arch. Ophthalmol. **96:**1043, 1978.

211. Wolter, J.R., Johnson, F.D., Meyer, R., and Watters, J.A.: Acquired autosensitivity to de-generating Descemet's membrane in a case with anterior uveitis in the other eye, Am. J. Ophthal-mol. **72:**782, 1971.

212. Wolter, J.R., and Larson, B.F.: Pathology of cornea guttata, Am. J. Ophthalmol. **48:**161, 1959.

213. Wolter, J.R., and Makley, T.A., Jr.: Cogan-Reese syndrome: formation of a glass membrane on an iris nevus clinically simulating tumor growth, J. Pediatr. Ophthalmol. **9:**102, 1972.

214. Yamaguchi, T., Kaufman, H.E., Fukushima, A., Safir, A., and Asbell, P.A.: Histologic and electron microscopic assessment of endothelial damage produced by anterior radial keratotomy in the monkey cornea, Am. J. Ophthalmol. **92:**313, 1981.

215. Zeporkes, J.: Glassy network in the anterior chamber: report of a case, Arch. Ophthalmol. **10:**517, 1933.

Ectatic dystrophies

216. Beardsley, S.L., and Foulks, G.N.: An associ-ation of keratoconus and mitral valve prolapse, Ophthalmology. **89:**35, 1982.

217. Biglan, A.W., Brown, S.I., and Johnson, B.L.: Keratoglobus and blue sclera, Am. J. Ophthal-mol. **83:**225, 1977.

218. Buxton, J.N.: Therapeutic use of contact lenses in keratoconus, Ophthalmol. Dig., p. 29, Jan., 1975.

219. Cavara, V.: Keratoglobus and keratoconus: a contribution to nasalogical interpretation of kera-toglobus, Br. J. Ophthalmol. **34:**621, 1950.

220. Copeman, P.W.M.: Eczema and keratoconus, Br. Med. J. **2:**977, 1965.

221. Davies, P.D., and Ruben, M.: The paretic pupil: its incidence and etiology after keratoplasty for keratoconus, Br. J. Ophthalmol. **59:**223, 1975.

222. Duke-Elder, S., and Leigh, A.G.: Corneal dystrophies: ectatic conditions. In Duke-Elder, S., editor: System of ophthalmology, vol. 8. Diseases of the outer eye, pt. 2. Cornea and sclera, St. Louis, 1965, The C.V. Mosby Co.

223. Gasset, A.R.: Fixed dilated pupil following penetrating keratoplasty in keratoconus (Castroviejo syndrome), Ann. Ophthalmol. **9:**623, 1977.

224. Geeraets, W.: Ocular syndromes, Philadelphia, 1976, Lea & Febiger.

225. Grayson, M.: Acute keratoglobus, Am. J. Ophthalmol. **56:**300, 1963.

226. Greenfield, G., Romano, A., Stein, R., et al.: Blue sclera and keratoconus: key features of a distinct heritable disorder of connective tissue, Clin. Genet. **4:**8, 1973.

227. Haney, W.P., and Falls, H.F.: The occurrence of congenital keratoconus posticus circumscriptus (in two siblings presenting a previously unrecognized syndrome), Am. J. Ophthalmol. **52:**53, 1961.

228. Hartstein, J., and Becker, B.: Research into pathogenesis of keratoconus, Arch. Ophthalmol. **84:**728, 1970.

229. Hoefle, F.B., Kooerman, J.J., and Buxton, G.: The use of contact lenses in patients with keratoconus, Contact Lens Med. Bull., Sept. 4, 1971.

230. Holtz, J.S.: Congenital ocular anomalies associated with Duane's retraction syndrome, Am. J. Ophthalmol. **77:**729, 1974.

231. Hyams, S.W., Kar, H., and Neuman, E.: Blue sclera keratoglobus, Br. J. Ophthalmol. **53:**53, 1969.

232. Iwamoto, R., and DeVoe, G.A.: Electron microscopic study of the Fleischer ring, Arch. Ophthalmol. **94:**1579, 1976.

233. Jacobs, D.S., Green, W.R., and Maumanee, D.: Acquired keratoglobus, Am. J. Ophthalmol. **77:**393, 1974.

234. Karlin, D.B., and Wise, G.N.: Keratoconus posticus, Am. J. Ophthalmol. **52:**119, 1961.

235. Lorfel, R.S., and Sugar, S.: Keratoconus associated with retrolental fibroplasia, Ann. Ophthalmol. **8:**449, 1976.

236. McKusick, V.A.: Heritable disorders of connective tissue, ed. 4, St. Louis, 1972, The C.V. Mosby Co.

237. Perry, H.D., Buxton, J.N., and Fine, B.S.: Round and oval cones in keratoconus, Ophthalmology **87:**905, 1980.

238. Pouliquen, Y., Graf, B., Kozak, Y. de, et al.: Étude morphologique de kératocône, Arch. Ophtalmol. (Paris) **30:**497, 1970.

239. Schocket, G.S., Phelps, W.L., and Pettit, T.H.: Bilateral posterior circumscribed keratoconus, Am. J. Ophthalmol. **57:**840, 1964.

240. Schwartz, D.E.: Noonan's syndrome associated with ocular abnormalities, Am. J. Ophthalmol. **73:**955, 1972.

241. Slusher, M.M., Laibson, P.R., and Mulberger, K.D.: Acute keratoconus in Down's syndrome, Am. J. Ophthalmol. **63:**1137, 1968.

242. Spencer, W.H., and Fisher, J.J.: The association of keratoconus with atopic dermatitis, Am. J. Ophthalmol. **47:**332, 1959.

243. Wolter, J.R.: Bilateral keratoconus in Crouzon's syndrome with unilateral hydrops, Ann. Ophthalmol. **14:**141, 1976.

ADDITIONAL READING
Epithelium and Bowman's layer

Alkemade, P.P.H., and Van Balen, A.T.M.: Hereditary epithelial dystrophy of the cornea, Meesmann type, Br. J. Ophthalmol. **50:**603, 1966.

Burke, E.: Zur Kenntnis der erblichen Epitheldystrophie der Hornhaut, Ophthalmologica **111:**134, 1941.

DeVoe, A.G.: Certain abnormalities of Bowman's membrane with particular reference to fingerprint lines in the cornea, Trans. Am. Ophthalmol. Soc. **60:**195, 1962.

Guerry, D., III: Fingerprint lines in the cornea, Am. J. Ophthalmol. **33:**724, 1950.

Guerry, D., III: Observations on Cogan's microcystic dystrophy of the cornea epithelium, Trans. Am. Ophthalmol. Soc. **63:**320, 1965.

Kornzweig, A.L.: Epithelial dystrophy of the cornea associated with macular degeneration of the retina, J. Pediatr. Ophthalmol. **1:**51, 1964.

Kuwabara, R., and Cicarelli, E.C.: Meesmann's corneal dystrophy, Arch. Ophthalmol. **71:**676, 1964.

Levitt, J.M.: Microcystic dystrophy of the corneal epithelium, Am. J. Ophthalmol. **72:**381, 1971.

Liakos, G.M., and Casey, T.A.: Posterior polymorphous keratopathy, Br. J. Ophthalmol. **62:**39, 1978.

Perry, H.D., Fine, B.S., Caldwell, D.R.: Reis-Bücklers' dystrophy, Arch. Ophthalmol. **97:**664, 1979.

Pinsky, A., and Irwin, E.S.: Hereditary epithelial dystrophy of the cornea, Am. J. Ophthalmol. **57:**996, 1964.

Snyder, W.B.: Hereditary epithelial corneal dystrophy, Am. J. Ophthalmol. **55:**56, 1963.

Stocker, F.W., and Holt, L.B.: Rare form of hereditary epithelial dystrophy. Arch. Ophthalmol. **53:** 536, 1955.

Yamaguchi, T., Polack, F.M., and Valenti, J.: Electron microscopic study of recurrent Reis-Bücklers' corneal dystrophy, Am. J. Ophthalmol. **90:**95, 1980.

Stromal dystrophies

Bowen, R.A., Hassard, D.T.R., Wong, V., et al.: Lattice dystrophy of the cornea as a variety of amyloidosis, Am. J. Ophthalmol. **70:**822, 1970.

Collyer, R.T.: Amyloidosis of the cornea, Can. J. Ophthalmol. **3:**35, 1968.

François, J., Hanssens, M., and Teuchy, H.: Ultrastructural changes in lattice dystrophy, Ophthalmic Res. **7:**321, 1975.

Frayer, W.C., and Blodi, F.: The lattice type of familial corneal degeneration, Arch. Ophthalmol. **61:**721, 1959.

Garner, A.: Amyloidosis of the cornea, Br. J. Ophthalmol. **53:**73, 1969.

Ghosh, M., and McCulloch, C.: Macular corneal dystrophy, Can. J. Ophthalmol. **8:**15, 1973.

Ghosh, M., and McCulloch, C.: Crystalline dystrophy of the cornea: a light and electron microscopic study, Can. J. Ophthalmol. **12:**321, 1977.

Karseras, A.G., and Price, D.C.: Central crystalline dystrophy of the cornea, Br. J. Ophthalmol. **5r:** 659, 1970.

Klintworth, G.: Primary familial corneal amyloidosis (lattice dystrophy), Ann. Intern. Med. **66:**1288, 1967.

Klintworth, G.K.: Current concepts of the ultrastructural pathogenesis of macular and lattice dystrophies, Birth Defects (original article series) **7:** 27, 1971.

Lempert, S.L., Jenkins, M.S., Johnson, B.L., and Brown, S.I.: A simple technique for removal of recurring granular dystrophy in corneal grafts, Am. J. Ophthalmol. **86:**89, 1978.

McPherson, S.D., Kiffney, G.T., and Freed, C.C.: Corneal amyloidosis, Am. J. Ophthalmol. **62:** 1025, 1966.

McTigue, S., and Drine, B.: The stromal lesion in lattice dystrophy of the cornea. A light and electron microscopic study, Invest. Ophthalmol. **3:**355, 1964.

Michaels, R.G.: Corneal crystalline dystrophy of Schnyder, Arch. Ophthalmol. **92:**64, 1974.

Pillat, A.: Zur Frage der familiären Hornhautentartung: ueber eine eigenartige tiefe schollige und periphere gitterförmige familiäre Hornhautdystrophie, Klin. Monatsbl. Augenheilkd. **104:**571, 1940.

Tremblay, M., and Dube, I.: Macular dystrophy of the cornea, ultrastructure of two cases, Can. J. Ophthalmol. **8:**37, 1973.

Endothelial dystrophies

Bourne, W.M., and Kaufman, H.E.: Cryopreserved endothelial cell survival in vivo, Am. J. Ophthalmol. **81:**685, 1975.

Brown, S.I., and McLean, J.M.: Peripheral corneal edema after cataract extraction, a new clinical entity, Trans. Am. Acad. Ophthalmol. Otolaryngol. **73:**465, 1969.

Cogan, D.G., and Kuwabara, R.: Growth and regenerative potential of Descemet's membrane, Trans. Ophthalmol. Soc. U.K. **91:**875, 1971.

Coles, W.H.: Effects of antibiotics on the in vitro rabbit corneal endothelium, Invest. Ophthalmol. **14:**246, 1975.

Freudenthal, O.: Veränderung an der Hornhauthinterfläche, Klin. Monatsbl. Augenheilkd. **74:**777, 1925.

Haddad, R., Font, R.L., and Friendly, D.S.: Cerebrohepata-renal syndrome of Zellweger: ocular histopathologic findings, Arch. Ophthalmol. **94:** 1927, 1976.

Kanai, A., Waltman, S., Polack, F.M., and Kaufman, H.E.: Electron microscopic study of hereditary corneal edema, Invest. Ophthalmol. **10:**89, 1971.

Keates, R.H., and Cvintal, T.: Congenital hereditary corneal dystrophy, Am. J. Ophthalmol. **60:**892, 1965.

Koeppe, L.: Klinische Beobachtungen mit der Nerst Spaltlampe und dem Hornhautmikroskop, Arch. Ophthalmol. **91:**375, 1916.

Laing, R.A., Sandstrom, M., Berrospi, A.R., and Leibowitz, H.M.: Morphological changes in corneal endothelial cells after penetrating keratoplasty, Am. J. Ophthalmol. **82:**459, 1976.

Norn, M.S.: Corneal thickness after cataract extraction with air in the anterior chamber, Acta Ophthalmol. **53:**747, 1975.

Pardos, G.J., Krachmer, J.H., and Mannis, M.J.: Posterior corneal vesicles, Arch. Ophthalmol. **99:**1981.

Rodrigues, M.M., Waring, G.O., Laibson, P.R., and Weinreb, S.: Endothelial alterations in congenital corneal dystrophies, Am. J. Ophthalmol. **80:**678, 1975.

Sanchez, J., and Polack, F.: The effect of topical steroids in the healing of corneal endothelium, Invest. Ophthalmol. **13:**17, 1970.

Schlichting, H.: Blasen und dellenförmige Endotheldystrophie der Hornhaut, Klin. Monatsbl. Augenheilkd. **107:**425, 1941.

Theodore, F.H.: Congenital type of endothelial dystrophy, Arch. Ophthalmol. **21:**626, 1939.

Triebenstein, O.: Veränderung an der Hornhauthinterfläche, Klin. Monatsbl. Augenheilkd. **74:**777, 1925.

Waring, G.O., III,: Posterior collagenous layer of the cornea: ultrastructural classification of abnormal collagenous tissue posterior to Descemet's membrane in 30 cases, Arch. Ophthalmol. **100:** 122, 1982.

Ectatic dystrophies

Aquavella, J.V.: Thermokeratoplasty, Ophthalmic Surg. **5:**39, 1974.

Arentsen, J.J., and Laibson, P.R.: Thermokeratoplasty for keratoconus, Am. J. Ophthalmol. **82:** 447, 1976.

Gasset, A.R., and Kaufman, H.E.: Thermokeratoplasty in the treatment of keratoconus, **79:**226, 1975.

Gasset, A.R., and Lobo, L.: Dura-T semiflexible lens for keratoconus, Ann. Ophthalmol. **7:**1353, 1975.

Keates, R.H.: Thermokeratoplasty for keratoconus, Ophthalmic Surg. **6:**89, 1975.

Kenyon, K.R., Fogle, J.A., and Stark, W.J.: Complications of thermokeratoplasty: persistent epithelial defects, Contact Lens **2:**33, 1976.

Krachmer, J.H.: Pellucid marginal corneal degeneration, Arch. Ophthalmol. **96:**1217, 1978.

12 Epithelial keratopathy

Punctate epithelial erosions (PEE)
Punctate epithelial keratopathy (PEK)
Superficial punctate keratitis of Thygeson
(TSPK)
Superior limbic keratoconjunctivitis (SLK)
Keratoconjunctivitis sicca (KCS)
Epidemic keratoconjunctivitis (EKC)
Staphylococcus aureus punctate keratopathy
Herpes simplex hominis keratitis
Trachoma
Molluscum contagiosum

Medications and physical agents
Neurotrophic keratopathy
Herpes zoster
Epidemic hemorrhagic keratoconjunctivitis
Vitamin A deficiency
Superficial epithelial keratopathy of vernal
catarrh
Filaments
Pannus
Subepithelial lesions

Diseases of the epithelium other than dystrophic entities are categorized in this chapter. Epithelial keratopathies are classified according to the following factors:

1. Etiologic agent (Table 12-1)
2. Location (Table 12-2)
3. Morphologic characteristics (Table 12-3)
4. Association with filamentary keratopathy (Table 12-4)
5. Association with lid and conjunctival diseases (Table 12-5)

Some distinctive superficial epithelial keratopathies may be identified on a purely morphologic basis and are described next in detail.

Text continued on p. 331.

Table 12-1. Etiologic agents of epithelial keratitis

General grouping	Specific disease
Viral	Herpes simplex Herpes zoster Molluscum contagiosum Measles Mumps Infectious mononucleosis Adenoviral disease
Chlamydial	Trachoma Inclusion conjunctivitis
Bacterial	Staphylococcic
Systemic immune disease	Keratoconjunctivitis sicca
Traumatic and mechanical	Posttraumatic erosion Exposure Trichiasis
Allergy	Vernal catarrh
Nutritional	Vitamin A deficiency
Toxic	Drug-induced disease[7, 10]
Neurologic	Neutrophic keratitis
Unknown	Superior limbic keratoconjunctivitis Superficial punctate keratitis of Thygeson

Table 12-2. Characteristic locations of superficial keratitis

Location	Etiologic factor
Lower third	Staphylococcic (neutralizing toxin)
	Exposure
	Entropion
	Drug toxicity[7, 10]
Lower two thirds	Keratitis sicca
	Neurotrophic keratitis
	Exposure keratitis
	Ultraviolet exposure
	X-ray exposure
Upper third	Trachoma
	Inclusion conjunctivitis
	Superior limbic keratoconjunctivitis
	Vernal catarrh
	Molluscum contagiosum
Central	Epidemic keratoconjunctivitis
	Superficial punctate keratitis
	Inclusion conjunctivitis (rare)
Diffuse	Verruca vulgaris
	Mumps
	Infectious mononucleosis
	Acute conjunctivitis: bacterial and hemorrhagic
	Drug toxicity[7, 10]
	Severe vernal
	Abrasion
	Keratoconjunctivitis sicca
	Vitamin A deficiency
	Edema of epithelium
Random	Erosion
	Trichiasis
	Foreign body
	Herpes simplex keratitis

Table 12-3. Morphologic characteristics of epithelial lesions

Type of lesion	Etiologic factor
Fine	Staphylococcal infection of lid margins Herpes simplex keratitis Measles keratitis Mumps keratitis Infectious mononucleosis Molluscum contagiosum Keratitis sicca Early exposure Drugs (topical) Neomycin Anesthetics (topical) Acute hemorrhagic conjunctivitis Adenoviral (early) disease Early edema of epithelium of cornea Early inclusion conjunctivitis
Coarse	Herpes simplex Vaccinia Varicella zoster Keratoconjunctivitis sicca Superficial punctate keratitis Superior limbic keratoconjunctivitis Exposure (late) X-ray exposure Chemical burns Adenoviral disease (late) Inclusion conjunctivitis (late)
Linear	Trichiasis

Characteristic forms	Syncytial: vernal
	Vitamin A deficiency
	   Keratinized epithelium
	   "Flour-sprinkled"
	Dendritic: herpes simplex and herpes zoster
	Stellate: herpes zoster and herpes simplex
	Pseudodendritic
	   Healing abrasion
	   Tyrosinosis

Table 12-4. Filaments

Etiologic group	Specific disease	Location and number of filaments
Viral	Herpes simplex (transitory)	Usually single filament
Surgical	After cataract After corneal surgery[4] Bullous keratopathy (transitory)	Diffuse if eye is occluded
Trauma	After corneal abrasion and erosion (transitory)	Usually single layer filaments
Systemic	Keratoconjunctivitis sicca Psoriasis (rare) Brain-stem injury[3]	Lower one third of cornea
Mechanical	Occlusion (including ptosis)	Diffuse
Unknown	Superior limbic keratoconjunctivitis	Upper one third of cornea

Table 12-5. Superficial epithelial keratopathy

Superficial punctate epithelial erosions	Morphologic characteristics	Associated lid disease	Associated conjunctival lesions
Bacterial: staphylococcal (most common)	Fine	Rosacea	Follicles
Viral	Staphylococcal disease	Ichthyosis	Adenovirus
Herpes simplex	Trachoma	Urbach-Wiethe disease	Trachoma
Exanthema (measles)	Molluscum contagiosum	Entropion	Molluscum
Chlamydial: trachoma	Herpes simplex	Ectropion	Primary herpes simplex
Drying	Vernal catarrh	Lid warts	Herpes zoster
Keratitis sicca	Drugs (toxicity)	Molluscum contagiosum	Giant papillae
Cicatricial conjunctivitis	Coarse and blotchy	Staphylococcal blepharitis	Vernal catarrh
Allergic: vernal catarrh	Vaccinia	Seborrhea of lids	Contact lens
	Keratitis sicca	Ulcers of vesicles of lid as seen in herpes simplex, vaccinia, zoster	Acute inflammation of conjunctiva:
	Superficial punctate keratitis	Meibomian keratoconjunctivitis	*Neisseria gonorrhoeae*
	Pemphigoid		Mucoid discharge:
	Exposure		Keratitis sicca
	X-ray exposure		Membrane (conjunctival)
	Vitamin A deficiency		Epidemic keratoconjunctivitis
	Chemical (alkali, acid) burns		Hyperacute inflammation
	Filamentous		Ligneous conjunctivitis
	Keratitis sicca		Stevens-Johnson syndrome
	Superior limbic keratoconjunctivitis		Scarring of conjunctiva
	Herpes simplex		Pemphigoid
	Vaccinia		Trachoma
	Adenoviral		Epidemic keratoconjunctivitis
	Occlusion (prolonged)		Atopic disease
	Postcorneal abrasion		Lye burns
	Postcataract surgery		Stevens-Johnson syndrome
	Trauma		Lyell's disease (Ritter) (toxic epidermal necrolysis)
	Combined with subepithelial lesions		
	Adenoviral disease		
	Inclusion conjunctivitis		
	Trachoma		
	Vaccinia		
	Herpes zoster		
	Reiter's disease		

PUNCTATE EPITHELIAL EROSIONS (PEE)

These lesions manifest themselves as fine, slightly depressed spots in the epithelium that are visible only with fluorescein staining and result from desquamation of the superficial epithelial cells. The patient complains of photophobia and irritation. The condition is associated with punctate epithelial keratopathy. A wide variety of causes for PEE includes vernal catarrh, exposure to ultraviolet rays, staphylococcal blepharitis, and keratoconjunctivitis sicca. Rarely one can see these erosions in seborrhea, verruca vulgaris, and molluscum contagiosum.

PUNCTATE EPITHELIAL KERATOPATHY (PEK) (Fig. 12-1)

These lesions are gray-white opacities in the epithelium that are visible without stain. They will stain with fluorescein but do so poorly; however, they take in rose bengal red rather well. The lesions may be fine or coarse and have a wide etiologic spectrum. They are the result of intraepithelial cellular infiltration or inflammation. The etiologic agents of PEK may include vernal catarrh, keratitis sicca, early exposure, and staphylococcal blepharitis. Coarser lesions may be seen in herpes zoster and herpes simplex vaccinia and late adenoviral or inclusion conjunctivitis.

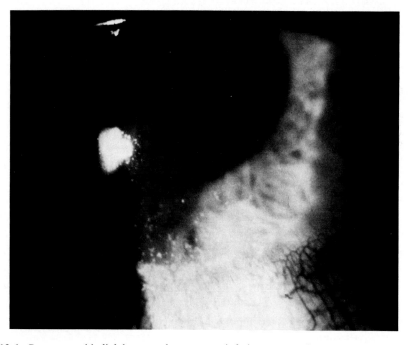

Fig. 12-1. Punctate epithelial keratopathy seen on inferior aspect of cornea. Some gray-white opacities are coarse; others are fine. The opacities stain with fluorescein.

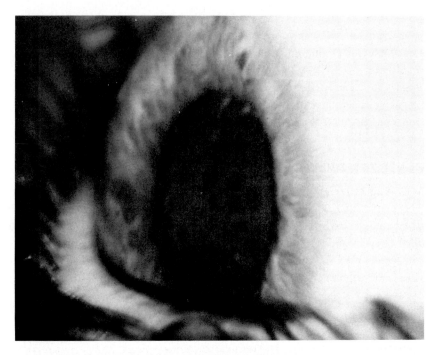

Fig. 12-2. Superficial punctate keratitis of Thygeson. Aggregates of intraepithelial dots. Some of these aggregates are raised and stain with fluorescein.

SUPERFICIAL PUNCTATE KERATITIS OF THYGESON* (TSPK) (Fig. 12-2)

The classic corneal sign of TSPK is a grouped punctate epithelial keratitis in an oval shape that stains with fluorescein. It is somewhat raised above the corneal surface and located in the pupillary axis, but it is not accompanied by subepithelial infiltration. However, this classic sign may not be observed in some patients who have a long history of recurrent corneal epithelial disease and keratitis sensitive to topical corticosteroids. The oval, grouped punctate epithelial keratitis is present during active phases of the disease. During inactive stages the lesions can be flat gray intraepithelial dots that do not stain, or they may present a stellate appearance that can be confused with herpes simplex keratitis. Topical corticosteroids can alter the epithelial lesions, and antiviral agents may increase the degree of subepithelial infiltration.[2]

Herpes simplex keratitis must be ruled out because it is treated with topical IDU and is aggravated by topical corticosteroids. The exact opposite is true of TSPK, which is worsened by topical IDU and improved by corticosteroids. Differentiating between TSPK and herpes simplex keratitis may be difficult when a few pseudodendritic corneal lesions are the initial sign.

---

*References 1, 2, 5, 6, 8, 9.

Although the combined epithelial and subepithelial opacities in TSPK are similar to those occurring with adenovirus and other viral infections,[2] they may be differentiated by retroillumination of the stromal disturbance of TSPK. The stromal component of TSPK is transparent, and all the opacity is in the epithelial lesion. In contrast, retroillumination reveals that the opacity in the stromal disturbance associated with adenovirus and other viral diseases is in the subepithelial component.[2]

Evidence supports the belief that subepithelial opacities are part of the natural history of TSPK and not the result of treatment with topical antiviral agents.[2] More than a fine diagnostic point is involved in determining whether subepithelial opacities can be a part of the TSPK complex. If the corneal lesions are strictly limited to the epithelium and associated only with anterior stromal edema and not with infiltration or opacity, then the corneal disease is unlike that of adenovirus, herpes simplex virus, variola virus, and varicella-zoster virus keratitis. On the other hand, if the corneal disease of TSPK does include subepithelial opacities and infiltrates, the corneal signs more closely resemble the keratitis produced by these viruses.

It is significant that an adenovirus had been isolated from a case of TSPK. The ability of some adenoviruses to persist over time and to recur must depend not only on the virulence of the virus but on the immune response of the host. Differences in the immune response may alter the course of a common viral infection of the cornea so that the same virus can produce different clinical syndromes in different persons.

Symptoms can be relieved and signs suppressed by using soft, extended wear, or hard contact lenses as well as by topical corticosteroids.

The concept that TSPK is caused by a virus is supported by the resemblance of the epithelial lesions of TSPK to those seen in variola and certain adenovirus infections, by electron microscopic evidence of virus particles in epithelial lesions, and by the isolation of both adenovirus and varicella-zoster virus from eyes of patients with TSPK. However, there is no definite proof that a certain virus plays any part in the etiology of this disease.

The frequency of histocompatability antigen HLA-DR3 is significantly increased in patients with TSPK. Because this antigen is associated with several autoimmune diseases, it is likely that immune mechanisms also play a role in TSPK. Further evidence for an immune mechanism is the lymphocytic response with corneal epithelial lesions and in conjunctival cytology, the dramatic response to topical corticosteroids, and the extended course of the disease.[2] Response to trifluorothymidine topically applied can be dramatic.

SUPERIOR LIMBIC KERATOCONJUNCTIVITIS (SLK)

This entity is characterized by papillary hypertrophy of the upper tarsus, superior conjunctival bulbar hyperemia with keratinization, and redundant epithelium at the limbus. One sees a punctate epithelial keratitis superiorly often with filament formation. SLK is described fully in Chapter 5.

KERATOCONJUNCTIVITIS SICCA (KCS)

This problem is characterized by deficient tear meniscus, which is filled with mucous secretions and debris. A nonspecific conjunctival injection and a blotchy epithelial keratitis with filaments are seen in the lower third of the cornea. KCS is fully covered in Chapter 13 and in the section on autoimmune diseases in Chapter 14.

EPIDEMIC KERATOCONJUNCTIVITIS (EKC)

Epidemic keratoconjunctivitis is characterized by the onset of diffuse epithelial keratitis, conjunctival follicles or pseudomembranes, focal epithelial keratitis in 8 to 10 days, and then by grossly visible subepithelial opacities. EKC should be differentiated from trachoma and inclusion conjunctivitis of acute onset, which also develop subepithelial opacities. Micropannus develops early in trachoma diseases but not in epidemic keratoconjunctivitis. EKC is described in detail in Chapter 8.

STAPHYLOCOCCUS AUREUS PUNCTATE KERATOPATHY

This disease is caused by a staphylococcal exotoxin. The lesions are microerosions and are similar to the type of epithelial lesions one may see in some cases of trachoma but with differing distribution.

HERPES SIMPLEX HOMINIS KERATITIS

Herpes simplex hominis keratitis is discussed in Chapter 8. However, the condition is characterized by initial linear or branching epithelial keratitis followed by ulceration and subepithelial opacification. If located near the limbus, this keratitis must be differentiated from catarrh with infiltrates, as well as from pseudodendrites of varicella-zoster ophthalmicus.

TRACHOMA

Trachoma with superficial epithelial keratitis is often characterized by punctate epithelial keratitis and gross pannus, mostly seen in the superior limbal area. One may also see subepithelial infiltrates that are occasionally nummular in shape.

MOLLUSCUM CONTAGIOSUM

Molluscum contagiosum may cause an epithelial keratopathy. The lesions are small microerosions mostly located in the upper one third of the cornea. It is believed that the toxic nature of the molluscum virus is the cause of these epithelial lesions rather than the molluscum virus itself.

MEDICATIONS AND PHYSICAL AGENTS

Medications such as IDU, neomycin, and topical anesthetics; prolonged use of steroids; and exposure to ultraviolet light are known to cause epithelial keratopathy. Drug preservatives such as benzalkonium chloride,[10] which has a lytic effect on plasma membranes, may cause an epitheliopathy. Often in these conditions one will see a focal edema and interepithelial cysts.

NEUROTROPHIC KERATOPATHY

A decrease in corneal sensation or innervation in the epithelium from fifth nerve disease is indicative of this disease. It may also be seen with herpes simplex and herpes zoster infection or in contact lens wearers.

HERPES ZOSTER

Herpes zoster results in epithelial and subepithelial opacities, which are described in full in Chapter 8.

EPIDEMIC HEMORRHAGIC KERATOCONJUNCTIVITIS

This condition exhibits a punctate epithelial keratopathy more often in the palpebral aperture zone associated with preauricular adenopathy and the follicular type of conjunctivitis. A characteristic sign is subconjunctival hemorrhage, as seen in the bulbar conjunctiva near the fornix, which may spread below. The condition is limited, lasting about 1 to 2 weeks. Occasionally one may note systemic signs. Epidemic hemorrhagic keratoconjunctivitis is described in Chapter 6.

VITAMIN A DEFICIENCY

Vitamin A deficiency may result in epithelial keratopathy. Deposits of keratin granules in the cytoplasm may cause a spotty type of epithelial opacity. The keratopathy at this stage, which may be considered a prexerosis stage, is reversible with no damage to the stroma if vitamin A is given in adequate doses. One may see a Bitot spot associated with the opacity. A Bitot spot is not necessarily pathognomonic of vitamin A deficiency. The Bitot spot is a limbus-based area of keratinization with a foamy secretion atop it. One may find keratin and xerosis bacilli from scrapings of the area. On occasion Bitot's spot can be confused with a leukoplakic plaque. With a leukoplakic plaque, however, the cornea is normal, whereas with a Bitot spot the cornea is usually dry and lacks luster.

SUPERFICIAL EPITHELIAL KERATOPATHY OF VERNAL CATARRH

This condition accompanies the palpebral and limbal types of vernal conjunctivitis. The morphologic characteristics of the keratitis are often diagnostic, consisting of intraepithelial opacification in syncytial formation. One may also see minute punctate epithelial erosions. The disease is described in full in Chapter 14.

FILAMENTS

Filaments should be considered a sign rather than a disease. One may see two types of filaments: mucous filaments, which are actually not true filaments, and epithelial filaments, which are considered true filaments. They are characteristically seen in Sjögren's syndrome and in other conditions that exhibit or are associated with keratoconjunctivitis sicca, as well as in SLK. One may also see filaments in recurrent erosion problems and in bullous keratopathy. In recurrent erosions of traumatic nature, the filament is usually unilateral. However, one may see filaments as part of a dystrophic type such as is seen in familial recurrent erosions of the corneas. In this instance the filaments are bilateral, usually milder, and often controlled by medical means. Some filaments are caused by prolonged occlusion for 2 or 3 weeks and are usually located in the superior aspect of the cornea. Filaments also can occur in ptosis and in both herpes simplex and herpes zoster infections. The filaments may be seen with the epithelial disease or just before the true dendritic figure appears in herpes simplex. They are thin and small and cause discomfort.

PANNUS

Pannus must be distinguished from the unusually wide normal limbus. In cases involving Asiatic persons, it should be recalled that the normal limbus is unusually wide; one will have to distinguish the normal variations from disease processes. Active pannus will demonstrate vascular and cellular elements, whereas inactive pannus will show fibrous tissue and obliterated blood vessels. One can see a pannus extending all around the limbal area. It may be much more extensive superiorly as is seen in trachoma. Sector pannus is seen in such diseases as rosacea or phlyctenulosis. Micropannus, which was at one time considered diagnostic of childhood trachoma, is also seen in inclusion conjunctivitis, molluscum contagiosum, vernal catarrh, SLK, and contact lens wearers. Micropannus is no longer considered to be a purely diagnostic sign as it once was thought to be in childhood trachoma. The pannus of trachoma is often considered a gross pannus and probably is more evident in chronic cases. Rarely a macropannus occurs in molluscum contagiosum. The pannus of phlyctenulosis is triangular, results from old limbal phlyctenules, and is sector in nature. The pannus sectorlike condition of rosacea occurs without a phlyctenulous scar at the limbus; one can also see extensive conjunctival and limbal vessel engorgement and tortuosity of the vessels. Herpes simplex keratitis, a potent imitator, can result in a pannus that is usually irregular in shape and that may even be fascicular in configuration. The pannus seen in leprosy may be similar in appearance to the phlyctenular pannus and is also associated with limbal granulomas.

Micropannus is considered to be one in which the length is 0.5 to 2 mm.

SUBEPITHELIAL LESIONS

Often one may see subepithelial lesions in association with epithelial disease. These conditions are listed in Table 12-6.

Table 12-6. Diseases that may cause subepithelial keratitis

Etiologic agent	Specific entity
Viral	Herpes simplex Herpes zoster (round irregular) Epidemic keratoconjunctivitis
Immunologic	Phlyctenulosis
Unknown	Nummular (Dimmer)[1] *Padi* keratitis
Rare forms	Leprosy (rare) Onchocerciasis (more common)
Chlamydial	Trachoma Inclusion conjunctivitis (round like EKC)

REFERENCES

1. Abbott, R.L., and Forster, R.K.: Superficial punctate keratitis of Thygeson associated with scarring and Salzmann's nodular degeneration, Am. J. Ophthalmol. **87:**296, 1979.
2. Darrell, R.W.: Thygeson's superficial punctate keratitis: natural history and association with HLA DR3, Tr. Am. Ophth. Soc. **79:**486, 1981.
3. Davis, W., Drewry, R.D., and Wood, T.O.: Filamentary keratitis and stromal vascularization associated with brain-stem injury, Am. J. Ophthalmol. **90:**489, 1980.
4. Dodds, T.H., and Laibson, P.R.: Filamentary keratitis following cataract extraction, Arch. Ophthalmol. **88:**609, 1972.
5. Forstot, S.L., and Bender, P.S.: Treatment of Thygeson's superficial punctate keratopathy with soft contact lenses, Am. J. Ophthalmol. **88:**186, 1979.
6. Goldberg, D.B., Schanzlin, D.J., and Brown, S.I.: Management of Thygeson's superficial punctate keratitis, Am. J. Ophthalmol. **89:**22, 1980.
7. Pfister, R.R., and Burnstein, N.: The effects of ophthalmic drugs, vehicles, and preservatives on corneal epithelium: a scanning electron microscopic study, Invest. Ophthalmol. **15:**246, 1976.
8. Tabbara, K.F., Ostler, H.B., Dawson, C., and Oh, J.: Thygeson's superficial punctate keratitis, Ophthalmology **88:**75, 1981.
9. Thygeson, P.: Superficial punctate keratitis, J.A.M.A. **144:**1544, 1950.
10. Tonjum, A.M.: Effects of benzalkonium chloride upon the corneal epithelium studied with scanning electron microscopy. Acta Ophthalmol. **53:**358, 1975.

CHAPTER

13 The dry eye

Aqueous deficiencies: keratoconjunctivitis sicca (KCS)
Mucin deficiencies
Lipid deficiencies
Diagnostic hints
Treatment

The tear film consists of three layers. The outermost layer, the lipid layer, consists of low polarity lipids such as waxy and cholesterol esters.[5] The middle layer consists of aqueous tear fluid and contains ions of inorganic salt, glucose, urea, and various biopolymers, such as enzymes, protein, and glycoproteins.[14] The third layer of the tear film is the mucous coat of the superficial epithelium and is very important to the stability of the tear film.[13] In the healthy eye the mucous layer is extremely thin and resembles the microvillous, ridged appearance of the superficial epithelial cells.

The meibomian gland is the source of the lipid layer. The glands of Zeis and Moll may also contribute to this layer. The accessory lacrimal gland and the main lacrimal gland contribute to the formation of the aqueous tears. The conjunctival goblet cells probably are the origin of the mucin layer.

Tear film abnormalities that contribute to aqueous deficiency (Table 13-1) are seen in disease conditions such as keratoconjunctivitis sicca (KCS), Riley-Day syndrome, congenital alacrima, and paralytic hyposecretions. Mucin deficiencies are noted in Stevens-Johnson disease, ocular pemphigoid, cicatricial conjunctivitis, hypovitaminosis A, chemical and thermal burns, trachoma, and drug-induced diseases. Lipid abnormalities are seen in chronic blepharitis and radiation complications of the lid. Tear film abnormalities, in addition to the preceding, may occur as a result of impaired lid function from exposure keratitis, pterygium, and other major epithelial elevations resulting in dellen formation in the sclera (Fig. 13-1) or cornea. Tear film abnormalities also occur in epithelial disease, causing irregularity of the surface, and in anesthetic corneas.

AQUEOUS DEFICIENCIES: KERATOCONJUNCTIVITIS SICCA (KCS)

This condition most frequently occurs in women in their forties and fifties. The patient complains of burning and irritation of both eyes. Occasionally, the complaint of

338

Table 13-1. Main causes of alteration in tear makeup

Layer	Thickness	Source	Cause
Outer (lipid)	0.1 μm	Meibomian glands; also minor contribution by glands of Zeis and Moll	Chronic blepharitis Radiation

Middle (aqueous)	6 to 7 μm	Accessory lacrimal and main lacrimal gland	Bilateral
			    Congenital absence of lacrimal gland
			    Cri du chat syndrome
			    KCS
			    Riley-Day syndrome
			    Multiple endocrine neoplasia
			    Congenital alacrima
			    Paralytic hyposecretion
			    Systemic disease, that is, rheumatoid arthritis and other collagen diseases
			Unilateral
			    Seventh cranial nerve paresis
			    Viral dacryoadenitis
			    Scarring of lacrimal glands and ducts after radiation or trauma
			    Anhidrotic ectodermal dysplasia

Inner (mucin)	0.02 to 0.05 μm	Goblet cells of conjunctiva	Hypovitaminosis A Ocular pemphigold Cicitricial conjunctivitis Stevens-Johnson syndrome Chemical and thermal burns Drug-induced Trachoma

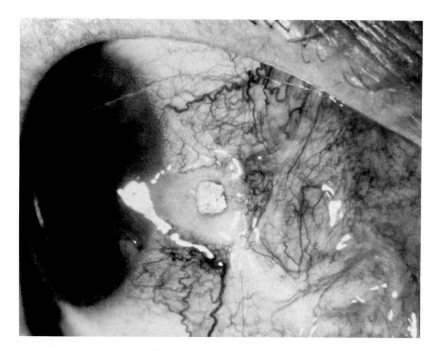

Fig 13-1. Dellen formation of sclera.

foreign body sensation is present; the whole picture may be very debilitating to the patient.

Examination of the eye with the slit lamp will reveal an increased amount of debris in the tear film that results from the poor tear flow and accumulation of epithelial cell debris. The tear meniscus for marginal tear strip is scant, and one might see increased amount of mucus threads in the tear film and in the inferior fornix. The exposed parts of the cornea and the conjunctiva stain with rose bengal red solution (Fig. 14-45). A filamentary keratitis (Fig. 14-46) is noted in a number of patients; the filaments are caused by breaks in the continuity of the normal corneal epithelial cell layer, probably secondary to drying, to which viscous mucin threads, containing desquamated epithelial debris as well as lipids, attach.[12] Until recently the thick mucin strands seen in KCS were thought to be a result of increased mucin production by the goblet cells; however, in KCS the mucin production may be decreased.[22] An abnormal accumulation of mucin results from impaired drainage secondary to reduced aqueous tear production.

Lysozyme and beta lysin are important components of the tear film because they possess antibacterial activity.[7, 8]

Hen egg white is a convenient and rich source of lysozyme. It is composed of 130 amino acids. Mammalian sources other than tears and nasal secretions include saliva, serum, and urine. High levels of lysozyme are present in cells, most importantly in polymorphonuclear leukocytes and macrophages, but also in basophils and eosinophils.

The antibacterial properties of lysozyme apparently lie in its ability to cleave to bacterial cell walls. These walls are composed of two aminosugars, N-acetylglucosamine and N-acetylmuramic acid, which alternately form a polysaccharide chain linked by intervening oxygen atoms. Lysozyme acts as the oxygen linkage of N-acetylmuramic acid and N-acetylglucosamine, breaking the bond and thus lysing the cell wall. Lysozyme accounts for 20% to 40% of the protein content of human tears and, together with secretory IgA complement, beta lysin, and lactoferrin, is responsible for defense of the external segment of the eye against bacterial invaders.

Lysozymes are markedly reduced in KCS. It should also be noted that the tear flow diminishes and the normal flushing action of the tears decreases as the aqueous tears diminish. This mechanical effect is also important in secondary infection. The dry eye is thus a compromised eye.

KCS can develop in the absence of systemic disease. However, there is a frequent association of this problem with systemic disease. As noted, KCS is seen more frequently in menopausal and postmenopausal women. The association with the menopausal era would suggest that lack of estrogen may play a part in the picture of the disease.

KCS is often associated with immune diseases and with collagen vascular disease, most frequently rheumatoid arthritis.[25] Other systemic disorders associated with KCS include systemic lupus erythematosus,[1] Waldenström's hyperglobulinemia, purpura,[22] progressive systemic sclerosis, lymphoproliferative disorders,[4] Hashimoto's thyroiditis, arthritis, celiac disease, pulmonary fibrosis, and sarcoidosis. When KCS occurs as a part of systemic involvement, it is called Sjögren's syndrome,[26] which is discussed in Chapter 14. Defective lacrimation can be seen in central autonomic dysfunction.[21, 23]

Histologically in KCS there are changes in the lacrimal gland consisting of lymphocytic and plasma cell infiltration with degeneration of glandular material. These changes resemble those seen in autoimmune disease in other tissues, giving rise to speculation that KCS has an autoimmune basis. Because of the frequent involvement of the labial glands of the mouth, biopsy of these glands has been used as a diagnostic test for Sjögren's syndrome.[6] The pathologic condition in these buccal glands is the same as that in the salivary glands.

In KCS the corneal and conjunctival surfaces appear lusterless; occasionally one will find corneal ulceration[21] and, as the most severe complication, perforation.[10] KCS is a bilateral disease, but it can be seen as a unilateral problem as a result of viral dacryoadenitis, surgical removal of lacrimal gland, irradiation to the eye, chemical burns, and mechanical trauma, as well as after seventh-nerve paresis (Table 13-1).

One of the leading causes of localized drying occurs in association with seventh cranial nerve paresis. The drying of the cornea may extend from a mild euperficial punctate erosion problem to an area of severe desiccation. Secondary keratinization may occur. Lid movements may be restricted by scars and symblepharons. Ocular pemphigoid, Stevens-Johnson syndrome, and chemical burns all may contribute to the drying effect.

Epitheliopathy may result in the alteration of the normal morphologic picture of the corneal epithelium and affect the corneal surface and the tear film, thus altering the stability of the tear film. Electron microscopic studies have shown that the normal microvillous structure of the corneal epithelium is associated with the presence of a normal mucous layer.[19]

It is seen that corneal anesthesia after damage to the fifth cranial nerve is frequently associated with epithelial break-down. The corneal epithelium is rich in acetylcholine and acetylcholinesterase[27]; such neurohumoral influences have been demonstrated to be important in the regulation of epithelial turnover.[17]

MUCIN DEFICIENCIES

Conditions that result in a decrease in mucin are listed in Table 13-1. The conjunctival mucin, spread by the action of the lid, forms a hydrophilic coating over the corneal epithelium and contributes to tear film stability.[11] Mucin plays an important role in removal of lipid contamination from the epithelial interface; interference with this by states or conditions that decrease the lipid removal activity will result in an abnormal breakup time of the tear film.[15] Normal tear breakup time ranges from 15 to 45 seconds.[16] The tear breakup time is the interval between complete blink and the development of the first dry spot on the cornea as evidenced by the pulling apart of the tear film, which has been stained with fluorescein.

Tear film instability occurs often in aqueous-deficient conditions and is present in all tear film abnormalities that have a significant epitheliopathy. In the absence of these other conditions, decreased tear breakup time is highly indicative of mucin-deficient dry eyes. Hypovitaminosis A results in a mucin-deficient state by virtue of a change of the mucous epithelium to a keratinized epithelium and the disappearance of conjunctival goblet cells in this clinical condition. In addition to vitamin A deficiency, other conditions that destroy the conjunctival goblet cells are pemphigoid, Stevens-Johnson syndrome, trachoma, chemical burns, and certain forms of drug-induced diseases such as the use of a beta-adrenergic receptor-blocking agent like practolol.

LIPID DEFICIENCIES

There is no specific cause of a deficiency of tear lipid film. However, it is often seen in alterations of lipid composition as a result of chronic blepharitis. It is suggested that some common microbes have enzymes such as lypases that hydrolize lipids with the release of free fatty acids. These substances are capable of triggering instant dry spot formation in the precorneal film.[18] This alteration in tear film lipids, in combination with blink abnormalities, leads to superficial punctate erosions of the corneal epithelium.

Periodic resurfacing of the tear film by the blinking reaction of the lid is necessary to remove lipid-containing mucous strands and thus maintain a vital role in rejuvenation of mucous layer of the tear film.

DIAGNOSTIC HINTS

The *slit-lamp examination* is very helpful. In aqueous tear deficiency, one may see a scanty appearance of the tear meniscus along the lid margin. This strip, which is nor-

TEAR FUNCTION TESTS

The Schirmer tests of tear quantity reflect the measurement of the aqueous layer only. The tests are performed with 5 × 30 mm strips of Whatman filter paper (available commercially from Smith Miller & Patch Laboratories). The paper is folded so that 5 mm of the strip will lie within the lower conjunctival sac, and the remaining 25 mm will project over the lower eyelid. The amount of moistening of the exposed paper is recorded at the end of 5 minutes. It is paramount to remember that these tests are rough measurements only. They are clinically useful as gross indicators of tear function.

Schirmer's test I *(measures total reflex and basic tear secretion)*

To minimize reflex tearing, avoid a brightly lit room and instillation of ocular medications prior to testing. The patient is to keep his eyes open and look forward. If paper is wetted completely before 5 minutes, note this time; if not, note the amount of wetting at the end of 5 minutes.

Results: Normals will wet approximately 10 to 30 mm at the end of 5 minutes. This amount decreases with age but probably should not be less than 10 mm. If wetting is greater than 30 mm, reflex tearing is intact but not controlled, or insufficient tear drainage is present. Tear secretion between 5 and 30 mm may be normal, or basal secretion may be low and compensated for by reflex stimulation. A value of less than 5 mm indicates hyposecretion.

Basic secretion test *(measures basic tear secretion)*

Instill topical anesthetic and wait until anesthesia is achieved. Only basic secretion is being measured. The difference between this test and the Schirmer I is the amount of reflex secretion.

Schirmer's test II *(measures reflex tear secretion)*

Instill topical ocular anesthetic and irritate unanesthetized nasal mucosa by rubbing it with a cotton swab. Measure wetting after 2 minutes. Less than 15 mm wetting represents failure of reflex secretion. This test is seldom employed, since reflex tearing is usually intact.

•　　•　　•

Many patients with minimal secretion of tears have few or no symptoms and require little treatment. In symptomatic patients, an attempt is made to replace the tear deficiency by topical agents (artificial tears). Lavage of the cul-de-sac and acetylcysteine may be helpful to remove excess mucus. Surgical closure of the punctate and tarsorrhaphy have been advocated in severe cases in an attempt to prolong contact time of the deficient tears. Transposition of the parotid duct to the lower cul-de-sac has been done in patients with xerophthalmia, but this treatment is not advised. Topical antibiotics may be needed if secondary infection occurs. Guibor shields have been most effective and are more comfortable than swimmer's goggles.

mally 1 mm in width, may show irregularity of the width of the strip or areas of discontinuity. In KCS a marked increase in the corneal tear film debris represents desquamated epithelium. In addition, one may see viscous mucin threads in the inferior cul-de-sac. The mucous threads are evidence of increased lipid contamination of the mucous layer facilitated by decreased tear flow.

Schirmer's test is used in KCS to determine the amount of tears that will wet a standardized strip of paper. The strip is usually left in place for 5 minutes while the patient looks straight ahead in dim light. Schirmer's test is done without anesthetic agents, is a valuable test of tear production, and is easily performed. Of course, results are significant if they are consistently below 5 mm of wetting at 5 minutes (p. 343).

Tear breakup time is a valuable test to use; although KCS can frequently cause an instability of the tear film, the unstable tear film is the hallmark of mucin-deficient dry eye. It should not be used in conjunction with topical anesthetic agents. The interval of time between a complete blink and the formation of the first randomly distributed dry spot is termed breakup time. An abnormally unstable tear film is associated with a breakup time of less than 10 seconds.

The *rose bengal stain* is valuable in eliciting devitalized cells and precipitative mucin, which are abundant in KCS. In the laboratory a lysozyme agar diffusion test can be performed. This test employs wetted Schirmer strips, which are placed on agar media that has been inoculated with a suspension of *Micrococcus lysodeikticus* bacteria. A zone of lysis around the strip at 24 hours indicates the antibacterial activity of tear lysozyme[2,3] (Fig. 13-2). The production of the lysozyme parallels tear secretion.

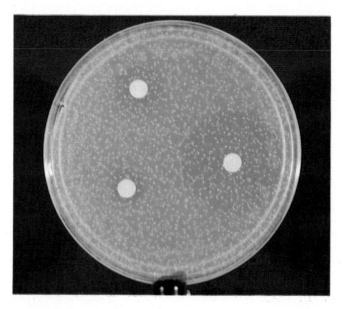

Fig. 13-2. Lysozyme activity assay. Note zone of lysis of agar medium inoculated with suspension of *Micrococcus lysodeikticus*.

TREATMENT

Treatment of the dry eye is extremely difficult and often without patient satisfaction, but the artificial tear appears to be the mainstay in treatment of tear deficiency. The dose schedule is usually left to the discretion of the patient. Medications that employ benzalkonium chloride should not be used because of the deleterious effect of the benzalkonium chloride on the tear film stability and possibly the surface epithelium. Those that do not contain benzalkonium should be used, that is, Liquifilm or Tears Plus.

Cauterization of the puncta has been advocated to preserve what little tears are available in a patient with severe dry eyes. This procedure should be done only on patients who show 1 mm or less of wetting of the Schirmer strip at 5 minutes and should be performed with extreme caution in the young, since KCS tends to wax and wane. If a patient begins to produce more tears, epiphora can result, which can be extremely annoying.

Synthetic plugs inserted in the inferior and superior puncta have been advocated and can test the effect of this type of treatment before permanent closure is anticipated. Inserts are also used and placed in the eyes for extended use.

The hydrophilic bandage lens is extremely useful in cases of KCS with filament keratitis, in mucin-deficient dry eyes that cannot be managed with artificial tears alone, and in certain cases of exposure keratitis. Patients with filamentary keratitis are relieved dramatically in some instances, with disappearance of the filaments after a short time of wearing the lens. However, if the lens is removed, the filaments reappear. These lenses must be kept moist; patients with dry eyes are prone to infection, and the insertion of a device like this lens probably increases the predisposition of the eye to infection.

In some cases of KCS, an extreme amount of tenacious mucin is present that attaches at certain points to the epithelium and can be pulled on by the lids. Such cases will be helped by the use of mucolytic agents such as 10% acetylcysteine solution three or four times a day.

Lysozyme is a sensitive test for diagnosing KCS. Bromhexine (Salvex) has little influence on tear secretion, but it does increase the level of lysozyme in Sjögren's syndrome. In patients with KCS the effect is less marked.

Dry eyes in patients with collagen disease are usually less symptomatic than those in patients with keratoconjunctivitis alone. Involvement of the lacrimal glands in the latter instance is more severe. This may explain the lesser response to bromhexine. It is a synthetic derivate of visicine, an alkaloid derived from a plant, and has been used in treating chronic bronchitis.[24]

The mean lysozyme level in normal eyes is 767 μg/ml. In patients with KCS the mean lysozyme level is 298 μg/ml. After treatment with bromhexine the lysozyme level can elevate to 772 μg/ml.[24]

Systemic treatment with bromhexine orally 24 to 28 mg/day divided into three doses is suggested in Sjögren's syndrome.[9]

Surgical methods to treat dry eye conditions are available, but in many instances they are too drastic, and their benefit is questionable. Surgical methods are usually advised only as a last resort.

In addition to the foregoing suggestions for treatment, it is important that the physician counsel the patient, explaining the situation and emphasizing the difficulty in treatment of dry eye. Other considerations for the physician are the avoidance of irritating topical medication, the use of swimmers' goggles[20] and in severe cases Guibor shields, the use of home humidification, the possible use of tear pumps, and the avoidance of secondary infection. The use of sustained-release inserts is a new approach.

The recognition that KCS can be made worse after cataract surgery and result in this severe corneal problem should prompt vigorous treatment for the dry eye.

REFERENCES

1. Alarcón-Segovia, D., Ibáñez, G., Velázquez-Forero, F., et al.: Sjögren's syndrome in systemic lupus erythematosus: clinical and subclinical manifestations, Ann. Intern. Med. **81:**577, 1974.
2. Bijsterveld, O.P. van: Diagnostic tests in the sicca syndrome, Arch. Ophthalmol. **82:**10, 1969.
3. Bijsterveld, O.P. van: Standardization of the lysozyme test for a commercial available medium, Arch. Ophthalmol. **91:**432, 1974.
4. Bolangenini, G., and Riva, G.: Lymphoproliferative diseases and paraproteinemias in Sjögren's syndrome, Schweiz. Med. Wochenschr. **105:**1493, 1975.
5. Brown, S.I., and Dervichian, D.G.: The oils of the meibomian glands: physical and surface characteristics, Arch. Ophthalmol. **82:**537, 1969.
6. Chisholm, D.M., and Mason, D.K.: Labial salivary gland biopsy in Sjögren's disease, J. Clin. Pathol. **21:**656, 1968.
7. Fleming, A.: On remarkable bacteriolytic elements found in tissue secretions, Proc. R. Soc. Lond. **93:**306, 1922.
8. Ford, L.C., DeLong, R.J., and Petty, R.W.: Identification of a nonlysosomal bacterial factor (beta lysin) in human tears and aqueous humor, Am. J. Ophthalmol. **81:**30, 1976.
9. Frost-Larsen, K., Isager, H., Manthrope, R., et al.: Sjögren's syndrome, Arch. Ophthalmol. **98:**836, 1980.
10. Gudas, P.O., Altman, B., Nicholson, D.H., and Green, W.R.: Corneal perforation in Sjögren's syndrome, Arch. Ophthalmol. **90:**470, 1973.
11. Holly, F.J.: Formation and rupture of the tear film, Exp. Eye Res. **15:**515, 1973.
12. Holly, F.J., and Lemp, M.A.: Tear physiology and dry eyes, Surv. Ophthalmol. **22:**69, 1977.
13. Holly, F.J., Patten, J.T., and Dohlman, C.H.: Surface activity of aqueous tear components in dry eye patients and normals, Exp. Eye Res. **24:**479, 1977.
14. Iwata, S.: Chemical composition of the aqueous phase. In Holly, F.J., and Lemp, M.A., editors: The preocular tear film and dry eye syndromes, Int. Ophthalmol. Clin. **13**(1):29, 1973.
15. Lemp, M.A.: Breakup of the tear film. In Holly, F.J., and Lemp, M.A., editors: The preocular tear film and dry eye syndromes, Int. Ophthalmol. Clin. **13:**(1):97, 1973.
16. Lemp, M.A., and Hamil, J.R.: Factors affecting the tear film breakup in normal eyes, Arch. Ophthalmol. **89:**103, 1973.
17. MacManus, J.P., and Whitfield, J.E.: In Braun, W., Lichtensteise, L.M., and Parker, C.W., editors: Cyclic AMP, cell growth and immune response, New York, 1974, Springer-Verlag New York, Inc.
18. McDonald, J.E.: Surface phenomena of tear films, Trans. Am. Ophthalmol. Soc. **66:**905, 1968.
19. Pfister, R.R.: The normal surface of corneal epithelium: a scanning electron-microscopic study, Invest. Ophthalmol. **12:**654, 1973.
20. Povier, R.H., Ryburn, F.M., and Israel, C.W.: Swimmers' goggles for keratoconjunctivitis sicca, Arch. Ophthalmol. **95:**1405, 1977.
21. Radtke, N., Meyer, S., and Kaufman, H.E.: Sterile corneal ulcers after cataract surgery in keratoconjunctivitis sicca, Arch. Ophthalmol. **96:**51, 1978.
22. Ralph, R.A.: Conjunctival goblet density in normal subjects and in dry eye syndrome, Invest. Ophthalmol. **14:**299, 1975.
23. Riley, C.M., Day, R.L., Greeleg, D.M., and Longford, H.S.: Central autonomic dysfunction with defective lacrimation. Pediatrics **3:**468, 1949.
24. Scharf, J.M., Obedeanu, N., Meshulam, T., et al.: Influence of bromhexine on tear lysozyme level in keratoconjunctivitis sicca, Am. J. Ophthalmol. **92:**21, 1981.
25. Sjögren, H., and Block, K.K.: Keratoconjunctivitis sicca and Sjögren's syndrome, Surv. Ophthalmol. **16:**145, 1971.
26. Talal, N.: Sjögren's syndrome, Bull. Rheum. Dis. **16:**404, 1966.
27. Van Alphen, G.: Acetylcholine synthesis in corneal epithelium, Arch. Ophthalmol. **58:**499, 1957.

14 Immune and mucous membrane diseases

Mucous membrane diseases
Ocular pemphigoid (cicatricial pemphigoid,
    essential shrinkage of conjunctiva)
    Signs and symptoms
    Management
Stevens-Johnson syndrome (erythema
    multiforme)
    Systemic involvement
    Ocular involvement
    Management
Toxic epidermal necrolysis (TEN) (Lyell's
    disease, scalded skin syndrome)
    Systemic involvement
    Ocular involvement
    Management
Exfoliative dermatitis
    Systemic involvement
    Ocular involvement
    Management

Behçet's syndrome
    Systemic involvement
    Ocular involvement
    Management
Reiter's syndrome
    Systemic involvement
    Ocular involvement
    Management
Cicatrizing conjunctival diseases
    Scars of pseudomembranous and
        membranous conjunctivitis
    Characteristic scarring in specific
        diseases
        Trachoma
        Atopic keratoconjunctivitis
        Others
Ligneous conjunctivitis

Immunologic diseases

T AND B LYMPHOCYTES

Lymphocytes involved in immunity and its disorders are known as thymus-derived (T) and bone marrow–derived (B) lymphocytes. The T lymphocytes are derived from the bone marrow and migrate to the thymus, where they develop the ability to respond to antigens. The T cell is active in delayed hypersensitivity; allograft rejection; graft-versus-host reaction; lymphokine production; defense against intracellular bacteria, fungi, and most viruses; immune surveillance against malignancy; and regulation of immunoglobulins and antibody production by B cells and plasma cells. B-lymphocytes similarly arise in the bone marrow and are concerned with humoral responses. The mature B cells are active in the defense against bacteria, in neutralizing some viruses, and in detoxifying toxins and are responsible for production of the five major antibodies.

The T-lymphocytes exhibit helper T cells, suppressor T cells, and null cells (Fig. 14-1). T cells show an interesting reaction in that they undergo spontaneous rosette formation in the presence of sheep red blood cells (Fig. 14-2). The sheep red blood cells form a circle around the T-lymphocyte, thus forming a rosette figure. However, neither B cells nor null T cells form rosettes. The B cells, on the other hand, exhibit surface immunoglobulins (Fig. 14-2). These can be seen by employing fluorescein-tagged, antihuman immunoglobulin antibodies raised in another species. The fluorescent antibody is seen with a fluorescence microscope and denotes that immunoglobulin is present on the surface of B cells. The T cells do not demonstrate this quality.

Antibodies

B cells mature and become the plasma cells. The plasma cells thus form the antibodies: IgG, IgA, IgD, IgE, and IgM.

There are thus five immunoglobulin classes, IgG, IgA, IgM, IgD, and IgE. Each class possesses specific antigenic properties that elicit specific antibodies. All five classes also have antigenic determinants in common.

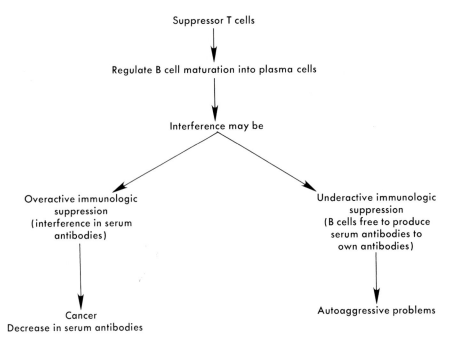

Fig. 14-1. Suppressor T cells may result in overactive immunologic suppression or underimmunologic suppression, as noted from outline.

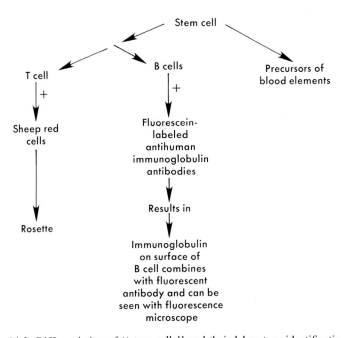

Fig 14-2. Differentiation of ''stem cells'' and their laboratory identification.

The immunoglobulin molecule is composed of two pairs of polypeptide chains co-valently bonded by disulfide bonds. Reducing agents may cleave these bonds, and enzymes digest the protein, producing light chains (L) and heavy chains (H). The light chains are divided into kappa (κ) and lambda (λ) subclasses. The heavy chain determines the class to which the immunoglobulin belongs, for example, alpha chains determine the class IgA.

Papain cleaves the immunoglobulin molecule into three large pieces. Two of the pieces are identical and are the antibody-containing fragments (Fab). They are composed of the light chains and the amino portion of a heavy chain. The third piece (Fc) possesses functional sites such as those determining complement fixation, macrophage and lymphocyte binding, rheumatoid factor binding, passive cutaneous anaphylaxis, and placental transport. This Fc portion tends to crystallize in some species.

IgA neither crosses the placenta nor fixes complement. IgA antibodies include the insulin antibody of diabetes mellitus, the thyroglobulin antibody of chronic thyroiditis, and the antibodies to red cell antigens. A special form of IgA is present in external secretions such as tears and saliva. This secretory antibody is supposed to provide the body with a first line of defense against microorganisms. IgA is produced by plasma cells under the conjunctiva and other mucosal surfaces. It is often reduced in auto-immune diseases.

IgA is also composed of two heavy and two light chains, with a molecular weight of 170,000. It activates the alternate complement pathway. Secretory IgA is found in the gastrointestinal and respiratory tracts, tears, urine, and colostrum. It possesses anti-bacterial properties and may neutralize viral replication.

IgE is the human anaphylactogenic skin-sensitizing antibody. It appears in tears and does not fix complement. IgE is responsible for the reactions seen in hay fever allergy. It is made mostly at mucosal surfaces and is found in increasing amounts in tears of the atopic conjunctivitides. IgE appears to produce its damage by causing degranulation of mast cells and basophils, with subsequent liberation of histamine, bradykinin, serotonin, and other mediators of anaphylactoid inflammation.

IgE thus plays a role in allergic reactions. Patients with extrinsic asthma and hay fever demonstrate elevated levels of IgE. The half-life of IgE is just over 2 days—even shorter than that of IgD.

IgG crosses the placenta. It fixes complement but is less efficient in doing so than is IgM. IgG antibody constitutes a major part of the body's immune response and is the principal antibody to bacteria and viruses. It has been detected in aqueous humor and in the cornea.

Antibody activity is most frequently demonstrated by the IgG class. The molecule is composed of two heavy and two light chains, with a molecular weight of 150,000. This immunoglobulin can cross the placenta and is involved in the transference of passive immunity to the fetus. In addition, it plays a role in the complement system.

IgM has been detected in the conjunctiva, in the cornea, and beneath the epidermis, but it is primarily intravascular. IgM molecules fix complement and are involved in the early primary antibody response.

IgM is composed of subunits held together by disulfide bonds at the Fc end of the heavy chain. It agglutinates red cells and bacteria more efficiently than IgG. IgM is primarily seen in a primary immune response. Cold agglutinins, rheumatoid factor, heterophile, and Wasserman antibodies are the IgM class.

IgD has been found to exist mostly within the intravascular spaces. Its antibody activity has been associated with thyroglobulin nuclear antigens and insulin. The half-life of IgD in the serum is less than 3 days.

B cells are influenced by the suppressor T cells and helper T cells. It is thought that the helper T cells must perform properly to form the serum antibodies; in addition it is believed that the suppressor T cells have a regulatory function to control this process. If something goes awry with the suppressor T cells, such as loss of suppressor T cells, regulation of B cells is removed; thus the B cells are free to produce serum antibody to an individual's own tissue and thus introduce autoimmune disease (Fig. 14-1). T cells may, on the other hand, produce a substance that may prevent maturation of the B cells into plasma cells and in this way interfere with the production of the serum antibodies. Thus diseases associated with decreased serum antibodies may occur.

Alterations in the proportions of T and B cells have been reported with systemic diseases.[106] A recent study of patients with Graves' disease showed that patients with infiltrative ophthalmopathy without previous antithyroid therapy and euthyroid patients with progressive ophthalmopathy had decreased percentages of T cells compared to thyrotoxic patients without ocular disease or to control patients.[125]

Patients with rheumatoid arthritis demonstrated a wide range of peripheral blood T cell values, with low percentages of peripheral blood T cells correlating to some extent with severe clinical disease.[142] Patients with systemic lupus erythematosus showed reduced percentages and absolute numbers of peripheral blood T cells that correlated with clinical disease activity.[97] There is a slight decrease in the proportion of T cells in the peripheral blood in patients with Werner's syndrome,[63] a condition characterized by accelerated aging. Goto et al.[63] found a similar pattern in healthy donors more than 90 years old. A decrease in T cells in patients with neoplasms and with certain viral illnesses has been noted.[148] Most patients with Sjögren's syndrome showed an increase in peripheral blood B cells, and there was a decrease in T cells in some.[135] Patients with lepromatous leprosy showed reduced percentages of both T and B peripheral blood lymphocytes.[95]

Decreased percentages and absolute numbers of T- and B-lymphocytes are immunologic abnormalities associated with ocular cicatricial pemphigoid. These lymphocytic abnormalities may have important implications in the immunopathogenesis of the disease. The reduction in T-lymphocytes may reflect a disproportionate loss of suppressor cells compared to helper T cells. Autoimmune diseases such as systemic lupus erythematosus and juvenile rheumatoid arthritis have been associated with a loss of suppressor cells.[62, 131]

With reduced numbers of suppressor T cells, T and B cell responses to host tissues such as the conjunctiva may not be properly regulated or suppressed so that destructive autoimmune phenomena develop. It is also possible that the reduction of circulating lymphocytes in this disease results from sequestration of these cells beneath the skin and mucous membranes. Specimens of skin and mucous membranes, including

Table 14-1. Significant lymphokines formed from interaction of T cells and antigen

Mediators of macrophage activity	Mediators of neutrophilic leukocyte activity	Mediators of lymphocyte activity	Mediators of basophil and eosinophil activity	Others
Migration-inhibit-ting factor (MIF) Macrophage-acti-vating factor Macrophage-aggregating factor	Leukocyte-inhibit-ing factor (LIF) Chemotactic factor	Mitogenic factor Helper and sup-pressor factor	Chemotactic factor	Transfer factor (TF) Interferon Growth-inhibiting factor Cytotoxic factors (lymphotoxins) Skin reactive factor

the conjunctiva, show an infiltration beneath the epithelium consisting primarily of lymphocytes and plasma cells, with occasional eosinophils and a few polymorpho-nuclear leukocytes. B-lymphocytes sequestered beneath the skin and mucous mem-branes may be converted to plasma cells, producing antibodies against these tissues.

Lymphokines

Following the reaction of antigen with T-lymphocyte is a series of events that results in the liberation of soluble substances known as lymphokines (Table 14-1). Transfer factor (TF) is one of these substances and has the capacity to transfer delayed hyper-sensitivity. Another lymphokine is migration-inhibiting factor (MIF), which is impor-tant as a substance that retains macrophages in an area of injury. It is involved in the formation of granulomatous lesions and in infectious diseases such as tuberculosis in which cell-mediated immunity and mononuclear infiltration are pathologic features. Another lymphokine is lymphotoxin. It seems to be associated with target cell injury and inhibits the capacity of the cell to divide. Chemotactic lymphokines also are re-leased after the reaction of antigens with lymphocytes. These factors cause migrations of monocytes, eosinophils, and neutrophils. Other lymphokines are mitogenic factors and interferon, which is an important effector molecule significant in the recovery mechanism of viral infections. It inhibits the ability of virus to infect more cells.

An individual will be susceptible to viral and fungal disease in the event of an ab-normality that results in an inability of the thymus to produce T cells. The inability for one reason or another to produce B cells will lead to an immunodeficiency with par-ticular susceptibility to bacterial infections.

IMMUNOLOGIC MECHANISMS

It is seen that proper regulation of the aforementioned immune systems will help the eye avoid infection. The eye, as will be seen, is peculiar in its responses to im-munologic and inflammatory mechanisms. The unique responses of the cornea, for example, are related to its avascularity and lack of lymphatic elements. The cornea is therefore a site of privilege as far as survival of a graft is concerned. However, this is changed if the cornea becomes vascularized. The corneal vessels act as the efferent limb of the immunologic effective system. In addition, lymphoid channels are produced along with the vascular response. The lymphoid channels thus formed are continuous with the conjunctival lymphatic vessels. If there is an antigenic insult to the cornea, vascularization and lymphatic infiltration of the cornea may occur; these channels form a continuous channel with those of the conjunctiva. Thus corneal antigen is recognized by the conjunctival lymphocytes, and conjunctival follicular hypertrophy and local and systemic sensitization occur.

Local immunity, as has been noted, must also be considered since secretory antibodies occur in the tears. Tears are rich in IgA, which provides the body with a first line of defense against microorganisms. Immunoglobulins are present in the conjunctiva and in the eye, though not in the lens. The highest concentrations are in the cornea, choroid, and conjunctiva.

HLA system

The human leukocyte antigen (HLA) system is the major histocompatibility system in humans. The human histocompatibility complex involving the HLA system is located on chromosome 6. The HLA antigens are genetically determined and are present on most of the tissues of the body. Multiple transfusions induce HLA antibodies, as do pregnancies. The frequency of appearance of the various human lymphocyte antigens varies with geographic location and race. It also appears that some diseases occur preferentially in individuals possessing certain HLA types. The presently known antigens fall into four groups that segregate together: A, B, C, and D, corresponding to the arrangement of genes within the HLA region on chromosome 6. More antigens of the B and A series have been defined than have antigens of the C and D series. The association of HLA-B27 with ankylosing spondylitis is very strong: HLA-B27 occurs in about 96% of individuals with this disease. In addition, about 40% of the individuals with ankylosing spondylitis have uveitis. Graves' disease shows an increased incidence of HLA-B8; multiple sclerosis, HLA-B7 and HLA-DW2; and Reiter's disease, HLA-B27. Of great importance to the ophthalmologist is HLA typing associated with herpes simplex keratitis. HLA-B5 is significantly increased in patients with herpes simplex keratitis, suggesting an altered immune state in patients with recurrent herpes keratitis.

Immune response genes

Immune response (IR) genes are also important in defense against microorganisms. The lack of an IR gene increases the risk of infection; on the other hand, a very aggressive immune response determinant might increase the risk of autoimmune phenomena developing.

Molecular mimicry

Another explanation for some of the associations between HLA antigens and specific diseases is molecular mimicry. Certain organisms may resemble human tissue

354   Diseases of the cornea

Table 14-2. Significant ophthalmic hypersensitivity reactions

Type I (anaphylactoid)	Type II (cytotoxic)	Type III (immune complex)	Type IV (cell mediated)
Complement not involved	Complement involved	Complement involved	Complement not involved
Hay fever	Perhaps long-standing corneal	Serum sickness	Phlyctenular disease
Vernal catarrh	allograft reaction	Marginal infiltrates associated	Allograft reaction
Atopic dermatitis with	Pemphigus vulgaris	with *Staphylococcus*	Allergic contact dermatoconjunctivitis
keratoconjunctivitis	Bullous pemphigoid	species and *Moraxella*	of lids
	Cicatricial pemphigoid	*lacunata*	Granulomatous diseases: lues,
	Mooren's ulcer	Marginal corneal infiltrates	tuberculosis, leprosy, and
		and melts in immune	toxoplasmosis
		diseases	Herpetic stromal keratitis
		Disciform keratitis, mumps,	Phacolytic glaucoma
		infectious mononucleosis,	Sympathetic ophthalmia (?)
		and subepithelial infiltrates	Vogt-Koyanagi-Harada (?)
		in adenoviral disease	Sjögren's syndrome (?)
		Padi keratitis	
		Wessely ring	
		Scleritis and scleromalacia	

antigens; this could lead to decreased attack against these organisms and an increased susceptibility to severe infections. This mimicry can also result in induced auto-immunity.

Classes of immunologic reactions

All immunologic mechanisms usually belong to one of the four types (Table 14-2) that follow.

Type I: anaphylactoid hypersensitivity. Antigen reacts with IgE antibody that is bound to mast cells or circulating basophils. This reaction leads to degranulation of the mast cells or basophils and to the release of various substances such as histamine, heparin, serotonin, eosinophil chemotactic factor, and slow-reacting substance of anaphylaxis (SRS-A). The levels of intracellular cyclic adenosine monophosphate (cyclic AMP) and cyclic guanine monophosphate (cyclic GMP) influence the release of these moderators from the mast cells and basophils. Elevated levels of cyclic AMP inhibit the release of the mediators. Elevated levels of cyclic GMP enhance the release of the histamine-like substances.

Type II: cytotoxic hypersensitivity. Type II hypersensitivity is caused by the action of antibodies directed against antigens present on cells. The cytotoxic anaphylaxis is thus caused by antitissue antibodies. Circulating immunoglobulins are usually combining, in the presence of complement, with antigens that are present already on the cell. The mechanism in this particular reaction is concerned with IgM and IgG.

Type III: immune-complex hypersensitivity. Type III hypersensitivity is concerned with antigen-antibody complexes. Antigen reacts in tissue spaces with antibody, thus forming microprecipitates in and around small blood vessels and causing damage to cells. Type III reactions may also occur when excess antigen reacts in the blood-stream with antibody. Soluble circulating complexes are formed, which are then deposited in blood vessel walls or in the basement membrane to cause local inflammation. In each instance complement is fixed to the antigen-antibody complex. This type of reaction is designated the *Arthus reaction*. Serum sickness is also considered to be a good example of immune-complex disease.

Type IV: cell-mediated hypersensitivity. Type IV reactions may be clearly differentiated from the other types by the time taken to mount the reaction after injection of antigen and by the fact that they occur in the absence of circulating antibody. Although it is not possible to transfer cell-mediated hypersensitivity passively by means of serum, it is possible with cells of its products. MIF can be used as a test of some relevance in certain immunologic diseases in the eye such as Sjögren's syndrome and Wegener's granulomatosis.

APPROACHES TO TREATMENT

The foregoing classes of immune reactions may be approached by various methods as far as treatment is concerned.

Type I

Desensitization. Treatment in the form of desensitization (1) results in reduction in level of IgE, (2) causes an induction of state of immune tolerance toward injected antigen, and (3) may result in mast cells being rendered insensitive to degranulating action of antigen combined with IgE on the cell membrane.

Surface-acting drugs. The interaction of the allergen with specific IgE on the mast cell surface interferes with adenyl cyclase activity and the synthesis of cyclic AMP. The reduced concentration of cyclic AMP results in loss of stability of lysosomal membranes and release of vasoactive amines.

1. Epinephrine (Adrenalin) reverses the inhibition of adenylcyclase so that cyclic AMP may carry on its action.
2. Aminophylline prevents destruction of cyclic AMP by phosphodiesterase.
3. Cromolyn sodium suppresses phosphodiesterase and prevents degranulation of the mast cell.

Drugs acting on the organelle system. Steroids are able to stabilize the lysosomal membrane and prevent the release of histamine-like substances from the activated mast cells.

Antilymphocytic globulin and transfer factor. Antibody is mainly of IgG class and is effective against circulating lymphocytes in the intravascular compartment. It can affect delayed hypersensitivity and allograft reactions, and it causes lysis of target lymphocytes. It should be used with caution in corneal graft reaction.

Immune deficiency has been treated with lymphocyte extracts containing transfer factor in T cell deficiencies such as Wiskott-Aldrich syndrome and in keratoconjunctivitis associated with mucocutaneous candidiasis.[146]

Antihistamines. These substances compete with histamines for reactive sites on the target cell.

Types II to IV

Corticosteroids. This treatment often results in or causes the following:
1. Lympholysis, especially of B cells
2. Inhibition of T cell cytotoxicity
3. Restriction of leukocytic migration from circulating blood
4. Inhibition of prostaglandin synthesis
5. Reduction of antibody synthesis

Antimitotic drugs

Folic acid analogues (methotrexate). Folic acids play an important role in formation of nucleotides. Methotrexate acts by competitive inhibition of the enzymes involved in folic acid production. DNA synthesis is impaired, as is the proliferation of B- and T-lymphocytes that follows contact with antigen. Antibody production is inhibited and inflammatory reactions curtailed.

Purine analogues (azathioprine, mercaptopurine). These compounds inhibit DNA synthesis by interfering with purine metabolism and are thus antinucleic acid metabolites.

Alkylating agents (chlorambucil, cyclophosphamide). These agents promote cross-linkage of double-stranded DNA in the nuclear chromatin and affect resting as well as dividing cells.

ALLERGIC CONTACT DERMATOCONJUNCTIVITIS
Etiologic factors

This condition is induced by the delayed hypersensitivity reaction (type IV) and is related to agents such as topical drugs. The reaction is a haptenic one, wherein the drug conjugates with tissue protein; this antigenic conjugate reacts with the sensitized T cell, which then elaborates lymphokines. The sensitization lasts for the lifetime of the patient; future exposure may result in dermatitis. Reexposure elsewhere may result in a flare-up of the reaction at the original site. The drug must pass through the epidermis or conjunctiva for the reaction to occur. The conjugation reaction takes place in the subepidermal dermis; since the conjunctiva and skin of the lid are thin, these areas are more vulnerable to this type of reaction than such areas as the palms or soles, where the skin is thick.

Agents commonly responsible for allergic contact dermatoconjunctivitis are neomycin, eserine, pilocarpine, penicillin, epinephrine, idoxuridine, topical anesthetic agents, nail polish, and mascara.

Symptoms

The conjunctiva, especially the inferior areas, may manifest redness, swelling, and thickening. The rest of the conjunctiva and the skin of the lids are then involved in the allergic contact dermatoconjunctival problem (Fig. 14-3). Crusting, flaking, thickening, scaling, and oozing of the skin of the lids occur. If the offending medication is continued for a long time, toxic reactions may occur in addition to the sensitivity reaction.

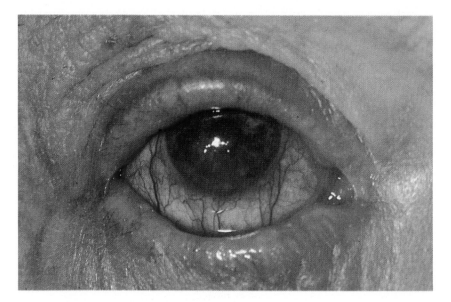

Fig. 14-3. Allergic contact dermatoconjunctivitis. Skin of lids is thick, crusting, flaking, and injected. Conjunctiva is also injected.

The cornea may show extensive epithelial defect with heaping up of the epithelium in toxic reactions; this element of the reaction must be differentiated from the allergic reaction. The complaints of itching and burning are quite common.

Management

Patch testing is used for confirmation of the diagnosis, as is discontinuation of the medication. Antihistamines have no effect, and desensitization is not of help. Topical steroids may be of value. One should watch for secondary infection.

VERNAL CATARRH (Table 14-3)

Vernal catarrh is a bilateral, seasonal inflammation caused by allergy and usually seen in young patients. It is one of three atopic ocular diseases that affect humans, the other two of which are hay fever conjunctivitis and atopic dermatitis with conjunctivitis. The word *atopy* is used to describe allergic individuals with a hereditary background of allergic diseases; atopy is also used to refer to a group of problems that include infantile eczema with atopic dermatitis, seasonal allergic rhinitis, conjunctivitis, bronchial asthma, urticaria, and certain forms of food allergy. IgE is elevated in the tears in vernal catarrh.[91]

Table 14-3. Major pathologic changes of cornea and conjunctiva occurring in hay fever, vernal catarrh, and atopic dermatitis with keratitis

	Hay fever	Vernal catarrh	Atopic dermatitis with keratitis
Immunity type	I	I	I
Scars	−	−	In conjunctiva and papillae
Edema	+ (Wheal)	+	−
Hyperplasia	−	+	+
Papillae Location	− −	Giant Upper lid	Small Lower lid
Corneal involvement	−	Micropannus Epithelial keratopathy "Shield" ulcer	Vacularization Opacification
Limbus	−	Trantas' dots Cysts Pseudogerontoxon	Trantas' dots Cysts
Eosinophils	+	+ (Fragmented)	+
Basophils	−	+ (Fragmented)	+

The incidence of atopy increases in vernal patients and their relatives; some patients may show an increased incidence of circulating antibodies to airborne pollens, although no evidence exists of any particular allergen that would cause the disease. These patients, like many other patients with allergies, show blood eosinophilia.

Incidence

Vernal catarrh is usually seen in males until puberty, when the incidence of females rises, so that by the age of 20 the sex incidence is about equal. The disease occurs most often between the ages of 6 and puberty[120]; it is occasionally seen in older age groups. A suggestion has been made that limbal vernal disease is more common in blacks. The disease is uncommon in the cooler, more temperate climates; there seems to be a high incidence of vernal catarrh in Mexico, the Middle East, and the Mediterranean areas. The seasonal variation is of importance, since the disease usually occurs with the onset of spring, continues through summer, and gradually decreases in the fall. During the colder months the symptoms decrease, but the proliferative changes may persist with only slight regression. The limbal form of the disease is more likely to show regression, which is often complete in mild cases.

Symptoms and clinical findings

The most outstanding symptom is itching; other symptoms include photophobia, burning lacrimation, and foreign body sensation. These are associated in many instances with a keratitis and a very thick, sticky, mucoid discharge, the pH of which is alkaline.

Vernal conjunctivitis is a simple hyperemic type of conjunctivitis that is followed by a tissue hyperplasia.[108] The palpebral form of the disease may demonstrate a dull, pale, milky-blue hue to the conjunctiva. A flat, focal or uniform widening of the limbus occurs when tissue hyperplasia is seen at the corneoscleral junction. Papillary hypertrophy is seen predominantly on the upper tarsal conjunctiva. These papillary vegetations are flat-topped, polygonal excrescences and give the classic cobblestone appearance to the upper tarsal conjunctiva (Fig. 14-4). The weight of the papillae may be so great that a pseudoptosis often occurs. The lower tarsus is usually free of giant papillae in vernal catarrh. The presence of giant papillae in this location is more often seen in atopic keratoconjunctivitis.

Limbal papillary hypertrophy may be seen in the interpalpebral area (Fig. 14-5). The gelatinous-appearing limbal hypertrophy may involve the peripheral cornea, often leaving focal areas of corneal opacity and micropannus after their regression. Micropannus is seen in a number of other conditions in addition to vernal catarrh (Fig. 14-6):

1. Contact lens wearers
2. Corneal arcus (rarely)
3. Superior limbic keratoconjunctivitis
4. Long-standing *Staphylococcus aureus* keratoconjunctivitis
5. Trachoma in children
6. Molluscum contagiosum (rarely a gross pannus may occur)
7. Inclusion conjunctivitis

Small, flat, or mildly elevated, grayish-white to yellow dots may be seen in the lim-

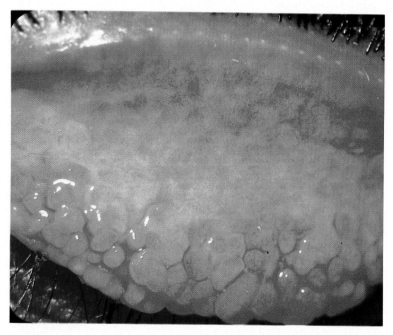

Fig. 14-4. Giant papillary hypertrophy (cobblestone appearance) of upper tarsal conjunctiva.

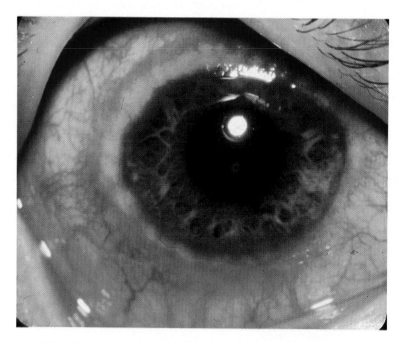

Fig. 14-5. Limbal vernal catarrh exhibiting papillary hypertrophy.

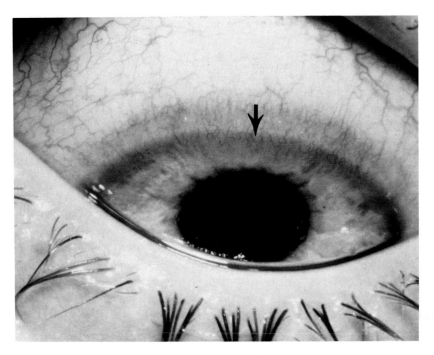

Fig. 14-6. Vernal catarrh with micropannus *(arrow).*

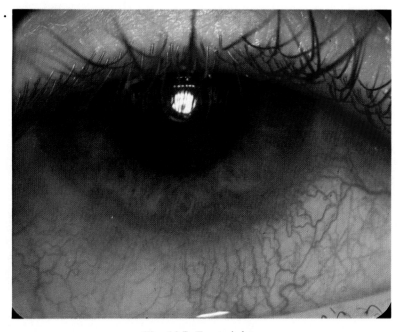

Fig. 14-7. Trantas' dots.

bal area. These are Trantas' dots (Fig. 14-7). Although Trantas' dots are usually confined to the upper limbus, they may appear on the bulbar conjunctiva and semilunar folds. Trantas' dots can occur in the center of the cornea. They are most often seen in vernal catarrh, but they can occur in chronic atopic dermatitis with keratoconjunctivitis as well. The dots consist of degenerated eosinophils and epithelial cells. These localized white dots are transient and usually do not last longer than a week. They may extend into the deep layers of the epithelium; however, they gradually become superficial and break through the epithelium. Trantas' dots have been seen in patients who wear soft contact lenses.[93] Epithelial inclusion cysts of the upper limbus may occur but are more common in atopic keratoconjunctivitis.

Corneal changes in addition to the micropannus include a farinaceous epithelial keratitis (keratitis epithelialis vernalis of Tobgy), which consists of tiny, gray-white intraepithelial corneal opacities (Fig. 14-8). These lesions are worse above and fewer in the periphery and will stain with fluorescein and rose bengal red. A more intense form of the farinaceous keratitis occurs when the epithelial cells degenerate and shrink, producing the appearance of a cobweb or syncytium.

Also appearing are vernal corneal ulcers, which are horizontal or shield-shaped ulcers usually occurring above. The ulcers have thickened opaque edges and an opaque base (Fig. 14-9). Less commonly, deep keratitis with vascularization and pseudogerontoxon may be seen. In addition, keratoconus and keratoglobus are occasionally associated with vernal keratoconjunctivitis.

The most characteristic feature of the conjunctival scrapings in vernal disease is the

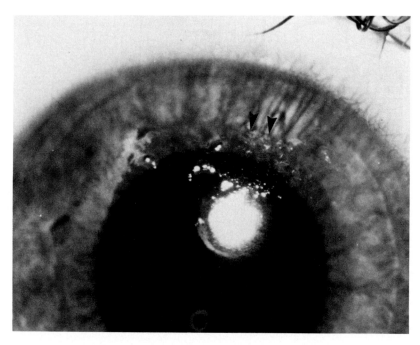

Fig. 14-8. Epithelial keratopathy seen in vernal catarrh *(double arrow)*.

presence of eosinophils and free eosinophilic granules (Fig. 14-10). In addition, basophils and free basophilic granules may be seen. Occasionally lymphocytes and monocytes occur. The histopathologic picture in general usually consists of a cellular infiltration of the substantia propia with eosinophils, hyperplasia of connective tissue that becomes hyalinized, and proliferative or degenerative changes of the epithelium. Secondary amyloidosis of the conjunctiva may occur occasionally.

Differential diagnosis

The papillae seen in atopic dermatitis with keratoconjunctivitis are usually small and involve the lower tarsal conjunctiva. The conjunctival discharge is meager and watery, and there are fewer eosinophils but no free granules.

Trachoma should also be considered in the differential diagnosis. Trachoma produces a follicular conjunctivitis with round, translucent bodies of uniform size; limbal trachoma follicles; Herbert's pits; and a fleshy, vascularized gross pannus. The course of trachoma is chronic and nonseasonal. Conjunctival scrapings reveal polymorphonuclear cells, plasma cells, Leber's cells, and epithelial inclusions but no eosinophils.

Phlyctenular conjunctivitis is another disease that must on occasion be differentiated from vernal disease. The isolated limbal vegetation of vernal catarrh may give the appearance of a phlyctenule. The phlyctenule, however, ulcerates and undergoes resolution in 10 days to 2 weeks, whereas the vegetation of limbal vernal disease persists longer. The follicular conjunctivitis associated with chlamydial infection and viral diseases does not offer a great difficulty in a differential diagnosis. The viral diseases are usually associated with a follicular response and preauricular adenopathy and exhibit a watery discharge. Mononuclear cells are found on conjunctival scrapings. Herpes simplex keratitis may occur in patients with vernal disease, and the differentiation of vernal ulcer from a herpes ulcer may become difficult. However, in herpes simplex infection, the sensitivity of the cornea is reduced, giant cells are seen in the scrapings, and there is a positive herpes FA test.

Management

Vernal disease, with a long but self-limited course, is normally benign. Poor treatment has included destruction of the conjunctival vegetations by (1) radiation (radium, beta radiation), (2) surgery (excision of papillae and even tarsectomy), and (3) carbon dioxide snow and, for the relief of symptoms, the continuous use of strong corticosteroid preparations both systematically and topically. Radiation treatment in particular has led to keratinization of the tarsal conjunctival epithelium and extensive cicatrization. Unwise steroid therapy has led to steroid cataract, steroid glaucoma, prolongation of the clinical course, and secondary infection with opportunist, particularly herpes simplex virus.

Treatment of vernal catarrh should include the following concepts:
1. Antihistamines are usually ineffective.
2. Vasoconstrictors are not as effective therapeutically as they are in hay fever conjunctivitis.
3. Mild or dilute steroid drops instilled three to four times a day afford relief.

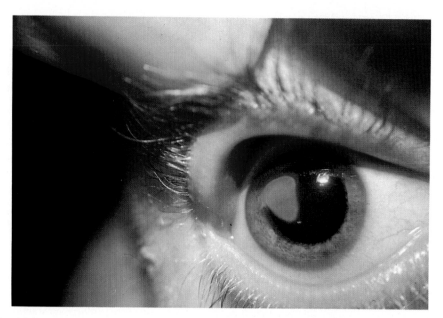

Fig. 14-9. Shieldlike ulcer of cornea occasionally seen in vernal catarrh. (From Grayson, M., and Keates, R.H.: Manual of diseases of the cornea, Boston, 1969, Little, Brown & Co.)

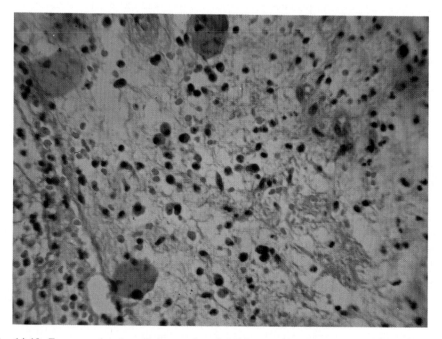

Fig. 14-10. Fragmented and nonfragmented eosinophils seen in conjunctival scrapings in case of vernal catarrh.

4. Cromolyn sodium drops, 4%,* one drop five times daily,[37, 38, 75] is effective. (The use of cromolyn sodium will help to decrease the amount of steroid that is used. Cromolyn sodium prevents the degranulation of mast cells and thus the release of the vasoactive amines that cause many of the symptoms. As the patient's symptoms improve, both the steroid and the cromolyn sodium drops may be titrated to the minimal effective dose.) Acute chemotic reaction has taken place after topical use of this medication. It should be looked for since it can cause signs that may be confused with the disease process.[111]

5. Cold compresses or air conditioning aids in relieving the symptoms.

6. Acetylcysteine (Mucomyst) 10%, decreases the thick, ropy, sticky discharge.

ATOPIC DERMATITIS WITH KERATOCONJUNCTIVITIS (Table 14-3)

Atopic dermatitis with keratoconjunctivitis is an allergic disease of the skin and conjunctiva mediated by IgE.[66, 84] Patients with this disorder have a decreased cellular immunity; a number of patients exhibit an increased susceptibility to seborrheic blepharitis and herpes simplex infections.[121] These patients also never seem to develop phlyctenular disease. They may give a positive family history of other manifestations of atopy such as hay fever, allergic rhinitis, urticaria, asthma, or anaphylaxis. It has been suggested that certain patients with atopic dermatitis exhibit contact hypersensitivity to human dander on patch test.[137]

Symptoms and clinical findings

The problem starts with infantile eczema and can be seen as a rather severe disease in the late teens.[36] The problem may persist until the forties or fifties. The primary skin lesions are pruritic, succulent, weeping, and crusting. In adolescence, the disease tends to involve the face, neck, and antecubital fossae (Fig. 14-11, *A*), as well as the hands, feet, and ears at times. These lesions are usually dry.

The eyelids may be severely affected. They may be quite thick and lichenified from constant rubbing (Fig. 14-11, *B*). Weeping fissures occur at the lateral canthi.

The conjunctiva appears often as hyperemic and chemotic in the acute state. The conjunctiva in the chronic case will show congestion. Conjunctival scarring is focal and tends to occur in the centers of the giant papillae (Fig. 14-12, *A*); in addition, shrinkage of the lower cul-de-sac (Fig. 14-12, *B*) can occur. Atopic keratoconjunctivitis is therefore a cicatrizing disease. Secondary *Staphylococcus* or *Streptococcus* infection may occur with resulting infectious eczematoid dermatitis. Recognition of this infectious extension of the disease is essential. It will respond to systemic antibiotics such as dicloxacillin.

Giant papillae are especially apparent on the lower lid. The upper tarsal area often appears milky but without much giant papillae formation. Clear inclusion cysts occur at the upper limbus (Fig. 14-13); on occasion they can be seen in the lower cul-de-sac (Fig. 14-14). In addition, symblepharon, entropion of the lids, and trichiasis are seen.

Trantas' dots have been found, but they do not occur as frequently as in vernal

---

*This medication is not available at present for commercial use. It may be developed by dissolving 60 capsules (20 mg each) of cromolyn sodium (Intal) in triple-distilled water (30 ml). This should then be filtered through a Milex filter. Proper adjustment for pH will be necessary.

Text continued on p. 372.

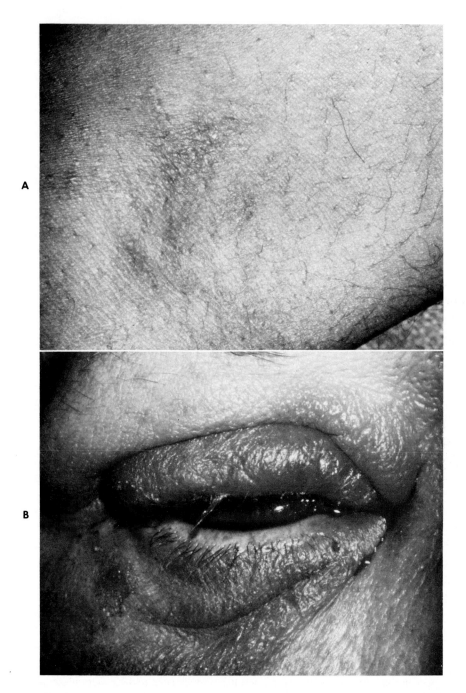

Fig. 14-11. A, Antecubital skin lesions as noted in atopic dermatitis. Eczematous skin lesion is on occasion a weeping, crusting lesion. It may also be dry and lichenified in nature. **B,** Eyelids may be thick and lichenified as result of constant rubbing in atopic dermatitis with keratoconjunctivitis.

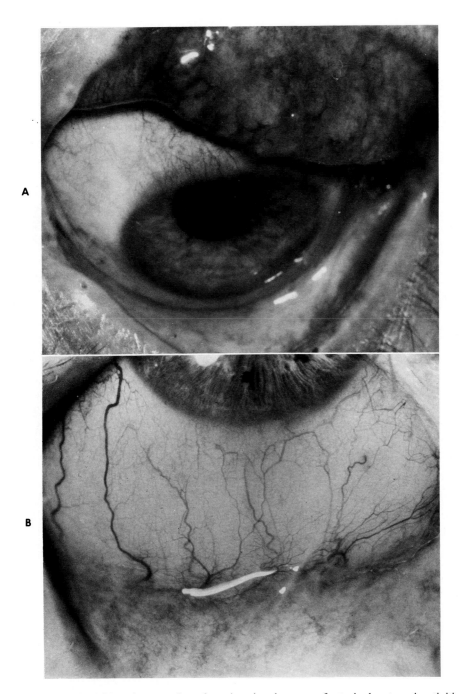

Fig. 14-12. A, Papillary hypertrophy of conjunctiva in case of atopic keratoconjunctivitis.
B, Atopic keratoconjunctivitis is cicatrizing disease. Small symblepharons are seen in lower
cul-de-sac.

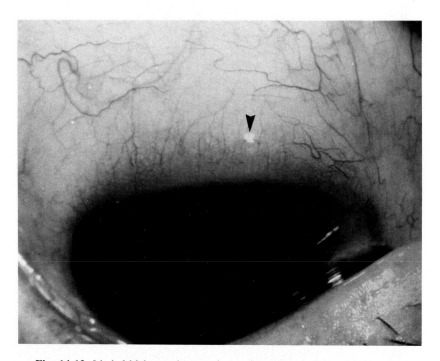

Fig. 14-13. Limbal bleb may be seen in atopic conjunctival keratitis *(arrow)*.

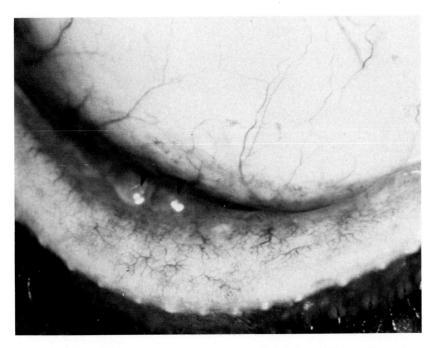

Fig. 14-14. Small cystic blebs may also be seen in inferior cul-de-sac *(arrows).*

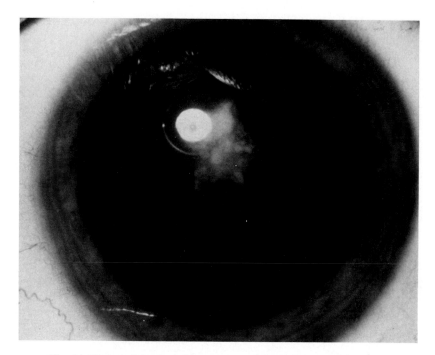

Fig. 14-15. Anterior subcapsular cataract of atopic keratoconjunctivitis.

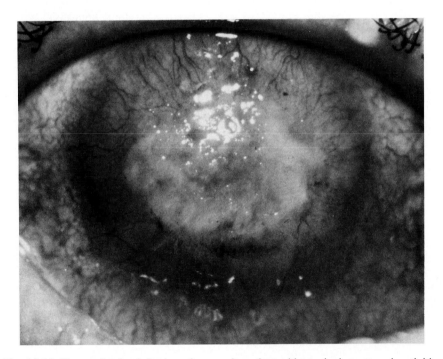

Fig. 14-16. Herpes simplex infection of cornea in patient with atopic dermatoconjunctivitis.

catarrh. The cornea may manifest an epithelial keratitis, marginal ulceration, vascularization, and stromal opacification.

Eosinophils and basophils may be found in the conjunctival scrapings, but usually there are no free granules.

Anterior and posterior subcapsular cataracts, retinal detachments, and keratoconus can be seen as complications of atopic keratoconjunctivitis (Fig. 14-15).

Management

A major problem of atopic dermatitis is the threat of superimposed herpes simplex or vaccinia infection (Kaposi's varicelliform eruption). It is important that these patients avoid contact with active herpes simplex lesions or individuals recently vaccinated. Herpes simplex virus is seen in Fig. 14-16 in association with atopic dermatitis. Smallpox vaccination should not be attempted. Sensitizing chemicals such as neomycin and systemic steroids should also be avoided.

Cromolyn sodium drops, 4%, applied four to five times a day are effective in relieving the symptoms.[111] Although steroids have been used, there is a poor overall response to them. Long-term use of steroids should be avoided.

HAY FEVER (Table 14-3)

This condition affects young people primarily and is a clear-cut antibody-antigen reaction to pollen and a number of ectodermal agents. One may see a jellylike clear conjunctival swelling that resembles a giant hive or wheal (Fig. 14-17). If the conjunc-

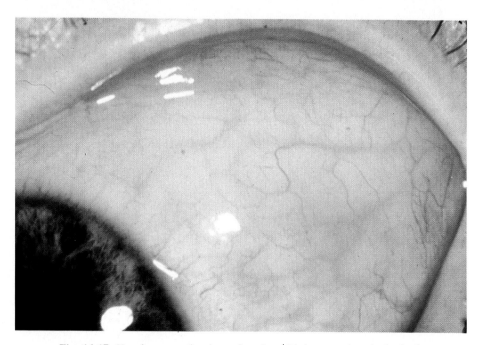

Fig. 14-17. Hay fever reaction in conjunctiva with large conjunctival wheal.

tival wheal or swelling is large enough, areas of corneal drying central to the wheal may cause drying out of the cornea with delle formation.

Severe itching of the lid, itching in the area of the inner canthi, hyperemia of the conjunctiva, and lid edema without redness or tenderness are the main external findings.

The corneas are always clear, and no scarring or giant papilla occurs.

Usually one can find the cause of hay fever, and desensitization treatment offers good results. Antihistamines and astringents applied topically may help.

GIANT PAPILLARY CONJUNCTIVITIS IN CONTACT LENS WEARERS

A syndrome exists in wearers of hard and soft contact lenses that consists of increased mucus, mild itching, and the development of giant papillae in the upper tarsal conjunctiva[1,65] (Fig. 14-18). The same findings are seen with a methyl methacrylate corneal shell, a postenucleation prosthesis, or a keratoprosthesis. Giant papillary conjunctivitis of the tarsus of the upper lids can develop after prolonged wear. In addition to the problem developing in contact lens and prosthesis wearers, one can encounter giant papillary conjunctivitis from 10-0 nylon sutures with exposed knots.[128]

An SLK-like condition may also be noted. Recognition of these contact lens–induced conditions is essential to proper treatment and care of contact lenses. Giant papillary conjunctivitis may occur in 10% of soft contact lens wearers and 1% of hard contact lens wearers. The problem may be caused by the preservatives used in cleaning the lens, the lypoproteins deposited on the lens, microbial adherence to the lens, or the monomers of polymers of the lens itself.

On occasion papillary keratoconjunctivitis associated with contact lenses may be confused with SLK.[145] In some cases, one can see a mucopurulent discharge from which *Staphylococcus aureus* grows. The syndrome develops in wearers of soft contact lens after a few weeks or after a long period of continuous wear.

Giant papillary conjunctivitis exhibits a strong clinical similarity to vernal conjunctivitis. Itching, which is severe in vernal conjunctivitis, is mild in contact lens wearers. Punctate keratitis is usually not seen in soft contact lens–wearing syndrome; it is routine in vernal conjunctivitis. There is no seasonal variation in the contact lens syndrome, whereas there is a definite seasonal variation in symptoms and findings in vernal catarrh. The histamine level of the tears is increased in vernal conjunctivitis but not in giant papillary conjunctivitis. The cytologic scrapings from the conjunctiva of subjects with the syndrome often show eosinophils, but these are few. Scrapings from the conjunctiva of patients with vernal conjunctivitis routinely contain many eosinophils, both whole and fragmented. Giant papillary conjunctivitis in contact lens wearers, which is relieved by the removal of the contact lens, is common; vernal conjunctivitis is relatively rare.

Floppy eyelid syndrome is a disorder of unknown origin manifested by an easily everted, floppy upper eyelid and papillary conjunctivitis of the upper palpebral conjunctiva. The upper eyelid everts during sleep, resulting in irritation, papillary conjunctivitis, and conjunctival keratinization. Effective treatment consists of preventing the upper eyelid from everting while the patient is sleeping.[34]

The cause of giant papillary conjunctivitis is probably immunologic because of the nature of the cellular infiltrate. The presence of lymphocytes, plasma cells, mast cells,

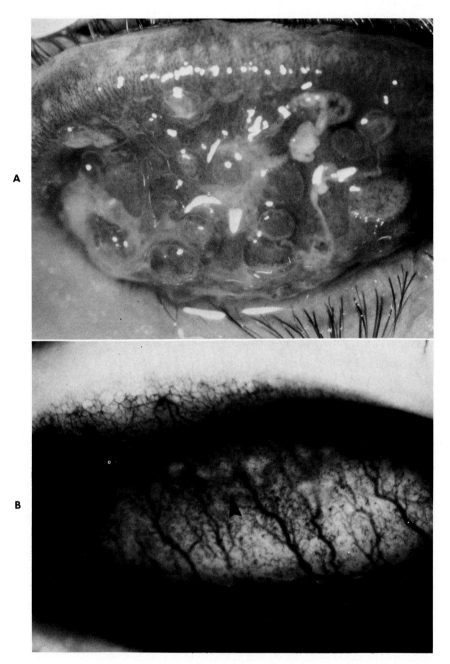

Fig. 14-18. A, Giant papillary reaction of upper tarsal plate in soft contact lens wearer. **B,** Early reaction of same pathologic condition in wearer of soft contact lens *(arrow).*

basophils, and eosinophils indicates a similarity between this syndrome and delayed hypersensitivity of the cutaneous basophilic type, as has been described in humans. Cutaneous basophilic hypersensitivity is an expression of cell-mediated immunity that has been separated from the classical tuberculin type of reaction. In the tuberculin type a predominant infiltration of lymphocytes occurs. Conditions that in addition to lymphocytic infiltration were found to have basophilic infiltration with some eosinophils are considered in humans to be an expression of cutaneous basophilic hypersensitivity. The presence of basophilic and eosinophilic mast cells suggest an antigen-antibody mechanism underlying the response.

PHLYCTENULOSIS

Sensitivity to the tuberculin antigen may cause phlyctenulosis and is an example of pure cellular immunity. Phlyctenulosis is often associated with poor hygienic conditions and poor nutrition, and its incidence in girls is high.

Symptoms and clinical findings

The attacks are usually self-limited, although some cases may persist for many weeks. A diffuse conjunctival injection is seen; in purely conjunctival cases the subjective symptoms are mild, but severe photophobia is characteristic when the cornea is involved. The first attack is usually always at the limbus; however, phlyctenulosis may be seen on the bulbar (Fig. 14-19) or tarsal conjunctiva.

The older the child, the larger the phlyctenule; the phlyctenules tend to be large and succulent if active tuberculosis is present. The lesions are pinpoint to several millimeters in size, and each follows a course of elevation, infiltration, ulceration, and resolution. The total process usually takes 6 to 10 days. The lesion itself is usually yellow-white, opaque, and surrounded with blood vessels.

Two thirds of the phlyctenule may be on the conjunctiva and one third on the cornea; the phlyctenule usually leaves a scar only on the corneal side (Fig. 14-20).

A corneal infiltrate may be noted (Fig. 14-21), or a fascicular corneal ulcer may extend centrally across the pupillary area (Fig. 14-22). The phlyctenular fascicular corneal ulcer resembles the "wandering" ulcer of herpes simplex. Herpes simplex should always be suspected. The decreased corneal sensitivity and the finding of multinucleated giant cells of herpes simplex aid in making a differentiation.

Miliary phlyctenules and deep or superficially infiltrated lesions may also be seen. Stromal involvement may be severe and may even lead to perforation, as has been noted in phlyctenular disease of staphylococcal origin.[110] A micropannus that is often noted in the lower part of the cornea is a response to necrosis in the cornea.

Phlyctenulosis may be a flare-up of childhood tuberculosis as indicated by an elevated sedimentation rate or by dilation of limbal vessels from superimposed bacterial infection.

Nontuberculous phlyctenular disease

A certain number of cases of phlyctenulosis appear in every nontuberculous population. Bacteria, fungi, and viruses are all capable of inducing delayed hypersensitivity reaction. Nontuberculous phlyctenular disease is associated with (1) *S. aureus,* (2) *Coc-*

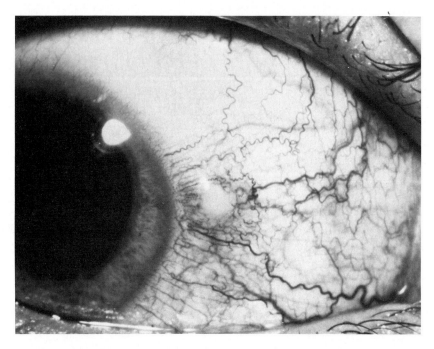

Fig. 14-19. Conjunctival phlyctenule.

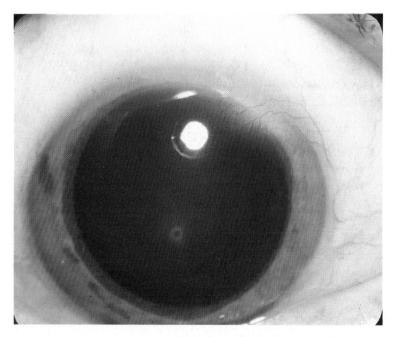

Fig. 14-20. Scarring of cornea with superficial vascularization residual reaction from limbal phlyctenular disease. (Courtesy F. Wilson II, M.D., Indianapolis, Ind.)

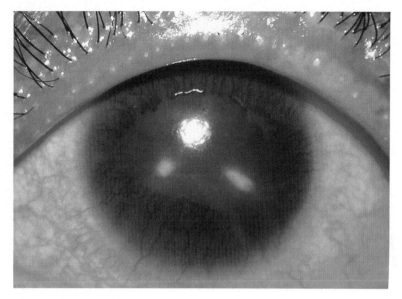

Fig. 14-21. Corneal infiltrate resulting from tuberculous phlyctenular disease.

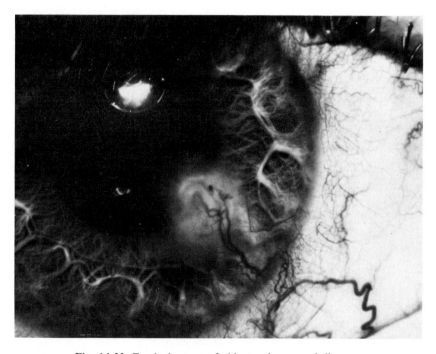

Fig. 14-22. Fascicular type of phlyctenular corneal disease.

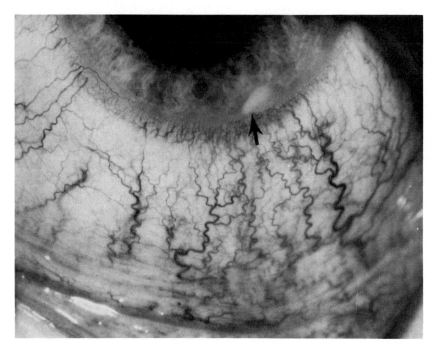

Fig. 14-23. *Candida albicans* phlyctenulosis *(arrow).*

cidioides immitis, (3) *Candida albicans* (Fig. 14-23), and (4) lymphogranuloma vene-reum. The greatest number of cases today, in fact, are caused by *S. aureus* and are always in association with staphylococcal blepharitis. Phlyctenulosis as part of the pa-tient's allergic manifestation during convalescence from coccidioidomycosis is not un-common. In coccidiomycosis there are no corneal stromal phlyctenules; the phlyctenules are confined to the limbal area. Therefore the visual disability so characteristic at times of tuberculous phlyctenulosis is not seen. The phlyctenulosis of cutaneous candidiasis is recurrent but usually not visually damaging.

Rabbit models now exist for phlyctenulosis and catarrhal infiltrates. After immuni-zation and challenge with *S. aureus,* rabbits developed lesions resembling phlyctenules and marginal infiltrates. The former consisted of polymorphonuclear leukocytes, mono-nuclear cells including plasma cells, lymphocytes, and macrophages. The catarrhal in-filtrates were composed of polymorphonuclear leukocytes and mononuclear cells.[105]

Old phlyctenular disease is a cause of Salzmann's nodular corneal degeneration.

Management

Tuberculous phlyctenulosis responds extremely well to topical steroids. However, this is not true of the staphylococcic type of phlyctenular disease. Steroids aggravate the underlying staphylococcal infection and therefore should not be used. Treatment of staphylococcal phlyctenulosis should be confined to control of the blepharitis and the eradication of the staphylococcal organism (Chapter 9).

Penetrating keratoplasty for corneal scarring and decreased vision caused by phlyc-tenulosis offers a favorable prognosis.[127]

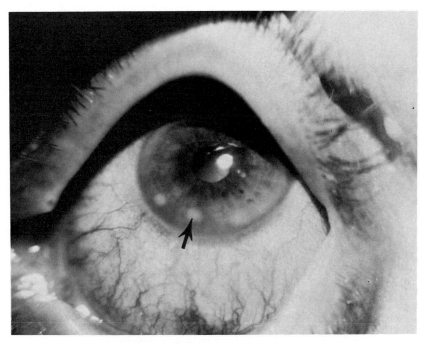

Fig. 14-24. Catarrhal ulcers of staphylococcal origin *(arrow)*.

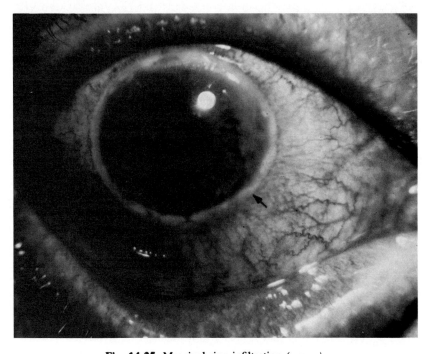

Fig. 14-25. Marginal ring infiltration *(arrow)*.

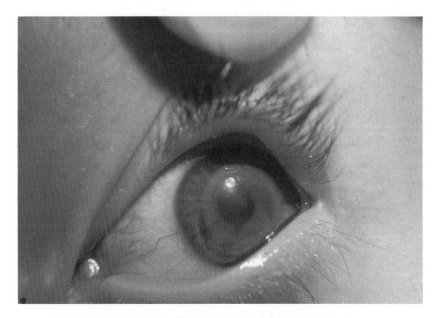

Fig. 14-26. Ring keratitis. Reaction is similar to Wessely ring.

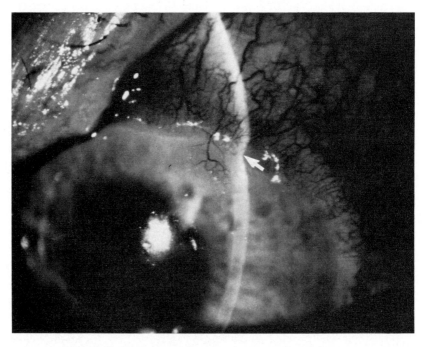

Fig. 14-27. Slit-lamp section of early Mooren's ulcer *(arrow)*.

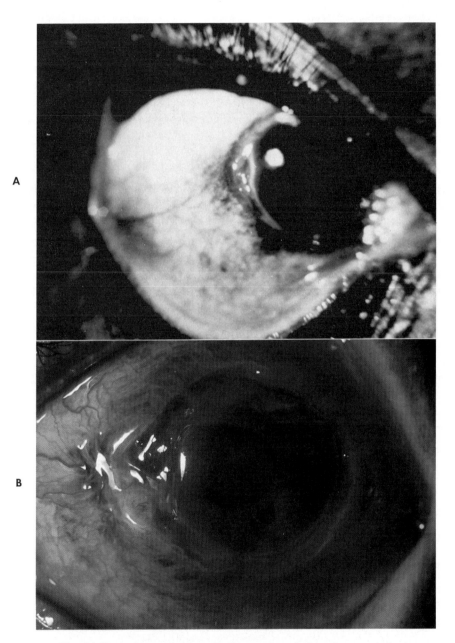

Fig. 14-28. A, Mooren's ulcer. **B,** Progression of ulceration as seen in **A.**

MARGINAL (CATARRHAL) INFILTRATES AND ULCERS

Catarrhal ulcers and infiltrates of the cornea are associated as a rule with chronic blepharoconjunctivitis resulting from *S. aureus* infection. It has not been entirely determined as to whether the catarrhal ulcers are caused by the staphylococcic toxin or by immune complex-mediated reactions. One or both of these modalities may be involved in the development of these lesions.

The catarrhal infiltrate or ulcer is a gray-white, painful lesion that is circumferential with the limbus. A lucid corneal interval occurs between the lesion and the limbus (Fig. 14-24).

In addition, a punctate epithelial keratopathy is often seen in the lower one third of the cornea when a staphylococcal etiologic agent is present.

Treatment

Treatment of staphylococcal catarrhal infiltrates and ulcers should be directed toward the infecting agent and the antigen-antibody reaction. Lid scrubs and applications of antibiotic ointment such as bacitracin, erythromycin, or gentamicin may help eliminate the staphylococcal infection. Corticosteroid drugs can reduce the catarrhal infiltration. The corticosteroids work in these antigen-antibody reactions by reducing inflammation. This lessens the amount of antigen and antibody presented to the target site by decreasing the number of lymphocytes present, which then lowers the number of antibody-producing cells at the target site.

Catarrhal infiltrates and ulcers, in addition, may be caused by (1) *Haemophilus aegyptius* (Koch-Weeks bacillus), (2) *Moraxella lacunata* (*H. duplex,* diplococcus of Morax-Axenfeld, Morax's diplobacillus), (3) β-hemolytic streptococcus, (4) bacillary dysentery, (5) allergy to food or drugs, (6) lymphogranuloma, and (7) peripheral corneal infiltrates from intravenous injection of a radiopaque dye containing iodide (meglumine diatrizoate).[8]

Marginal infiltrates may be caused by herpes simplex, but with herpes there is little pain and decreased corneal sensitivity. In addition, with herpes simplex the epithelium is involved first, and subsequently the stroma becomes involved. With staphylococcal catarrhal ulcers, the stroma is involved first.

It is also essential to differentiate the catarrhal infiltrate from the infiltrates of a polymorphonuclear nature at the tips of blood vessels in any hyperacute conjunctivitis. In these instances, there is no lucid corneal interval.

Corneal infiltrates caused by soft contact lenses

Conjunctival hyperemia and anterior stromal infiltrates of the cornea may develop in contact lens wearers who chemically disinfect their lenses. Delayed hypersensitivity to thimerosal may play a role in this condition.[104] Chlamydial infection and cultures for bacteria and adenovirus should be undertaken because they may result in a similar-appearing lesion of the cornea. If indeed the lesions are caused by the chemicals, the lens wearing should be discontinued and heat sterilization and saline without preservative should be employed when wearing is resumed.[104]

Ring infiltrates and ulcers

Ring ulcers and infiltrates (Fig. 14-25) usually occur bilaterally. They consist of infiltrates occurring in a continuous ring, or they may represent a confluence of multiple individual lesions. No lucid interval occurs. Ring ulcers or marginal corneal infiltration can be seen in the following conditions, which will be discussed in detail in appropriate sections of the chapter: acute leukemia, scleroderma, systemic lupus erythematosus, polyarteritis nodosa, Wegener's granulomatosis, rheumatoid arthritis, relapsing polychondritis, gonococcal arthritis, dengue, tuberculosis, and gold poisoning.

A special form of ring infiltration is the classical corneal ring reaction of Wessely (a white ring in the peripheral cornea), which can occur from 10 to 12 days after the experimental introduction of antigen into a cornea. The ring, which consists primarily of antigen-antibody complex, complement, and polymorphonuclear leukocytes, slowly migrates centripetally and diminishes in intensity until the cornea is clear. Occasionally pannus may persist as a sequela of this phenomenon. A Wessely type of ring (Fig. 14-26) has been seen in patients with severe corneal burns, antigenic corneal foreign bodies, chronic herpetic and fungal keratitis, and abuse of topical anesthetic agents.

Mooren's ulcer

The corneal periphery receives its nourishment from (1) the aqueous humor, (2) the limbal arteries, and (3) the tear film. The cornea is in close proximity to both the subconjunctival lymphoid tissue and lymphatic limbal arcades. These anatomic features provide the corneal periphery with adequate humoral and cellular immunologic defense mechanisms, protecting it against various offending agents, but at the same time such mechanisms might contribute to immunologically mediated diseases that could lead to tissue damage and destruction. The perilimbal conjunctiva appears to play an important role in the pathogenesis of several corneal lesions resulting from local or systemic disorders. The limbal capillaries have both uniform endothelium and a well-defined basement membrane. The capillaries form loops at the limbus and have a marked morphologic resemblance to renal glomerular capillaries. Immune complexes in the bloodstream may therefore be deposited by entrapment on the endothelial basement membranes of the limbal or renal glomerular capillaries.

The periphery of the cornea is frequently the site of pathologic changes caused by certain degenerative, immunologic, and infectious diseases. Such diseases may lead to infiltration, ulceration, thinning, and in certain instances, perforation of the cornea. Mooren's ulcer is a localized disease of the cornea characterized by chronic ulceration.

This slowly progressive marginal ulcer begins in the teens or twenties and is bilateral in 25% to 50% of cases. The relatively benign, unilateral form of Mooren's ulcer usually occurs in older people, and this form of the disease responds to such procedures as conjunctival resection. The more severe, atypical, bilateral form found in younger people is much more difficult to treat and may not respond at all. The eye becomes red and painful. The deep marginal ulcer with overhanging edges gradually spreads circumferentially to include the entire cornea (Figs. 14-27 and 14-28, *A*), extending from the periphery to central cornea (Fig. 14-28, *B*). Periods of remission are not uncommon, but ultimately the entire cornea is usually involved. Perforations can occur.

Etiologic factors. The occurrence of physical or chemical trauma may antedate the development of Mooren's ulcers. It is possible that the inflammation associated with an antecedent injury alters the epithelial antigens of the cornea and conjunctiva and initiates the development of autoantibodies in an individual prone to their development. Infectious agents have also been implicated in the development of Mooren's ulcer. Infectious agents such as herpes zoster may initiate the autoimmune process in a manner similar to physical and chemical trauma, and the autoimmune phenomena may perpetuate and intensify rather than initiate corneal destruction, which is mediated through the conjunctiva.

Pathologic findings. It has been demonstrated that the metabolic products from tissue culture of the conjunctiva adjacent to Mooren's ulcers are able to degrade collagen and corneal proteoglycan.[18] Histologic examination of the excised conjunctiva shows that the excised tissue is heavily infiltrated with plasma cells and lymphocytes. The presence of many plasma cells in the conjunctiva[144] and circulating antibodies against the conjunctival and corneal epithelium, as well as the association of the tissue-fixed immunoglobulins with complement in the conjunctival epithelium, suggests that immunopathologic phenomena are involved in Mooren's ulcers. Direct immunofluorescent techniques demonstrate immunoglobulins localized to the conjunctival epithelium of Mooren's ulcers; complement is found in association with the immunoglobulins in some

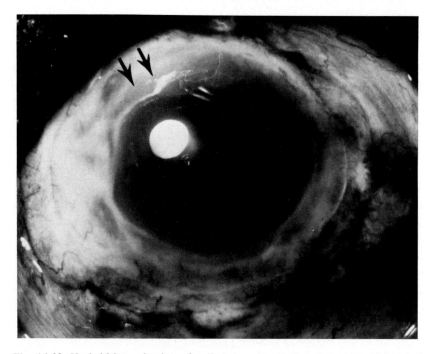

Fig. 14-29. Healed Mooren's ulcer after limbal conjunctival resection *(double arrow)*.

cases. Circulating antibodies to the conjunctival and corneal epithelium can be seen by indirect immunofluorescent techniques.[21] It also has been shown that positive macrophage migration inhibition occurs in response to corneal antigen, suggesting that a cell-mediated immunity may play a role in Mooren's ulcer.[102] In addition, specific stimulation to blastogenic transformation and proliferation of the lymphocyte by normal corneal stroma has been demonstrated.[53]

Treatment. Radiation, penetrating keratoplasty,[22] lamellar keratoplasty, conjunctival flaps, corticosteroids, and subconjunctival heparin have all been tried with generally poor results. Resection of the conjunctival in the area of the ulcer has met with some success[19, 20, 29, 144] (Fig. 14-29); this treatment is by no means ideal but has offered some hope in some cases. Methotrexate has been tried with some success. However, long-term observation of medical treatment will have to be studied in more detail.[52]

CORNEAL GRAFT REJECTION
Etiologic factors

Graft survival is greatest in corneas that are avascular before surgery.

Not all failed grafts are the result of immunologic rejection. The first 3 weeks of corneal graft failure is more likely to result from defective donor endothelium or from surgical trauma. Therefore the criteria for clinical diagnosis of allograft reaction would involve (1) a preceding period of at least 3 weeks during which the graft was technically successful and clear, (2) a line of opacity corresponding to the interface between rejected endothelium and the advancing inflammatory infiltrate, (3) a favorable response to steroids, and (4) an inflammation confined to the donor tissue nearest to blood vessels.

Allograft rejection caused by histoincompatibility depends on the recognition of the foreign antigens by thymus-dependent host lymphocytes, stimulation of the lymphoid tissues in the draining lymph nodes, and destruction of donor tissue by sensitized lymphocytes and their products.

In corneal allograft rejection, the cell-mediated immune response plays a significant role.

A long-standing allograft reaction that has withstood the cell-mediated immunity reaction can evoke humoral antibodies in the host that are directed against surface-transplantation antigens on the graft. Immunologic reactions that are directly cytotoxic (type II) may cause adherence of phagocytic cells, may evoke attack by "killer" lymphocytic cells, and may evoke the complement system.

Sensitization of the recipient by previous grafting or the use of large grafts increases the incidence of corneal graft rejection. The presence of preformed anticorneal antibodies and the vascularity of the donor tissue bed increase the rejection rate. Vascularized acute corneal herpes simplex, trauma, and grafts placed eccentrically toward the limbus are associated with increased rejection; in these situations, both sensitization and vascularization may play a role. Graft procedures in response to chemical burns, inflammatory disease, and rosacea keratitis in which there is an inordinate amount of vascularization tend to do poorly. Grafts for conditions that have an immunologic basis, such as pemphigoid and Stevens-Johnson syndrome, also give poor results. It should be borne in mind that the recurrences of dystrophies and failure of grafts in herpetic keratitis are factors that may have nothing to do with histoincompatibility. Neither cryopreservation nor culturing of the cornea alters significantly the antigenicity of the donor tissue.

Signs and symptoms

The initial signs of graft rejection are a faint flare, a few cells in the anterior chamber, and mild ciliary flush. The patient complains of decreased vision. To become aware of the latter sign quickly, patients with a corneal graft should test their vision daily by whatever means advised by their surgeon. Any change noted should be investigated, since it may be the first sign of a corneal graft rejection that the patient perceives.

Epithelial rejection begins in the vicinity of congested vessels, especially when extension of the vessel into the rim of the recipient cornea has occurred, followed by replacement with host epithelium. The intervening necrotic zone between the rejected and host epithelium is infiltrated with inflammatory cells that give rise to a fine line of opacity that may not always be detected clinically.

Stromal rejection is manifested by an advancing band of haziness attributed to pleomorphic leukocytic infiltration, which includes polymorphonuclear cells as well as lymphocytes and plasma cells.

Endothelial rejection usually begins in the proximity of invading blood vessels with the formation of keratotic precipitates. Destruction of donor endothelium spreads across the graft as the fine keratotic precipitate advances from its origin, giving a progressive edema to the stroma. Since endothelial rejection is usually associated with a variable degree of anterior uveitis, it has been suggested that the leukocytes extend from the iris vessels and reach the cornea by the aqueous, but evidence also exists that the leukocytes may originate in the limbal vessels and reach the endothelium by the unhealed Descemet membrane. The distribution of the lymphocytes corresponds to the rejection line that is seen clinically. Retrocorneal membranes may arise from the endothelial rejection as a result of the graft reaction.

Management

Treatment should be started as soon as possible. High steroid doses are immunosuppressive and anti-inflammatory, whereas low doses are probably only anti-inflammatory. Both effects are essential. Instillation of steroid eye drops such as prednisolone acetate (1% Pred-Forte) every half hour and subconjunctival injections of dexamethasone sodium phosphate (Decadron Phosphate), 4 mg/ml daily, are essential. Oral steroids such as 80 to 120 mg of prednisone (Deltasone) every other day at breakfast should also be considered, depending on case severity and response. Cycloplegics are used for the accompanying iritis. The patient should be seen every day, and the vision, corneal edema, appearance of corneal endothelial surface, and inflammatory reaction evaluated.

At the moment, histocompatibility antigen typing certainly cannot be done in all instances of corneal grafting; however, it may be of great importance in instances in which the individual has a mark of the vascularized cornea and certainly in instances in which three or four previous grafts have failed because of immunologic problems and the patient has received previous blood transfusions.

AUTOIMMUNE DISEASES (Table 14-4)
Systemic lupus erythematosus (SLE)

Systemic lupus erythematosus is characterized by the abnormality of the body's immune makeup and the production of a number of autoantibodies. It is seen more frequently in females, with the peak age of onset in the twenties to thirties. SLE can occur after ingestion of drugs such as penicillin, sulfonamides, iodides, gold, isoniazids, and methyldopa. It may be associated with impaired cell-mediated immunity.[115] In addition, SLE has been seen in several members of the same family and may be found in patients who have other connective tissue diseases such as Sjögren's syndrome.[130]

Pathogenesis. The events in the evolution of SLE clearly have an immunologic basis. Some immunologic abnormality results in the production of autoantibodies, which form immune complexes with the antigen and fixed complement. The results of this reaction are a deposition of complement in the blood vessel walls and the accumulation of neutrophils. The final result is the damaging of basement membranes with splitting and fragmentation.

Signs and symptoms. The most common cutaneous features of SLE are erythematous rash, commonly called a butterfly rash, located on the face and a rash of the neck

Table 14-4. Infiltrative and noninfiltrative corneal lesions

	Corneal reaction			
	Infiltrative, with ulceration	Noninfiltrative, with ulceration	Superficial	Deep
Phlyctenule	+	−	+	−
Catarrhal ulcer	+	−	+	−
Trachoma pustule	+	−	+	−
Gold hypersensitivity	+	−	+	−
Vernal ulcer	−	+	+	−
Neurotrophic ulcer	−	+	+	−
Wegener's granulomatosis	+	−	−	+
Polyarteritis nodosa	+	+	−	+
Ulcerative colitis	+	−	−	+
Crohn's disease	+	−	−	+
Psoriasis	+	+	−	+
Bacillary dysentery	+	+	+	+
Rheumatoid ulcer	+	+	−	+
Lupus erythematosus	+	+	−	+
Diffuse systemic sclerosis	−	+	−	+
Mooren's ulcer	−	+	−	+
Stevens-Johnson syndrome	−	+	−	+
Pemphigoid	−	+	−	+
Rosacea	+	+	−	+
Vitamin A deficiency	+	+	−	+
Relapsing polychondritis	+	+	−	+

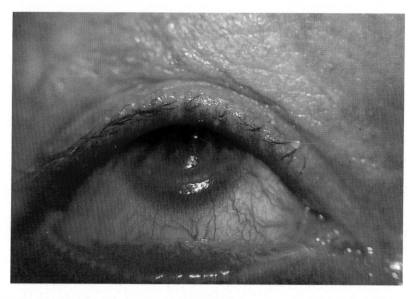

Fig. 14-30. Noninfiitrative marginal melt of cornea seen in case of lupus erythematosus. The eye, in addition, is dry with totally lusterless appearance.

and extremities, especially the tips and dorsa of the fingers, palms, and areas of skin above the elbows. Discoid rashes can also be seen. Alopecia may be part of the picture. Involvement of mucous membranes is marked by shallow, painful ulcers in the mouth, pharynx, and sometimes the vagina. Recurrent herpetic dermatitis or monilial infection may occur.

Arthritis, polyarthralgia, or both occur in many patients. Pleuritis, pericarditis, lymphadenopathy, and splenomegaly are seen. In addition, symptoms and signs related to the gastrointestinal and nervous systems occur.

The most common findings in the eye are confined to the retina with the appearance of cotton-wool spots, retinal hemorrhages, and edema of the retina and disc. Involvement of the retinal vascular tree is also noted.

The lids may exhibit telangiectasia just above the lid margins, and one may find persistent conjunctival injection. Episcleritis, scleritis, and anterior uveitis are also seen in some cases.

Keratoconjunctivitis sicca, epithelial keratitis, stromal infiltration, and vascularization may be seen. In addition, the cornea may exhibit quiet, relatively noninfiltrative marginal melts (Fig. 14-30). Infiltrative lesions also occur and respond to topical steroid therapy (Fig. 14-31).

Discoid lupus erythematosus

In discoid lupus erythematosus, the disease is confined to the skin, but it can progress to the full-blown picture of SLE. Some patients with discoid lupus may exhibit lupus erythematosus (LE) cells and antinuclear antibodies.[118] One may find on the eye-

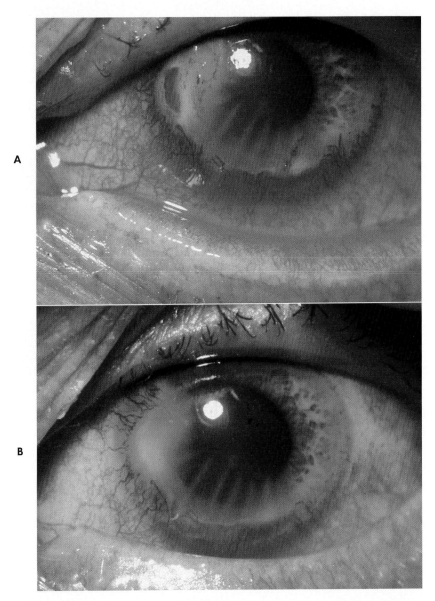

Fig. 14-31. A, Infiltrative marginal melt in case of lupus erythematosus. **B,** Its response to topical steroid medication.

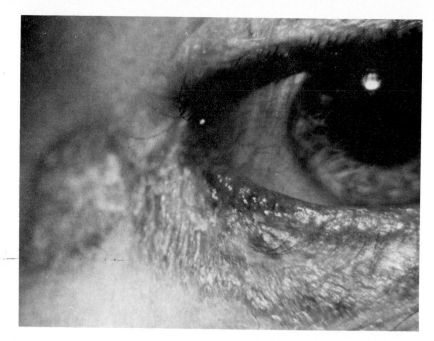

Fig. 14-32. Discoid lupus. (From Grayson, M., and Keates, R.H.: Manual of diseases of the cornea, Boston, 1969, Little, Brown & Co.)

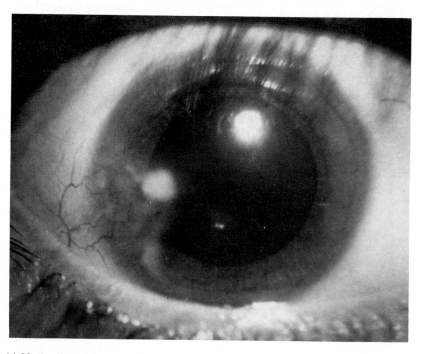

Fig. 14-33. In discoid lupus scarring and vascularization of cornea occurs occasionally. (From Grayson, M., and Keates, R.H.: Manual of diseases of the cornea, Boston, 1969, Little, Brown & Co.)

lid red, scaly plaques with follicular plugging, atrophic areas of skin, and scarring (Fig. 14-32). Examination of the skin may show fixed-tissue antibodies, whereas in SLE fixed-tissue antibodies and circulating antibodies are found.

This type of photosensitive skin lesion of lupus may extend over the lid margins and into the conjunctival sac. Conjunctival scarring and lid margin distortion may occur as a result of discoid lupus erythematosus.

Patients with discoid lupus may show corneal changes. Superficial corneal lesions may progress to deep parenchymatous involvement. Epithelial keratitis and marginal corneal infiltrations with vascularization may also be seen (Fig. 14-33).

Rheumatoid arthritis

Rheumatoid arthritis is a chronic, progressive polyarthritis and multisystem disease that is found more frequently in women, with the age of onset between 30 and 40 years.

The onset of the arthritis is gradual, although acute cases occur. Involvement of the elbows, ankles, feet, fingers, and knees is noted, but characteristic involvement of the joints of the hand is seen (Fig. 14-34). The condition, in reality, should be named rheumatoid disease because many extra-articular manifestations are noted: the disease may affect the heart, lungs, lymphatic system, spleen, and muscles of the body. Rheumatoid vasculitis is associated with peripheral neuropathy and various cutaneous lesions.[46]

The ocular complications usually occur in patients with severe disease, especially

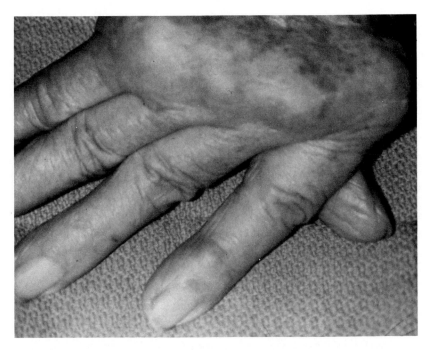

Fig. 14-34. Characteristic appearance of hands in rheumatoid arthritis.

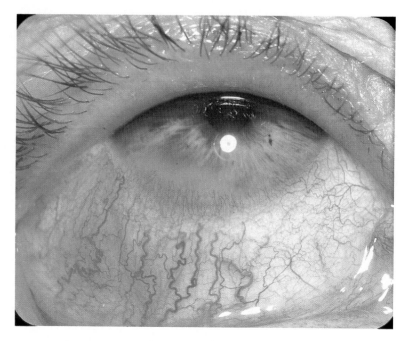

Fig. 14-35. Nodular sclerokeratitis of rheumatoid arthritis.

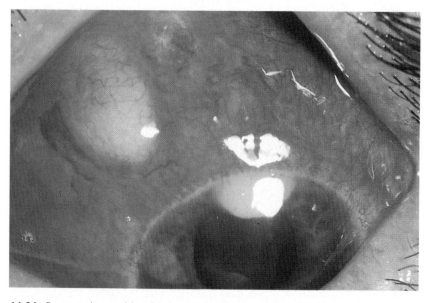

Fig. 14-36. Severe sclerouveitis with large necrotizing granulomas. One of lesions extends into anterior chamber.

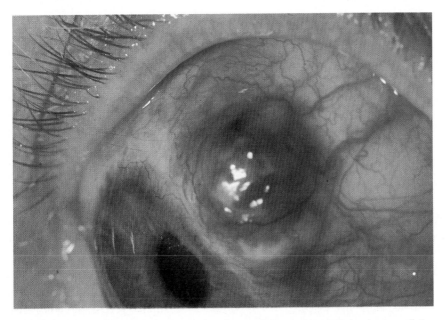

Fig. 14-37. Large area of scleral melting without much inflammatory reaction in case of rheumatoid arthritis.

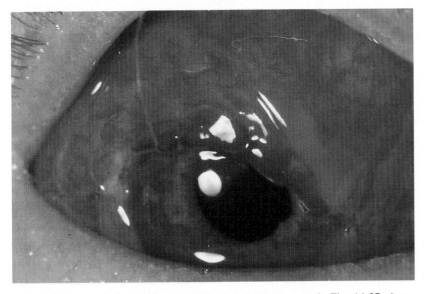

Fig. 14-38. Periosteal graft from tibia used with success in case seen in Fig. 14-37. Autogenous tissue is used.

those who develop extra-articular complications. One of the most common ophthalmic findings in rheumatoid arthritis is keratoconjunctivitis sicca.

Scleritis and sclerokeratitis are also seen[74] (Fig. 14-35). Nodules may form on the sclera (Fig. 14-35), which histopathologically demonstrate fibrinoid necrosis of the sclera with varying degrees of inflammation. Anterior scleritis may be diffuse, nodular, or necrotizing. The latter may be with or without inflammation. The anterior scleritis may be associated with severe pain and redness and may be found unilaterally or bilaterally (Fig. 14-36). Necrotizing scleritis (Fig. 14-37) occurs and may result in loss of the eye. The large defect may be treated with a periosteal graft taken from the anterior surface of the tibia[16] (Fig. 14-38). Bone formation has been reported in a periosteal graft.[28]

With extensive involvement of the anterior sclera, one may find extension of the pathologic condition onto the surface of the cornea; in this instance a sclerokeratitis exists. The cornea becomes deeply infiltrated and vascularized in the areas adjacent to the scleritis.

If the posterior region of the globe is involved in severe scleritis (posterior scleritis), the proliferative scleritis may involve the orbital tissues, with proptosis resulting, and also can result in exudation and retinal and choroidal detachment. In the latter instance, it has been mistaken for a melanoma. However, a normal choroidal vascular pattern will favor the diagnosis of a posterior scleritis.[45]

Peripheral corneal melting is not uncommon in severe rheumatoid arthritic disease.[20] The cornea may show a noninfiltrative, slowly melting lesion either at the limbus or 1 or 2 mm inside the limbus (Fig. 14-39). However, infiltrative peripheral corneal lesions also occur (Fig. 14-40). Occasionally the furrows or melting areas may perforate (Fig. 14-41). The perforation may be treated with surgical adhesive and soft contact lenses (Fig. 14-42). In addition, surgical adhesive may be used effectively to interrupt progressive corneal melting in this and various other disorders before anticipated perforation could occur.[51]

Some of the drugs used in treating rheumatoid arthritis, such as systemic steroids, gold salts, and antimalarials, may produce a variety of ocular problems. The corneal toxicity to some of the antimalarials is manifested by a whorl-like pattern of intraepithelial deposits in the interpalpebral zone. The whorl-like pattern resembles the keratopathy seen in Fabry's disease. The involvement of the macula and perimacular areas can be seen with the administration of chloroquine, which may result in irreversible retinal degeneration. Severe visual impairment results when the typical bull's-eye macular lesion is seen, which is well revealed with fluorescein angiography. It is interesting that the advanced retinopathy may continue to progress even though the drug has been stopped. On the other hand, the electroretinographic changes, which may be abnormal, may revert to normal after the cessation of the drug.

Although gold is employed in the treatment of rheumatoid arthritis, it is not without toxic manifestations. Blepharitis and conjunctivitis are manifestations of intolerance to gold. Its use may result in peripheral corneal infiltration (Fig. 14-43) and ulceration, as well as pulmonary fibrosis in some instances.[57]

Extended use of steroid drugs may result in lenticular opacities and increased intraocular pressure.

Juvenile arthritis[30] may be of interest to the ophthalmologist because of the common occurrence of nongranulomatous iridocyclitis and its complications. The iritis is dangerous because the disease may go unrecognized for a long while.[83] The chronic iritis may result in cataract, anterior or posterior synechia, and secondary glaucoma.

One of the most common complications of rheumatoid arthritis in childhood is the development of band keratopathy. Keratoconjunctivitis sicca has also been reported in this disease.[73]

Sjögren's syndrome

This entity consists of the combination of any two of the following: (1) KCS, (2) dryness of the mouth or other nonocular mucous membranes, and (3) rheumatoid arthritis or other autoimmune connective tissue disease. The onset of the disease occurs in the thirties to fifties; however, it has been seen in children. It is more frequently found in women. In addition to rheumatoid arthritis, this problem has been found in association with psoriatic arthritis, polyarteritis nodosa, progressive systemic sclerosis, SLE, Hashimoto's thyroiditis, and chronic hepatobiliary disease.

Systemic manifestations. In Sjögren's syndrome, one may see involvement of not only the lacrimal and salivary glands but also the mucus-secreting glands, the respiratory and gastrointestinal tracts, and the vagina. Xerostomia[126] (Fig. 14-44) may cause difficulty in swallowing and chewing, and the patient may suffer the development of ulcers of the tongue and buccal mucous membrane. Dryness may involve the mucous membrane, the lining of the nose, and the upper and lower respiratory tract. This dryness can account for the development of bronchitis, pneumonia, pulmonary fibrosis, hoarseness, and epitaxis. In addition, one may find hypergammaglobulinemia, Raynaud's phenomenon, neuropathies, renal dysfunction, impaired lymphocyte function, liver disease, gastrointestinal disease, lymphoreticular neoplasms,[3] a positive LE cell test in 10% of cases, and numerous antibodies, such as rheumatoid factor, antisalivary and lacrimal gland, antisalivary duct, antilacrimal duct, anti-DNA, and antithyroglobulin. Indeed, Sjögren's syndrome may also be associated with other collagen diseases such as scleroderma.[78]

The KCS of Sjögren's syndrome results from what might well be an immune attack on the lacrimal glands. The glandular insufficiency of this disease is associated with lymphocytic and plasma cell infiltration of the gland.[143] Areas of mononuclear cell infiltrate are associated with focal degeneration of the glandular acini. Cellular infiltration and glandular atrophy increase, and proliferating ductal epithelial cells form myoephithelial islands. The gland eventually will be replaced by connective tissue. Biopsy of accessible minor glands of the lip and palate will demonstrate changes similar to those noted in the lacrimal gland. Thus an easy and accessible method of diagnosis is available.[133]

Ocular manifestations. Patients with Sjögren's syndrome usually complain of itching, burning, dryness, photophobia, and foreign body sensation. The symptoms are worse in the later afternoon and in conditions of low humidity.

One may find a ropy mucous discharge that can be extremely annoying. The eyes are red, and the patient may complain of decreased vision, possibly as a result of the presence of extensive discharge or epitheliopathy. There is a scant tear meniscus and

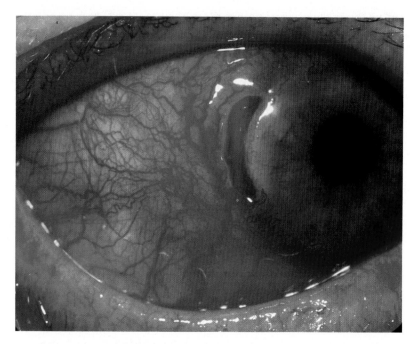

Fig. 14-39. Marginal noninfiltrative melting of limbal tissues in rheumatoid arthritis.

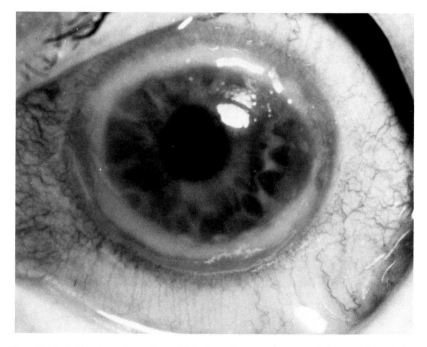

Fig. 14-40. Infiltrative circumferential lesion of cornea in case of rheumatoid arthritis.

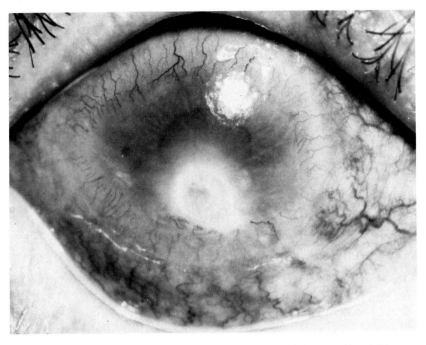

Fig. 14-41. Central corneal perforation seen in case of rheumatoid arthritis.

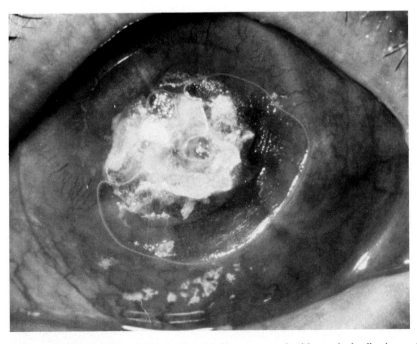

Fig. 14-42. Central perforation shown in Fig. 14-41 was treated with surgical adhesive and soft contact lens applied over area of adhesive.

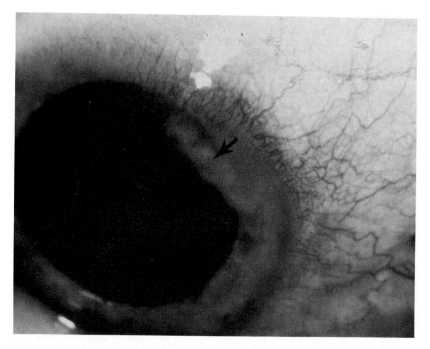

Fig. 14-43. Marginal infiltration noted in patient treated with gold for rheumatoid arthritis *(arrow)*.

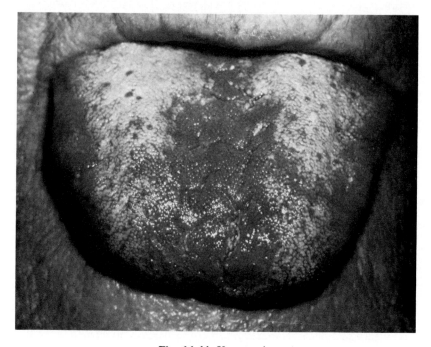

Fig. 14-44. Xerostomia.

debris-laden tear film. The tear film breakup time is markedly reduced. A reduced Schirmer time occurs with anesthetic agents, and a variable reduced Schirmer time without the instillation of anesthetic agents.

Interpalpebral staining of the conjunctiva and the cornea occurs with rose bengal red (Fig. 14-45). The cornea will also stain with fluorescein. In rare cases, I as well as others[59,80] have observed perforation of the cornea. Corneal filaments occur, and keratinization of the conjunctiva and lid margins may be seen in severe cases (Fig. 14-46).

Polyarteritis

Polyarteritis (periarteritis nodosa) occurs most often in men of ages 20 to 50. The cause is obscure, but the disease is considered one of collagen nature, and the pertinent pathologic condition resembles the angiitis seen in rheumatoid vasculitis, giant cell arteritis, and Wegener's granulomatosis. Polyarteritis is also seen in association with allergic reactions to drugs such as penicillin, arsenicals, phenytoin, and iodides. In addition, multisystem vasculitis is seen in the Churg-Strauss syndrome, in which bronchial asthma, fever, eosinophilia, and allergic granulomatosis are found. Amyloidosis of the upper tarsal conjunctiva has been reported in this syndrome.[94]

Systemic manifestations. Since the blood vessels of any organ system of the body may be involved, the systemic manifestations are varied. One can see involvement of the central nervous, renal, gastrointestinal, cardiovascular, and respiratory systems, as well as the skin.

Ocular involvement. Retinopathy such as hemorrhages, exudates, and cotton-wool spots occurs. In addition, an exudative retinal detachment may be seen.[76]

The conjunctivae of patients with polyarteritis may be hyperemic and may exhibit subconjunctival hemorrhages. As previously noted, Sjögren's syndrome with KCS may be noted in association with polyarteritis. Nodular episcleritis, nodular scleritis, and more severe forms of scleritis and sclerokeratitis can be seen.

Melting of the margins of the cornea, which may be noninfiltrative or infiltrative, can be seen to spread circumferentially around the eye to form a ring ulcer[107] (Fig. 14-47). This is associated with marked injection of the eye and severe pain. The process may extend centrally, and the final result may be one of scarring, vascularization, and finally perforation of the globe.

Cogan's syndrome is believed to be associated with polyarteritis.[88] In this particular condition one sees interstitial keratitis characterized by deep stromal infiltration with corneal vascularization. The keratitis may occur bilaterally with pain, photophobia, and redness. A yellowish infiltrate is seen in the corneal stroma. Eighth-nerve involvement in association with vertigo and total deafness occurs in some cases.

Management. The prognosis is usually poor, although corticosteroids may result in remissions. Immunosuppressive drugs may be of limited value.

Wegener's granulomatosis

This disease occurs in the middle-aged adult but may be seen at any age. Here again the prominent feature is vasculitis. Lethal midline granuloma may be related to this granulomatosis but is confined to the midline facial structures and upper respiratory

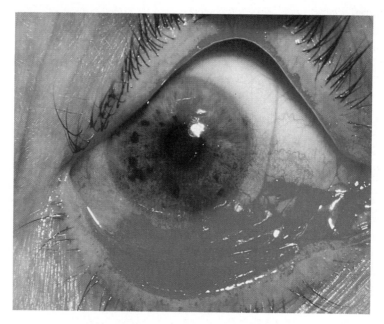

Fig. 14-45. Rose bengal red staining of cornea and conjunctiva in Sjögren's syndrome. Note extensive amount of stained mucoid material.

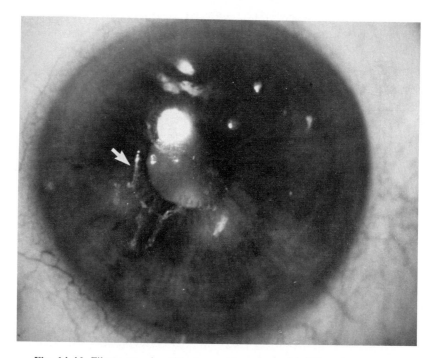

Fig. 14-46. Filamentary keratitis *(arrow)* in patient with Sjögren's syndrome.

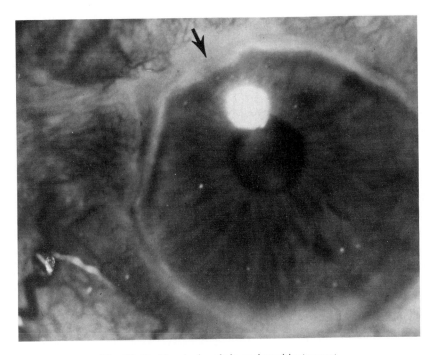

Fig. 14-47. Marginal melt in periarteritis *(arrow).*

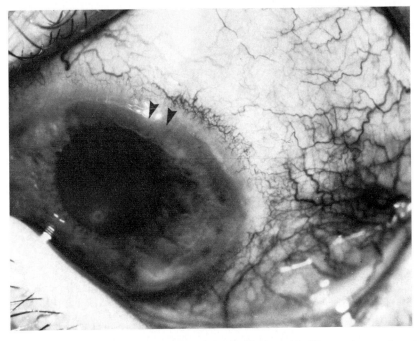

Fig. 14-48. Infiltrative peripheral corneal lesion *(double arrow)* in Wegener's granulomatosis.

tract[27]; often persons with this problem will later develop the features of Wegener's granulomatosis. Patients with Wegener's granulomatosis may exhibit fever, arthritis, myocardial dysfunction, skin rashes, renal diseases, peripheral and central nervous system disease, and necrotizing granulomas involving the upper and lower respiratory tracts.[31,33]

Retinal hemorrhages, cotton-wool spots,[119] and papilledema may occur. Orbital edema with proptosis may also be a part of the picture. Neovascular glaucoma and uveitis are also found.

If the exposure as a result of the proptosis is great, chemosis and keratitis may result. The proptosis may appear as a pseudotumor of the orbit.[141]

Episcleritis, scleritis, sclerokeratitis, and scleromalacia are also noted.[61]

The cornea in patients with Wegener's granulomatosis may exhibit a necrotizing infiltrative marginal ulcer[15,47] (Fig. 14-48). These ulcers may spread peripherally as well as centrally, producing vascularization and scarring of the cornea, and may also perforate. The observation that occlusive vasculitis of the anterior ciliary vessels occurs in some patients gives credence to the contention that ischemia may play a part in the peripheral marginal degeneration of the cornea.[5]

Cyclophosphamide combined with prednisone may at this time be the recommended treatment for Wegener's granulomatosis.[26]

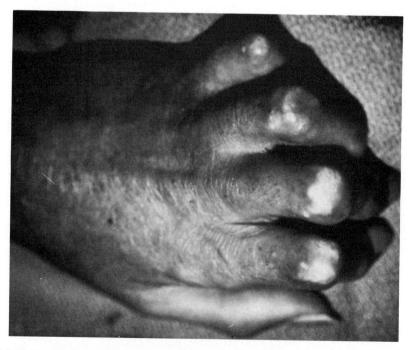

Fig. 14-49. Progressive systemic sclerosis. Tightening of skin and contraction of fingers with Raynaud's phenomenon is seen. (From Grayson, M.: The cornea in systemic disease. In Duane, T.D. [ed.]: Clinical Ophthalmology. Hagerstown, Md.: Harper & Row, 1976, vol. 4, chap. 15.)

Progressive systemic sclerosis (scleroderma)

This chronic disease of connective tissue, characterized by inflammatory, fibrotic, and degenerative changes, is associated with vascular lesions in the skin, the internal organs of the body, and the esophagus. The disorder may appear initially as an acrosclerosis or a diffuse scleroderma. Acrosclerosis is characterized by Raynaud's phenomenon and sclerosis of the digits, whereas diffuse scleroderma more often begins with hardening of the skin and the trunk. Visceral involvement is the same in both varieties. Thickening of the skin (Fig. 14-49), loss of skin folds, and contraction of the lips occur.

Cotton-wool spots, hemorrhages, and exudates may be found in the retina. Focal chorioretinitis and iridocyclitis also occur.[35]

One might find lid distortions from involvement of the lid of the skin and lid telangiectasis. The fornices may also be shallow.

Corneal involvement is rare, but when it occurs, one may find an infiltration of the cornea with opacities, vascularizations (Fig. 14-50), and KCS.

Crohn's disease

Crohn's disease primarily affects the gastrointestinal system by segmental infiltration of granulomatous and fibrous tissue into all layers of the bowel.[70,88]

One may see retinal edema, neuroretinitis, periorbital edema, and recurrent iridocyclitis. Episcleritis, scleritis, sclerokeratitis, and scleromalacia[43] have been reported.

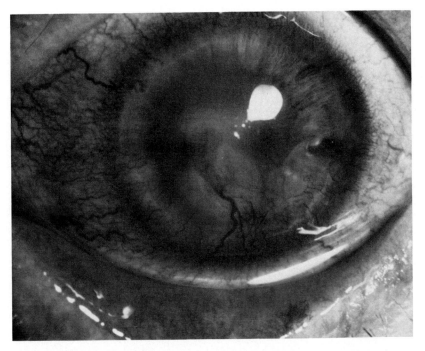

Fig. 14-50. Marked injection, vascularization, and infiltration of cornea in progressive systemic sclerosis. (From Grayson, M.: The cornea in systemic disease. In Duane, T.D. [ed.]: Clinical Ophthalmology. Hagerstown, Md.: Harper & Row, 1976, vol. 4, chap. 15.)

Infiltrative marginal ulcerations of the cornea occur. In addition, small white non-fluorescein-staining opacities can be seen in the midperipheral superficial stroma.[79, 124]

Ulcerative colitis

In this condition one may note various eye complications such as edema, orbital congestion, and iritis, as well as episcleritis and scleritis. Necrotizing infiltrative marginal corneal melting and marginal infiltrates may be present.[40]

Temporal arteritis

Giant cell arteritis, an inflammatory disorder of large- and medium-size arteries, occurs mostly in older people. The aortic, iliac, renal, and temporal arteries may be involved. Ocular findings include central retinal artery and choroidal infarction, ischemic optic neuropathy, cranial nerve palsies, uveitis, and scleritis.

Although it is rarely found, marginal corneal ulceration has been reported in this condition. In addition, conjunctival and scleral ulceration was seen in the same patient.[58]

Relapsing polychondritis[72]

This disease is characterized by recurrent inflammation of cartilage tissue in the body. Occurring equally in both sexes, relapsing polychondritis has its onset between 20 and 50 years of age. Anticartilage antibodies have been found in patients with this disorder.

Inflammation of the pinnae of the ears occurs, as well as of the nose cartilage, larynx, and other areas of the body.[7]

Conjunctivitis, episcleritis, and scleritis play a prominent part in eye involvement.[92] Infiltrative lesions of the peripheral cornea and areas of necrotizing corneal involvement

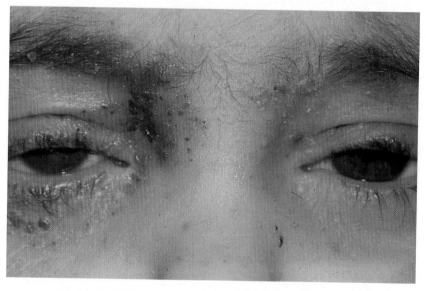

Fig. 14-51. Wiskott-Aldrich syndrome with ulcerative lid lesions.

occur. The latter may progress to perforation of the globe.[7,149]

Prednisolone, in combination with azathioprine, may be of value in the treatment of this disease. Dapsone has been used by Martin et al.[90] with some success.

Wiskott-Aldrich syndrome

This sex-linked inherited immune disease results in susceptibility to bacterial, viral, fungal, and protozoal infections. Elements of the efferent limb of the immune system, immunoglobulin production, and lymphocyte transformation are normal. It is postulated that the basic defect may lie in the afferent limb or immunity, such as in the recognition and processing of antigen. Most patients die in the first decade of life from bleeding or infection.[117] The findings of thrombocytopenia, eczema, and infection are classic. In addition, lymphoma and leukemia appear to develop with increased frequency.

Conjunctivitis, conjunctival bleeding, necrotizing lid ulcers, blepharoconjunctivitis, and episcleritis are not uncommon (Fig. 14-51). In addition, ulcerative keratitis may be seen.

Discussion

The recurring findings of episcleritis, scleritis, sclerokeratosis, and marginal corneal ulcers of a noninfiltrative or infiltrative nature play an important role in the autoimmune diseases (Table 14-4). Tables 14-5 and 14-6 summarize the scleritis problem in these diseases as to etiologic factors, types, treatment, and necessary investigative laboratory work.[140]

It must be stressed, however, that posterior scleritis may cause a diagnostic dilemma, and the external disease specialist must be aware of this. Mistaken diagnoses such as intraocular neoplasm, retrobulbar tumors, choroiditis, and idiopathic central serous

Table 14-5. Episcleritis

Possible etiologic factors	Types	Symptoms and signs	Treatment	Routine investigation for repetitive case
Rheumatoid arthritis (common) Rosacea Tuberculosis Syphilis Herpes simplex Herpes zoster Gout Collagen diseases (rarely occur other than in rheumatoid arthritis) Allergic diseases (atopic history)	Simple (78%) Nodular (22%)	May have pain localized to area of injection Nodular type may last for several weeks	Usually needs no therapy; however, if injection and pain are present for 10 days, topical steroids every 2 hours may be used until injection has ceased and then three times a day for 1 week	No investigation is necessary for mild and simple attack. If recurrent and persistent, obtain the following: Sedimentation rate Rheumatoid factor Antinuclear antibody Serology— FTA-ABS Uric acid Medical examination

Table 14-6. Scleritis and sclerokeratitis

Etiologic factor	Types	Symptoms and signs	Treatment	Recommended routine investigation

Rheumatoid arthritis and related arthritis such as psoriatic arthritis
Cogan's interstitial keratitis
Polyarteritis
Wegener's granulomatosis
Lupus erythematosus
Crohn's disease
Ulcerative colitis
Herpes zoster
Herpes simplex
Tuberculosis
Leprosy
Syphilis
Pyoderma gangrenosum
Gout
Ophthalmia nodosum (caterpillar hair)
	Anterior
	  Diffuse (40%)
	  Nodular (44%)
	  Necrotizing (14%)
	    With inflammation
	    Without inflammation
	Posterior (2%)
		Signs and symptoms may be related to diseases listed under etiologic factors column
		Anterior
		  May exhibit secondary glaucoma, scleral necrosis with thinning, deep infiltration into cornea; necrotizing process in sclera may be a slow one also, as is often seen in rheumatoid arthritis
		Posterior
		  Pain, proptosis, exudative choroiditis, optic nerve edema
			Medical
			  Serious collagen disease should be treated. Drugs employed today that treat severe scleritis and sclerokeratitis include the following:
			    Oxyphenbutazone
			    Indomethacin
			    Prednisolone
			    Immunosuppressive drugs such as azathioprine
			Surgical
			  In case of scleral thinning to point at which integrity of eye is threatened, one may have to employ patch graft of periosteum from anterior tibial surface or sclera from eye bank specimen
				Sedimentation rate
				Serum complement (C3)
				Rheumatoid factor
				Antinuclear antibody
				LE preparation
				FTA-ABS test
				Uric acid test
				PPD
				X-ray study of chest
				Thorough systemic examination for evidence of vasculitis and multisystem organ disease

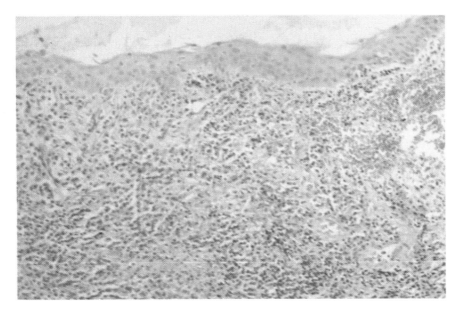

Fig. 14-52. Conjunctivectomy exhibiting plasma cell and lymphocytic infiltration.

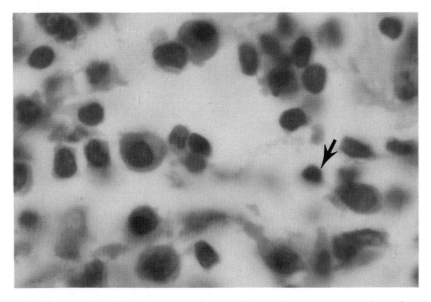

Fig. 14-53. Plasma cell is indicated at end of arrow. These cells are seen in sections of conjunctiva in marginal corneal ulcer.

choroidopathy have been made. Features that help to make a correct assessment are the presence of a fundus mass the same color as normal adjacent pigment epithelium, choroidal folds, serous retinal detachment with cloudy fluid and shifting subretinal fluid, early pinpoint leaking spots seen by fluorescein angiography, thickening of the posterior coats of the eye on ''B'' scan, retrobulbar edema with low reflectivity, and high internal reflectivity of the mass on ultrasonography.[13] Corticosteroids retrobulbarly or systemically are effective.

The conjunctiva may be a source of collagenase and proteoglycanase enzymes, which are capable of causing corneal ulcerations by producing destruction of corneal collagen and ground substance.[18,25] The exact origin of conjunctival or corneal collagenase is not certain; however, epithelium in contact with wounded stroma,[24] PMNs,[21,23] and fibroblasts[14] have all been found capable of producing collagenase under various experimental circumstances. It is presumed that immunologic or traumatic stimuli call forth and activate one or more of the cell types just listed.

The presence of plasma cells (Figs. 14-52 and 14-53) and lymphocytes in the conjunctival tissue of excised specimens that were located adjacent to the peripheral marginal ulcer suggests that humoral or cellular immune phenomena are operative, although most of these cell types are not infrequently found in subepithelial conjunctival inflammation of various causes and may be nonspecific findings.

Conjunctivectomy has been advocated as a treatment for marginal corneal ulceration; however, it is not advocated as a primary treatment in every case of marginal corneal ulceration.[144] Marginal ulcers develop from a varied group of diseases, as was noted in the preceding paragraphs, and many cases respond to other modes of therapy. Some types are self-limited and do not require specific treatment. The superficial infiltrative ulcers listed in Table 14-4 are self-limited or may respond reasonably well to topical therapy with antibiotics or corticosteroids. Corticosteroids are generally effective for the noninfectious types of deep infiltrative ulcers, whereas these drugs tend to worsen most of the ulcers of the deep noninfiltrative group.[144] This latter group tends to respond best to the use of collagenase inhibitors, such as L-cysteine, but not invariably so. If L-cysteine drops are given, they may be used every 4 to 6 hours and replaced every 4 days.

The results of conjunctivectomy appear to be encouraging for the deep noninfiltrative group. Mooren's ulcer is notorious for frequently resisting all medical therapy. The excision of limbal conjunctiva as a treatment for Mooren's ulcer[23,144] has been advocated, and excision of overlying conjunctiva has been successfully used for some cases of scleromalacia. The limbal conjunctivectomy is a simple procedure and may be performed in the office with the use of topical anesthetic drops and a subconjunctival injection of 1% lidocaine in the area of the limbal melt. A 4 to 5 mm strip of limbal conjunctiva (or larger, depending on the ulcer size) adjacent to the ulcer is resected. The conjunctiva is not sutured.

Occasionally this method is not successful and the cornea may go on to perforation. In this instance, one may apply a surgical adhesive to a small perforation, which in turn is covered with a soft contact lens, allowing for the reformation of the collapsed anterior chamber. The anterior chamber usually reforms within minutes. In a week or so the surgical adhesive detaches and reveals a vascularized scar over the site of the perforation.

The surrounding epithelium must be removed before the application of the surgical adhesive.

Immunosuppressive therapy[52] in life-threatening diseases with destructive ocular lesions, such as severe rheumatoid arthritis, SLE, and polyarteritis nodosa, is advisable. Cyclophosphamide, at present, is considered an effective drug for this purpose.

Immunosuppressive treatment for non-life-threatening situations may be less convincing. However, immunosuppression is an acceptable therapy for cicatricial pemphigoid. Mooren's ulcer, in addition, is another severe sight-threatening problem in which immunosuppression appears to exert some beneficial effect on the progressive ocular destruction.

Mucous membrane diseases

OCULAR PEMPHIGOID (CICATRICIAL PEMPHIGOID, ESSENTIAL SHRINKAGE OF CONJUNCTIVA)[6, 69] (Table 14-7)

Ocular pemphigoid is an autoimmune, cicatricial disease of the conjunctiva and, to a lesser extent, other mucous membranes and skin.[6] It is generally believed to exhibit type II hypersensitivity reactions. IgG and IgA and complement can be demonstrable along the epithelial basement membrane of the conjunctiva by direct immunofluorescence[55] (Fig. 14-54); circulating autoantibodies have been detected by indirect immunofluorescence.[138] HLA-B12[103] and HLA-B3 have been demonstrated in ocular pemphigoid. Fixed-tissue and circulating antibodies are found by immunofluorescence in pemphigus vulgaris and bullous pemphigoid.[9-11, 98, 99] The antibodies of pemphigus vulgaris are localized to the epithelial intercellular spaces (Fig. 14-55) rather than to the

Table 14-7. Features of the pemphigoid bullous diseases

	Benign mucous membrane pemphigoid (BMMP)	Bullous pemphigoid (BP)	Pemphigus vulgaris (PV)
Ocular involvement	+	Probably not	Probably not
Oral involvement	+	+	+
Site of bulla formation	Subepithelial	Subepithelial	Intraepithelial
Scarring	+	+	−
Direct immunofluorescence*	Sometimes −; not infrequently + to epithelial basement membrane	+ (To epithelial basement membrane)	+ (To intracellular areas within epithelium)
Indirect immunofluorescence†	Usually −; occasionally + to epithelial basement membrane	+ (To epithelial basement membrane)	+ (To intercellular areas within epithelium)

*This test is used to demonstrate the presence and the localization of tissue fixed immunoglobulins or complement.
†This test is used to demonstrate the presence of circulating antibodies in the sera of patients with pemphigus, bullous pemphigoid, and ocular pemphigoid.

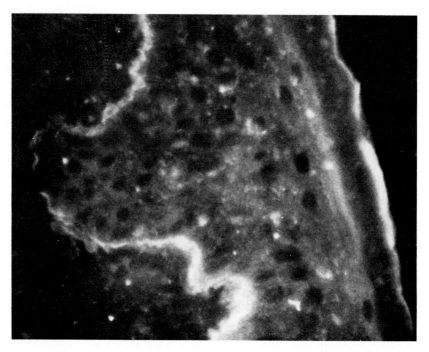

Fig. 14-54. Direct immunofluorescence of epithelial basement in case of ocular pemphigoid. (Courtesy S.F. Bean, M.D., Houston, Tex.)

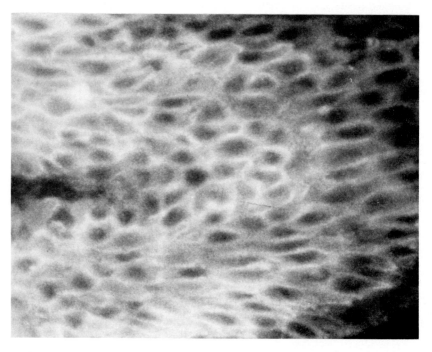

Fig. 14-55. Indirect immunofluorescence intercellular staining in pemphigus vulgaris. (Courtesy S.F. Bean, M.D., Houston, Tex.)

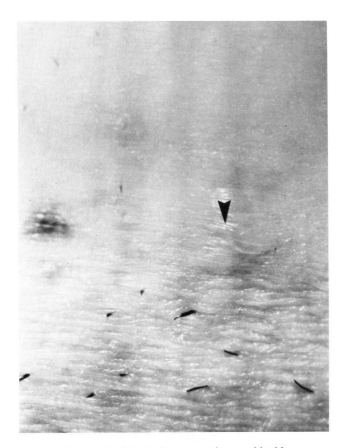

Fig. 14-56. Skin bulla *(arrow)* in pemphigoid.

epithelial basement membrane.[9-11,68] The bullae of pemphigus vulgaris, which are non-cicatrizing because of their intraepithelial location, can easily be enlarged by pressure (Nikolsky's sign).[67,81] Ocular involvement in pemphigus vulgaris is rare; however, inflammatory bullae have occurred in the conjunctiva.

In bullous pemphigoid, fixed-tissue and circulating autoantibodies, like those of ocular pemphigoid, are directed against the epithelial basement membrane. Now that such antibodies have been detected in cases of ocular pemphigoid, although less predictably than in bullous pemphigoid, these two disorders can be considered to be variants of the same disease, differing only in the likelihood of antibody detection and in the presence or absence of ocular involvement. Indeed, about 50% of cases of ocular pemphigoid show vesiculobullous involvement of skin and nonocular mucous membranes (Fig. 14-56).

Ocular and bullous pemphigoid are relenting cicatrizing diseases in keeping with the subepithelial location of the antibody response, and thus the Nikolsky sign is absent. Fatalities are not to be expected in ocular and bullous pemphigoid, although esophageal involvement has occasionally led to perforation.[81] Pemphigus vulgaris can be fatal.

Signs and symptoms

Ocular pemphigoid is a disease of older people, is more common in women, and is seldom seen before age 50. Oral mucosal lesions (Fig. 14-57) as well as lesions of the nose, larynx, and anus are seen. Ocular involvement occurs in the majority of cases and in fact may be the only visible manifestation of the disease. The onset is usually insidious with recurrent attacks of mild and clinically nonspecific conjunctival inflammation. On occasion, mucopurulent discharge occurs, and erroneous diagnoses of bacterial conjunctivitis are not uncommon.

In the early stages of ocular pemphigoid, conjunctival hyperemia, edema, tear dysfunction, conjunctival ulceration, and vesicles are noted. The first clinical clue as to the true nature of the problem, other than coexisting vesiculobullous inflammation of the skin and nonocular mucosae, usually is slight foreshortening of the inferior conjunctival fornices (Fig. 14-58). Gossamer subepithelial scarring of the conjunctiva may also be found. These subtle conjunctival signs should be sought in any older patient with chronic or recurrent red eyes of unknown origin. Further support of the diagnosis can often be obtained by the finding of a few eosinophils in the conjunctival scrapings (Fig. 14-59). The eosinophils are seldom numerous, but the presence of even a single eosinophil in the absence of conjunctival bleeding is considered to be significant; eosinophils are more likely to be found during acute inflammatory exacerbations of the disease. Ocular pemphigoid occasionally appears with severe and acute inflammation. The patient thus sud-

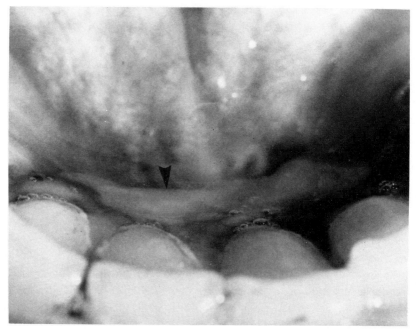

Fig. 14-57. Ulcer of oral mucous membrane *(arrow)* of floor of mouth in pemphigoid.

denly develops lid swelling, intense conjunctival hyperemia and edema, and infiltration with rapid scarring of the subepithelial conjunctiva. Bullae are encountered only rarely.

The late complications of ocular pemphigoid are related to extensive conjunctival scarring and consist of symblepharons, misdirected lashes (Fig. 14-60), KCS, lid margin keratinization, and conjunctival and lid scarring (Fig. 14-61). The cornea is remarkably spared except in the late stages, when it may be seriously compromised by the secondary effects of cicatrization, drying, and trichiasis (Fig. 14-62). The compromised cornea is subject to bacterial ulceration (Fig. 14-63). In the acute florid form of the disease, however, involvement with moderately thick, circumferential pannus extending into the peripheral 1 to 3 mm of the cornea may be seen.

It should be emphasized that ocular pemphigoid is a bilateral disease. One eye may be more severely involved, but the second eye nearly always shows some early signs of the disease. One should think twice before making the diagnosis of unilateral pemphigoid, since some cases have later turned out to be diffuse, cicatrizing, epithelial carcinomas of the conjunctiva (Fig. 14-64). Chronic cicatrization of the conjunctiva also may occur as a result of toxicity from prolonged topical administration of such medications as echothiophate iodide, pilocarpine, and IDU.[114] Practolol has been shown to cause the mucocutaneous syndrome with progressive sicca, conjunctival scarring, corneal thinning, opacification, and perforation.[147] Intercellular and antinuclear antibodies can be demonstrated in sera of patients with practolol-induced mucocutaneous syndrome.[147]

Text continued on p. 419.

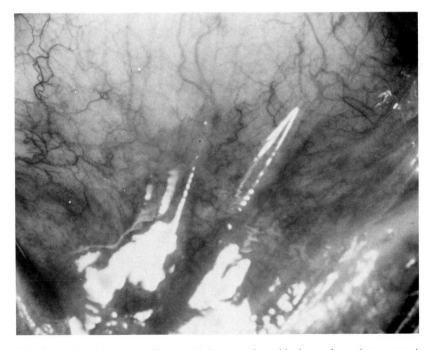

Fig. 14-58. Early foreshortening of lower cul-de-sac and symblepharon formation as seen in ocular pemphigoid.

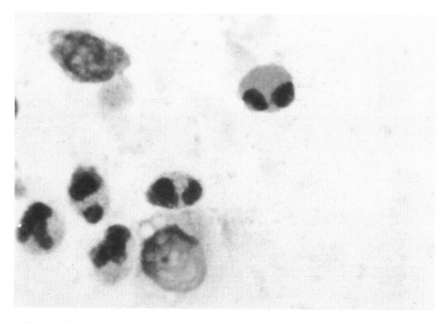

Fig. 14-59. Conjunctival scraping in case of ocular pemphigoid reveals eosinophils.

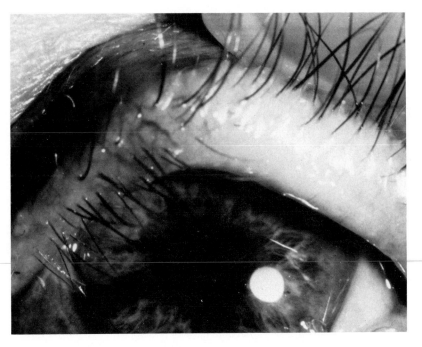

Fig. 14-60. Secondary distichiasis in benign mucous membrane pemphigoid.

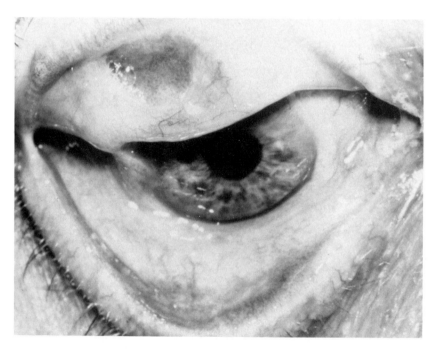

Fig. 14-61. Extensive scarring of upper tarsal conjunctiva in ocular pemphigoid.

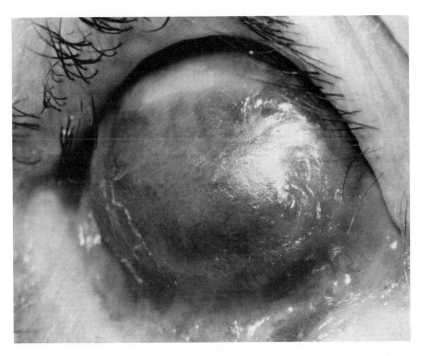

Fig. 14-62. Advanced ocular disease in benign mucous membrane pemphigoid. Foreshortening of lower cul-de-sac and drying and keratinization of corneal and conjunctival epithelium are noted.

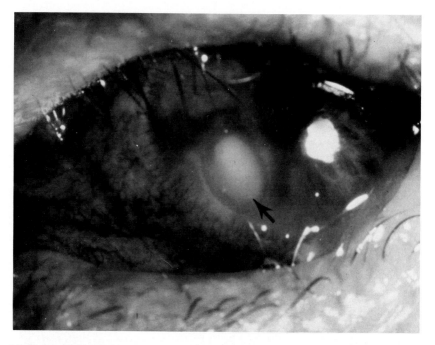

Fig. 14-63. Dry and compromised cornea of pemphigoid is subject to bacterial invasion. *Staphylococcus aureus* ulcer of cornea has occurred *(arrow)*.

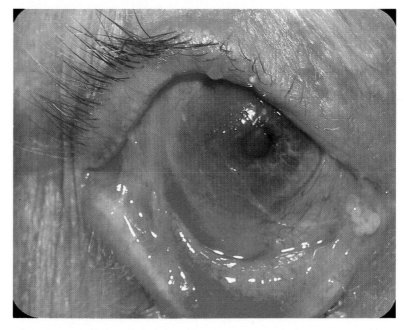

Fig. 14-64. Conjunctival pathologic condition resembling ocular pemphigoid. This case, however, is one of conjunctival carcinoma masquerading as ocular pemphigoid.

Management

The treatment of ocular pemphigoid is disappointing. Corticosteroids have been administered by various routes without significant or beneficial effect on the ocular pathologic condition, although systemic corticosteroids seem to have been beneficial for lesions of mucous membranes in areas other than the eye and the skin.[136] Topical corticosteroids can be employed in the hyperacute form of ocular pemphigoid with what appears to be some beneficial effect in decreasing inflammation and in making the patient more comfortable; the formation of extensive symblepharons, however, may not be prevented. Furthermore, the possible ameliorative effect of the steroids must be evaluated in view of the knowledge that acute exacerbations of ocular pemphigoid are normally of self-limited duration. The role of noncorticosteroid immunosuppressive therapy has yet to be clarified.

In view of the possible immunologic origin of the disease, it would seem to be not unreasonable to try intensive corticosteroids for a short time in the hyperacute form of the disease. Beyond this rather questionable therapy, there are available only palliative treatments for the dry eye and distorted lids. Hydrophilic contact lenses may offer some help in the early dry eye periods, but it must be noted that there is a constant threat of infection in this compromised host.

Although lid surgery may occasionally be indicated, intraocular procedures should be undertaken only in rare and desperate circumstances. The trichiasis may very well be helped with cryosurgery of the lid margins. I have seen more than one eye progress to atrophy bulbi after otherwise uncomplicated cataract extraction in pemphigoid patients.

Table 14-7 summarizes the features of ocular pemphigoid and related diseases.

STEVENS-JOHNSON SYNDROME (ERYTHEMA MULTIFORME)
(Table 14-8)

Erythema multiforme is a mucocutaneous hyperreactivity that some patients manifest after exposures to various triggers such as drug ingestion or topical administration of ophthalmic sulfonamide ointment,[64, 112] proparacaine hydrochloride, herpes simplex infection,[17, 87] Stevens-Johnson syndrome,[77] smallpox vaccination, measles, physical agents, and malignancy.[112] Some cases arise in the absence of any apparent predisposing cause. Stevens-Johnson syndrome is a clinical entity and has not been defined with regard to specific etiologic factors or pathogenesis.

It is important to realize that not all cases are drug induced. Cases of erythema multiforme were were known prior to the advent of antibiotics or sulfonamides. Because of the prodrome of fever and respiratory symptoms, these patients frequently receive antibiotics prior to the onset of skin disease, and the antibiotics subsequently are blamed for the mucocutaneous eruption. On the other hand, it is clear that drugs, particularly sulfonamides, topical or systemic, sometimes cause the disease.

Systemic involvement

Erythema multiforme occurs most commonly in children and in young or middle-aged adults and is seldom encountered in the elderly. Onset is usually sudden and stormy

Table 14-8. Differential diagnosis of Stevens-Johnson syndrome

Lyell's disease	Stevens-Johnson syndrome	Exfoliative dermatitis
Prodrome of toxemia begins abruptly and subsides quickly after skin eruption	Fever persists with severe systemic picture	May be associated with other skin or systemic disease
Maximum severity at 48 hours and levels in 2 to 4 weeks	Crops of new lesions appear for 4 to 6 weeks (15 days for lesion to complete cycle)	May be a feature of Lyell's disease
Flaccid bullae—intradermal	Tense bullae—erythematous, subepidermal	Marked desquamation and erythroderma
Skin is painful and peels; skin lesions heal after shedding of epidermis	Mucous membrane affected first, then skin is affected	Conjunctiva affected by desquamation process
Scalded skin appearance	Self-limited attack	Cornea not affected
Positive Nikolsky's sign	Negative Nikolsky's sign	Shrinkage of lower cul-de-sac
Conjunctiva and cornea are affected	Conjunctiva and cornea also affected	Slate-gray appearance to skin
Conjunctiva, mouth, vagina, penis, and rectum may be involved	Pseudomembrane formation	Loss of hair and nails
Purulent conjunctivitis and in some cases a pseudo-membrane	Scarring, sicca, symblepharon formation, etc.	Mortality, 20%
Scarring trichiasis, sicca; eyelashes may shed	Mortality, 20%	
Staphylococcal infections	Etiologic origin is not sure	
Mortality, 20%		

with fever, malaise, arthralgia, and respiratory symptoms. A few days later, the skin eruption appears, consisting of macules, papules, "target" lesions of alternating red and white rings, and bullae. The arms and legs, trunk, and face are frequently involved, often with a strikingly symmetric distribution[71, 116] (Fig. 14-65). Occasionally permanent anonychia is seen.[139] The mucous membranes, especially of the eyes, mouth, genitalia, and arms, may be affected by bullous and erosive lesions with membranes and crusting. This form of erythema multiforme with severe, extensive mucous membrane and systemic involvement has been referred to as the Stevens-Johnson syndrome. The bullous changes of the skin can occasionally be so severe as to cause hemorrhagic and necrotic lesions (Fig. 14-66). Individual skin lesions tend to have life cycles of about 2 weeks; the entire disease usually has a duration of about 6 weeks.[112] Mortality rates between 5% and 20% have been reported.

Ocular involvement

Diffuse, bilateral conjunctivitis is a characteristic finding of severe erythema multiforme (Fig. 14-67). The conjunctivitis may be catarrhal, mucopurulent, hemorrhagic, or membranous and ultimately cicatrizing. There is a tendency for relative sparing of the cornea until the late problems of scarring and drying of the cornea ensue. However, one may see cases of corneal ulceration, drying, and peripheral vascularization during the acute phase of the disease. Unlike ocular pemphigoid, the corneal and conjunctival

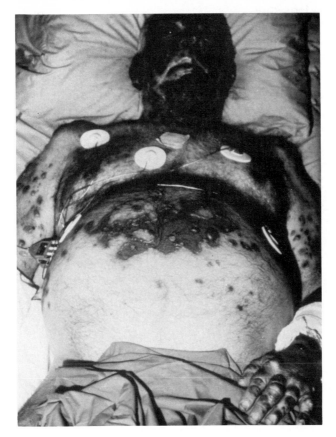

Fig. 14-65. Involvement of arms, trunk, and face in Stevens-Johnson syndrome.

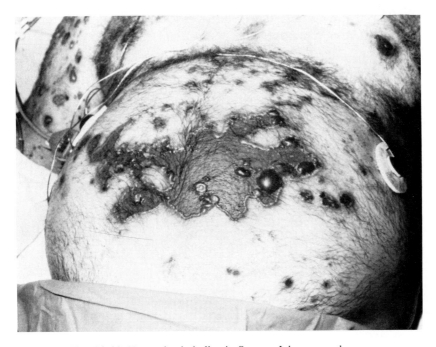

Fig. 14-66. Hemorrhagic bullae in Stevens-Johnson syndrome.

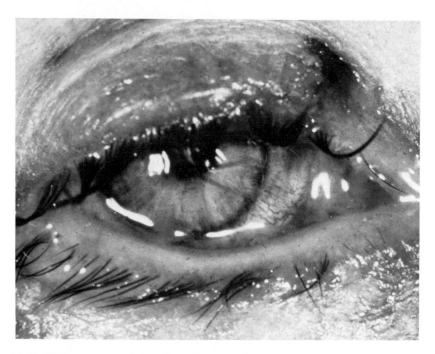

Fig. 14-67. Diffuse mucopurulent and membranous conjunctivitis in Stevens-Johnson syndrome.

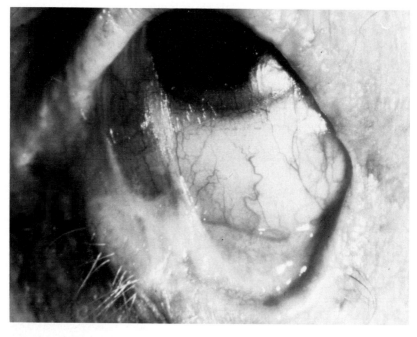

Fig. 14-68. Corneal keratinization, symblepharon formation, dry eye, and corneal vascularization as complications from Stevens-Johnson syndrome.

pathologic conditions of erythema multiforme does not progress indefinitely. Once the systemic disease has resolved, the ocular findings stabilize. The final result can vary from minimal conjunctival scarring to severe scarring, severe KCS, corneal vascularization, keratinization of lid margins (Fig. 14-68), symblepharons, and lid distortions with trichiasis and entropion.[4] Erythema multiforme can recur; the recurrences would be expected to be accompanied by reactivation of ocular involvement. Iridocyclitis and even panophthalmitis can occur.

Included in the differential diagnosis of erythema multiforme should be Kawasaki's disease or mucocutaneous lymph node syndrome. This syndrome exhibits a fever that lasts 1 to 2 weeks and does not respond to antibiotics, injection of the conjunctiva, reddening of oral and pharyngeal mucosae, dryness and fissuring of the lips and tongue, reddening of palms and soles with fingertip desquamation, polymorphous exanthem of trunk without crust or vesicles, and acute nonsuppurative swelling of cervical nodes.[60]

Conjunctival scrapings reveal a predominantly polymorphonuclear response with fibrin. Eosinophils are not characteristically present. The level of cleavage in the bullae can be subepithelial or intraepithelial. The subepithelial lesions result in the scarring.

Management

The treatment of erythema multiforme is primarily supportive. Systemic corticosteroids are frequently used, and they seem clinically to be of some benefit for the systemic

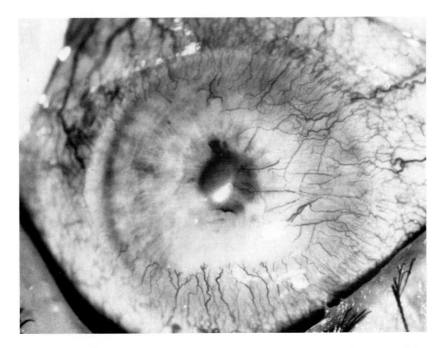

Fig. 14-69. Perforation of cornea after treatment of vascularized and dry cornea of Stevens-Johnson syndrome with frequent application of topical steroids.

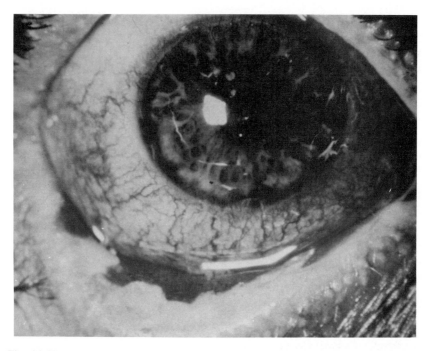

Fig. 14-70. Keratinization of lid margin as complication of Stevens-Johnson syndrome.

condition; such therapy appears to have no beneficial or harmful effect on the ocular problem. Topical and systemic corticosteroids have been advocated for ocular therapy in the early stages of the problem, but their benefits may be questioned.

Secondary infection must be watched for, and stromal destruction and corneal perforation can occur in patients with erythema multiforme who are treated with topical corticosteroids[134] (Fig. 14-69). It should be remembered that secondary bacterial and fungal infections of the conjunctiva and cornea can occur and should be sought and treated appropriately. Periodic irrigation of the eyes to cleanse them of exudate, along with gentle stripping of easily removed membranes, is perhaps of some benefit. Daily lysis of symblepharons appears to have little effect on their development. Insertion of a scleral shell in the hope of maintaining the conjunctival fornices might sometimes be indicated. Cycloplegia and perhaps topical corticosteroids would seem to be indicated in the presence of moderate to severe iridocyclitis.

Late management is that of the dry eye.[1] Plastic surgery on the lid margins is in order if there is severe keratinization of the margins (Fig. 14-70). Cryosurgery of the lid margins is suggested in cases of trichiasis.[30]

TOXIC EPIDERMAL NECROLYSIS (TEN) (LYELL'S DISEASE, SCALDED SKIN SYNDROME)

Toxic epidermal necrolysis (TEN) may represent a variant of erythema multiforme in which there is sloughing of large sheets of skin.[85,86] The inciting factors for the

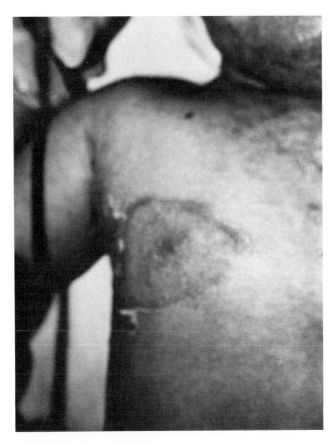

Fig. 14-71. Skin bullae become flaccid, and large areas of epidermis fall away, leaving ''scalded skin'' areas.

two diseases appear to be the same, and some patients may show admixtures of the clinical features of both illnesses.

Systemic involvement

TEN begins with a prodrome like that of erythema multiforme. A few days later erythema and bullae of the skin and mucous membranes appear.[2] The bullae become flaccid, and large areas of epidermis fall away, leaving an appearance of scalded skin (Fig. 14-71). Remaining areas of skin are often wrinkled and can be made to slide away like a ''slipped rug'' when pressure is applied. Mucous membranes of the mouth, genitalia, and rectum may be affected. The disease exhibits maximum severity in 24 hours and levels in about 2 to 4 weeks. Mortality is about 20%.

A staphylococcal form occurs almost always in children and has been referred to as Ritter's disease or scalded skin syndrome (SSS). However, it may occur in adults in whom a compromised immune status is seen or in patients with an overwhelming infection.[42] The rarity of SSS in adults can be attributed to immunologic competence or enhanced capacity of the adult to metabolize the staphylococcal exfoliation toxin. SSS in adults is often called *bullous impetigo*.[39, 132] This specific form of TEN is caused by a septicemia with *S. aureus* of phage group II, especially type 71.[82, 85, 86, 122] A nursery outbreak of SSS has been reported as caused by a group I staphylococcus rather than the group II organisms previously associated with SSS.[44] The staphylococcus produces the exfoliative skin exotoxin in humans and in addition can produce an identical syndrome in experimental animals.[96] TEN has been associated with administration of allopurinol for treatment of gout.[12, 41]

Intraepithelial cleavage accounts for the skin sloughing. The cleavage occurs superficially in the granular layer of the skin in Ritter's disease, whereas in the drug-induced forms, cleavage occurs in the area of the basal layer of the epidermis. Basal cell immunofluorescence has been demonstrated in this area in drug-induced cases.[129] Some epithelial cleavage also occurs, especially in the conjunctiva, where scarring may consequently result.

Ocular involvement

Ocular findings are the same as those of erythema multiforme, except that they perhaps tend to be somewhat milder in TEN. One can see trichiasis, lid distortion, and corneal opacification, vascularization, and drying.

Management

Treatment is no different from that described for erythema multiforme, except that intensive and immediate therapy with penicillinase-resistant penicillin should be instituted for the staphylococcal form of disease. Systemic corticosteroids can be harmful in staphylococcal cases, particularly if not covered by antibiotic therapy, but corticosteroid therapy is beneficial in the drug-induced forms, as noted.

EXFOLIATIVE DERMATITIS

Exfoliative dermatitis is characterized by chronic diffuse erythroderma and desquamation of the epidermis (Fig. 14-72). Its causes are multiple; it often represents the late chronic stage of any number of chronic dermatoses, including psoriasis, atopic dermatitis, pityriasis rubra pilaris, and ichthyosis.

Systemic involvement

There usually is no acute, systemic illness, as occurs in erythema multiforme and TEN, although secondary infections can occur because of the compromised state of the integument. Patients with exfoliative dermatitis show the general appearance of a chronically reddened skin that is covered by many tiny, white scales from the epidermis (Fig. 14-72). The patient's clothing and the examining room chair may be covered with thousands of these small flakes. The pathogenesis of the disease is not known.

Ocular involvement

Nonspecific conjunctival irritation can be caused by desquamation of scales from adjacent skin into the conjunctival sacs. Chronic inflammatory skin changes can pro-

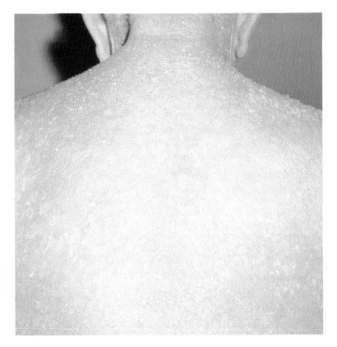

Fig. 14-72. Exfoliative dermatitis with chronic erythroderma and extensive skin scaling.

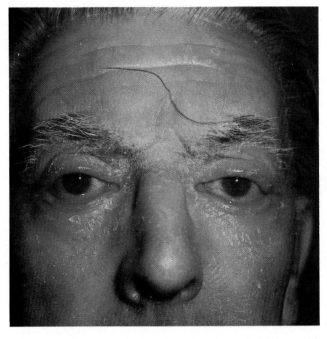

Fig. 14-73. Severe ectropion with injection of conjunctiva and shrinkage of lower fornix.

duce contractural ectropion of the lower eyelid. Some shrinkage of the lower conjunctival fornix may be seen. The cornea is not affected except secondarily from the effects
of the scales and ectropion (Fig. 14-73).

Management

Therapeutic measures include the cleansing away of periocular scales, the application of corticosteroid preparations to the skin, and the topical use of ocular lubricants
for nonspecific conjunctival irritation or exposure keratopathy. Surgical correction of
ectropion can be helpful. The management of any underlying disease is, of course,
within the realm of the dermatologist.

Table 14-8 charts the differential points between Stevens-Johnson syndrome, Lyell's
syndrome, and exfoliative dermatitis.

BEHÇET'S SYNDROME

Behçet's syndrome is a rare, relapsing mucocutaneous ocular condition of unknown
cause. Altered humoral and cellular reactions in patients with this syndrome suggest the
presence of autoimmunity. Histocompatibility antigen (HLA-B5) is present in Behçet's
disease.[123]

Circulating antibodies to oral mucous membrane antigens are present in most affected
individuals. Destruction of mucous membranes by the patient's lymphocytes has been
demonstrated in vivo.

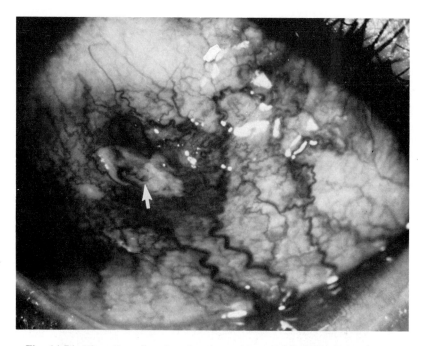

Fig. 14-74. Ulceration of conjunctiva *(arrow)* as noted in Behçet's syndrome.

Systemic involvement

Behçet's syndrome has been described as a triple-system complex consisting of recurrent aphthous stomatitis, genital ulceration, and iritis. This disorder is twice as common in men as it is in women, appears to be worldwide in distribution, and occurs with particularly high incidence in the eastern Mediterranean basin, Japan, and Italy. Added to the original triad, one may find pustular skin lesions, polyarthritis, thrombophlebitis, involvement of the central nervous system, and gastrointestinal disturbances. The underlying pathologic condition appears to be an inflammatory obliterative vasculitis, particularly involving the venous system.

Ocular involvement

Uveitis is a prominent feature in Behçet's syndrome. The retina may show signs of retinitis, neuroretinitis, retinal hemorrhages, optic neuritis, and cloudy vitreous with serious diminution of vision.

The conjunctiva may exhibit inflammation, ulcerations (Fig. 14-74), edema, and hemorrhages. These lesions may be recurrent.

The cornea may show opacification, vascularization, ulceration, and punctate keratopathy.

Management

Encouraging results from treatment with chlorambucil have been obtained. Azathioprine, which suppresses both cellular and humoral responses, has been tried with some success.[89, 109]

REITER'S SYNDROME

This disease was first reported in 1916; its cause is unknown. Mycoplasma and chlamydial origins have been proposed, but contradictory and inconclusive evidence prevails.

Young men are mainly affected[113]; the disease is extremely rare in women and in children.

More than 76% of patients with Reiter's syndrome have the histocompatibility antigen HLA-W27, which has an incidence of less than 10% in the general population.

Systemic involvement

Reiter's syndrome is characterized by the presence of urethritis, arthritis, circinate balanitis, shallow ulcerations of the buccal mucosa, and a characteristic dermatitis: keratoderma blennorrhagicum.[101]

The lesions of keratoderma blennorrhagicum consist of painless hyperkeratotic pustules, which may occur on the palms and soles but may also appear elsewhere, as on the nails. The mucosal erosions and balanitis are painless and may be overlooked. Arthritis and periostitis are also a part of the picture. The disease can be serious if and when pericardial and cardiac involvement occur. A small number of patients may develop aortic insufficiency as a result of dilation of the root of the aorta.

It is interesting that there may be a possible relationship between Reiter's syndrome

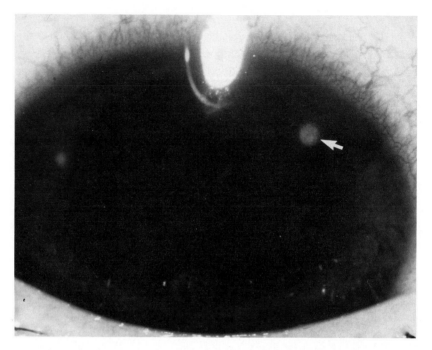

Fig. 14-75. Subepithelial lesions *(arrow)* of cornea in Reiter's syndrome.

and psoriatic arthritis. The keratoderma blennorrhagicum is similar in both instances, as is the spondylitis found in both conditions. More significant still are a number of well-documented instances in which patients with typical Reiter's syndrome gradually developed unquestionable psoriatic arthritis. It should be noted that the eye may also be involved in psoriasis. This is reviewed in Chapter 23.

Reiter's syndrome is usually self-limited, subsiding in 6 weeks to 6 months, and complete remission with full recovery of the joints is the rule. Skin and mucous membrane lesions heal without a trace.

Ocular involvement

The main ocular sign of Reiter's syndrome is a nonbacterial, mucopurulent papillary conjunctivitis. Episcleritis and scleritis occur rarely. The keratitis is variable. Punctate epithelial lesions, erosions, edema, subepithelial keratopathy, stromal infiltration, interstitial keratitis, and corneal ulcerations may be seen in some cases (Fig. 14-75).

Management

Treatment of Reiter's syndrome with systemic tetracyclines, 250 mg four times a day, and topical tetracycline drops has offered good results in some cases.

CICATRIZING CONJUNCTIVAL DISEASES

Cicatrization of the conjunctiva with associated corneal complications has been a prominent finding of a number of the diseases discussed previously. It is apropos, at this point, to include a summary of the differential diagnoses of this feature. Scarring of the conjunctiva associated with corneal involvement occurs in the following disorders:

1. Pseudomembranous and membranous conjunctivitis (hyperacute disease)
2. Stevens-Johnson syndrome
3. Ocular pemphigoid
4. Exfoliative dermatitis, dermatitis herpetiformis, epidermolysis bullosa
5. Trachoma, lymphogranuloma venereum
6. Atopic keratoconjunctivitis
7. Lye burns
8. Medication toxicity
    a. Topical (for example, echothiophate iodide drops)
    b. Systemic (practolol)
9. Sarcoidosis[50]

The ordinary acute or chronic conjunctivitis of bacterial origin heals without cicatrization. The epithelium can, in fact, be severely damaged without provoking the formation of scar tissue. Scars form only to replace necrotic stromal tissue, and there may be severe infiltration and edema of the stroma, as in gonococcal ophthalmia of the adult, without scar formation.

Every possible effort should be made to prevent conjunctival cicatrization because of its long-term complications, such as entropion and trichiasis. Atrophy of goblet cells and closure of lacrimal secreting tubules may occur, both of which lead to KCS.

Conjunctival scarring varies in its location, extent, and morphologic characteristics in the various cicatrizing diseases; for this reason it has great diagnostic value.

Any conjunctival disease sufficiently severe to produce either a pseudomembrane or a true membrane can lead to nonspecific scar formation, for example, the scars occasionally seen in EKC, inclusion conjunctivitis, and gonorrheal blennorrhea. This type of cicatrization is diffuse, amorphic, and entirely nonspecific.

Scars of pseudomembranous and membranous conjunctivitis

A variety of infectious agents can produce pseudomembranous or membranous conjunctivitis, but, from whatever cause, this type of conjunctivitis is now rare. Formerly it was caused principally by the diphtheria organism *(Corynebacterium diphtheriae)* and β-hemolytic streptococci. But now, in western areas of the country, adenovirus 8 (EKC) has become the most common cause, with HSV (primary herpetic conjunctivitis in children) second in frequency. Membranes are also seen in the rare cases of erythema multiforme (Stevens-Johnson syndrome).

Any inflammation severe enough to produce pseudomembranes can cause conjunctival cicatrization of the diffuse type. In this type, there seems to be no predilection for the conjunctiva of either lid, upper or lower.

Characteristic scarring in specific diseases

Special types of scarring, with characteristic morphologic features and location, are seen in trachoma, ocular pemphigoid, and atopic keratoconjunctivitis. Severe shrinkage such as in ocular pemphigoid also occurs occasionally in a few other diseases.

Trachoma. The scar pathognomonic of trachoma is at the limbus. It is the so-called Herbert's peripheral pit and consists of the cicatricial remains of a limbal follicle. Less characteristic, but still diagnostically important, are the so-called stellate scars resulting from cicatrization of necrotic conjunctival follicles. Diffuse scarring may also occur, leading to bowling of the upper tarsus with subsequent ectropion formation. Arlt's line (the cicatricial line near the lid border of the upper tarsus) has some diagnostic value, as does the S curve of the upper lid border, which is a cicatricial complication. In trachoma, cicatrization is always more prominent on the upper lid than on the lower lid.

Atopic keratoconjunctivitis. The scars of this disease are focal and tend to occur in the centers of the giant papillae. There is also a diffuse shrinkage of the lower fornix, but in this instance there is less tendency for symblepharon or entropion and trichiasis to occur. Vernal keratoconjunctivitis does not normally scar the conjunctiva, but radical treatment of the disease frequently does so.

Others. Severe conjunctival scarring can occur in dermatitis herpetiformis, epidermolysis bullosa, and lymphogranuloma venereum, as well as from ingesting drugs such as practolol,[56, 147] which is a β-adrenergic receptor-blocking drug. Scarring has also been noticed in sarcoidosis.[50]

Ligneous conjunctivitis

Ligneous conjunctivitis (a special membranous conjunctivitis)[48,49,54] is a bilateral membranous conjunctivitis seen in childhood. It is more frequent in females and may persist for years. It may be associated with membranous tracheal obstruction,[32] vulvovaginitis, and other systemic findings. It is also characterized by a chronic phase that affects the upper tarsal area with a form of inflammation nasally in both eyes. The membranes are thick and exhibit a hard and boardlike appearance (Fig. 14-76). If the membranes are scraped, the area bleeds and they regrow readily.

Occasionally ligneous conjunctivitis is associated with corneal involvement that may lead to perforation and loss of the globe.

This membranous conjunctivitis has been resistant to treatment, although the following therapy has been claimed to be effective[48]; 1/5000 dilution of α-chymotrypsin in hyaluronidase, 35 to 175 IU/ml every hour for 2 to 3 months, then reduced to six times daily, then three times daily.

However, a histopathologic section of the membrane reveals eosinophils (Fig. 14-77), mononuclear cells, neutrophils, and mast cells. The presence of mast cells and eosinophils prompted the use of 4% cromolyn sodium. Mast cells are seen well with Unna's stain (Fig. 14-78). Cromolyn sodium interferes with the release of mediators from mast cells by inhibiting cyclic AMP phosphodiesterase or by inhibiting calcium uptake in the mast cell. Cromolyn sodium is effective in vernal catarrh and atopic disease of the conjunctiva and cornea. It is also used for systemic diseases such as bronchial asthma.

It may be necessary to excise the boardlike membrane and apply cryotherapy to the areas of excision. The combination of this surgical treatment with cromolyn sodium is effective.[54]

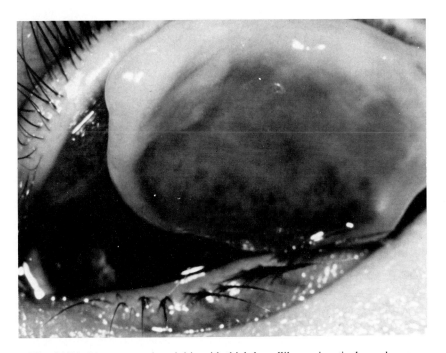

Fig. 14-76. Ligneous conjunctivitis with thick boardlike conjunctival membrane.

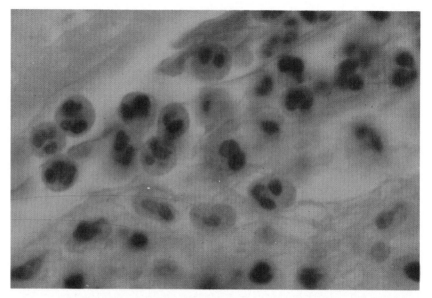

Fig. 14-77. Eosinophils noted in smear in ligneous conjunctivitis.

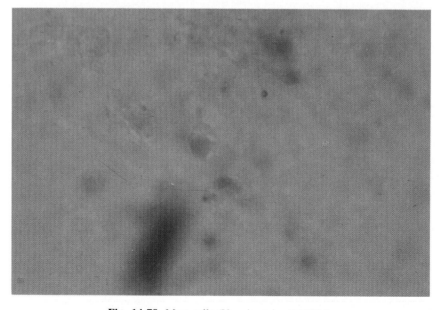

Fig. 14-78. Mast cells (Unna's stain; ×1000.)

REFERENCES

1. Allansmith, M.R., Greiner, J.V., Henriquez, A.S., et al.: Giant papillary conjunctivitis in contact lens wearers, Am. J. Ophthalmol. **83:**697, 1977.
2. Amon, R.B., and Dimond, R.L.: Toxic epidermal necrolysis, Arch. Dermatol. **111:**1433, 1975.
3. Anderson, L.G., and Talal, N.: The spectrum of benign to malignant lymphoproliferation in Sjögren's syndrome, Clin. Exp. Immunol. **9:**199, 1971.
4. Arstikoitis, M.J.: Ocular aftermath of Stevens-Johnson syndrome, Arch. Ophthalmol. **90:**376, 1973.
5. Austin, P., Green, W.R., Sallyer, D.C., et al.: Peripheral corneal degeneration and occlusive vasculitis in Wegener's granulomatosis, Am. J. Ophthalmol. **85:**311, 1978.
6. Bairstow, B.: Cicatricial pemphigoid, Arch. Dermatol. **104:**454, 1971.
7. Barth, W.F., and Berson, E.F.: Relapsing polychondritis, rheumatoid arthritis and blindness, Am. J. Ophthalmol. **66:**890, 1968.
8. Baum, J.L., and Bierstock, R.S.: Peripheral corneal infiltrates following intravenous injection of diatrizoate meglumine, Am. J. Ophthalmol. **85:**613, 1978.
9. Bean, S.F.: Cicatricial pemphigoid, Int. J. Dermatol. **14:**23, 1975.
10. Bean, S.F., Furey, N., West, C., Andres, T., and Esterly, N.: Ocular cicatricial pemphigoid, Trans. Am. Acad. Ophthalmol. Otolaryngol. **81:**806. 1976.
11. Bean, S.F., Holubar, K., and Gillett, R.B.: Pemphigus involving the eyes, Arch. Dermatol. **11:**1484, 1975.
12. Bennett, T.O., Sugar, J., and Sudarchan, S.: Ocular manifestations of toxic necrolysis associated allopurinol ulcers, Arch. Ophthalmol. **95:**1362, 1977.
13. Benson, W.E., Shields, J.A., Tasman, W., et al.: Posterior scleritis: a cause of diagnostic confusion, Arch. Ophthalmol. **97:**1482, 1979.
14. Bloomfield, S.E., and Brown, S.I.: Treatment of corneal ulcers with collagenase inhibitors, Int. Ophthalmol. Clin. **13:**225, 1973.
15. Brady, H.R., Israel, M.R., and Lewin, W.H.: Wegener's granulomatosis and corneoscleral ulcer, JAMA **193:**148, 1965.
16. Breslin, C.W., Katz, J.I., and Kaufman, H.E.: Surgical management of necrotizing scleritis, Arch. Ophthalmol. **95:**2038, 1977.
17. Britz, M., and Sibulkin, D.: Recurrent erythema mulltiforme and herpes genitallis (type 2), JAMA **233:**812, 1975.
18. Brown, S.I.: Mooren's ulcer: histopathology and proteolytic enzymes of adjacent conjunctiva, Br. J. Ophthalmol. **59:**670, 1975.
19. Brown, S.I.: Mooren's ulcer. Treatment by conjunctival excision, Br. J. Ophthalmol. **59:**675, 1975.
20. Brown, S.I., and Grayson, M.: Marginal furrows: a characteristic corneal lesion of rheumatoid arthritis, Arch. Ophthalmol. **79:**563, 1968.
21. Brown, S.I., and Hook, C.W.: Isolation of stromal collagenase in corneal inflammation, Am. J. Ophthalmol. **72:**1139, 1971.
22. Brown, S.I., and Mondino, B.J. Penetrating keratoplasty in Mooren's ulcer, Am. J. Ophthalmol. **89:**255, 1980.
23. Brown, S.I., Mondino, B.J., and Rabin, B.S.: Autoimmune phenomenon in Mooren's ulcer, Am. J. Ophthalmol. **82:**835, 1976.
24. Brown, S.I., and Weller, C.A.: Cell origin of collagenase in normal and wounded corneas, Arch. Ophthalmol. **83:**74, 1970.
25. Brown, S.I., Weller, C.A., and Akiya, S.: Pathogenesis of ulcers and alkali burns, Arch. Ophthalmol. **83:**205, 1970.
26. Brubaker, R., Font, R.L., and Sheperd, E.M.: Granulomatous sclerouveitis: regression of ocular lesions with cytophosphamide and prednisone, Arch. Ophthalmol. **86:**517, 1971.
27. Byrd, L.J., Shearn, M.A., and Tu, W.: Relationship of lethal midline granuloma to Wegener's granulomatosis, Arthritis Rheum. **12:**247, 1969.
28. Carroll, C.P., Keates, R.H. Bone formation in a periosteal graft, Arch. Ophthalmol. **97:**916, 1979.
29. Christiansen, J.M., and Arentsen, J.J.: Surgical therapy of Mooren's ulcer: report of two cases successfully treated, Ann. Ophthalmol. **7:**1507, 1975.
30. Chylack, L.T., Jr., Bienfang, D.C., Bellows, A.R., and Stillman, J.S.: Ocular manifestations of juvenile rheumatoid arthritis, Am. J. Ophthalmol. **79:**1026, 1975.
31. Cogan, D.G.: Corneoscleral lesions in periarteritis and Wegener's granulomatosis, Trans. Am. Ophthalmol. Soc. **53:**321, 1955.
32. Cooper, T.J., Kazdan, J.J., and Cutz, E.: Ligneous conjunctivitis with tracheal obstruction: a case report, with light and electron microscopy findings, Can. J. Ophthalmol. **14:**57, 1979.
33. Coutu, R.E., Klein, M., Lessell, S., Friedman, E., and Snider, G.L.: Limited form of Wegener's granulomatosis: eye involvement as a major sign, JAMA **122:**868, 1975.
34. Culbertson, W.W., and Ostler, H.B.: The floppy eyelid syndrome, Am. J. Ophthalmol. **92:**568, 1981.

35. David, R., and Ivry, M.: Focal chorioretinitis and iridocyclitis associated with scleroderma, Ann. Ophthalmol. **8:**199, 1976.

36. Dobson, R.L.: Diagnosis and treatment of eczema, JAMA **235:**2228, 1976.

37. Easty, D.L., Rice, N.S.C., and Jones, B.R.: Disodium cromoglycate (Intal) in the treatment of keratoconjunctivitis, Trans. Ophthalmol. Soc. U.K. **91:**491, 1971.

38. Easty, D.L., Rice, N.S.C., and Jones, B.R.: Clinical trial of topical disodium cromoglycate in vernal keratoconjunctivitis, Clin. Allergy **2:**99, 1972.

39. Elias, P.M., and Levy, W.: Bullous impetigo. Occurrence of localized scaled skin syndrome in adults, Arch. Dermatol. **112:**850, 1976.

40. Ellis, P.P., and Gentry, J.H.: Ocular complications of ulcerative colitis, Am. J. Ophthalmol. **58:**779, 1964.

41. Ellman, M.H., Fretzan, D.F., and Olson, W.: Toxic epidermal necrolysis associated with allopurinol administration, Arch. Dermatol. **11:**986, 1975.

42. Epstein, E.H., Flynn, P., and Davis, R.S.: Adult toxic epidermolysis necrolysis with fatal staphylococcal septicemia, JAMA **229:**425, 1974.

43. Evans, J.P., and Eustace, P.: Scleromalacia perforans associated with Crohn's disease treated with sodium versenate (EDTA), Br. J. Ophthalmol. **57:**330, 1973.

44. Faden, H.S.: Nursery outbreak of scalded skin syndrome, Am. J. Dis. Child. **130:**265, 1976.

45. Feldon, S.E., Sigelman, J., Albert, D.M., and Smith, T.R.: Clinical manifestations of brawny scleritis, Am. J. Ophthalmol. **85:**781, 1978.

46. Ferry, A.P.: The histopathology of rheumatoid episcleral nodules: an extra-articular manifestation of rheumatoid arthritis, Arch. Ophthalmol. **82:**77, 1969.

47. Ferry, A.P., and Leopold, I.H.: Marginal (ring) corneal ulcer as a presenting manifestation of Wegener's granuloma: a clinicopathologic study, Trans. Am. Acad. Ophthalmol. Otolaryngol. **74:**1276, 1970.

48. Firat, T.: Ligneous conjunctivitis, Am. J. Ophthalmol. **78:**679, 1974.

49. Firat, T., and Tinaztepe, B.: Histochemical investigations on ligeneous conjunctivitis and a new method of treatment, Acta Ophthalmol. **48:**3, 1970.

50. Flach, A.: Symblepharon in sarcoidosis, Am. J. Ophthalmol. **85:**210, 1978.

51. Fogle, J.A., Kenyon, K., and Foster, C.S.: Tissue adhesive arrests stromal melting in the human cornea, Am. J. Ophthalmol. **89:**795, 1980.

52. Foster, C.S.: Immunosuppressive therapy for external ocular inflammatory disease, Ophthalmology **87:**140, 1980.

53. Foster, C.S., Kenyon, K.R., Greiner, J., et al.: The immunopathology of Mooren's ulcer, Am. J. Ophthalmol. **88:**149, 1979.

54. Friedlander, M., and Ostler, H.B.: Treatment of ligneous conjunctivitis with cromolyn: a case report, presented at a meeting of the American Academy of Ophthalmology, Dallas, Oct., 1977.

55. Furney, N., West, C., Andrews, T., Paul, P.D., and Bean, S.E.: Immunofluorescent studies of ocular cicatricial pemphigoid, Am. J. Ophthalmol. **80:**825, 1975.

56. Garner, A., and Rahi, A.H.S.: Practolol and ocular toxicity: antibodies in serum and tears, Br. J. Ophthalmol. **60:**684, 1976.

57. Geddes, D.M., and Brostoff, J.: Pulmonary fibrosis associated with hypersensitivity to gold salts, Br. Med. J. **1:**444, 1976.

58. Gerstle, C.S., and Friedman, A.H.: Marginal corneal ulceration (limbal guttering) as a presenting sign of temporal arteritis, Ophthalmology **87:**1173, 1980.

59. Girdas, P.P., Altman, B., Nicholson, D.H., and Green, W.R.: Corneal perforations in Sjögren's syndrome, Arch. Ophthalmol. **90:**470, 1973.

60. Glanzer, J.M., Galbraith, W.B., and Jacobs, J.P.: Kawasaki disease in a 28 year old man, JAMA **244:**1604, 1980.

61. Goder, G., and Dolter, J.: Wegener's granulomatosis of conjunctival origin, Ophthalmologica **162:**321, 1971.

62. Goodwin, J.S., and Williams, R.C.: Suppressor cells: a recent conceptual epidemic, J. Clin. Lab. Immunol. **2:**89, 1979.

63. Goto, M., Horiuchi, Y., Okumura, K., Tada, T., and Ohmori, K.: Immunological abnormalities of aging: an analysis of T lymphocyte subpopulations of Werner's syndrome, J. Clin. Invest. **64:**695, 1979.

64. Gottschalk, H.R., and Stone, O.J.: Stevens-Johnson syndrome from ophthalmic sulfonamide, Arch. Dermatol. **112:**513, 1976.

65. Greiner, J.V., Covington, H.I., and Allansmith, M.R.: Giant papillary conjunctivitis, Am. J. Ophthalmol. **85:**242, 1978.

66. Hanifin, J.M., and Lobitz, W.C.: Newer concepts of atopic dermatitis, Arch. Dermatol. **113:**663, 1977.

67. Hardy, K.M., Perry, H.O., Pengree, G.C., and Kirby, T.J.: Benign mucous membrane pemphigoid, Arch. Dermatol. **104:**467, 1971.

68. Herron, B.E.: Immunologic aspects of cicatricial pemphigoid, Am. J. Ophthalmol. **79:**271, 1975.

69. Hood, C.I.: Essential shrinkage of conjunctiva, chronic cicatrizing conjunctivitis, and benign mucous membrane pemphigoid, Invest. Ophthalmol. **12:**308, 1973.

70. Hopkins, D.J., Horan, E., Burton, I.L., Clamp, S.E., DeDombal, F.T., and Goligher, J.C.: Ocu-

lar disorders in a series of 332 patients with Crohn's disease, Br. J. Ophthalmol. **58:**732, 1974.

71. Howard, G.M.: The Stevens-Johnson syndrome, Am. J. Ophthalmol. **55:**893, 1963.

72. Hughes, R.A.C., Berry, C.L., Seifert, M., and Lessof, M.H.: Recurrent polychondritis: three cases with a clinocopathological study and literature review, Q.J. Med. **41:**363, 1972.

73. Jackson, J., Anderson, L., Schur, P.H., and Stillman, H.S.: Sjögren's syndrome in juvenile rheumatoid arthritis (JRA), abstracted, Arthritis Rheum. **16:**122, 1973.

74. Jayson, M.I., and Jones, D.E.P.: Scleritis and rheumatoid arthritis, Ann. Rheum. Dis. **30:**343, 1971.

75. Kazdan, J.J., Crawford, J.S., Langer, H., and MacDonald, A.L.: Sodium cromoglycate (Intal) in the treatment of vernal keratoconjunctivitis and allergic conjunctivitis, Can. J. Ophthalmol. **11:**300, 1976.

76. Kielar, R.A.: Exudative retinal detachment and scleritis in polyarteritis, Am. J. Ophthalmol. **82:**695, 1976.

77. Kiernan, J.P., Schanzlin, D.J., and Leveille, A.S.: Stevens-Johnson syndrome associated with adenovirus conjunctivitis, Am. J. Ophthalmol. **92:**543, 1981.

78. Kirkham, T.: Scleroderma and Sjögren's syndrome, Br. J. Ophthalmol. **53:**131, 1969.

79. Knox, D., Snip, R.C., and Stark, W.J.: The keratopathy of Crohn's disease, Am. J. Ophthalmol. **90:**862, 1980.

80. Krachmer, J.H., and Laibson, P.R.: Corneal thinning and perforation in Sjögren's syndrome, Am. J. Ophthalmol. **78:**917, 1974.

81. Lever, W.F.: Pemphigus and pemphigoid, Springfield, Ill., 1965, Charles C Thomas, Publisher.

82. Levine, G., Norden, C.W.: Staphylococcal scalded-skin syndrome in an adult, N. Engl. J. Med. **287:**1339, 1972.

83. Lipton, N.L., Crawford, J.S., Greenberg, M.L., Boone, J.E., and Stein, H.B.: The risk of iridocyclitis in juvenile rheumatoid arthritis, Can. J. Ophthalmol. **11:**26, 1976.

84. Luckasen, J.R., Sabad, A., Goltz, R.W., and Kersey, J.H.: T and B lymphocytes in atopic eczema, Arch. Dermatol. **110:**375, 1974.

85. Lyell, A.: Toxic epidermal necrolysis: an eruption resembling scalding of the skin, Br. J. Dermatol. **68:**355, 1956.

86. Lyell, A., Dick, H.M., and Alexander, J.O.D.: Outbreak of toxic epidermal necrolysis associated with staphylococci, Lancet **1:**787, 1969.

87. MacDonald, A., and Feiwel, M.: Isolation of herpes virus from erythema multiforme, Br. Med. J. **2:**570, 1972.

88. Macoul, K.L.: Ocular changes in granulomatous ileocolitis, Arch. Ophthalmol. **84:**95, 1970.

89. Mamo, J.G., and Azzam, S.A.: Treatment of Behçet's disease with chlorambucil, Arch. Ophthalmol. **84:**446, 1970.

90. Martin, J., Roenigk, H.H., Lynch, W., and Tingwald, F.R.: Relapsing polychondritis treated with dapsone, Arch. Dermatol. **112:**1272, 1976.

91. McClellan, B.H., Whitney, C.R., Newman, L.P., and Allansmith, M.R.: Immunoglobulins in tears, Am. J. Ophthalmol. **76:**89, 1973.

92. McKay, D.A.R., Watson, P.G., and Lyne, A.J.: Relapsing polychondritis and eye disease, Br. J. Ophthalmol. **58:**600, 1974.

93. Meisler, D.M., Stock, L.E., Wertz, R.D., et al.: Conjunctival inflammation and amyloidosis in allergic granulomatosis and angiitis (Churg-Strauss syndrome), Am. J. Ophthalmol. **91:**216, 1981.

94. Meisler, D.M., Zaret, C.R., and Stock, E.L.: Trantas' dots and limbal inflammation associated with soft contact lens wear, Am. J. Ophthalmol. **84:**66, 1980.

95. Mendes, N.F., Kopersztych, S., and Mota, N.G.S.: T and B lymphocytes in patients with lepromatous leprosy, Clin. Exp. Immunol. **16:**23, 1974.

96. Melish, M.E., and Glasgow, L.A.: The staphylococcal scalded-skin syndrome: development of an experimental model, N. Engl. J. Med. **282:**1114, 1970.

97. Messner, R.P., Lindstrom, F.D., and Williams, R.C.: Peripheral blood lymphocyte cell surface markers during the course of systemic lupus erythematosus, J. Clin. Invest. **52:**3046, 1973.

98. Michel, B., Thomas, C.I., Levine, M., Waisman, M., and Bean, S.M.: Cicatricial pemphigoid and its relationship to ocular pemphigus and essential shrinkage of the conjunctiva, Ann. Ophthalmol. **7:**11, 1975.

99. Michel, B., Waisman, M., Thomas, C.I., and Levine, M.: Immunofluorescent test in bullous diseases of skin and mucous membranes, Ann. Ophthalmol. **6:**1311, 1974.

100. Michelson, J.B., and Chisari, F.V.: Behçet's disease, Surv. Ophthalmol. **26:**190, 1982.

101. Mills, R.P., and Kalina, R.E.: Reiter's keratitis, Arch. Ophthalmol. **87:**447, 1972.

102. Mondino, B.J., Brown, S.I., Robin, B.S., and Lemp, M.A.: Autoimmune phenomena of the conjunctiva and cornea: a case report, Arch. Ophthalmol. **95:**468, 1977.

103. Mondino, B.J., and Brown, S.I.: Ocular cicatricial pemphigoid, Ophthalmology **88:**95, 1981.

104. Mondino, B.J., and Groden, L.R.: Conjunctival hyperemia and corneal infiltrates with chemically disinfected soft contact lenses, Arch. Ophthalmol. **98:**1767, 1980.

105. Mondino, B.J., Kowalski, R., and Rotajczak, H.V.: Rabbit model phlyctenulosis and catarrhal infiltrates, Arch. Ophthalmol. **99:**891, 1981.

106. Mondino, B.J., Rao, H., and Brown, S.I.: T and B lymphocytes in ocular cicatricial pemphigoid, Am. J. Ophthalmol. **92:**536, 1981.

107. Moore, J.G., and Sevel, D.: Corneoscleral ulceration in periarteritis nodosa, Br. J. Ophthalmol. **50:**651, 1966.

108. Morgan, G.: Pathology of vernal conjunctivitis, Trans. Ophthalmol. Soc. U.K. **91:**467, 1971.

109. Nethercott, J., and Lester, R.S.: Azathioprine therapy in incomplete Behçet's syndrome, Arch. Dermatol. **110:**432, 1976.

110. Ostler, H.B.: Corneal perforation in nontuberculous (staphylococcal) phlyctenular keratoconjunctivitis, Am. J. Ophthalmol. **79:**446, 1975.

111. Ostler, H.B.: Acute chemotic reaction to cromolyn, Arch. Ophthalmol. **100:**412, 1982.

112. Ostler, H.B., Conant, M.A., and Groundwater, J.: Lyell's disease, the Stevens-Johnson syndrome, and exfoliative dermatitis, Trans. Am. Acad. Ophthalmol. Otolaryngol. **74:**1254, 1970.

113. Ostler, H.B., Dawson, C.R., Schachter, J., and Engleman, E.P.: Reiter's syndrome, Am. J. Ophthalmol. **71:**986, 1971.

114. Patten, J.T., Cavanagh, D.H., and Allansmith, M.R.: Induced ocular pseudopemphigoid, Am. J. Ophthalmol. **82:**212, 1976.

115. Paty, J.G. Jr., Sienknecht, C.W., Townes, A.S., et al.: Impaired cell-mediated immunity in systemic lupus erythematosus (SLE): a controlled study of 23 untreated patients, Am. J. Med. **59:**769, 1975.

116. Patz, A.: Ocular involvement in erythema multiforme, Arch. Ophthalmol. **43:**244, 1950.

117. Podos, S.M., Albert, R.B., and Blaese, R.M.: Wiskott-Aldrich syndrome, Arch. Ophthalmol. **82:**322, 1969.

118. Prystorwsky, S., and Gilliam, J.N.: Discoid lupus erythematosus as a part of a larger disease spectrum, Arch. Dermatol. **111:**1448, 1975.

119. Reza, M.J., Dornfeld, L., Goldberg, L.S., et al.: Wegener's granulomatosis: long-term follow-up of patients treated with cyclophosphamide, Arthritis Rheum. **18:**501, 1975.

120. Rice, N.S.C., and Jones, B.R.: Vernal keratoconjunctivitis: an allergic disease of the eyes of children, Clin. Allergy **3:**629, 1973.

121. Rogge, J.L., and Hanifin, J.N.: Immunodeficiencies in severe atopic dermatitis: depressed chemotaxis and lymphocyte transformation, Arch. Dermatol. **112:**1391, 1976.

122. Rothenberg, R., Renna, F.S., Drew, T.M., et al.: Staphylococcal scalded skin syndrome in an adult, Arch. Dermatol. **108:**408, 1973.

123. Scharf, Y., and Zonis, S.: Histocompatibility antigens (HLA) and uveitis, Surv. Ophthalmol. **24:**220, 1980.

124. Schulman, M.F., and Sugar, A.: Peripheral corneal infiltrates in inflammatory bowel disease, Ann. Ophthalmol. **13:**109, 1981.

125. Sergott, R.C., Felberg, N.T., Savino, P.J., Blizzard, J.J., and Schatz, N.J.: E-rosette formation in Graves' ophthalmolopathy, Invest. Ophthalmol. Vis. Sci. **18:**1245, 1979.

126. Sjögren, H., and Block, K. J.: Keratoconjunctivitis sicca and Sjögren's syndrome, Surv. Ophthalmol. **16:**145, 1971.

127. Smith, R.E., Dippe, D.W., and Miller, S.D.: Phlyctenular keratoconjunctivitis: results of penetrating keratoplasty in Alaskan natives, Ophthalmic Surg. **6:**62, 1975.

128. Srinivasan, D.B., Jakobiec, F.A., Iwanoto, T., et al.: Giant papillary conjunctivitis with ocular prosthesis, Arch. Ophthalmol. **97:**892, 1979.

129. Stein, K.M., Schlappner, O.L., Heaton, C.L., and Decherd, J.W.: Demonstration of basal cell immunofluorescence in drug-induced toxic epidermal necrolysis, Br. J. Dermatol. **86:**246, 1972.

130. Sternberg, A.D., and Talae, N.: Coexistence of Sjögren's syndrome and systemic lupus erythematosus, Ann. Intern. Med. **74:**55, 1971.

131. Strelkauskas, A.J., Callery, R.T., McDowell, J., Borel, Y., and Schlossman, S.F.: Direct evidence for loss of human suppressor cells during active autoimmune disease, Proc. Natl. Acad. Sci. USA **75:**5150, 1978.

132. Sturman, S.W., and Malkinson, F.D.: Staphylococcal scalded-skin syndrome in an adult and a child, Arch. Dermatol. **112:**1275, 1976.

133. Tabbara, K.F., Ostler, H.B., Daniels, T.E., Sylvester, R.A., Greenspan, J.S., and Talae, N.: Sjögren's syndrome: a correlation between ocular findings and labial salivary gland histology, Trans. Am. Acad. Ophthalmol. Otolaryngol. **78:**467, 1974.

134. Tabbara, K.F., and Shammas, H.F.: Bilateral corneal perforations in Stevens-Johnson syndrome, Can. J. Ophthalmol. **18:**514, 1975.

135. Talal, N., Sylvester, R.A., Daniels, T.E., Greenspan, J.S., and Williams, R.C.: T and B lymphocytes in peripheral blood and tissue lesions in Sjögren's syndrome, J. Clin. Invest. **53:**180, 1974.

136. Thomas, C.I., Michel, B., Waisman, M., Levine, M., and Bean, S.: Treatment of shrinkage diseases of the conjunctiva, Ann. Ophthalmol. **6:**1289, 1974.

137. Uehara, M., Shigeo, O.: Patch test reactions to human dander in atopic dermatitis, Arch. Dermatol. **112:**951, 954, 1976.

138. Waltman, S.R., and Yarran, D.: Circulating autoantibodies in ocular pemphigoid, Am. J. Ophthalmol. **77:**891, 1974.

139. Wanscher, B., and Thorman, J.: Permanent anonychia after Stevens-Johnson syndrome, Arch. Dermatol. **113:**970, 1977.

140. Watson, P.G., and Hazelman, B.L.: The sclera and systemic disorders, Philadelphia, 1976, W.B. Saunders Co.

141. Weith, J., and Farkos, T.G.: Pseudotumor of the orbit as a presenting sign in Wegener's granulomatosis, Surv. Ophthalmol. **17:**106, 1970.

142. Williams, R.C., DeBoard, J.R., Mellbye, O.J., Messner, R.P., and Lindström, F.D.: Studies with T- and B-lymphocytes in patients with connective tissue diseases. J. Clin. Invest. **52:**283, 1973.

143. Williamson, J.: Keratoconjunctivitis sicca, histology of lacrimal gland, Br. J. Ophthalmol. **57:**852, 1973.

144. Wilson, F.M., Grayson, M., and Ellis, F.D.: Treatment of peripheral corneal ulcers by limbal conjunctivectomy, Br. J. Ophthalmol. **60:**713, 1976.

145. Wilson, F.M. II: Differential diagnosis of superior limbic keratoconjunctivitis and papillary keratoconjunctivitis associated with contact lenses. In Hughes, W.F., editor: The yearbook of ophthalmology, 1981, Chicago, 1981, Year Book Medical Publishers, Inc.

146. Wong, V.G., and Kirkpatrick, C.H.: Immune reconstitution in keratoconjunctivitis and superficial candidiasis: the role of immunocompetent lymphocyte transfusion and transfer factor, Arch. Ophthalmol. **92:**335, 1974.

147. Wright, P., and Fraunfelder, F.T.: Practolol induced oculomucocutaneous syndrome. In Leopold, I.H., and Burns, R.P., editors: Symposium on Ocular Therapy, vol. 9, New York, 1976, John Wiley & Sons, Inc.

148. Wybran, J., and Fudenberg, H.H.: Thymus-derived rosette-forming cells in various human disease states: cancer, lymphoma, bacterial and viral infections, and other diseases, J. Clin. Invest. **52:**1026, 1973.

149. Zion, V.M., Brackup, A.H., and Weingeist, S.: Relapsing polychondritis, erythema nodosum and sclerouveitis: a case report with anterior segment angiography, Surv. Ophthalmol. **19:** 107, 1974.

ADDITIONAL READING

Allansmith, M., Halin, G.S., and Simon, M.A: Tissue, tear and serum IgE concentrations in vernal conjunctivitis, Am. J. Ophthalmol. **81:**506, 1976.

Allansmith, M., and McClellan, B.H.: Immunoglobulins in the human cornea, Am. J. Ophthalmol. **80:**123, 1975.

Andersen, S.R., Jensen, O.A., Kristensen, E.B., and Norn, M.S.: Benign mucous membrane pemphigoid. III. Biopsy, Acta. Ophthalmol. **52:**455, 1974 1974.

Arbesman, C.E., Wypych, J.I., Reisman, R.E., and Beutner, E.H.: IgE levels in sera of patients with pemphigus or bullous pemphigoid, Arch. Dermatol. **110:**378, 1974.

Barker, C.F., and Billingham, R.E.: The lympatic status of hamster check pouch tissue in relation to its properties as a graft and as a graft site, J. Exp. Med. **133:**620, 1971.

Bean, S.F., Waisman, M., Michel, B., Thomas, C.E., Knox, J.M., and Levine, M.: Cicatricial pemphigoid, Arch Dermatol. **106:**195, 1972.

Eiferman, R.A., Carothers, D.J., and Yankeelov, J.A., Jr.: Peripheral rheumatoid ulceration and evidence for conjunctival collagenase production, Am. J. Ophthalmol. **87:**703, 1979.

Foster, C.S., and Duncan, J.: Randomized clinical trial of topically administered cromolyn sodium for vernal keratoconjunctivitis, Am. J. Ophthalmol. **90:**175, 1980.

Inomata, H., Smelser, G.K., and Polack, F.M.: Fine structure of regenerating endothelium and Descemet's membrane in normal and rejecting corneal grafts, Am. J. Ophthalmol. **70:**48, 1970.

Jones, B.R.: Allergy of the outer eye, Trans. Ophthalmol. Soc. U.K. **91:**441, 1971.

Kanai, A., and Polack, F.M.: Ultramicroscopic changes in the corneal graft stroma during early rejection, Invest. Ophthalmol. **10:**415, 1971.

Khodadoust, A.A.: The allograft rejection reaction: the leading cause of late failure of clinical corneal grafts. In Corneal graft failure, Ciba Found. Symp. **15:**151, 1973.

Korb, D.R., Allansmith, M.R., Greiner, J.V., Henriquez, A.S., Herman, J.P., Richmond, P.P., and Finnemore, V.M.: Biomicroscopy of papillae associated with hard contact lens wearing, Ophthalmology **88:**1132, 1981.

Maumanee, A.E.: Clinical patterns of corneal graft failure. In Corneal graft failure, Ciba Found. Symp. **15:**5, 1973.

Mondino, J.B., Brown, S.I., and Rabin, B.S.: Autoimmune phenomenon of the external eye, Am. Acad. Ophthalmol. Otolaryngol. **85:**801, 1978.

Norn, M.S., and Kristensen, E.B.: Benign mucous membrane pemphigoid. II. Cytology, Acta. Ophthalmol. **52:**282, 1974.

Penneys, N.S., Eaglstein, W.H., and Frost, P.: Management of pemphigus with gold compounds, Arch. Dermatol. **112:**185, 1976.

Pfister, R., and Murphy, G.E.: Corneal ulceration and perforation associated with Sjögren's syndrome, Arch. Ophthalmol. **98**:89, 1980.

Price, M.J., Morgan, J.F., Willis, W.E., and Wasan, S.: Tarsal conjunctival appearance in contact lens wearers, Contact Lens, p. 16, Jan./March 1982.

Rook, A., Wilkinson, D.S., and Ebling, F.J.G.: Textbook of dermatology, Oxford, Blackwell Scientific Publications, **2**:1182, 1968.

Rycroft, P.N.: Corneal graft membranes, Trans. Ophthalmol. Soc. U.K. **85**:317, 1963.

Tabbara, K.F.: Extralimbal Trantas' dots: report of a case, Am. Ophthalmol. **14**:458, 1982.

Ward, B., McCulley, J.P., and Segal, R.J.: Dermatologic reaction in Stevens-Johnson syndrome after ophthalmic anesthesia with proparacaine hydrochloride, Am. J. Ophthalmol. **86**:133, 1978.

Watson, P.G., McKay, D.A.R., Clemett, R.S., and Wilkinson, P.: Episcleritis (treatment), Br. J. Ophthalmol. **57**:866, 1973.

Wood, W.J., and Nicholson, D.H.: Corneal ring ulcer as the presenting manifestation of acute monocytic leukemia, Am. J. Ophthalmol. **76**:69, 1973.

15 Diseases of protein and amino acid metabolism

Corneal involvement in several amino acid abnormalities is illustrated in Table 15-1.

ALKAPTONURIA

One of the prominent clinical features of this autosomal recessive inborn error of metabolism is a characteristic bluish-gray or black pigmentation of the cartilaginous and fibrous tissues of the body known as *ochronosis*.[26] The disease affects individuals between the ages of 20 and 40 years. Homogentisic acid is excreted in the urine as a result of the deficiency of homogentisic acid oxidase, an enzyme that is normally present in the liver and kidneys. This enzyme normally converts homogentisic acid to maleylacetoacetic acid. Thus the deficiency of homogentisic acid oxidase causes an accumulation of homogentisic acid, a product of phenylalanine and tyrosine metabolism. The oxidation of homogentisic acid produces a black-brown polymer that is closely related to melanin and may account for pigmentation of the tissues.

Ochronotic pigment is seen in light microscopy as amber globules or fiberlike structures in the cornea, conjunctiva, and sclera combined with degenerated collagen. Ultrastructurally, most of the pigment is extracellular, partly altering the fibrocytes and collagen.[21] The tissues most often affected are the cartilaginous tissues, ligaments, tendons, and degenerated collagen and elastic fibers.

Ultrastructurally the pigment appears to be similar to melanin, but the chemical behavior is different and seems similar to elastin.[21]

Clinitest reagent tablets and Benedict's sugar reagent[26] are used for simple and ready tests on the urine to detect homogentisic acid. A more sophisticated and complicated test for quantitative determination of this acid is achieved by spectrofluorometric measurements.

Table 15-1. Corneal involvement in amino acid abnormalities

Disease	Deficiency	Corneal involvement
Tyrosine aminotransferase deficiency	Aminotransferase Paraphenylhydroxypyruvate oxidase	Tyrosine crystals in epithelium Dendriform figure in epithelium Sunburst ulcer
Oculocerebrorenal (Lowe's) syndrome	Unknown	Cloudy cornea (may be caused by increased intraocular pressure)
Hypophosphatasia	Alkaline phosphatase	Band keratopathy
Familial dysautonomia (Riley-Day syndrome)	Dopamine β-hydroxylase	Alacrima Corneal ulcers Decreased corneal sensation
Cystinosis	Unknown	Corneal crystals
Alkaptonuria	Homogentisic acid oxidase	"Melanin-like deposits" in limbal area
Porphyria		Keratomalacia Crystals in cornea (rare)

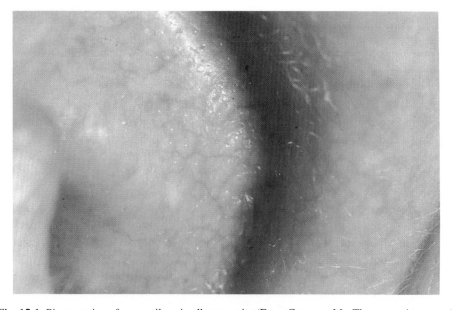

Fig. 15-1. Pigmentation of ear cartilage in alkaptonuria. (From Grayson, M.: The cornea in systemic disease. In Duane, T.D. [ed.]: Clinical Ophthalmology. Hagerstown, Md.: Harper & Row, 1976, vol. 4, chap. 15.)

Systemic involvement

One can see pigmentation of cartilages of the ears (Fig. 15-1), nose, cerumen, and urine in alkaptonuria.[18] Degenerative arthropathy of the spine and large joints, cardiac disease, and genitourinary stones are not uncommon findings. The urine at times darkens on standing as a result of the oxidation of homogentisic acid; however, in the presence of reducing agents or if the urine has an acid pH, darkening does not occur.

Ocular involvement

Ocular pigmentation occurs in the interpalpebral fissure zone. The conjunctiva, episclera, sclera, and tendons of the horizontal recti are pigmented with this material (Fig. 15-2). In addition, the cornea immediately inside the limbus may exhibit areas of pigmentation. The pigment is usually of a brownish-black nature and is located in the area of Bowman's layer and deep epithelium. Pigmentation of the tarsal plates and lid may also be seen.

CYSTINOSIS (INFANTILE NEPHROPATHIC CYSTINOSIS, FANCONI'S DISEASE, DE TONI-FANCONI-LIGNAC DISEASE)

This disorder is characterized primarily by the intracellular deposition of crystalline cystine in the reticuloendothelial cells of the bone marrow, liver, spleen, and lymphatic system. Crystal deposits are also found in the kidney.[29, 41] The cystine can be found in the leukocytes and cultured fibroblasts, but in these instances the cystine has an amorphous and noncrystalline appearance.

Cystine and cysteine levels in plasma are not elevated, but intracellular concentra-

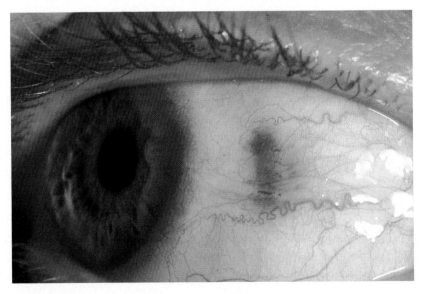

Fig. 15-2. Pigmentation of lateral rectus tendon (alkaptonuria). (From Grayson, M.: The cornea in systemic disease. In Duane, T.D. [ed.]: Clinical Ophthalmology. Hagerstown, Md.: Harper & Row, 1976, vol. 4, chap. 15.)

tions of cysteine are elevated in the leukocytes, macrophages, and fibroblasts.[23] The cystine is compartmentalized within lipid-storing membranes, suggesting localization in lysosomes.[40]

Systemic involvement

Growth retardation, decreased pigmentation of skin and hair, rickets, and progressive renal failure occur in Fanconi's syndrome[36]; the specific enzyme defect is not known.

Ocular involvement

Crystals are found in the cornea in the following conditions (Table 15-1):
Lipid disturbances
    Schnyder's crystalline dystrophy
    Lecithin cholesterol–acyltransferase deficiency
    Tangier disease
    Secondary lipid keratopathy
Calcium disturbances
    Band keratopathy
Protein disturbances
    Cystinosis
      Infantile
      Adolescent
      Adult
    Gout
    Tyrosinosis
    Multiple myeloma and other dysproteinemias
    Porphyria
Unknown
    Marginal crystalline dystrophy of Bietti

These glistening, polychromatic, needlelike to rectangular corneal crystals are distributed throughout the anterior stroma with a slight increase in concentration peripherally (Fig. 15-3). The corneal crystals first appear at the age of 6 to 15 months. These crystals may cause a rather intense photophobia but do not actually decrease the vision. In addition to being found in the cornea, the crystals occur in the conjunctiva,[48] sclera, aqueous humor, uvea, extraocular muscles, and retinal pigment epithelium.[47] The retinal pigmentary changes may precede the changes found in the cornea or conjunctiva and rarely may be seen as early as the fifth week of life.[42] The retinopathy is one of the patchy depigmented areas alternating irregularly with clumped pigmented regions[47] (Fig. 15-4). The electroretinogram may be abnormal, as is the fluorescein angiogram.

A conjunctival biopsy specimen may be taken fairly easily and should be fixed or stored in absolute ethanol. The specimen can be examined under polarized light, without staining, for detection of typical crystals, or it can be analyzed for cystine content[48] (Fig. 15-5).

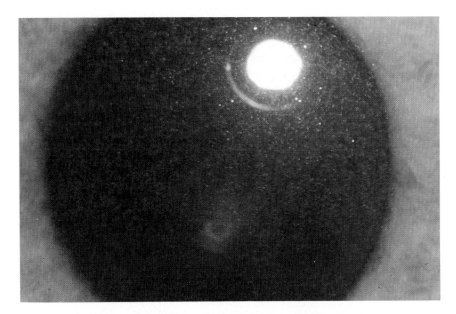

Fig. 15-3. Corneal crystals in cystinosis.

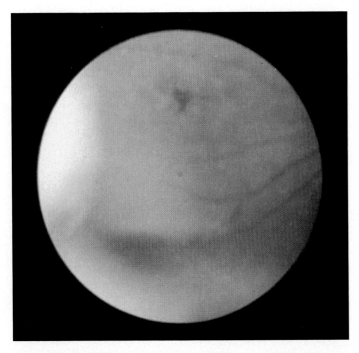

Fig. 15-4. Patchy areas of depigmentation irregularly spaced with clumped retinal pigmentation in cystinosis. (From Grayson, M.: The cornea in systemic disease. In Duane, T.D. [ed.]: Clinical Ophthalmology. Hagerstown, Md.: Harper & Row, 1976, vol. 4, chap. 15.)

Infantile cystinosis

The infantile form of cystinosis is often fatal, but recently renal transplant has been successful in prolonging life, although not in improving the cystine storage.

Two other forms[16] of cystinosis are an adult benign form and an adolescent form.[49]

Adult cystinosis

In the adult form of cystinosis the patients are in good health. They are usually free of symptoms except perhaps for photophobia. There are no systemic problems or retinopathy, and the renal function is normal. The age of onset is usually from the teen years to 50 years of age. There is no pattern of inheritance, although it might be recessive.

Adolescent cystinosis

Adolescent cystinosis usually is noted in the teens and exhibits varying combinations of rickets, retinopathy, renal failure, and conjunctival and corneal crystals. No growth impediment or hypopigmentation occurs. Adolescent cystinosis is probably an autosomal recessive disease.[41]

Corneal conjunctival crystals occur and are distributed in the same manner as in the infantile form of cystinosis. The crystals are also needlelike or rectangular. In adolescent cystinosis varying combinations of corneal conjunctival crystals with rickets and renal failure occur. Rarely one may see retinopathy, but neither growth retardation nor systemic hypopigmentation problems occur.

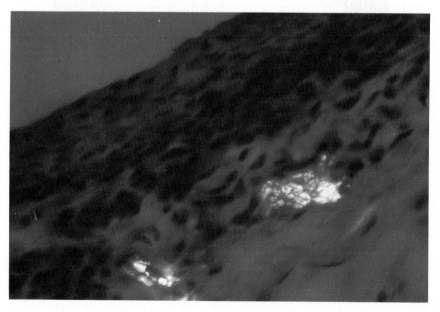

Fig. 15-5. Typical crystals seen with polarized light in biopsy specimen of conjunctiva (cystinosis).

GOUT AND URATE KERATOPATHY

Gout can be an insidious disease. In the young adult or middle-aged patient no greater symptom picture may occur than nonspecific manifestations such as myositis and vague knee or elbow pains. Of course, the disease can be much more serious than this; hidden under the joint pain one may find hyperuricemia; uricosuria; vascular disease, including hypertension; hyperlipidemia; cerebral vascular disease; liver disease; diabetes; and renal calculi. No relationship exists between the intensity of overt gout attacks and the degree of hyperuricemia, but the diagnosis cannot be made unless the serum uric acid level is elevated.

Ocular involvement

Conjunctival hyperemia can be severe (Fig. 15-6). In addition, one may find a scanty foaming discharge along the lid margins; with this symptom the patient complains of photophobia, discomfort, and pain.

Monosodium urate crystals are deposited in superficial stroma and epithelium of the conjunctiva and cornea.[43] This deposition may occur in cases of hyperuricemia with or without gouty symptoms or in cases without hyperuricemia or gout (cornea urica). In the latter instance, it would appear that there is a local disturbance of uric acid metabolism. The corneal disease may be accompanied by a band-shaped keratopathy; instead of being the whitish-gray lesion as seen with calcium deposition, the band keratopathy is brown (Fig. 15-7) and may result in ulceration of the epithelium. In addition, the urate crystals may be multicolored, punctate or needlelike, and located in the stroma.

Text continued on p. 452.

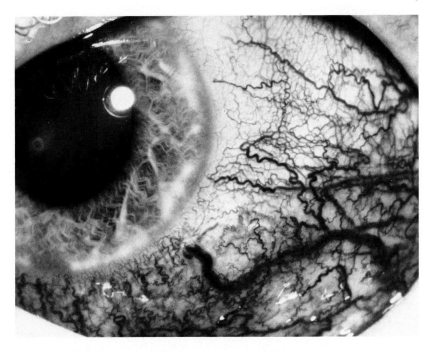

Fig. 15-6. Severe hyperemia of conjunctiva and episclera seen in gout.

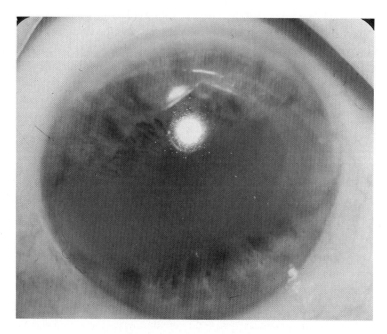

Fig. 15-7. Urate band keratopathy (gout).

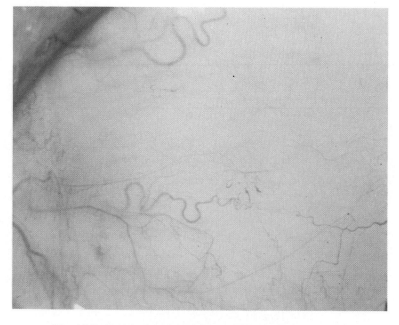

Fig. 15-8. Conjunctival vessel tortuosity in multiple myeloma.

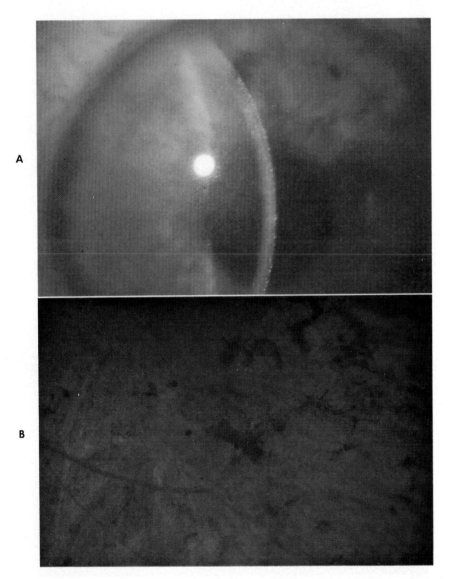

Fig. 15-9. Multiple myeloma. **A,** Corneal crystals in epithelium and stromal haze **B,** Retinal crystals.

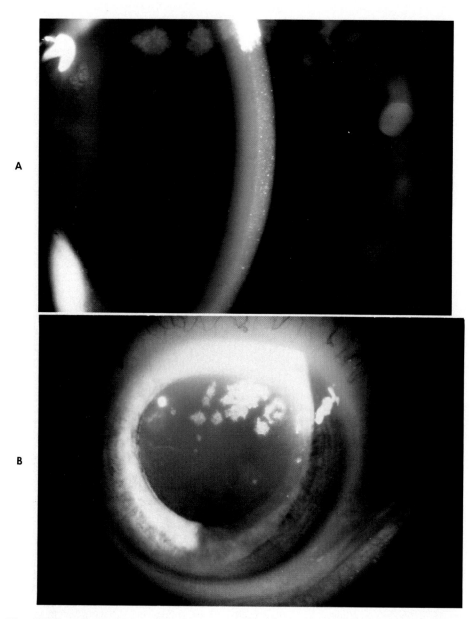

Fig. 15-10. A, Appearance of subepithelial glistening deposits. **B,** Large geographic crystalline patches involving full thickness of cornea of right eye. (From Miller, K.H., et al.: Ophthalmology **87:**944, 1980.)

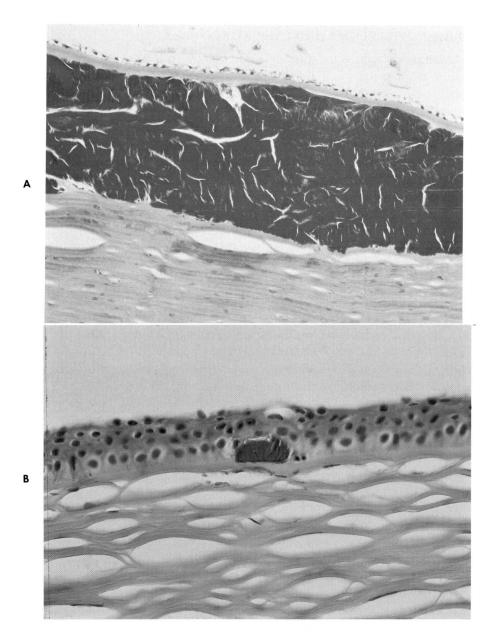

Fig. 15-11. A, Large deposits in posterior corneal stroma. Descemet's membrane and endothelium are normal. (Masson's trichrome, original magnification × 400.) **B,** Subepithelial corneal deposit and surrounding normal epithelium, Bowman's membrane, and stroma. (Van der Grift, original magnification × 100.) (From Miller, K.H. et al.: Ophthalmology **87:**944, 1980.)

These may cause irritation with vascularization. The uric acid crystals in the cornea have been demonstrated with the electron microscope.

MULTIPLE MYELOMA AND DYSPROTEINEMIAS

Multiple myeloma is a disease associated with the proliferation of abnormal plasma cells in the bone marrow.[33] The disease results in bone pain, depression of bone elements, hypercalcemia, uremia, paramyloidosis, and immunologic abnormalities; it usually becomes evident between the ages of 50 and 70 years.

Ocular involvement

Lytic lesions of the orbital bone, nerve palsies, papilledema, and visual field defects occur in multiple myeloma. In addition, one may find infiltration of adnexal tissue by myeloma cells, proteinaceous cysts of the nonpigmented ciliary epithelium, and hyperviscosity retinopathy.

A marked tortuosity of the conjunctival vessels may occur with sludging of circulation in the conjunctival blood vessels resulting from increased blood viscosity (Fig. 15-8).

Corneal crystal changes are seen.[34] These fine, punctate or needlelike, multicolored crystals occur in the corneal epithelium[1]; in addition, a stromal haze is noted (Fig. 15-9, A). The crystals, which may also be seen in the conjunctiva and in the retina (Fig. 15-9, B) may consist of abnormal immunoglobulins. The polychromatic corneal crystals in the dysproteinemia states are found within the cytoplasm of the keratocytes.[2] Histochemical studies of the corneal crystals attest to their proteinaceous state. Often patients afflicted with this problem exhibit a monoclonal gammopathy with an elevated IgG level and increased kappa light chains. Immunoperoxidase stains have been most strongly positive for IgG and also for IgA kappa and lambda light chains in certain cases of immune-complex diseases.[30] Neoplastic processes such as Hodgkin's and lymphoproliferative diseases are not infrequently found in such patients. In cases of benign monoclonal gammopathy, corneal crystals have been found in the posterior cornea and in the epithelium[38] (Figs. 15-10 and 15-11).

A polychromatic, dustlike deposition of copper occurs in Descemet's membrane of the central cornea with sparing of the peripheral cornea. This deposition also occurs in the anterior lens capsule[27] when the myeloma tracings have shown copper binding properties.

"Dystrophic" corneal changes have been reported in multiple myeloma, Waldenström's macroglobulinemia, and cryoglobulinemia.[15,32] These dystrophic changes appear as reticulated and undulating patterns of opacification in the posterior stroma.[32] Patches of myeloma and plasma cells may be deposited on the endothelium as well as in almost all ocular tissues; in addition, a calcific band keratopathy may result from the hypercalcemia in multiple myeloma.

AMYLOIDOSIS

Amyloidosis occurs as a primary or secondary phenomenon. Secondary amyloid disease may occur as a localized or systemic condition. Secondary generalized amyloidosis does not usually cause an ophthalmic problem. The primary form of the disease may also be divided into a primary localized amyloidosis and a primary systemic amyloidosis.

Amyloid stains with hematoxylin and eosin stain and is eosinophilic and hyaline in appearance. It is PAS positive and stains mahogany brown with iodine, changing to blue with the addition of sulfuric acid. Amyloid stains brown with Congo red (Fig. 11-18) and exhibits dichroism with polarized light (Fig. 11-19). After staining with Congo red, the color of the amyloid preparation varies from red to green with the rotation of the polarizing filters. Birefringence is noted with polarized light. Metachromasia occurs; that is, staining with methylene blue demonstrates a purple rather than the blue color of the stain. Amyloid fluoresces yellow-green with thioflavine T. By electron microscopy, it exhibits filaments that are 80 Å in length. Amyloid consists of immunoglobulins or their light chains.

Primary localized amyloidosis

Primary localized amyloidosis can affect the bulbar or palpebral conjunctiva, Tenon's capsule, tarsus, limbus, lacrimal gland, or orbit.[25] The conjunctival involvement is usually subepithelial; the cornea may be involved.[4, 13] This condition may appear as tapioca-like white nodules or as gelatinous droplike corneal excrescences.[14, 31, 35] In addition, lattice corneal dystrophy can be classified as a special type of primary localized amyloidosis of the cornea.[29, 44]

Primary systemic amyloidosis

Primary systemic amyloidosis may exhibit purpuric and papillary lesions of the eyelids and conjunctiva. Primary systemic amyloidosis is sometimes familial and autosomal dominant; the findings are the same as those seen in the nonfamilial form, but vitreous veils and opacities and retinal periphlebitis are more common.[22]

Extensive systemic involvement of the muscles, skin, nerves, and blood vessels is seen. Ocular involvement includes ptosis, pupillary abnormalities, hemorrhages into the conjunctiva, external ocular movement involvement, retinal perivasculitis, glaucoma, neuroparalytic keratitis, and vitreous opacities.[10, 11]

Sporadic reports suggest that rare cases exhibiting lattice dystrophy may involve a familial primary systemic amyloidosis.[24] These individuals develop lattice dystrophy in early adulthood and later develop skin changes, cranial nerve palsy, peripheral neuropathy, and visceral complaints. The lattice dystrophy with systemic involvement is milder with regard to visual loss but more extensive in that it extends to the corneal periphery without the peripheral clear interval as seen in the primary lattice dystrophy.

Secondary localized amyloidosis

Secondary localized amyloidosis of the anterior segment may occur after a chronic ocular systemic disorder. Sarcoidosis, lipid proteinosis (Urbach-Wiethe disease), retrolental fibroplasia, phlyctenular disease, trachoma, interstitial keratitis, uveitis, glaucoma, and trauma are all possible etiologic factors in secondary localized amyloidosis. The cornea and the conjunctival lid may become involved. Such amyloid deposits in secondary amyloidosis are usually insignificant clinically and are most often found only on histologic examination.

Conjunctival inflammation and amyloidosis of the upper tarsal conjunctiva have been reported in Churg-Strauss syndrome.[28] These lesions are yellow, waxy, and nodular. Churg-Strauss syndrome is a severe multisystem angiitis and allergic granulomatosis. Bronchial asthma, fever, and eosinophilia are also a part of the syndrome. This entity belongs to the polyarteritis group of systemic necrotizing vasculitides.[9]

Secondary systemic amyloidosis

Secondary systemic amyloidosis for all practical purposes does not involve the eye. About 10% of patients with multiple myeloma develop amyloidosis.

RICHNER-HANHART SYNDROME (TRYOSINEMIA TYPE 2)

In this condition, also called tyrosinosis, there is an increase in serum tyrosine[3] and urinary tyrosine. Hyperkeratotic lesions of the skin are limited to the palms, soles, and elbows[17] (Fig. 15-12). Current research suggests that tyrosine may cause these lesions by its direct action on lysosomal membranes, thereby resulting in a release of lysosomal enzymes. Occasionally mental retardation occurs; it is believed that the disease is transmitted as an autosomal recessive trait. Tyrosinemia is associated with a deficiency of soluble tyrosine aminotransferase or parahydroxyphenylpyruvate hydroxylase.[5]

Ocular involvement

The patient exhibits marked photophobia and tearing, subcapsular lens opacities, conjunctival thickening, and an extensive papillary hypertrophy of the tarsal conjunctiva.

It is interesting that corneal opacification occurs with intraepithelial and subepithelial opacities and ulceration.[14, 37, 39] The corneal lesions may be dendritic in nature or superficial with the characteristic sunburst type of configuration (Fig. 15-13) perhaps as a result of the deposition of tyrosine crystals. The lesion may heal spontaneously in months to years.

The following are distinctive features of the pseudodendrite: (1) the lesions in tyrosinemia II are thick and plaquelike; (2) the dendritic figure does not exhibit the fine and delicate club-shaped edges seen in herpetic dendritic keratitis; rather the lesions resemble more the dendritic pattern seen with herpes zoster; and (3) the lesions are bilateral, whereas bilateral herpetic keratitis is quite rare. It should be remembered that the most consistent finding of tyrosinemia type II is the pseudodendrite, and it is here that the alert ophthalmologist can aid the pediatrician in making a proper assessment of the problem.[6]

Tyrosine-fed rats develop corneal disease that mimics that found in the human metabolic disorder of tyrosinosis. Crystals in the cornea appear as negative images by electron microscopy. The crystals are limited to the epithelial areas. It is hypothesized that the crystals are tyrosines and crystal growth in cells initiates lesions and subsequent formation.

Treatment

Corticosteroids prevent the tyrosine-induced corneal opacification, edema, and vascularization; it is suggested that this change in keratopathy results from stim-

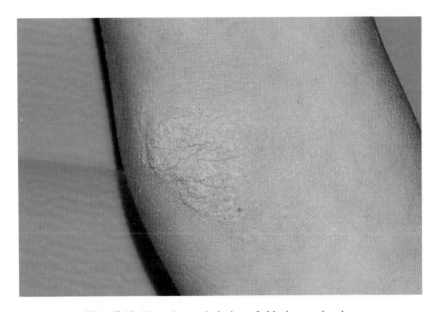

Fig. 15-12. Hyperkeratotic lesion of skin in tyrosinosis.

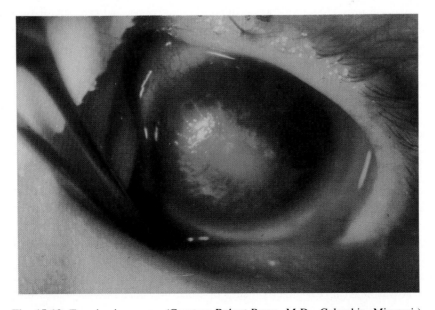

Fig. 15-13. Tyrosine in cornea. (Courtesy Robert Burns, M.D., Columbia, Missouri.)

ulation of hepatic production of tyrosine aminotransferase.

A low-tyrosine and low-phenylalanine diet is the basis of therapy for this disease. After the skin and eye manifestations have been brought under control, the diet can be liberalized.

Differential diagnosis

Tyrosine increases of the extent seen in this syndrome occur in three conditions:
1. Tyrosinemia I
2. Tyrosinemia II
3. Neonatal tyrosinemia

In neonatal tyrosinemia the problem is transient, especially in those born prematurely. It is usually associated with some lethargy but no skin or eye involvement. Neonatal tyrosinemia responds well to ascorbic acid therapy.

Tyrosinemia I is a rare metabolic defect of recessive inheritance with enlargement of the spleen, liver cirrhosis, fever, renal glycosuria, aminoaciduria, phosphaturia, and renal rickets. Tyrosine and methionine are increased in the blood, and liver function tests are abnormal. These patients do not have the characteristic skin and eye lesions of tyrosinemia II.

In Richner-Hanhart syndrome (tyrosinemia II) a deficiency of soluble tyrosine aminotransferase converts tyrosine to parahydroxyphenylpyruvic acid.

WILSON'S HEPATOLENTICULAR DEGENERATION

Wilson's disease is characterized by progressive neurologic impairment, ataxia, hepatosplenomegaly, and cirrhosis of the liver. Copper is deposited in almost all body tissues, especially the liver, basal ganglia of the brain, kidney, and cornea. Biochemical changes occur, including reduction in both serum copper and ceruloplasmin, with a rise in copper excretion. The ceruloplasmin binds copper, but since the ceruloplasmin is deficient, the copper is free to go into the tissues, causing the blood level of copper to fall.

The disease is usually transmitted as an autosomal recessive trait. The enzyme defect is essentially unknown.

Ocular involvement

The Kayser-Fleischer copper ring, a characteristic finding in Wilson's disease, occurs in the corneal periphery and is usually yellow-brown but may be red, blue, green, or a mixture of any of these colors. The Kayser-Fleischer ring is about 1 to 3 mm in width and extends to the limbus without a lucid interval except when a posterior embryotoxon is present (Fig. 15-14). In this instance, the interval is to be expected, since Descemet's membrane and the ring of Schwalbe are placed more anteriorly. The copper is deposited at the level of the posterior portion of Descemet's membrane.[8, 19] The Kayser-Fleischer ring is often absent in patients younger than 10 years of age. In addition to involvement of Descemet's membrane, one may find anterior subcapsular sunflower cataracts.

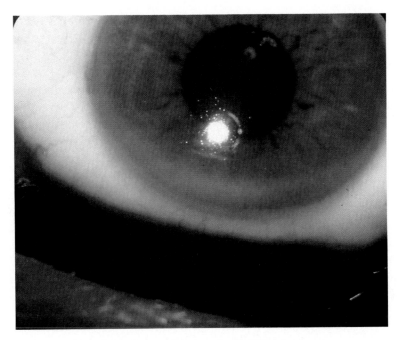

Fig. 15-14. Kayser-Fleischer ring in Wilson's disease.

Treatment

Only by treatment with chelating agents and a highly restricted copper intake can patients be kept in negative copper balance; under these circumstances clinical improvement usually occurs.[46]

Differential diagnosis

Pigmented corneal rings clinically identical to Kayser-Fleischer rings have been reported in primary biliary cirrhosis, progressive intrahepatic cholestasis of childhood, and chronic active hepatitis.[12] These diseases have in common elevated levels of copper in the blood, urine, and liver. Only Wilson's disease has subnormal levels of ceruloplasmin. The combination of pigmented corneal rings in hepatic diseases therefore is not pathognomonic of Wilson's disease. Kayser-Fleischer rings in combination with neurologic disease with or without evidence of hepatic disease, however, remains suggestive of Wilson's disease (Fig. 15-14).

Wilson's disease is also discussed in Chapter 22.

LOWE'S OCULOCEREBRORENAL SYNDROME[20]

This problem includes congenital bilateral cataracts, nystagmus, glaucoma, oculodigital sign of Franceshetti, hypotonia, areflexia, renal tubular acidosis, vitamin D–resistant rickets, proteinurea, and aminoaciduria. Aminoaciduria is seen in a number of corneal problems (Table 15-1). Most of the patients with Lowe's syndrome have been fair-haired boys; however, the disease has now been described in four females and one black individual. The disease is often transmitted as a sex-linked recessive trait; however, this is not a consistent finding.

Ocular involvement

A mild haze occurs in the cornea; however, this may be associated with glaucoma. The female carrier may show white, punctate, anterior and posterior lens opacities. Rubella can cause both cataract and glaucoma but usually not together in the same patient. It may be wise to check the mother of a boy with cataracts and glaucoma.

PORPHYRIA (Table 15-2)
Congenital erythropoietic porphyria

This type of porphyria is rather rare. It has its onset at birth or in infancy and is recognized by the excretion of red-colored urine accompanied by hemolytic anemia, splenomegaly, and photosensitivity causing bullous eruptions of skin. Optic nerve atrophy and retinal hemorrhages are found on fundus examination.

Conjunctival and scleral necrosis, depigmentation of the eyelids, and corneal scarring occur. The metabolic defect does not seem to be entirely worked out.

Porphyria variegata

This form of porphyria is transmitted as an autosomal dominant trait and is seen among the Afrikaner community of South Africa. The clinical signs are similar to the congenital type. In addition to the photosensitivity, patients with porphyria variegata suffer from severe attacks of abdominal pain and associated neurologic crisis that may be associated with barbiturates and sulfonamides.

The eye may be involved through conjunctival and scleral necrosis and corneal scarring in addition to optic neuritis, optic atrophy, and retinal hemorrhaging.

Acute intermittent porphyria

Acute intermittent porphyria is the only disorder of porphyrin metabolism not associated with cutaneous sensitivity. In this particular problem the major clinical signs are abdominal pain, sensual neuropathy, peripheral neuropathy, and hypertension. The ocular signs include retinal edema and occasionally hemorrhage, papilledema, and optic atrophy.

Cases of porphyria that manifest ulcers of the sclera are rare; the ulcers usually occur in the horizontal meridian, extending to the limbus and peripheral corneal areas. The progress of these ulcers is rather slow; however, they may perforate. They are bilateral and show pink fluorescence with ultraviolet light.

The cornea may reveal crystals in Bowman's layer[7] and deep stromal opacification. The nature of these crystals is unknown.

PHENYLKETONURIA (PHENYLPYRUVIC OLIGOPHRENIA)

Phenylketonuria is usually diagnosed soon after birth. Nonspecific spotty corneal opacities with other ocular signs such as cataracts, photophobia, partial albinism, mental retardation, and extrapyramidal neurologic signs are seen. In addition, one can see a

Table 15-2. Porphyria

Type	Systemic involvement	Urine and stool	Scleromalacia	Cornea
Adults				
Acute intermittent porphyria (Swedish type)	After puberty Hyperpigmentation "Acute abdomen" Central nervous system Excess of hepatic enzyme, δ-aminolevulinic synthetase, leading to porphyria precursors	Excretion in urine of precursor of porphyria	None	None
Porphyria variegata (South African type)	Seen at puberty May show acute symptoms Skin changes same as in cutanea tarda variety	High level of porphyria in stool	Rare	Not reported
Porphyria cutanea tarda symptomatica*	Seen in forties Excessive alcohol intake Bullae produced by trauma or light Increased serum ion due to lack of transferrin Hyperpigmentation Bushy eyebrows Lacrimal obstruction[45] Cicatricial ectropion[45]	High level of porphyria in urine Little or no increase in stool porphyria	Rare Usually in horizontal meridian Melting may extend into cornea May show brawny scleritis in other quadrants	Two cases revealed white-tan nonrefractive crystals in Bowman's layer at peripheral cornea Opacification of Bowman's layer Lamella of opacification in deep stroma
Children				
Congenital erythropoietic porphyria	Infancy and childhood Itching and swelling of skin after light exposure, which leads to blisters and hydroa aestivale Splenomegaly Skin discoloration Loss of hair Some red blood cells may fluoresce	Burgundy red urine	Ulcers of sclera (rare)	Leukoma (rare)

*Area of pink fluorescence with ultraviolet light around edges of the scleral ulcer.

diffuse hypopigmentation of the skin, very light blue eyes, and light-colored hair and irides, which are said to be caused by the lack of the enzyme, L-phenylalanine hydroxylase.

Phenylketonuria is transmitted as an autosomal recessive trait.

The biochemical defects may result in a variety of neurologic abnormalities, including mental retardation and seizures. Eczema is found in some cases, and photophobia and photosensitivity are secondary complicating factors.

REFERENCES

1. Baker, T.R., and Spencer, W.H.: Ocular findings in multiple myeloma: a report of two cases, Arch. Ophthalmol. **91**:110, 1974.
2. Barr, C.C., Gelender, H., and Font, R.: Corneal crystalline deposits associated with dysproteinemia: report of two cases and review of literature, Arch. Ophthalmol. **98**:884, 1980.
3. Bienfang, D.C., Kuwabara, T., and Pueschel, S.M.: The Richner-Hanhart syndrome: report of a case with associated tyrosinemia, Arch. Ophthalmol. **94**:1133, 1976.
4. Brownstein, M.H., Elliott, R., and Helwig, E.B.: Ophthalmologic aspects of amyloidosis, Am. J. Ophthalmol. **69**:423, 1970.
5. Burns, R.P.: Soluble tyrosine aminotransferase deficiency: an unusual cause of corneal ulcers, Am. J. Ophthalmol. **73**:400, 1972.
6. Charlton, K.H., Binder, P.S., Wozniak, L., and Digby, J.D.: Pseudodendritic keratitis and systemic tyrosinemia, Ophthalmology **88**:355, 1981.
7. Chumbley, L.C.: Scleral involvement in symptomatic porphyria, Am. J. Ophthalmol. **84**:729, 1977.
8. Ellis, P.P.: Ocular deposition of copper in hypercupremia, Am. J. Ophthalmol. **68**:423, 1969.
9. Fauci, A.S., Haynes, B.F., and Katz, P.: The spectrum of vasculitis: clinical, pathologic, immunologic, and therapeutic considerations, Ann. Intern. Med. **89**:660, 1978.
10. Ferry, A.P., and Lieberman, T.W.: Bilateral amyloidosis of the vitreous body: report of a case without systemic or familial involvement, Arch. Ophthalmol. **94**:982, 1976.
11. Fishman, R.S., and Sunderman, F.W.: Band keratopathy in gout, Arch. Ophthalmol. **75**:367, 1967.
12. Fleming, C.R., Dickson, E.R., Wahner, H.W., Hollenhorst, R.W., and McCall, J.T.: Pigmented corneal rings in non-Wilsonian liver disease, Ann. Intern. Med. **86**:285, 1977.
13. Garner, A.: Amyloidosis of the cornea, Br. J. Ophthalmol. **53**:73, 1969.
14. Gipson, I.K., Burns, R.P., and Wolfe-Lande, J.D.: Crystals in corneal epithelial lesions of tyrosine-fed rats, Invest. Ophthalmol. **14**:937, 1975.
15. Gloor, B.: Diffuse corneal degeneration in case of Waldenström's macroglobulinemia, Ophthalmologica **155**:449, 1968.
16. Goldman, H., Scriver, C.K., Aaron, K., Delvin, E., and Canlos, Z.: Adolescent cystinosis: comparison with infantile and adult forms, Pediatrics **47**:979, 1971.
17. Goldsmith, L.A., and Reed, J.: Tyrosine-induced eye and skin lesions: a treatable genetic disease, JAMA **236**:382, 1976.
18. Grayson, M., and Keates, R.H.: Manual of diseases of the cornea, Boston, 1969, Little, Brown & Co.
19. Johnson, B.L.: Ultrastructure of the Kayser-Fleischer ring, Am. J. Ophthalmol. **76**:455, 1973.
20. Johnson, B.L., and Hiles, D.A.: Ocular pathology of Lowe's syndrome in a female infant, J. Pediatr. Ophthalmol. **13**:204, 1976.
21. Kampik, A., Sani, J.N., and Green, W.R.: Ocular ochronosis: clinicopathological, histochemical and ultrastructural studies, Arch. Ophthalmol. **98**:1441, 1980.
22. Kaufman, H.E., and Thomas, I.B.: Vitreous opacities diagnostic of familial primary amyloidosis, N. Engl. J. Med. **261**:1267, 1959.
23. Kenyon, K.R., and Sensenbrenner, J.A.: Electron microscopy of cornea and conjunctiva in childhood cystinosis, Am. J. Ophthalmol. **78**:68, 1974.
24. Kirk, H.Q., Rabb, M., Hattenhauer, J., and Smith, R.: Primary familial amyloidosis of the cornea, Trans. Am. Acad. Ophthalmol. Otolaryngol. **77**:411, 1973.
25. Knowles, D.M., II, Jakobiec, F.A., Rosen, M., and Howard, G.: Amyloidosis of the orbit and adnexae, Surv. Ophthalmol. **19**:367, 1975.
26. La Du, D.B.: Alkaptonuria. In Stanburg, J.B., Wyngaarden, J.B., and Fredrickson, D.S., editors: The metabolic basis of inherited disease, ed. 3, New York, 1972, McGraw-Hill Book Co.
27. Lewis, R.A., Falls, H.F., and Troyer, D.O.: Ocular manifestations of hypercupremia associated with multiple myeloma, Arch. Ophthalmol. **93**:1050, 1975.

28. Meisler, D.M., Stock, L.E., Wertz, R.D., et al.: Conjunctival inflammation and amyloidosis in allergic granulomatosis and angiitis (Churg-Strauss syndrome), Am. J. Ophthalmol. **91:**216, 1981.

29. Meretoja, J.: Comparative histopathological and clinical findings in eyes with lattice corneal dystrophy of two different types, Ophthalmologica **165:**15, 1972.

30. Miller, K.H., Green, W.R., Stark, W.J., et al.: Immunoprotein deposition in the cornea, Ophthalmology **87:**944, 1980.

31. Nagataki, S., Tanishima, T., and Sakimoto, T.: A case of primary gelatinous drop-like corneal dystrophy, Jpn. J. Ophthalmol. **16:**107, 1972.

32. Oglesby, R.B.: Corneal opacities in a patient with cryoglobulinemia and reticulohistiocytosis, Arch. Ophthalmol. **65:**63, 1961.

33. Orellana, J., and Friedman, A.H.: Ocular manifestations of multiple myeloma, Waldenström's macroglobulinemia and benign monoclonal gammopathy, Surv. Ophthalmol. **26:**3, Nov./Dec., 1981.

34. Pinkerton, R.M.H., and Robertson, D.M.: Corneal and conjunctival changes in dysproteinemia, Invest. Ophthalmol. **8:**357, 1969.

35. Ramsey, M.S., and Fine, B.S.: Localized corneal amyloidosis: case report with electromicroscopic findings, Am. J. Ophthalmol. **75:**560, 1972.

36. Read, J., Goldberg, M.F., Fishman, G., and Rosenthal, I.: Neophrotic cystinosis, Am. J. Ophthalmol. **76:**791, 1971.

37. Richner-Hanhardt syndrome: case report with associated tyrosinemia, Arch. Ophthalmol. **94:**1133, 1976.

38. Rodrigues, M.M., Krachmer, J.H., Miller, S.D., et al.: Posterior corneal crystalline deposits in benign monoclonal gammopathy: a clinicopathologic case report, Arch. Ophthalmol. **97:**124, 1979.

39. Sandberg, H.O.: Bilateral keratopathy in tyrosinosis, Acta Ophthalmol. **53:**760, 1975.

40. Sanderson, P.O., Kuwabara, T., Stark, W.J., Wong, V.G., and Collins, E.M.: Cystinosis: a clinical, histopathologic, and ultrastructural study, Arch. Ophthalmol. **91:**270, 1974.

41. Schneider, J.A., and Seegmiller, J.E.: Cystinosis and Fanconi syndrome. In Stanburg, J.B., Wyngaarden, J.B., and Fredrickson, D.S., editors: The metabolic basis of inherited disease, ed. 3, New York, 1972, McGraw-Hill Book Co.

42. Schneider, J.A., Wong, V.G., and Seegmiller, J.E.: The early diagnosis of cystinosis, J. Pediatr. **74:**114, 1969.

43. Slansky, H.H., and Kuwabara, T.: Intranuclear urate crystals in corneal epithelium, Arch. Ophthalmol. **80:**338, 1968.

44. Smith, M.E., and Zimmerman, L.E.: Amyloid in corneal dystrophies: differentiation of lattice from granular and macular dystrophies, Arch. Ophthalmol. **79:**407, 1968.

45. Sober, A.J., Grove, A.S., Jr., and Muhlbauer, J.E.: Cicatricial ectropion and lacrimal obstruction associated with sclerodermoid variant of porphyria cutanea tarda, Am. J. Ophthalmol. **91:**400, 1981.

46. Strickland, G.T., Blackwell, Q.T., and Watten, R.H.: Metabolic studies in Wilson's disease: evaluation of efficiency of chelating therapy in respect to copper metabolism, Am. J. Med. **51:**31, 1971.

47. Wong, V.G., Lietman, P.S., and Seegmiller, J.E.: Alterations of pigment epithelium in cystinosis, Arch. Ophthalmol. **77:**361, 1967.

48. Wong, V.G., Schulman, J.D., and Seegmiller, J.E.: Conjunctival biopsy for the biochemical diagnosis of cystinosis, Am. J. Ophthalmol. **70:**278, 1970.

49. Zimmerman, T.J., Hood, C.I., and Gasset, A.R.: "Adolescent" cystinosis: a case presentation and review of the recent literature, Arch. Ophthalmol. **92:**265, 1974.

ADDITIONAL READING

Barnes, H.D., and Boshoff, P.H.: Ocular lesions in patients with porphyria, Arch. Ophthalmol. **48:**567, 1952.

Dobyns, W.B., Goldstein, N.P., and Gordon, H.: Clinical spectrum of Wilson's disease (hepatolenticular-degeneration), Mayo Clin. Proc. **54:**35, 1979.

Dodd, M.J., Pusen, S.M., Green, W.R.: Adult cystinosis, Arch. Ophthalmol. **96:**1054, 1978.

Klentworth, G.K., Bredehoeft, S.J., and Reed, J.W.: Analysis of corneal crystalline deposits in multiple myeloma, Am. J. Ophthalmol. **86:**303, 1978.

Sevel, D., and Burger, D.: Ocular involvement in cutaneous porphyria: a clinical and histological report, Arch. Ophthalmol. **85:**580, 1971.

Wolter, J.R., Clark, R.L., and Kallet, H.A.: Ocular involvement in acute intermittent porphyria, Am. J. Ophthalmol. **74:**666, 1972.

16 Endocrine diseases

HYPERTHYROIDISM (GRAVES' DISEASE)

Graves' disease includes ophthalmopathy, goiter, and a hypermetabolic state. The eye changes in Graves' disease may be seen in the hypothyroid state, or they may appear after a hypothyroid or euthyroid state has been reached. However, it should be noted that in a number of patients with ophthalmopathy no clinical history of thyroid dysfunction can be elicited. The more severe eye changes seem to follow the treatment of hyperthyroidism in about 10% of the cases (with a higher incidence of ophthalmopathy in patients who have become hypothyroid). However, an inconsistent relationship exists between the ocular changes and the metabolic state. The ocular manifestations appear to be independent of thyroid activity; the active phase may span several months to several years; eyes seldom return to the normal state, but they may improve.

Laboratory tests

Thyroid-stimulating hormone (TSH), long-acting thyroid stimulator (LATS), and exophthalmos-producing substance (EPS) all appear to play a questionable role in the production of the ocular complications of Graves' disease. It is thought by some that an immune problem involving immunoglobulins E, M, and G and complement may be factors in the pathogenesis of this disease or that a cell-mediated immunity may be involved.[35] The serum T_4 level is a useful screening test for both mild hyperthyroidism and hypothyroidism. Determination of serum LATS levels are significant if positive, but they are rarely positive in any patient with a history of ophthalmopathy of more than 12 months' duration. One of the most useful laboratory tests is the thyroid-uptake suppression test (Werner's test) (p. 464). In euthyroid and hypothyroid subjects with Graves' disease, the thyroid becomes autonomous of pituitary control over the thyroid iodine-trapping mechanism and hence fails significantly to decrease ^{131}I uptake after thyroid hormone administration. A positive Werner test, which is found in 75% to 86% of euthyroid patients with progressive ophthalmopathy, indicates failure of thyroid suppression. If this test is normal and the eye changes are severe, or if the Werner test is negative, endocrine origin of proptosis is unlikely.

Ophthalmic involvement

In thyroid exophthalmos, a marked increase occurs in the tissue bulk of the orbit because of an increase in the mucopolysaccharide content, specifically hyaluronic acid.[45] The hydroscopic nature of the mucopolysaccharide results in an increase in the water content of orbital tissue, the orbital fat, and connective tissue of the extraocular muscles.[42] The hyaluronic acid may be a product of fibroblast and lymphocyte interaction.

The extraocular muscles may become involved in the inflammatory cell infiltration

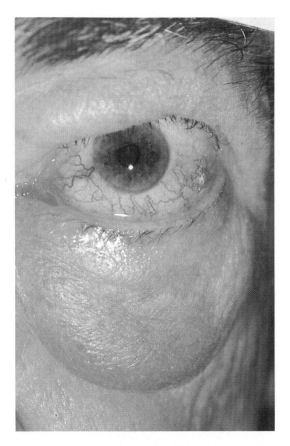

Fig. 16-1. Edema of lids, proptosis, conjunctival injection, and exposure keratitis of lower one fourth of cornea in hyperthyroid exophthalmopathy.

T₃ (WERNER) SUPPRESSION TEST

First day. The patient takes a dose of radioactive iodine (RA$_I$) (^{131}I or ^{123}I). A 6-hour RA$_I$ uptake test may be done, but it is not essential.
Second day. A 24-hour RA$_I$ uptake (baseline) test. The patient begins receiving liothyronine sodium (Cytomel), 25 μg three times daily for 7 days, which blocks the TSH.

One week later

First day. The patient takes another dose of RA$_I$.
Second day. Do a 24-hour RA$_I$ uptake test. If the thyroid is autonomous, it will take up more RA$_I$. It should be lower than its baseline to be normal.
Normal gland is suppressed.
Normal gland increase in thyroid-releasing hormone.

Table 16-1. Classification of eye changes in Graves' disease (American Thyroid Association)

Class	Ocular change
0	No signs or symptoms
1	Only signs, no symptoms (stare, upper lid retraction with or without lid lag and proptosis)
2	Soft tissue involvement (symptoms and signs), chemosis
3	Proptosis
4	Extraocular muscle involvement
5	Corneal involvement
6	Vision loss (optic nerve involvement)

and edema. The enlargement of these muscles is seen well in an EMI scan and is most helpful as a diagnostic measure. These changes are confined to the interstitial areas, thus sparing the muscle fibers. Degenerative changes in the muscle cells seem to be secondary to the edema, resulting in fibrosis, contracture, and atrophy. Progressive orbital involvement and enlargement of the extraocular muscles may lead to increased proptosis (Fig. 16-1), conjunctival chemosis, restriction of ocular movement, and lagophthalmos. The severity of the changes is classified by the American Thyroid Association (Table 16-1). The optic nerve can exhibit papilledema, papillitis, and/or retrobulbar neuropathy. Choroidal folds as well as dilation of retinal vessels and retinal hemorrhages have been observed.

A false increase in intraocular tension occurs secondarily to a fibrotic inferior rectus muscle restricting the elevation of the eye to the primary position; this effect can account for a rather severe rise in intraocular pressure between the primary position and a slight elevation of the eye.

Patients may complain of a sandy feeling in the eyes, lacrimation, photophobia, and double vision. The latter is especially marked when arising in the morning. The lacrimal gland may be palpable. There is a fullness and edema of the lids (Fig. 16-1), and

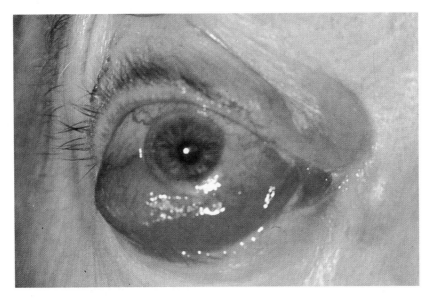

Fig. 16-2. Marked chemosis of lower conjunctiva in Graves' disease.

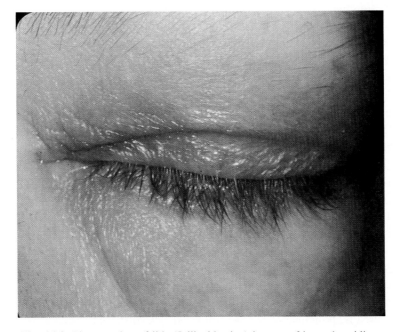

Fig. 16-3. Pigmentation of lids (Jellinek's sign) in case of hyperthyroidism.

the gross dilation of bulbar conjunctival vessels, most marked temporally, causes a chronic hyperemia or chemosis of the conjunctiva (Fig. 16-2). The lids occasionally may show increased pigmentation (Fig. 16-3).

Corneal exposure (Fig. 16-1) and drying with secondary infection and possible perforation is a complication that can occur in severe cases. In the average case, an exposure keratitis occurs in the inferior cornea with varying degrees of conjunctival chemosis. It is interesting that hyperthyroidism may be associated with superior limbic keratoconjunctivitis,[12] the corneal changes of which are discussed in Chapter 5.

HYPOTHYROIDISM

Epithelial keratopathy can be seen on occasion in hypothyroidism. It is also said that hypothyroidism can cause an increase in tear production.

MULTIPLE ENDOCRINE NEOPLASIA*

Multiple endocrine neoplasia (MEN) type I[47] includes the following:
1. Autosomal dominant inheritance
2. Parathyroid adenoma or hyperplasia
3. Pancreatic adenomas
4. Thyroid adenomas
5. Adrenocortical adenomas
6. Subcutaneous lipomas
7. Visual field defect caused by pituitary adenomas

MEN type II or IIa (Sipple's syndrome) includes:
1. Medullary carcinoma of the thyroid
2. Pheochromocytomas (tend to be intra-adrenal)
3. Parathyroid hyperplasia or adenoma
4. Autosomal dominant inheritance
5. Multiple mucosal neuromas
6. Rare occurrence of prominent corneal nerves
7. Marfanoid habitus

Gorlin et al.[24,25] and Baum, Tannenbaum and Kolodny[3] have also described similar syndromes. MEN type IIb (Froboese's syndrome) includes:
1. Medullary carcinoma of the thyroid
2. Parathyroid adenomas
3. Pheochromocytomas
4. Skeletal anomalies
5. Thick lips, soft tissue prognathism (Fig. 16-4)
6. Intestinal ganglioneuromatosis
7. Sporadic or autosomal dominant inheritance
8. Neuromas on the tongue
9. Prominent corneal nerves (Fig. 16-5), thick eyelids, nasal displacement of puncta, especially at the limbus (Fig. 16-6), everted eyelids, mucosal and subconjunctival neuromas, decreased tear function, poor pupillary dilation, thickened nerves in the iris, prominent eyebrows, and prominent perilimbal blood vessels.

---

*References 2, 9, 15, 24, 25, 30-32, 37, 44, 46.

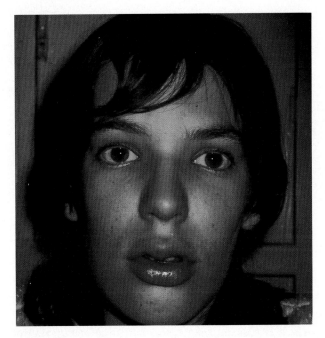

Fig. 16-4. Marfanoid habitus and facies in multiple endocrine neoplasia.

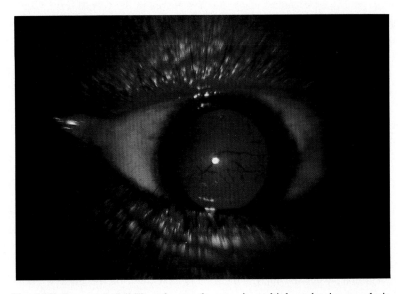

Fig. 16-5. Increased visibility of corneal nerves in multiple endocrine neoplasia.

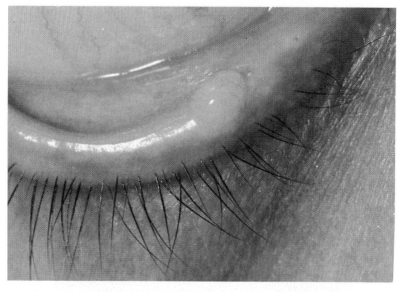

Fig. 16-6. Neuromas of conjunctival lid margin in multiple endocrine neoplasia. (From Grayson, M.: The cornea in systemic disease. In Duane, T.D. [ed.]: Clinical Ophthalmology. Hagerstown, Md.: Harper & Row, 1976, vol. 4, chap. 15.)

In MEN type IIb the patients develop a wheal without flare on intradermal injection of histamine. Normal patients develop a flare and wheal. This abnormal response to intradermal histamine probably does not result from increased levels of histaminase in the circulation, which is seen in some cases, but to an abnormality of the cutaneous nerves. The anomalous reaction to histamine still occurs after surgical removal of the medullary carcinoma of the thyroid.[4]

Electron microscopic studies show that the nerves in the cornea do not appear to be myelinated. They appear to be numerous closely packed axons and Schwann cells. The latter have abundant basal lamina material but almost no tendency to ensheathe the axons with myelin.

The nodules of the conjunctiva and lid are composed of coiled myelinated nerves with thickened perineurium and may also contain few ganglion cells. Thickened nerves in the iris are also seen.

Patients with MEN type IIb have diffuse thickening of the nerves with many ganglion cells within the enlarged nerves (ganglioneuromatosis) in the gastrointestinal tract. This can be seen on rectal biopsy. Discrete neurofibromas or schwannomas can be seen in the gastrointestinal tract in von Recklinghausen's disease.

The ophthalmologist may be the first physician to have the opportunity to make a diagnosis in MEN, once the prominent corneal nerves have been recognized[43]; investigation for medullary thyroid carcinoma and MEN is very important. The prominent corneal nerves, which form an irregular lattice pattern across the entire cornea, are relatively large in size (Fig. 16-5). The corneal nerve fibers are seen entering the midstroma as large white trunks, whereas small branches enter the anterior and posterior stroma. Enlarged prominent nerves can be seen in the subconjunctival region, where they raise the overlying tarsal or bulbar conjunctiva. The nerves frequently appear as flat, poorly cir-

Table 16-2. Comparison of MEN type IIb and neurofibromatosis

	MEN type IIb	Von Recklinghausen's neurofibromatosis
Basic defect	Disorder of neural crest derivatives	Disorder of neural crest derivatives
Mode of inheritance	Sporadic or autosomal dominant	Autosomal dominant
General appearance	Marfanoid habitus Characteristic facies	Hemihypertrophy of face or extremity (occasional) Lip hypertrophy (occasional)
Skeleton	Various anomalies	Various anomalies
Mucocutaneous	Multiple mucosal neuromas Café-au-lait spots	Multiple neurofibromas Café-au-lait spots Molluscum fibrosum Freckling, especially in armpits General hyperpigmentation
Alimentary tract	Ganglioneuromatosis (diffuse hyperplasia of nerves)	Neurofibromas (specific localized tumors)
Neural	Thickened peripheral nerves	Increased incidence of tumors of the central and peripheral nervous systems (neurofibromas, gliomas, meningiomas, ependymomas)
Other tumors	Increased incidence of pheochromocytomas (56%)*	Increased incidence of pheochromocytomas (1% to 5%)
Ophthalmic symptoms	Prominent corneal nerves	Prominent corneal nerves (questionable)
	Ocular neuromas	Ocular neurofibromas
	Thickened eyelids	Thickened eyelids
	Increased intraocular pressure (rare)	Congenital glaucoma
	Impaired pupillary dilation	Melanocytic hamartomas of iris
	Thickened conjunctiva of white lines in the area of the corneoscleral limbus	Hamartomas of retina and choroid Melanocytosis of choroid
	Decreased tear formation	Retinal detachment (secondary to choroidal neurofibromatosis)
	Nasal displacement of lacrimal puncta	Optic nerve gliomas and meningiomas
	Prominent orbital ridges	Ectopic neurons in optic nerve
	Heavy eyebrows	Orbital bone defects Nonexpansile pulsating exophthalmos
	Medullary carcinoma of thyroid	Myelinated retinal nerve fibers

From Spector, B., Klintworth, G.K., and Wells, S.A.: Am. J. Ophthalmol. **91**:204, 1981. Published with permission from the American Journal of Ophthalmology. Copyright by the Ophthalmic Publishing Co.
*The pheochromocytomas appear to develop relatively late and are found in 90% of patients more than 20 years old.[2]

cumscribed bundles. The lesions may be smooth, yellow, and elevated within the palpebral fissure and may resemble pingueculae. Multiple white cords in the conjunctiva radiating from the cornea are also apparent. The paralimbal neuromas are generally associated with dilated perilimbal conjunctival vessels; the patient may complain of chronically red eyes. The chronically red eyes are in part caused by keratoconjunctivitis sicca and punctate epitheliopathy. However, this chronic condition is more commonly found in the older patient. Less common or gross alterations of the lids such as thickening or irregular prominences along the free margins are seen and are caused by abnormal nerves.

MEN type IIb and neurofibromatosis have many similarities and differences in their clinical picture. Table 16-2 lists these differences and similarities.

Differential diagnosis

Increased visibility of the corneal nerves[34] occurs in several other clinical conditions:
1. Fuchs' dystrophy
2. Keratoconus
3. Neurofibromatosis*
4. Refsum's syndrome[3]
5. Ichthyosis
6. Leprosy
7. Congenital glaucoma
8. Failed graft
9. Multiple endocrine neoplasia
10. Use of *Cannabis sativa* (marijuana)[18]
11. Deep filiform dystrophy
12. Aging[15]

Corneal nerves may become secondarily thickened (hyperregeneration) following keratoplasty or as a consequence of local inflammation. Hyperregeneration of the corneal nerves was described at length by Wolter[50-52] and is seen after trauma, keratoplasty, and granulomatous uveitis; with congenital glaucoma, retrolental fibroplasia, and congenital cataract; and secondary to intraocular foreign body, phthisis bulbi, band keratopathy, and increasing age. In these conditions, the nerve fibers are irregular and take an irregular course through the stroma and into the epithelium.

There is a possibility that a relationship exists between phakomatosis and MEN. Von Hippel-Lindau disease and multiple neurofibromatosis have been seen with pheochromocytomas. Physical similarities exist between multiple endocrine neoplasia and Marfan's syndrome. Features common with Riley-Day[16] syndrome can also be seen.[2]

Laboratory test

Measurement of the plasma calcitonin concentration is important. Calcitonin is secreted by the C cells that comprise medullary thyroid carcinoma.[16, 17] Excess calcitonin induces a decrease in plasma calcium and in organic phosphorus and an increase in parathyroid hormone concentration. Parathyroid hyperplasia may occur secondarily to calcitonin release. High concentrations of calcitonin are diagnostic for the medullary thyroid carcinoma. Calcitonin can be used as a diagnostic measure as well as an indicator of residual metastasis after primary surgery.

Calcitonin is increased in medullary thyroid carcinoma. It has a hypocalcemic effect. Basal concentrations are usually high, but in instances in which there is some question, an abnormal increase in response to addition of calcium will confirm the diagnosis.

---

*Thickened corneal nerves may really have been cases of MEN type IIb,[46] since it is rare to find this in neurofibromatosis.

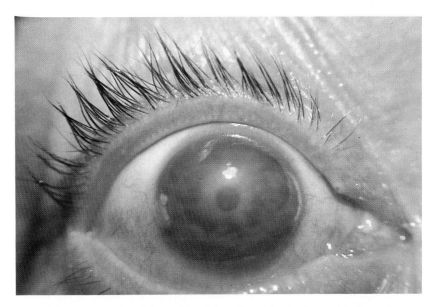

Fig. 16-7. Hyperparathyroidism with calcium deposition in deep epithelium of cornea.

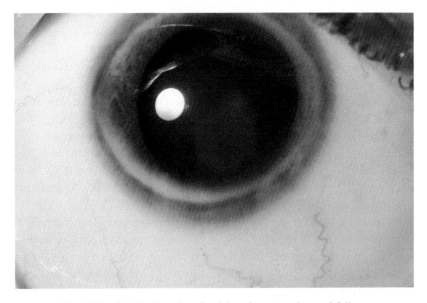

Fig. 16-8. Calcific deposits of calcium in cornea in renal failure.

PARATHYROID DISORDERS
General considerations

The primary role of the parathyroid gland is to assist in the control of calcium metabolism. The parathyroid hormone is the agent that causes a release of calcium and phosphorus from the bone, increased reabsorption of calcium from the renal tubule, and increased renal excretion of phosphate.[8] The hypercalcemia produced by this stimulates secretion of calcitonin, which is manufactured by cells located in the thyroid gland. Calcitonin acts by returning calcium back to normal calcemic levels. Therefore a feedback system is developed. The importance of the parathyroid gland is shown in its influence on structure of bone, regulation of neuromuscular activity, and concern with cardiac electric impulses and coagulation of the blood; in addition, parathyroid hormone appears to have a direct effect on the respiration of mitochondria.

Hyperparathyroidism[29]

The diagnosis of hyperparathyroidism is based primarily on the findings of hypercalcemia and hypophosphatemia. The clinical manifestations of hyperparathyroidism include muscular weakness, renal stones, gastrointestinal upset, pseudogout, and signs of increased bone absorption.

Calcification of the tympanic membrane with bilateral deafness has been seen in several cases. Electrocardiographic changes as well as mental changes are seen.

Papilledema may also be seen.[36] Ocular signs are directly related to hypercalcemia.[5] In hyperparathyroidism, one may see positive staining for calcium in the conjunctival epithelium, corneal epithelium (Fig. 16-7), and endothelium, as well as in the anterior sclera. An abundance of calcium is usually seen in conjunctival cells. With the transmission electron microscope, calcium is seen as intracellular deposits of needlelike structures in the nuclei and cytoplasm of the cells. In epithelial cells of the cornea, the crystals are often confined to the nucleus. The calcium is deposited as hydroxyaptite crystals, $Ca_{10}(PO_4)_6(OH)_2$.

Chronic kidney failure. Subepithelial calcifications and epithelial deposits have been seen in conjunctival biopsy specimens taken from patients with renal failure.[6] Electron microscopic examination demonstrates that the calcium appears to be deposited extracellularly and in spherical globules.

Limbal and conjunctival deposition of calcium salt is a frequent occurrence in advanced acute and chronic renal failure[11, 28, 40] (Fig. 16-8). Conjunctival metastatic calcification can be seen in uremic patients with a low or normal serum calcium level. The reason for this phenomenon is an elevated calcium-phosphorous product usually in the neighborhood of 70 mg/dl in such patients.[28] It is interesting that a kidney transplant will result in resolution of conjunctival and corneal calcification, although the corneal decalcification may take longer, but hemodialysis does not produce such results.

Limbal deposits are seen and may resemble Vogt's white limbal girdle. However, the limbal girdle is usually yellowish white, whereas the lesions of calcium are chalky white. Limbal calcification in uremic patients is distinguished from Vogt's white limbal girdle by its presence in young patients and by its large coarse nature as well as by the absence of a clear area of cornea at the limbus.[19] The patients, in addition, exhibit the red eye of renal failure with dense large conjunctival and corneal deposits in the form of crystals.[7]

Idiopathic hypercalcemia of infancy.[21, 27] Idiopathic hypercalcemia of infancy, with an onset between 3 and 9 months of age, should be included in this group, since one can see hypercalcemia associated with corneal disease. This is a somewhat rare disease resulting perhaps from vitamin D intoxication or the possibility of an unusual sensitivity to this vitamin. Failure to thrive, apathy, polyuria, and muscular weakness become manifest. Severe forms of the disease usually show an individual with dwarfed habitus who has a "peculiar facies" that is often described as "elfin" (Fig. 16-9).

Hypertension and mental retardation as well as osteosclerosis are seen. Stabismus and papilledema have also been described. Persons with idiopathic hypercalcemia of infancy may show, in addition to these general eye findings, nystagmus, pupillary changes, lenticular opacities, craniostenosis, and otosclerosis.

Deposits of calcium in the cornea may be seen ultrastructurally to be deposited intracellularly as precursors of calcium hydroxyapatite and are often confined to the nucleus, making the methodology indistinguishable from that of cases of hyperparathyroidism. Extracellular deposits have also been seen similar to those found in renal failure.

Idiopathic hypercalcemia is probably a disease of inborn error of metabolism.

Hypophosphatasia.[10, 20] This rare familial disease is characterized by multiple skeletal abnormalities and malformations, failure to thrive and often early death from nephrocalcinosis, and the sequelae caused by hypercalcemia and increased intracranial pressure. An inability of osteoblasts to incorporate calcium into an otherwise normal bone matrix thus prevents bone maturation. The pathologic condition is indistinguishable from that

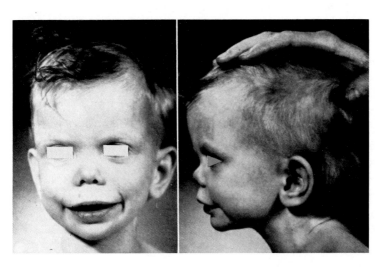

Fig. 16-9. Elfinlike face as seen in idiopathic hypercalcemia of infancy. (From Harley, R.D., DiGeorge, A.M., Mabry, C.C., and Apt, L.L.: Trans. Am. Acad. Ophthalmol. Otolaryngol. **69:** 997, 1965.)

of rickets. There is a low level of serum alkaline phosphatase in addition to excretion of phosphorethanolamine in the urine.

Prominent eyes result from malformation of the orbits (harlequin orbits); in addition, one sees cataracts, papilledema, and optic atrophy. Pathologic lid retraction and craniostenosis also occur.

Band keratopathy and conjunctival calcification are noted together with blue sclera. Early recognition is relatively important because one may be able to prevent the ocular and neurologic complications.

Band-shaped keratopathy and corneal calcium deposition. As is seen, band-shaped keratopathy and corneal calcium deposition occur in a variety of conditions:

Hypercalcemia[13, 14]

    Hyperparathyroidism[39]

    Hypophosphatasia

    Idiopathic hypercalcemia of infancy

    Vitamin D intoxication[1]

    Milk-alkali syndrome

    Renal failure

    Multiple myeloma

    Sarcoid[16]

    Malignancy with and without bone metastasis

    Immobilization of children or adults with Paget's disease of bone

Increased phosphorous product with normocalcemia

    Renal failure

Ocular diseases

    Idiopathy

    Corneal scars or old (long-standing) infection

    Iridocyclitis

    Norrie's disease

    Long-term miotic therapy[31]

    Phthisis or atrophy bulbi

    Interlamellar corneal membrane

    Leprosy

    Toxoplasmosis

    Interstitial keratitis

    Still's disease associated with iridocyclitis

    Progressive hemifacial atrophy[26]

    Rapid development of dry eyes[33]

Dermatologic disease

    Ichthyosis

Toxic effect

    Exposure to mercurial dust and vapors[22]

    Phenylmercuric nitrate (as a preservative in ocular medications such as pilocarpine and sulfisoxazole [Fig. 16-10])

In band keratopathy without hypercalcemia, the calcium is extracellular and confined

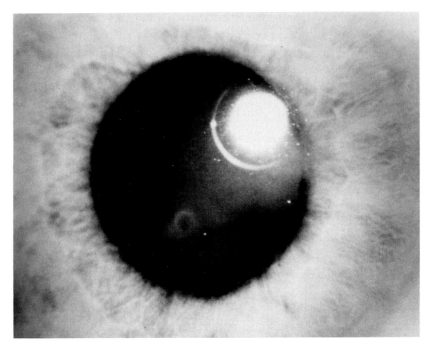

Fig. 16-10. Mercurial-induced, calcific band keratopathy.

to the subepithelial zone and Bowman's layer and takes the shape of spheres of tiny crystals in concentric circles. The calcific lesion of band keratopathy usually starts out as a haziness at the level of Bowman's membrane, which becomes dense until the area of the cornea exposed between the lids takes on a granular white appearance, with small round Swiss-cheese holes in the opacity. Close examination will show the calcium is located in the basement membrane as well as in Bowman's layer.

The calcium that is deposited is in the form of hydroxyapatite crystals. It is often asked why the anterior layers and the intrapalpebral tissue are involved. Gases exchanged at the surface of the exposed cornea with subsequent loss of carbon dioxide and a localized elevation of pH are thought to be significant in the precipitation of calcium.[38] It may be that the basement membrane and epithelium with its peculiar irregular thickening and hemidesmosomes may act as a lattice on which crystal structures are built. The reasons for anterior location of calcium deposits in bullous surface keratopathy may be related to the pH; that is, anaerobic glycolysis is the principal mode of metabolism on the deep corneal stroma.[38] If slightly lactic acid accumulates in the deep stroma, a lower pH exists than that in the superficial layers. The difference might be sufficient to render the deeper layers clear and the subepithelial layers opaque.[38]

When the corneal opacity from calcific deposits impedes the visual acuity, the cornea is treated with the chelating agent, 0.05 M 1.7% neutral solution of ethylenediamine tetraacetic acid (EDTA). Anesthetic agent is applied to the cornea (usually 4% cocaine). The epithelium is removed gently prior to the continuous dropping of the EDTA. Scraping away of the calcium deposits should be performed carefully so that no further damage is done to Bowman's layer. Scraping and EDTA drops are alternated. Simple scraping away of the calcium without application of EDTA has also been successful. The visual acuity can be increased considerably in some cases. However, if there is a fibrous pannus, it cannot be chelated and should not be scraped.

Hypoparathyroidism

Simple hypoparathyroidism. In this condition, there is a decrease in the level of calcium in the blood associated with elevation of phosphorus. The clinical aspects of the disease are those of hypocalcemia. Patients with simple hypoparathyroidism have symptoms associated with the neuromuscular system, the intestinal tract, and the ectodermal system: maculopapular eruptions occur,[48] as do a variety of ocular problems such as lenticular opacities, blepharospasm, strabismus, nystagmus, papilledema,[36] and ptosis. Photophobia is often a complaint.

Only infrequently will one find corneal vascularization and epithelial keratopathy.

Multiple endocrinopathy.[41] Chronic candidiasis has been described with functional failure of one or more endocrine glands.[49] Multiple endocrinopathy, which is often transmitted as an autosomal recessive trait, can be manifested by hypoparathyroidism, hypoadrenalism, gonadal failure, diabetes mellitus, hypothyroidism, thymic dysplasia, and pernicious anemia.

Moniliasis is not responsible for the endocrine disease. It is postulated that the endocrine problem and the candidiasis may be an immunologic deficiency disorder. It is interesting that an association with oral squamous cell carcinoma has been seen. Malignancy has been reported[23] in other immunodeficient syndromes, including ataxic telangiectasia and Wiskott-Aldrich syndrome. The latter disease presents conjunctival and corneal signs that are of interest to the ophthalmologist. (See Chapter 14.)

In multiple endocrinopathy associated with hypoparathyroidism, corneal findings such as ulcerating vascularization and opacification occur and may indeed result from a "phlyctenular" response to candidiasis.

Following are other conditions of hypoparathyroidism that do not manifest any corneal disease (however, numbers one, two, and four produce ophthalmic findings such as zonular tetany, cataracts, and papilledema):

1. Pseudohypoparathyroidism
2. Pseudo-pseudohypoparathyroidism
3. DiGeorge's syndrome (congenital thymic aplasia)
4. Secondary hypoparathyroidism (after thyroid surgery)

REFERENCES

1. Bauer, J.M., and Freybert, R.H.: Vitamin D intoxication, JAMA **130:**204, 1946.
2. Baum, J.L., and Adler, M.E.: Pheochromocytomas, medullary thyroid carcinoma, and multiple mucosal neuroma: a variant of the syndrome, Arch. Ophthalmol. **87:**574, 1972.
3. Baum, J.L., Tannenbaum, M., and Kolodny, E.H.: Refsum's syndrome with corneal involvement, Am. J. Ophthalmol. **60:**699, 1965.
4. Baylin, S.B., Beaven, M.A., Engelman, K., and Sjoerdsma, A.: Elevated histaminase activity in medullary carcinoma of the thyroid gland, N. Engl. J. Med. **283:**1239, 1970.
5. Berkow, J.W., Fine, S.B., and Zimmerman, L.E.: Unusual ocular calcification in hyperparathyroidism, Am. J. Ophthalmol. **66:**812, 1968.
6. Berlyne, G.M.: Microcrystalline conjunctival calcification in renal failure, Lancet **2:**366, 1968.

7. Berlyne, G.M., and Shaw, A.B.: Red eyes in renal failure, Lancet **1:**4, 1967.

8. Borle, A.B.: Calcium metabolism in HeLa cells and the effects of parathyroid hormone, J. Cell. Biol. **36:**567, 1968.

9. Braley, A.E.: Medullated corneal nerves and plexiform neuroma associated with pheochromocytoma, Trans. Am. Ophthalmol. Soc. **52:**189, 1954.

10. Brenner, R.L., Smith, J.L., Cleveland, W.W., Bejar, R.L., and Lockhart, W.S.: Eye signs of hypophosphatasia, Arch. Ophthalmol. **81:**614, 1969.

11. Caldeira, J.A.F., Sabbaga, E., and Ianhez, L.E.: Conjunctival and corneal changes in renal failure, Br. J. Ophthalmol. **54:**399, 1970.

12. Cher, I.: Clinical features of superior limbic keratoconjunctivitis in Australia: a probable association with thyrotoxicosis, Arch. Ophthalmol. **82:** 580, 1969.

13. Cogan, D.G., Albright, F., and Bartter, F.C.: Hypercalcemia and band keratopathy, Arch. Ophthalmol. **40:**624, 1948.

14. Cogan, D.G., and Henneman, P.H.: Diffuse calcification of the cornea in hypercalcemia, N. Engl. J. Med. **257:**451, 1957.

15. Colombo, C.G., and Watson, A.G.: Ophthalmic manifestations of multiple endocrine neoplasia, type three, Can. J. Ophthalmol. **11:**290, 1976.

16. Crick, R.P., Hoyle, C., and Smellie, H.: The eyes of sarcoid, Br. J. Ophthalmol. **45:**461, 1961.

17. Cunliffe, W.J., Hall, R., Hudgson, P., et al.: A calcitonia-secreting thyroid carcinoma, Lancet **2:**63, 1968.

18. Dawson, W.W.: Cannabis and eye function, Invest. Ophthalmol. **15:**243, 1976.

19. Demco, T.A., McCormick, A.Q., and Richards, J.S.F.: Conjunctival and corneal changes in chronic renal failure, Can. J. Ophthalmol. **9:**208, 1974.

20. Fraser, D.: Hypophosphatasia, Am. J. Ophthalmol. **22:**730, 1957.

21. Fraser, D., Kidd, B.S., Kooh, S.W., and Paumei, L.: A new look at infantile hypercalcemia, Pediatr. Clin. North Am. **13:**503, 1966.

22. Galin, M.A., and Obstbaum, S.A.: Band keratopathy in mercury exposure, Am. J. Ophthalmol. **12:**517, 1974.

23. Gatti, R.A., and Good, R.A.: Occurrence of malignancy in immunodeficient diseases: a literary review, Cancer **28:**89, 1971.

24. Gorlin, R.J., and Menkin, B.L.: Multiple neuromas, pheochromocytoma, medullary carcinoma of the thyroid and marfanoid body build with muscle wasting, Z. Kinderheilk. **113:**313, 1972.

25. Gorlin, R.J., Sedano, H.O., Vickers, R.A., et al: Multiple mucosal neuromas, pheochromocytoma and medullary carcinoma of thyroid—a syndrome, Cancer **22:**293, 1968.

26. Grayson, M., and Pieroni, D.: Progressive facial hemiatrophy with bullous and band-shaped keratopathy, Am. J. Ophthalmol. **40:**42, 1970.

27. Harley, R.D., DiGeorge, A.M., Mabry, C.C., and Apt, L.: Idiopathic hypercalcemia of infancy: optic atrophy and other ocular changes, Trans. Am. Acad. Ophthalmol. Otolaryngol. **69:**977, 1965.

28. Harris, L.S., Cohn, K., Toyofuku, H., Lonegran, E., and Galin, M.A.: Conjunctival and corneal calcific deposits in uremic patients, Am. J. Ophthalmol. **72:**130, 1971.

29. Jensen, O.A.: Ocular calcification in primary hyperparathyroidism, Acta Ophthalmol. **53:**173, 1971.

30. Keiser, H.R., Beaven, M.A., Doppman, J., et al.: Sipple's syndrome: medullary thyroid carcinoma, pheochromocytoma, and parathyroid disease: studies in a large family, Ann. Intern. Med. **78:** 561, 1973.

31. Kennedy, R.E., and Roca, P.: Atypical band keratopathy in glaucomatous patients, Am. J. Ophthalmol. **72:**917, 1971.

32. Khairi, R.A., Dexter, R.N., Burzynski, N.J., and Johnston, C.C.: Mucosal neuroma, pheochromocytoma and medullary carcinoma: multiple endocrine neoplasia type III, Medicine **54:** 89, 1975.

33. Lemp, M.A., and Ralph, R.A.: Rapid development of band keratopathy in dry eyes, Am. J. Ophthalmol. **83:**657, 1977.

34. Mensher, J.H.: Corneal nerves, Surv. Ophthalmol. **19:**1, 1974.

35. Munro, R.E., Lamki, L., Row, V.V., and Volpe, R.: Cell-mediated immunity in the exophthalmos of Graves' disease as demonstrated by the migration inhibition factor (MIF) test, J. Endocrinol. Metab. **37:**286, 1973.

36. Murphy, K.J.: Papilledema due to hyperparathyroidism, Br. J. Ophthalmol. **58:**694, 1974.

37. Norton, J.A., Froome, L.C., Farrell, R.E., and Wells, S.A.: Multiple endocrine neoplasia type IIb: the most aggressive form of medullary thyroid carcinoma, Surg. Clin. North Am. **59:**109, 1979.

38. O'Connor, G.R.: Calcific band keratopathy, Trans. Am. Ophthalmol. Soc. **58:**81, 1974.

39. Porter, R., and Crombie, A.L.: Corneal calcification as a presenting and diagnostic sign in hyperparathyroidism, Br. J. Ophthalmol. **57:**665, 1973.

40. Porter, R., and Crombie, A.L.: Corneal and conjunctival calcification in chronic renal failure, Br. J. Ophthalmol. **57:**339, 1973.

41. Richman, R.A., Rosenthal, I.M., Solomon, L. M., and Karachorlu, K.V.: Candidiasis and multiple endocrinopathy, Arch. Dermatol. **111:**625, 1975.
42. Riley, F.C.: Orbital pathology in Graves' disease, Mayo Clin. Proc. **4:**975, 1972.
43. Robertson, D.M., Sizemore, G.W., and Gordon, H.: Thickened corneal nerves as a manifestation of multiple endocrine neoplasia, Trans. Am. Acad. Ophthalmol. Otolaryngol. **79:**772, 1975.
44. Sipple, J.H.: The association of pheochromocytoma with carcinoma of the thyroid gland, Am. J. Med. **31:**163, 1961.
45. Sisson, J.C.: Hyaluronic acid in localized myxedema, J. Clin. Endocrinol. Metab. **28:**443-436, 1968.
46. Spector, B., Klintworth, G.K., and Wells, S.A.: Histologic study of the ocular lesions in multiple endocrine neoplasia syndrome type IIb, Am. J. Ophthalmol. **91:**204, 1981.
47. Steiner, A.L., Goodman, A.D., and Powers, S. R.: Study of a kindred with pheochromocytoma, medullary thyroid carcinoma, hyperparathyroidism, and Cushing disease: multiple endocrine neoplasia, type 2, Medicine **47:**371, 1968.
48. Waisman, M., and O'Regan, S.: Maculopapular eruption in hypoparathyroidism, Arch. Dermatol. **112:**991, 1976.
49. Whitaker, J., Landing, B.H., Esselborn, V.M., et al.: The syndrome of juvenile hypoadrenocorticism, hypoparathyroidism and superficial moniliasis, J. Clin. Endocrinol. Metab. **16:**1374, 1956.
50. Wolter, J.R.: Regeneration and hyper-regeneration of corneal nerves, Ophthalmologica **151:**588, 1960.
51. Wolter, J.R.: Hyper-regeneration of corneal nerves in bullous keratopathy, Am. J. Ophthalmol. **58:**31, 1964.
52. Wolter, J.R.: Hyper-regeneration of corneal nerves in a scarred transplant, Am. J. Ophthalmol. **61:**880, 1966.

ADDITIONAL READING

Glushien, A.S., Mansury, M.M., and Littman, D.S.: Pheochromocytoma: its relationship to the neurocutaneous syndromes, Am. J. Med. **14:**318, 1953.
Schimke, R.N., Hartman, W.H., Pront, E., et al.: Syndrome of bilateral pheochromocytoma, medullary thyroid carcinoma and multiple neuromas, N. Engl. J. Med. **279:**1, 1968.
Steiglitz, L.N., et al.: Keratitis with hypoparathyroidism, Am. J. Ophthalmol. **84:**467, 1977.
Walsh, F.B., and Howard, J.E.: Conjunctival and corneal lesions in hypercalcemia, J. Clin. Endocrinol. **7:**644, 1947.
Walsh, F.B., and Murray, R.G.: Ocular manifestations of disturbances in calcium metabolism; ninth Stanford R. Gifford lecture, Am. J. Ophthalmol. **36:**1657, 1953.
Wolter, J.R.: Corneal innervation after ocular evisceration, Arch. Ophthalmol. **68:**404, 1971.

17 Diseases of lipid metabolism

CORNEAL ARCUS

The corneal arcus is a deposition of phospholipids, cholesterol esters, and triglycerides[17] in the peripheral areas of Bowman's layer, Descemet's membrane, and the intervening cornea. A deposit of lipid material in younger people in the same area is called a juvenile arcus.[13] Corneal arcus is probably related to age, serum cholesterol, and heredity.

Corneal arcus is seen as a normal aging process (Fig. 10-5). However, if the lipid deposits are seen in young patients, it would be wise to obtain a serum lipid profile. It can be significant when a corneal arcus is seen in blacks before the age of 40 years and in whites before the age of 30.[14] About one third of patients with such findings in these groups will have an abnormality of their lipoproteins.

The incidence of coronary heart disease in patients with arcus probably relates to patients under 50 years of age.[12, 15] Unilateral arcus as a sign of occlusion disease of the carotid artery on the side contralateral to the arcus may occur.

A classification of the systemic lipid problems is essential to appreciate the eye findings. Therefore the following paragraphs are devoted to a description of the alterations in blood lipids together with the systemic and ophthalmic findings.

Table 17-1. Blood lipids and their relation to ophthalmic disease

Fredrickson type	Involved appearance		Triglyceride level*	Cholesterol level†	Hereditary frequency	Xanthomata	Eye and skin changes
	Lipoprotein level	Serum					
Type I recessive	Chylomicrons elevated	Creamy	Elevated	Normal or slightly elevated	2%	Eruptive	Lipid keratopathy (rare) Lipemia retinalis
Type II‡ dominant	β-Lipoproteins elevated	Clear	Normal or slightly elevated	Elevated	42%	Tendinous and tuberous	Corneal arcus Lipid keratopathy Xanthelasma
Type III§ recessive	Broad elevations of β-lipoproteins	Creamy	Elevated	Elevated	7%	Tendinous and tuberous	Corneal arcus Xanthelasma Lipemia retinalis
Type IV§ dominant	Pre-β-lipoproteins elevated	Creamy	Elevated	Normal or slightly elevated	42%	Eruptive	Lipemia retinalis Xanthelasma (sometimes)
Type V	Pre-β-lipoproteins and chylomicrons elevated	Creamy	Elevated	Normal or slightly elevated	7%	Eruptive	Lipemia retinalis

*Elevated triglyceride level can produce lipemia retinalis and eruptive xanthomata.
†Elevated cholesterol level may cause corneal arcus, lipid keratopathy, and xanthelasma.
‡Low-density lipoprotein (LDL).
§Very low-density lipoprotein (VLDL).

TYPE I[8, 18] (HYPERCHYLOMICRONEMIA, BUERGER-GRÜTZ DISEASE)

This type of lipoproteinemia is a rare condition and is transmitted as an autosomal recessive trait. Most patients are clinically well, but abdominal crises with vomiting and prostration may occur. Eruptive xanthomata, which are small, yellow-orange papules, may be found on the face, buttocks, and limbs. Cardiovascular complications and tendinous, tuberous xanthomata are seen. "Creamy" serum is noted, however, and the greatest part of the increased total serum lipid is triglyceride. Sugar tolerance is normal.

Occasionally eruptive xanthomata of the eyelid, lipid keratopathy (rare), and lipemia retinalis are seen. Corneal arcus usually does not occur (Table 17-1).

TYPE II (HYPERBETALIPOPROTEINEMIA,[8,18] ESSENTIAL FAMILIAL HYPERCHOLESTEROLEMIA)

This problem is transmitted as an autosomal dominant trait. The heterozygously involved patient may exhibit xanthomatous lesions in the tendinous areas (knuckles and Achilles tendon). Peripheral vascular disease is not found, but coronary disease can be seen. The serum is clear, and there is an elevated cholesterol level. Glucose tolerance tests are normal.

The homozygous individual exhibits the same problem; however, it occurs earlier in life, and the systemic disease is more severe.

Corneal arcus, xanthelasma (Fig. 17-1), conjunctival xanthomata, and lipid keratopathy (Fig. 10-6) occur in this type of lipoproteinemia.

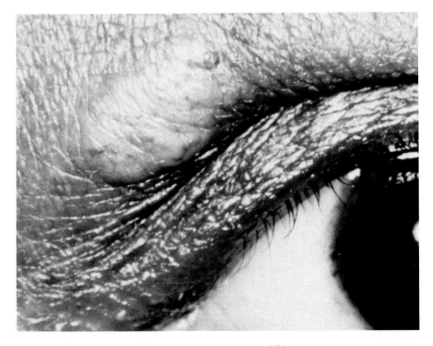

Fig. 17-1. Xanthelasma of lid.

TYPE III[8, 18] (DYSBETAPROTEINEMIA, IDIOPATHIC HYPERLIPEMIA)

This type is rare and is inherited as an autosomal recessive trait. Triglyceride, cholesterol, and β-lipoprotein levels are elevated. The serum is creamy; the glucose tolerance test is abnormal in 40% of the cases.

Tuberous and tendinous xanthomata are seen. Coronary and peripheral vascular disease is noted in men at 45 years of age and in women at 55. Diabetes and gout may occur.

Corneal arcus, xanthelasma, and lipemia retinalis may involve the eye.

TYPE IV[8, 18] (HYPERPREBETALIPOPROTEINEMIA, IDIOPATHIC HYPERLIPEMIA)

This problem, usually of autosomal dominant inheritance, is seen in young adults. The serum cholesterol level may be normal or slightly elevated, but the triglyceride level is elevated, and the serum is creamy. The glucose tolerance test is abnormal in 90% of the cases.[3] Peripheral vascular disease, coronary disease, and eruptive xanthomata on the buttocks, arms, and legs are seen. Gout, diabetes, and abdominal pain can accompany this type of lipoproteinemia.

Xanthelasma, corneal arcus, and lipemia retinalis can be seen.

TYPE V[8, 18] (HYPERPREBETALIPOPROTEINEMIA AND HYPERCHYLOMICRONEMIA)

This type of lipoproteinemia occurs in the 20- to 30-year-old group. The serum is creamy. The cholesterol level may be normal to high. The triglyceride level is elevated. Peripheral vascular disease has not been reported, and coronary disease is less significant. Abdominal pain may be severe. Occurring are eruptive xanthomata on the buttocks, arms, and legs; xanthelasma; corneal arcus; and lipemia retinalis.

Many patients, at least two thirds of whom have corneal arcus or xanthelasma, have no detectable systemic abnormality of lipoproteins.

FAMILIAL PLASMA–CHOLESTEROL ESTER DEFICIENCY (LECITHIN CHOLESTEROL–ACYLTRANSFERASE DEFICIENCY)

This entity is transmitted as an autosomal recessive trait. There is a marked reduction of the plasma cholesterol esters and plasma lysolecithin and an increase in the level of unesterified cholesterol, triglycerides, phospholipids, and plasma lecithin. The homozygote shows a deficiency in the ability to manufacture plasma lecithin–cholesterol acyltransferase. This prevents the maintenance of the normal balance between cholesterol and cholesterol esters in cell membranes.

One may see proteinuria, milky plasma, and normochromic anemia.

Corneal opacities consisting of many small gray dots appear throughout the stroma. The opacities may become dense at the periphery and resemble a corneal arcus.[9] Occasionally crystals, presumably cholesterol, appear near Descemet's membrane peripheral to the arcus if present.

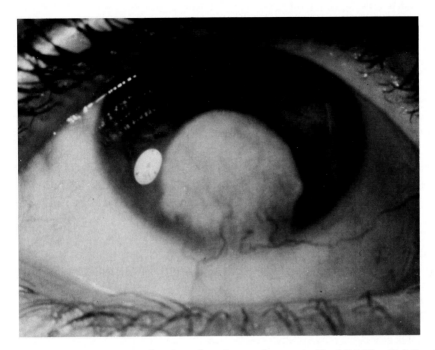

Fig. 17-2. Yellow infiltrate extending throughout layers of cornea in Hand-Schüller-Christian disease. (Courtesy L. Calkins, M.D., Kansas City, Mo.)

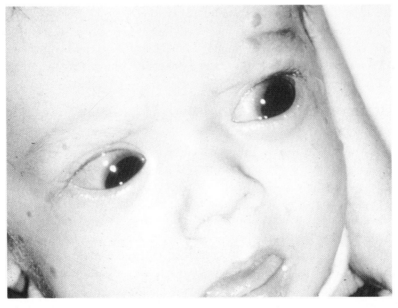

Fig. 17-3. Yellow-red papular lesions of skin in juvenile xanthogranuloma. These may be seen as epibulbar lesions that can extend onto cornea.

TANGIER DISEASE (HIGH-DENSITY α-LIPOPROTEIN DEFICIENCY)

This disease is transmitted as an autosomal recessive trait.[11] A complete absence of plasma high-density α-lipoprotein is noted; in its place an abnormal high-density lipoprotein is found. There may be an abnormally low level of cholesterol and phospholipids with normal or elevated concentrations of triglycerides in the plasma; however, an increase in the cholesterol esters in the tissues occurs. It is noteworthy to keep in mind several clues as to the diagnosis. Hypocholesterolemia in the absence of any malabsorption problem is an important clue.

One sees yellowish tinge to the tonsils, tonsil beds, rectal mucosa, and conjunctiva. Enlargement of the liver or lymph nodes occurs. There may also be a moderate hyperuricemia without any evidence of renal abnormality. Anemia and maculopapular rash may also be a part of the picture. Neurologic signs and coronary artery disease are seen in a number of patients.

The cornea shows stromal clouding caused by the deposition of cholesterol esters.[11] Many small dots in the posterior stroma may be distributed in a whorllike fashion.[11] There is an increased density or haze in the peripheral horizontal meridian. No arcus is seen.

HISTIOCYTOSIS X (HAND-SCHÜLLER-CHRISTIAN DISEASE, LETTERER-SIWE DISEASE)

In this group one may see disseminated xanthomata, lytic lesions of the bones, maculopapular skin rash, and diabetes insipidus if the pituitary area is involved. Histiocytosis X is not a true lipoidosis. The serum proteins are normal; however, an abnormal deposition of lipid-laden histiocytes is present.

Large xanthelasma of the lids may be seen. Proptosis and choroidal involvement may occur as a result of infiltration of the orbit and choroid with cholesterol-laden cells.

Although the cornea is not characteristically involved in any of the histiocytoses or related diseases, it may show an infiltration of the limbus and stroma with the same type of cell. This yellow-white infiltration extends throughout the layers of the cornea (Fig. 17-2) and may represent a nodular xanthoma.

JUVENILE XANTHOGRANULOMA (NEVOXANTHOENDOTHELIOMA)
(Fig. 17-3)

This disease, which may be grouped with the preceding entities, is a dermatologic problem seen in infants and children 8 to 10 years of age. Yellow-red papular skin lesions occur and may ultimately resolve. The iris and the ciliary body are infiltrated with histiocytes. The iris lesions can cauee spontaneous anterior chamber hemorrhages, and secondary glaucoma may ensue.

Multiple phlyctenular-like epibulbar lesions occasionally occur and may extend to the cornea. Corneal blood staining from hemorrhages and corneal edema and enlargement may be encountered from glaucoma. The epibulbar histiocytic lesions are yellow-white to pink and may resemble the salmon-pink infiltration of lymphoma lesions.

When one sees a spontaneous anterior chamber hemorrhage in children, one must keep in mind the possibility of retrolental fibroplasia, persistent hyperplastic vitreous, leukemia, lymphoma, retinoblastoma, and trauma.

IDIOPATHIC LIPID KERATOPATHY

This problem, which is manifested by deposition of lipid in the cornea, can occur with no apparent etiologic association. However, if diligent search is made, often an injury, a foreign body, herpes simplex, herpes zoster, or another entity can be elicited as the precipitating factor.

REFSUM'S DISEASE
(PHYTANIC ACID STORAGE DISEASE,
HEREDOPATHIA ATACTIA POLYNEURITIFORMIS)

It is presumed that phytanic acid accumulation in the tissues leads to the clinical manifestations of Refsum's disease. The enzymatic step at fault is the alpha oxidation of phytanic acid (C_{20} branched-chain fatty acid) to the corresponding hydroxy derivative. Dietary restrictions of phytanic acid in some patients has favorably influenced this autosomal recessive problem.[2] The acid originates mainly from dietary sources and from phytol, a component of leafy vegetables. Phytanic acid levels in the blood may be studied by gas chromatography. The most convenient method for detecting Refsum's disease is to examine the production of radioactive carbon dioxide from phytanic acid tagged with radioactive carbon in cultured skin fibroblasts.[10] Fibroblasts from heterozygotes oxidize phytanic acid at about one half the rate found in normal control cultures.[10]

One finds pigmentary retinal degeneration, peripheral neuropathy, cerebellar ataxia, nerve deafness, anosmia, pupillary abnormalities, and nystagmus. Skeletal and nonspecific electrocardiographic changes have been reported. Some patients have ichthyotic skin problems on the trunk, palms, and soles. There is an increase in the spinal fluid protein levels.[16]

Cataracts may be noted in some patients.

Irregular thick hazy corneal epithelium, fibrovascular pannus, and increased visibility of the corneal nerve are all seen. Cornea guttata and edema may be a part of the corneal disturbance.

URBACH-WIETHE DISEASE

This condition, which is probably transmitted as an autosomal recessive trait, at one time was thought to consist of deposition of a complex glycolipoprotein. There is little evidence to support this today. Direct chemical analysis of cutaneous lesions has shown that the lesions contain neither an excess nor a deficiency of glycolipids or phospholids when compared with the normal skin. Chemical and electron microscopic studies suggest the presence of protein deposits with a fine granular or filamentous hyaline-like appearance. The deposition increases until early adult life and then remains stable. The clinical picture depends on where the abnormal substance is deposited and how much is deposited. One finds most of the involvement in the skin, oropharynx,[4] tongue (Fig. 17-4), salivary glands, and central nervous system.[5] Short stature, hoarseness, photosensitivity, neurologic signs, and skin eruptions are seen.

Yellowish-colored papules, which are either verrucous or dome shaped, are noted on the lid margins (Fig. 17-5) and cause much irritation.

Corneal changes result from irritation by these lid lesions.[13]

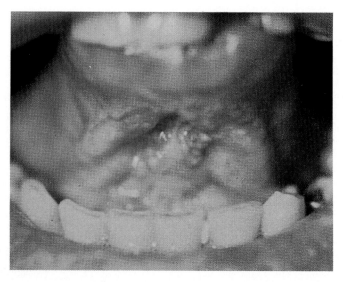

Fig. 17-4. Mucous membrane of mouth involved in Urbach-Wiethe disease. (From Muirhead, J.F., and Jackson, P.: Arch. Ophthalmol. **69:**174; copyright 1963, American Medical Association.)

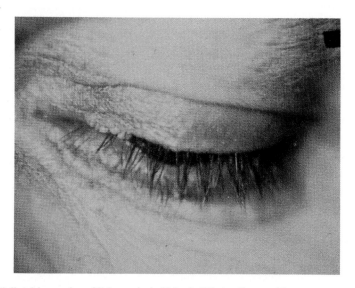

Fig. 17-5. Yellowish papules of lid margin in Urbach-Wiethe disease. These may cause secondary corneal changes by virtue of irritation from these lid lesions. (From Muirhead, J.F., and Jackson, P.: Arch. Ophthalmol. **69:**174; copyright 1963, American Medical Association.)

CHÉDIAK-HIGASHI SYNDROME

This syndrome is transmitted as an autosomal recessive trait and is associated with partial cutaneous and retinal albinism, photophobia, and nystagmus. Systemic involvement is noted with anemia, fever, convulsions, jaundice, hepatosplenomegaly, neuropathy, and lymphoreticular malignancy.[6] Giant azurophilic granules occur in the granulocytes, lymphocytes, and monocytes. The Chédiak-Higashi syndrome exhibits a disorder of white blood cell organelles, that is, enlarged, abnormal, and fragile lysosomes.[7]

The serum triglyceride and lecithin levels are increased. A decrease in lipoprotein and lysolecithin levels occurs.

The cornea may show noncharacteristic stromal opacities.

SCHNYDER'S CRYSTALLINE DYSTROPHY (Fig. 11-27)

This disorder is transmitted as an autosomal dominant trait. It is a slowly progressive or stationary bilateral problem with needle-shaped crystals in the subepithelial region of the cornea. The crystals occur centrally or paracentrally in a circle or disc-shaped form. Usually no loss of vision occurs, and irritation is minimal.

SECONDARY LIPID KERATOPATHY (CHOLESTEROL KERATOPATHY)
(Fig. 10-21)

Lipid deposits that appear as dense, yellow-white infiltrate can be seen in the cornea as a result of local corneal disease, especially that associated with vascularization. Chemical burns, long-standing herpes simplex, zoster scars, and interstitial keratitis may result in local deposits of cholesterol crystals.

In some instances no disease or history of trauma can be determined, but there are infiltrations of multicolored needlelike crystals in the cornea that probably are cholesterol in nature.[1]

It should be remembered that corneal crystals can be seen in entities other than lipid infiltration in the cornea. One must consider cystinosis, benign adult cystinuria, multiple myeloma, crystalline dystrophy, gout, marginal crystalline dystrophy of Bietti, Tangier disease, and porphyria.

PRIMARY LIPOIDAL DEGENERATION

The diagnosis of primary lipoidal degeneration is based on the presence of lipid deposits in a cornea that has not been previously vascularized or altered by inflammation. In addition, there should be no elevation of the serum lipid level. Primary lipoidal degeneration of the cornea is usually bilateral and may be a gross variation of a corneal arcus, an unusual variant of Schnyder's dystrophy, or both.[7]

REFERENCES

1. Baum, J.L.: Cholesterol keratopathy, Am. J. Ophthalmol. **67:**372, 1969.
2. Baum, J.L., Tannenbaum, M., and Kolodny, E.H.: Refsum's syndrome with corneal involvement, Am. J. Ophthalmol. **60:**699, 1965.
3. Bierman, E.L., and Porte, D.J., Jr.: Carbohydrate intolerance and lipemia, Ann. Intern. Med. **68:**926, 1968.
4. Burnett, J.W., and Marcy, S.M.: Lipid proteinosis, Am. J. Dis. Child. **105:**81, 1963.
5. Caplan, R.M.: Visceral involvement in lipoid proteinosis, Arch. Dermatol. **95:**149, 1967.

6. Dent, P.B., Fish, L.A., White, L.G., and Good, R.A.: Chédiak-Higashi syndrome: observations on the nature of the associated malignancy, Lab. Invest. **15**:1634, 1966.

7. Fine, B.S., Townsend, W.M., Zimmerman, L., and Lasahakari, M.H.: Primary lipoidal degeneration of the cornea, Am. J. Ophthalmol. **78**:12, 1974.

8. Fredrickson, D.S., Levy, R.I., and Lees, R.S.: Fat transport in lipoproteins: an integrated approach to mechanisms and disorders, N. Engl. J. Med. **276**:34, 1967.

9. Gjone, E., and Bergaust, B.: Corneal opacity in familial plasma cholesterol ester deficiency, Acta Ophthalmol. **47**:222, 1969.

10. Herdon, J.H., Steinberg, D., and Uhlendorf, B.W.: Refsum's disease: defective oxidation of phytanic acid in tissue cultures derived from homozygotes and heterozygotes, N. Engl. J. Med. **281**:1034, 1969.

11. Hoffman, H., II., and Fredrickson, D.S.: Tangier disease (familial high density lipoprotein deficiency): clinical and genetic features in two adults, Am. J. Ophthalmol. **39**:582, 1965.

12. Macaraey, P.V.J., Lasagna, L., and Snyder, B.: Arcus not so senilis, Ann. Intern. Med. **68**:345, 1968.

13. Newton, F.H., Rosenberg, R.N., Lampert, P.W., and O'Brien, J.S.: Neurologic involvement in Urbach-Wiethe's disease (lipid proteinosis): a clinical, ultrastructural, and chemical study, Neurology **21**:1205, 1971.

14. Press, M.: The significance of the corneal arcus, Practitioner **212**:75, 1974.

15. Roseman, R.H.: Corneal arcus in coronary heart disease, N. Engl. J. Med. **291**:1322, 1974.

16. Steinberg, D., Vroom, F.Q., Engel, W.K., et al.: Refsum's disease: a recently characterized lipidosis involving the nervous system, Ann. Intern. Med. **66**:365, 1967.

17. Tschetter, R.: Lipid analysis of the human cornea with and without arcus senilis, Arch. Ophthalmol. **76**:403, 1966.

18. Vinger, P.F., and Sacks, B.A.: Ocular manifestations of hyperlipoproteinemia, Am. J. Ophthalmol. **70**:563, 1970.

18 Mucopolysaccharidoses

Systemic mucopolysaccharidoses
    Hurler's syndrome
    Scheie's syndrome
    Hunter's syndrome
    Sanfilippo's syndrome
    Morquio's syndrome
    Maroteaux-Lamy syndrome
    β-Glucuronidase deficiency
    Differential diagnosis
    Tests
    Management

Local corneal mucopolysaccharide diseases
    Macular corneal dystrophy (MCD)
    Mucopolysaccharidoses of Bowman's
      layer
Other corneal conditions
    Winchester's syndrome
    Diabetes mellitus
    Glycogen storage disease type I
      (von Gierke's disease)
    Dermachondrocorneal dystrophy of
      François

The human body is composed primarily of three elements: (1) the cell, (2) cell fibrils, and (3) the surrounding extracellular matrix, or ground substance. The extracellular matrix plays a vital role in the maintenance and regulation of cellular function, as well as in intercellular support. The substance is composed primarily of macromolecules of carbohydrate and protein. *Acid mucopolysaccharide* is the term employed when a preponderance of carbohydrate is present; the term *glycoprotein* is used when a preponderance of protein is present in the extracellular matrix. The nomenclature for acid mucopolysaccharides suggested today is listed in Table 18-1.[10]

Three major acid mucopolysaccharides are found in the corneal stroma:

1. Keratan sulfate I (50%)
2. Chondroitin (25%)
3. Chondroitin 4 sulfate (25%)

Keratan sulfate I is found exclusively in the cornea.

The organelle system of the cell, consisting of the Golgi apparatus, mitochondria, and smooth and rough endoplasmic reticulum, is the site of cellular metabolism. The core protein and glycosyltransferases are synthesized by membrane-bound ribosomes in the rough endoplasmic reticulum of the cell. The initiation of acid mucopolysaccharide chains and synthesis of the linkage region occur predominantly in the cisternae of the rough endoplasmic reticulum. These macromolecules pass from the rough into the smooth endoplasmic reticulum and Golgi apparatus. Completion of the chain synthesis and sulfation occur to a large extent in the smooth endoplasmic and Golgi vesicles.[16, 24] The product is released by secretion vacuoles to the exterior. Thus it is seen that single membrane-bound vacuoles in the cytoplasm contain acid hydrolases to metabolize biochemical products of the cell. Any alteration in these factors or a missing enzyme may result in a modified final product with specific characteristics, either histochemically, structurally, or both. Degradation of the polysaccharide chain is catalyzed by glycosidases, hydrolytic enzymes present in lysosomes.[32] These enzymes are of particular interest because an absence of, or inactive form of, different lysosomal hydrolases is the cause of several mucopolysaccharide storage diseases, which are transmitted as autosomal recessive traits.

SYSTEMIC MUCOPOLYSACCHARIDOSES[7, 18]
Hurler's syndrome

Hurler's syndrome (MPS IH) (Tables 18-1 and 18-2) is characterized by a gargoyle-like facies and marked skeletal abnormalities such as reduced joint mobility, lumbar gibbus, chest abnormalities, dwarfism (Fig. 18-1), and deformities of the fingers (Fig. 18-2). Hepatic and cardiac problems are common features. Mental retardation is severe.

Pigmentary retinopathy with optic atrophy is found commonly.[12] A subnormal or external electroretinographic finding is also seen.

The cornea may be clear at birth but soon after becomes cloudy (Fig. 18-3). There is an avascular noninflammatory clouding. The fine, gray, punctate opacities are first seen in the anterior stroma, then in the posterior stroma and endothelium.

Scheie's syndrome

Scheie's syndrome (MPS IS) (Tables 18-1 and 18-2) has the same enzymatic defect as Hurler's syndrome. It exhibits the claw hand, moderate dwarfism, stiff joints, and facial coarseness, as well as cardiac disease. Mental retardation does not occur.

Pigmentary disease of the retina and optic atrophy appear. Acute narrow-angle glaucoma has been seen in MPS IS as a result of limbal thickening from acid mucopolysaccharide deposition.[25]

Severe progressive corneal clouding is seen.

In MPS IH[27] diffuse stromal haze appears as a myriad of minute opacities in the stroma reaching to the limbus. In MPS IS the cloudiness of the cornea is more marked peripherally.

Hunter's syndrome

Hunter's syndrome[1] (MPS II) (Tables 18-1 and 18-2) is transmitted as a sex-linked recessive trait and tends to be milder than does Hurler's syndrome. Severe and mild forms of MPS II occur, and in both forms skeletal dysplasia, mental retardation, and cardiovascular changes are seen. Retinal pigmentary changes and optic atrophy are also noted. There may be an involvement of the sclera and cilia in this form of mucopolysaccharidosis.[3, 14, 30]

In the mild form, a cornea opacity occurs that may manifest itself later in life and is mild compared with other mucopolysaccharidoses. In the severe form of Hunter's syndrome subclinical corneal clouding can be demonstrated histochemically.

Table 18-1. Ocular and systemic features of mucopolysaccharidoses (MPS)

Disease nomenclature	Cornea opacifi-cation	Retina (pigmentary degener-ation)	Optic atrophy	Mental retardation	Cardio-vascular	Skeletal dysplasia
MPS IH Hurler's syndrome	+	+	+	+	+	+
MPS IS Scheie's syndrome	+	+	+	−	+	+
MPS IH/S Hurler's Scheie syndrome	+	+	+	±	+	+ +
MPS IIA Hunter's syndrome, severe*	±	+	+	+	+	+
MPS IIB Hunter's syndrome, mild†	+	+	+	±	+	+
MPS IIIA Sanfilippo's syndrome A	−	+	+			
MPS IIIB Sanfilippo's syndrome B	−	−	+	+	−	+
MPS IVA Morquio's syndrome, severe	+‡	−	+	−	+	+
MPS IVB Morquio's syndrome, mild	+‡	−	+	−	+	+
MPS V Vacant						
MPS VIA Maroteaux-Lamy syndrome, severe†	+	−	+	−	+	+
MPS VIB Maroteaux-Lamy syndrome, mild	+	−	−	−	−	−
MPS VII β-Glucuronidase deficiency	−	?	?	+	?	+

*Ciliary body involved. Subclinical corneal clouding is demonstrable histochemically.
†Sclera involved.
‡Corneal clouding may not be grossly evident until after age 10.

Table 18-2. Heredity and enzymatic defects in systemic mucopolysaccharidosis

Disease nomenclature		Enzymatic defect	Excessive urinary MPS	Inheritance
MPS IH	Hurler's syndrome	α-L-Iduronidase	Dermatan sulfate* Heparan sulfate	Recessive
MPS IS	Scheie's syndrome	α-L-Iduronidase	Dermatan sulfate Heparan sulfate	Recessive
MPS IIA	Hunter's syndrome, severe	Sulfoiduronate sulfatase	Dermatan sulfate Heparan sulfate	X-linked recessive
MPS IIB	Hunter's syndrome, mild	Sulfoiduronate sulfatase	Dermatan sulfate Heparan sulfate	Recessive
MPS IIIA	Sanfilippo's syndrome A	Heparan sulfate sulfatase	Heparan sulfate	Recessive
MPS IIIB	Sanfilippo's syndrome B	N-Acetyl-α-D galactosaminidase	Heparan sulfate	Recessive
MPS IVA	Morquio's syndrome, severe	Hexosamine-6-sulfatase	Keratan sulfate	Recessive
MPS IVB	Morquio's syndrome, mild	Hexosamine-6-sulfatase	Keratan sulfate	Recessive
MPS V	Vacant			
MPS VIA	Maroteaux-Lamy syndrome, classic	Unknown	Dermatan sulfate*	Recessive
MPS VIB	Maroteaux-Lamy syndrome, mild	Unknown	Dermatan sulfate	Recessive
MPS VII	β-Glucuronidase deficiency	β-Glucuronidase	Dermatan sulfate	Recessive

*Dermatan sulfate was previously called chondroitin sulfate B.

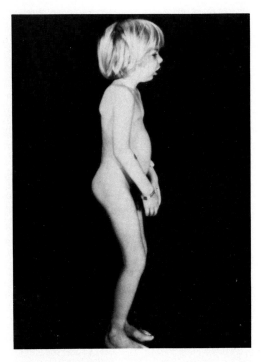

Fig. 18-1. Physical stature in Hurler's disease. (From Grayson, M., and Keates, R.H.: Manual of diseases of the cornea, Boston, 1969, Little, Brown & Co.)

It has been stated that corneal clouding that appears later can be used to discriminate clinically between Hurler's and Hunter's syndromes.[6] This, however, may not always be true; there are case reports of Hurler's syndrome (MPS IH) with clear corneas up to 14 years of age.[10]

Sanfilippo's syndrome

Sanfilippo's syndrome (MPS III) (Tables 18-1 and 18-2) manifests no corneal opacity. These patients exhibit severe mental retardation but less severe hepatosplenomegaly and skeletal and facial abnormalities (Fig. 18-4). The hand shows changes similar to those seen in Hurler's syndrome. Retinal pigmentary degeneration and optic atrophy occur.

Morquio's syndrome

Morquio's syndrome (Tables 18-1 and 18-2) may be mild or severe. Corneal clouding may not be grossly evident until after 10 years of age; it may only have a mild diffuse stromal haze; or it may be severe at any age.[33] Marked retardation of growth and skeletal dysplasia occurs. Neurosensory deafness is seen in the teens. Retinopathy is not present.

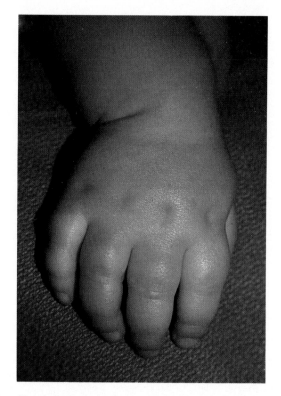

Fig. 18-2. Deformity of hands in Hurler's disease. (From Grayson, M., and Keates, R.H.: Manual of diseases of the cornea, Boston, 1969, Little, Brown & Co.)

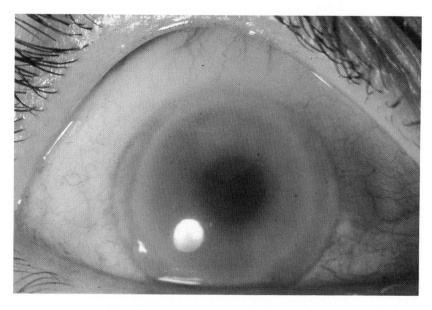

Fig. 18-3. Cloudy cornea in Hurler's disease.

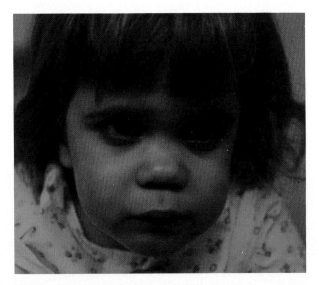

Fig. 18-4. Characteristic facial appearance in case of Sanfilippo's disease. (From Grayson, M., and Keates, R.H.: Manual of diseases of the cornea, Boston, 1969, Little, Brown & Co.)

Maroteaux-Lamy syndrome

Maroteaux-Lamy syndrome (Tables 18-1 and 18-2) exhibits many of the skeletal anomalies seen in Hurler's syndrome with claw fingers, skeletal dysplasia, and restricted joint mobility. Cardiac complications may be found, but there is no retinal pigmentary degeneration. Optic atrophy and hydrocephalus may be seen.[15] Corneal opacities are present in all cases, although a slit lamp is sometimes needed to see them.[15]

β-Glucuronidase deficiency

β-Glucuronidase deficiency (MPS VII) (Tables 18-1 and 18-2) exhibits mental retardation, skeletal dysplasia, and hepatosplenomegaly. Eye findings have not been reported.

Differential diagnosis

Great variation exists in the clinical appearance of the corneal opacification in the mucopolysaccharidoses; typical clinical corneal features are not characteristic enough to diagnose the specific mucopolysaccharidoses.

The ultrastructural findings in the conjunctiva, cornea, and sclera exhibit some characteristics.[20] In the conjunctiva, intracytoplasmic vacuoles limited by single-unit membranes derived from the golgi apparatus containing fibrillogranular substances are seen. Occasionally membranous lamellar inclusions occur. In the cornea, intraepithelial vacuoles limited by a single-unit membrane and containing fibrillogranular material are found. The keratocytes contain intracytoplasmic vacuoles (Fig. 18-5) with fibrillogranular material limited by a single membrane as well as extracellular fine granular material and small membrane-limited vacuoles (Fig. 18-6).

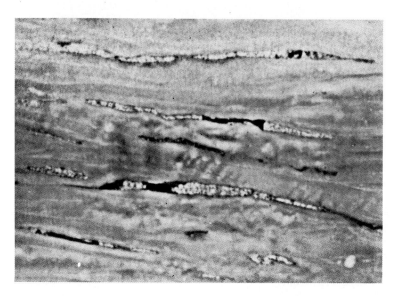

Fig. 18-5. In some mucopolysaccharide diseases, as in this case of Maroteaux-Lamy syndrome, keratocytes are swollen by foamy-appearing cytoplasm. (From Kenyon, K.R., Topping, T.M., Green, W.R., and Maumanee, A.E.: Am. J. Ophthalmol. **73:**718, 1972.)

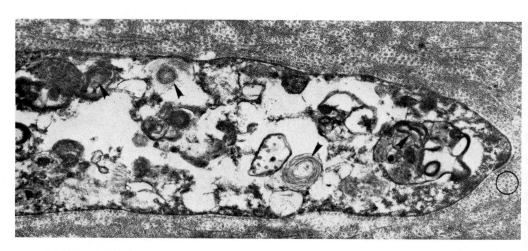

Fig. 18-6. Corneal stroma may show keratocytes containing membranous lamellar inclusions and fibrillogranular material. (From Kenyon, K.R., Topping, T.M., Green, W.R., and Maumanee, A.E.: Am. J. Ophthalmol. **73:**718, 1972.)

In clinically clear corneas these same microscopic findings may be seen in MPS IIB and very rarely in MPS III. In the sclera, fibrillogranular material in vacuoles is seen in MPS VIA and MPS IIB.

Therefore the common thread of the ultrastructural change in systemic MPS is the presence of single membrane-limited intracytoplasmic vacuoles containing fibrillogranular material. Occasionally membranous lamellar inclusions are seen.

These storage vacuoles containing the fibrillogranular material originate from lysosome, the cellular organelles responsible for enzymatically mediated degradative processes. The intracytoplasmic vacuoles may be considered as altered lysosomes that have become filled with acid mucopolysaccharide and glycolipid storage substances.

The enzymatic defect in each systemic MPS is shown in Table 18-2.

Tests

Several simple tests are presently available for the detection of excess urinary mucopolysaccharides.[13] A new test* uses a specially treated filter paper impregnated with azure A that is fast and reliable. Complete chemical analysis of urinary mucopolysaccharides should be carried out on all individuals with positive screening tests. The detection of heterozygotes (carriers) is not as simple. Metachromasia of cultured skin fibroblasts under carefully controlled conditions has been used for the detection of heterozygotes. However, the results should be interpreted cautiously, and diagnosis of the heterozygotes confirmed by an independent method. At the present time the most reliable method is direct chemical analysis of cultured skin fibroblast.[6] The methods of choice for in utero detection of the mucopolysaccharidoses are the measurement of labeled sulfate uptake and cultured amniotic cells or the assay for Hurler correction factor (α-L-iduronidase). Specific tests to differentiate the mucopolysaccharidoses can be found.

Management

Penetrating keratoplasty has been reported with both favorable and unfavorable results in the mucopolysaccharidoses. Unsuccessful results with penetrating keratoplasty in patients with Scheie's syndrome[9] have been experienced; however, a clear graft of 4 years has survived in a patient with MPS IH/S (Hurler-Scheie syndrome).[27]

Normal human plasma has been infused into patients with Hurler's and Hunter's syndromes in the hope of supplying the deficient enzyme.[5, 19] The first reports are encouraging; however, further study is necessary.[6, 8]

LOCAL CORNEAL MUCOPOLYSACCHARIDE DISEASES

The following two entities, macular dystrophy and mucopolysaccharidoses of Bowman's layer, are examples of a local corneal condition without any systemic enzymatic defects.

---

*MPS papers, Ames Co., Division of Miles Laboratories, Inc., Elkhart, Ind.

Macular corneal dystrophy[11] (MCD)

Macular dystrophy of the cornea is an isolated metabolic, genetically determined disorder of corneal fibroblast. These corneal opacities, which are thought to be secreted into the stroma by the corneal fibroblasts, have been identified as consisting of keratan sulfate; hexose-rich, periodic acid–reacting glycoproteins; or both.[21]

Hereditary transmission is usually considered autosomal recessive. The clinical appearance usually starts in the first decade of life and is progressive. A diffuse opacity occurs with grayish-white spots that have indistinct edges. Diffuse cloudiness of the stroma appears between the opacities. The opacities begin in the center of the cornea and at the superficial stromal layers but usually progress until they affect the proximities of the limbus and the entire thickness of the stroma. Subepithelial deposits frequently cause irregular astigmatism and recurrent epithelial erosions. The endothelium is frequently involved and forms excessive basement membranes (Descemet's membrane) in the form of clinical corneal guttata. Even if the opacities become very dense, the cornea is not usually thicker and can even be thinner than normal. The patient is plagued by photophobia and irritation, and the corneal opacities become so dense by the ages of 30 to 40 that visual acuity is markedly decreased. These corneas do not display increased vascularization but have a decreased corneal sensitivity.

MCD is a primary metabolic disorder of keratocytes and endothelium. The deficiency of lysosomal D-galactosidase in MCD cornea and conjunctival fibroblasts contributes to the inclusion of MCD among the inborn errors of lysosomal disorders.

Penetrating keratoplasty is frequently necessary for visual improvement in MCD. There have been several reports of opacification of the corneal graft in MCD that was thought to be a recurrence of excessive mucopolysaccharide accumulation.[17, 22, 23]

Mucopolysaccharidoses of Bowman's layer

Several cases of conjunctival and corneal clouding caused by AMP deposition limited to Bowman's layer, without systemic mucopolysaccharidoses, have been seen in infants.[26] Similar corneal involvement with additional anterior stromal involvement has been seen in a 20-year-old patient.

One of the cases with conjunctival corneal clouding involved anomalies of the cardiovascular system and telangiectasia of the face, scalp, trunk, bones, meninges, and mucosa. In addition, peripheral edema, cyanosis, and inguinal hernia have been seen.

OTHER CORNEAL CONDITIONS
Winchester's syndrome[2, 31]

The Winchester syndrome, a rare inherited disorder, is characterized by dwarfism, carpotarsal osteolysis, rheumatoid-like small joint destruction, and thickening and hypertrichosis of the skin. In addition to these features, a peculiar annular opacification, vascularization, and thinning of the peripheral cornea occur.

Brown and Kuwabara[2] considered the constellation of features comprising this disorder to represent a new acid mucopolysaccharide storage disease. These conclusions were based on cellular metachromasia and a twofold increase in cellular uronic acid in cultured fibroblasts. However, these criteria are not specific for making a diagnosis of lysosomal storage disease. It was shown that 27% of cell lines from control individuals demonstrate metachromasia.[29] In cases of mucopolysaccharidosis, the usual increase in intracellular uronic acid is in the fivefold to tenfold range rather than the twofold increase reported.[25]

It appears now that Winchester's syndrome is a disorder characterized partially by ultrastructural abnormalities of fibroblasts. The basic defect may be an abnormality of fibroblasts that, by proliferation, leads to thickened skin, peripheral opacities of the cornea, and joint contracture and that may be related to the osteolysis observed in Winchester's syndrome. Despite the familial nature of this disease and its clinical resemblance to some of the lysosomal storage diseases, no morphologic evidence exists at present for considering Winchester's syndrome to be a mucopolysaccharidosis or other lysosomal storage disorder.[3]

Diabetes mellitus

No specific corneal changes can be definitely related to diabetes mellitus. However, central corneal opacities, keratoconjunctivitis sicca, filamentary keratitis, decreased corneal sensitivity, wrinkling of Descemet's membrane, and pigmentation of endothelium have been reported.[4]

Laboratory studies of patients with diabetes indicate that significant amounts of glucose, fructose, and sorbitol, along with two other unidentified sugars, are present in the corneal epithelium of diabetic patients and are not present in nondiabetic patients. The significance of this observation with regard to the pathophysiology of corneal disease is speculative, but it is possible that intracellular accumulations of sorbitol in sufficient quantities could produce overhydration of epithelial cells. This also suggests that sorbitol accumulation in corneal epithelium may indeed have clinical significance with respect to the various forms of keratopathy seen in diabetic patients.[28]

Glycogen storage disease type I (von Gierke's disease)

A faint brown peripheral corneal clouding is reported that may resemble the clouding seen in the mucopolysaccharidoses. Other ocular abnormalities consist of multiple yellowish, discrete, paramacular lesions that appear to be unique to this syndrome.

Dermochondrocorneal dystrophy of François

This condition is transmitted as an autosomal recessive trait. Deformities of the hands and feet occur in the first 5 years of life. Xanthoma-like nodules appear in the skin of the nose, ears, and extensor aspects of elbows and joints of fingers.

By the end of the first decade white or brownish, irregular subepithelial opacities appear. The corneal periphery is clear, and the stroma and endothelium are normal. Vision is somewhat decreased, but the corneal changes do not advance.[9]

REFERENCES

1. Bach, G., Eisenberg, F., Cantz, M., and Neufeld, E.F.: The defect in Hunter syndrome: deficiency of sulfoiduronate sulfatase, Proc. Natl. Acad. Sci. U.S.A. **70:**2134, 1973.

2. Brown, S.I., and Kuwabara, T.: Peripheral corneal opacification and skeletal deformities: a newly recognized acid mucopolysaccharidoses simulating rheumatoid arthritis, Arch. Ophthalmol. **83:**667, 1970.

3. Cohen, A.H., Hollester, D.W., and Reed, B.: The skin in the Winchester syndrome. Arch. Dermatol. **111**:230, 1975.
4. Collier, M.: La pathologie cornéene des diabetiques, Bull. Soc. Ophthalmol. Fr. **67**:105, 1967.
5. DiFerrante, H., Nichols, B.L., Donnelly, P.V., Neri, G., Hrgovcic, R., and Berglund, R.K.: Induced degradation of glycosamino-glycans in Hurler's and Hunter's syndromes by plasma infusion. Proc. Natl. Acad. Sci. U.S.A. **68**:303, 1971.
6. DiFerrante, H., Nichols, B.L., Knudson, A.G., McCredie, K.B., Singh, J., and Donnelly, P.V.: Mucopolysaccharide storage diseases: corrective activity of normal human serum and lymphocyte extracts. Birth Defects **9**:31, 1973.
7. Dorfman, A., and Matalon, R.: The mucopolysaccharidoses. In Stanburg, J.B., Wyngaadern, J.B., and Fredrickson, D.S., editors: The metabolic basis of inherited disease, ed. 3, New York, 1972, McGraw-Hill Book Co.
8. Erickson, R.P., Sandman, R., Robertson, W.B., and Epstein, C.J.: Inefficiency of fresh frozen plasma therapy of mucopolysaccharidosis II, Pediatrics **50**:693, 1972.
9. François, J.: Heredo-familial corneal dystrophies, Trans. Ophthalmol. Soc. U.K. **86**:367, 1966.
10. Gardner, R.J.M., and Hay, J.R.: Hurler's syndrome with clear corneas (letter), Lancet **2**:845, 1974.
11. Garner, A.: Histochemistry of corneal macular dystrophy, Invest. Ophthalmol. **8**:475, 1969.
12. Gills, P.J., Hobson, R., Hanley, B., and McKusick, V.: Electroretinography and fundus oculi findings in Hurler's disease and allied mucopolysaccharidoses, Arch. Ophthalmol. **74**:596, 1965.
13. Goldberg, M.F.: Genetic and metabolic eye disease, Boston, 1974, Little, Brown & Co.
14. Goldberg, M.F., and Duke, J.R.: Ocular histopathology in Hunter's syndrome: systemic mucopolysaccharidosis, type II, Arch. Ophthalmol. **77**:503, 1967.
15. Goldberg, M.F., Scott, C.I., and McKusick, V.A.: Hydrocephalus and papilledema in Maroteaux-Lamy syndrome (mucopolysaccharidosis type VI), Am. J. Ophthalmol. **69**:969, 1970.
16. Goodman, G.C., and Lane, N.: On the site of sulfation in the chrondrocyte, J. Cell Biol. **21**:353-366, 1964.
17. Herman, S.J., and Hughes, W.F.: Recurrences of hereditary corneal dystrophy following keratoplasty, Am. J. Ophthalmol. **75**:689, 1973.
18. Jeanloz, R.W.: The nomenclature of acid mucopolysaccharides, Arthritis Rheum. **3**:323, 1960.
19. Kajii, T., Matsuda, I., Osawa, T., Katsunuma, H., Ichida, T., and Arashima, S.: Hurler/Scheie genetic compound (mucopolysaccharidoses IH/IS) in Japanese brothers, Clin. Genet. **6**:394, 1974.
20. Kenyon, K.R., Quigley, H.A., Hussels, I.E., and Wyllie, R.G.: The systemic mucopolysaccharidoses: ultrastructural and histological studies of conjunctiva and skin, Am. J. Ophthalmol. **73**:811, 1972.
21. Lamberg, S.I., and Stoolmiller, A.C.: Glycosaminoglycans: a biochemical and clinical review, J. Invest. Dermatol. **63**:433, 1974.
22. Lorenzetti, D.W.C., and Kaufman, H.E.: Macular and lattice dystrophies and their recurrences after keratoplasty, Trans. Am. Acad. Ophthalmol. Otolaryngol. **71**:112, 1967.
23. Morgan, G.: Macular dystrophy of the cornea, Br. J. Ophthalmol. **50**:57, 1966.
24. Neutra, M., and Leblond, C.P.: Radioautographic comparison of the uptake of galactose-H and glucose-H3 in the golgi region of various cells secreting glycoproteins or mucopolysaccharides, J. Cell. Biol. **30**:137, 1966.
25. Quigley, H.A., Maumanee, A.E., and Stark, W.J.: Systemic mucopolysaccharidosis, Am. J. Ophthalmol. **80**:1, 1975.
26. Rodrigues, M.M., Calhoun, J., and Harley, R.D.: Corneal clouding with increased acid mucopolysaccharide accumulation in Bowman's membrane, Am. J. Ophthalmol. **79**:916, 1975.
27. Scheie, H.G., Hambrick, G.W., and Barnes, L.A.: A newly recognized form of Hurler's disease (gargoylism), Am. J. Ophthalmol. **53**:753, 1962.
28. Schultz, R.O., Van Horn, D.L., Peters, M.A., Klewin, K.M., and Schutten, W.H.: Diabetic keratopathy, Trans. Am. Ophthalmol. Soc. **79**:180, 1981.
29. Taysi, K., Kistenmacher, M.L., Punnett, H.H., et al.: Limitations of metachromasis as a diagnostic aid in pediatrics, N. Engl. J. Med. **281**:1108, 1969.
30. Topping, T.M., Kenyon, R.K., Goldberg, M.F., and Maumanee, E.A.: Ultrastructural ocular pathology of Hunter's syndrome, Arch. Ophthalmol. **86**:164, 1971.
31. Winchester, P., Grossman, H., Lim, W.N., and Danes, B.S.: A new acid mucopolysaccharidosis with skeletal deformities simulating rheumatoid arthritis, Am. J. Roentgenol. Radium Ther. Nucl. Med. **106**:121, 1961.
32. Van Hoof, F., and Hers, H.G.: The abnormalities of lysosomal enzymes in mucopolysaccharidoses, Eur. J. Biochem. **7**:34, 1968.
33. Van Noorden, G.K., Zellweger, H., and Ponseti, I.: Ocular findings in Morquio-Ullrich's disease, Arch. Ophthalmol. **64**:585, 1960.

19 Mucolipidoses

Diseases of combined carbohydrate and lipid metabolism
GM_1 gangliosidosis I
Mucolipidosis I
Mucolipidosis II
Mucolipidosis III
Mucolipidosis IV
Goldberg-Cotlier syndrome
Metachromatic leukodystrophy (MLD)
Mannosidosis
Fucosidosis

DISEASES OF COMBINED CARBOHYDRATE AND LIPID METABOLISM

Table 19-1 compares the basic features or characterizations of mucopolysaccharidoses, sphingolipidoses, and mucolipidoses. One should review Table 19-1 before proceeding with the sphingolipidoses and mucolipidoses; it will aid in putting these disease groups in their proper perspective.

Patients with these diseases, who have been described as "Hurler variants," exhibit many of the features of Hurler's syndrome and related mucopolysaccharidoses but excrete normal amounts of urinary mucopolysaccharides.[15] In addition to the Hurler-like characteristics, symptoms of visceral and mesenchymal sphingolipid and/or glycolipid storage are present.[15] These diseases are now classified as a separate group—the *mucolipidoses*[1] (Table 19-2)—which is thought of as mucopolysaccharidoses (MPS) of the viscera with variable involvement of the cornea and as sphingolipidoses (SLS) of the central nervous system. Thus there is a combination of cloudy cornea seen in the MPS together with the macular cherry-red spot seen in the SLS, MLS I, MLS IV, generalized gangliosidosis, Goldberg-Cotlier syndrome, and metachromatic leukodystrophy (Austin variant).

Corneal opacities have been described in some of these mucolipidoses: generalized (GM_1) gangliosidosis I, mucolipidoses I to IV, and the Goldberg-Cotlier syndrome. Superficial opacities are seen occasionally in fucosidosis and mannosidosis.

Table 19-1. Features of mucopolysaccharidoses, sphingolipidoses, and mucolipidoses

Carbohydrate (mucopolysaccharidoses)	Lipid (sphingolipidoses)	Carbohydrate and lipid (mucolipidoses)
Prenatal diagnosis accomplished at present in Hurler's and Hunter's syndromes	Prenatal diagnosis accomplished at present in Tay-Sachs, Niemann-Picket, and Fabry's diseases	Prenatal diagnosis accomplished in metachromatic leukodystrophy
Lysomal storage material consists of mostly fibrillogranular (carbohydrate) and some lamellar membranous material (glycolipid)	Lysosomal storage material consists of lamellar membranous material (glycolipid)	Lysosomal storage material consists of fibrillogranular and membranous material
Ocular features variable	Ocular features variable	Ocular features variable
Optic atrophy	Optic atrophy	Optic atrophy
Retinal pigmentary degeneration	Cherry-red spot	Cherry-red spot
Corneal clouding	Corneal clouding	Corneal clouding
Mental retardation variable	Mental retardation variable	Mental retardation variable
Skeletal dysplasia	Skeletal dysplasia	Skeletal dysplasia
Gargoyle-like features	No gargoyle-like features	Gargoyle-like features
Abnormal mucopolysacchariduria	Normal mucopolysacchariduria	Normal mucopolysacchariduria, except juvenile sulfatidosis (Austin type)
Visceral storage of acid mucopolysaccharides	Visceral storage of glycolipids	Visceral storage of acid mucopolysaccharides and glycolipids

GM$_1$ GANGLIOSIDOSIS I

Corneal opacities described as mild, diffuse corneal clouding are only occasionally found in this disease, which results from the accumulation of keratan sulfate because of absent β-galactosidase.[5, 6] These corneal opacities are associated with a cherry red–spot lesion of the retina, hepatosplenomegaly, psychomotor retardation, and skeletal changes resembling gargoylism.[11, 16] The infant is affected at birth or shortly thereafter. β-Galactosidase, the missing enzyme, breaks down the ganglioside GM$_1$ and leads to accumulation of ganglioside of keratan sulfate. The physical appearance of these children resembles that of individuals with Hurler's syndrome.

MUCOLIPIDOSIS I

Corneal opacities, which may be associated with cherry-red macular spots, are seen rarely in this disease.[7] Physical growth is usually normal at first but slow after about age 10. The mental development is slow, but the children usually learn to walk, to play, and to say single words. Herniae and hepatic or splenic enlargement are inconsistently present.[8, 9]

MLS type	Corneal clouding	Enzyme defect	Excessively stored substance	Optic atrophy	Gray macular and/or cherry-red spot	Heredity
MLS I (lipomucopolysaccharidosis)	±	Unknown	Acid MPS and glycolipids	−	+	Recessive
MLS II (I cell disease)	±	β-Galactosidase	Acid MPS and glycolipids	−	+†	Recessive
MLS III (pseudo-Hurler polydystrophy)	+	Unknown	Acid MPS and glycolipids	−	−	Recessive
MLS IV	+	Unknown	Presumably MPS and lipids	−	+	Recessive (probably)
GM_1 gangliosidosis, type I	±	β-Galactosidases A, B, and C	Keratan sulfate in cornea GM_1 ganglioside in retinal ganglion cells and viscera	+	+	Recessive
GM_1 gangliosidosis, type II	−	β-Galactosidases B and C	Keratan sulfate in cornea GM_1 ganglioside in retinal ganglion cells and viscera	+	−	Recessive
Metachromatic leukodystrophy‡ (Austin variant)	±	Arylsulfatases A, B, and C	Sulfated mucopolysaccharides and sulfatide	+ +	+	Recessive
Mannosidosis	Bowman's layer (rare)	α-Mannosidase	Mannose-rich oligosaccharides	−	−	Unknown
Fucosidosis	Bowman's layer (opacity) +	α-Fucosidase	Fucose-containing glycolipids	−	−	Unknown
Goldberg-Cotlier syndrome	+	β-Galactosidase (uraminadase ?)	Unknown	−	+	Recessive
Farber's granulomatosis	−	Ceramidase	Acid MPS and ceramide	−	+	Recessive

*It should be noted that as enzyme assay tests and more patients are seen and diagnosed, additional information will come about. Occasionally one case shows up with a new finding that has not been previously reported—even changes in enzyme defects may be anticipated; therefore one can anticipate changes in this table.

†One case described.

‡Mucopolysaccharide in urine.

MUCOLIPIDOSIS II

This disease is characterized by gargoyle-like facies, severe growth and psychomotor retardation, thickened skin, and skeletal dysplasia; mild hepatomegaly, corneal clouding, glaucoma, and megalocornea occur as well. Cherry-red spots have never been seen.[4,7]

MUCOLIPIDOSIS III

Slit-lamp examination of the cornea may reveal fine corneal opacities in mucolipidosis III. The first symptoms usually originate from the skeletal muscular system. After the second year of life, restricted joint mobility, small stature, short necks, scoliosis, and hip dysplasia are noted. Mild gargoyle-like symptoms appear in some patients but may be absent in others. Moderate mental retardation is present. With advancing age, mentality seems to regress.[12]

MUCOLIPIDOSIS IV

This disease is a variant of the mucolipidosis that exhibits bilateral corneal opacities by 6 weeks of age.[2] Both corneas are opaque, the haziness being diffuse and homogenous from the center to the periphery. Slit-lamp examination reveals multiple opaque dots throughout all layers of the stroma with no obvious signs of edema. Normal fundi are seen. Intraocular pressure is normal. No skeletal or neurologic abnormalities occur up to the age of 5 months, but later signs of mild motor retardation can be detected. Another new mucolipidosis with psychomotor retardation, cloudy cornea, retinal degeneration, optic atrophy, and extinguished electroretinogram (ERG) has been described and may be a variant of mucolipidosis IV. Ultrastructural studies have shown single-membraned vacuoles containing laminated material and a polymorphous material in tissue-cultured cells and conjunctiva.[10]

GOLDBERG-COTLIER SYNDROME

Goldberg-Cotlier syndrome has many clinical features in common with both lipid and mucopolysaccharide storage diseases. These include coarse facies, mental and physical retardation, seizures, and skeletal anomalies. Hepatomegaly may be seen, as well as cherry-red spots and corneal clouding.

METACHROMATIC LEUKODYSTROPHY (MLD)

Metachromatic leukodystrophy[13] (MLD variant), with onset at 1 and 2 years of age, exhibits slow mental and physical development with progressive neurologic deterioration. In addition to these neurologic signs, there are signs of mucopolysaccharide storage disease such as skeletal abnormalities, splenomegaly, and deafness. The cornea shows cloudiness by 2 years of age, and the fundus may show grayness in perifoveal area similar to that seen in the late infantile MLD.

The total deficiency of arylsulfatase activity accounts for the failure to degrade both mucopolysaccharides and sulfatides. In contrast to the classic form of MLD in which only arylsulfatase A is deficient, mucopolysaccharides are found in the urine of the variant form of MLD but not in the classic form.

MANNOSIDOSIS

Mannosidosis is a lysosomal storage disorder clinically resembling Hurler's syndrome (MPS IH). Because of a deficiency of α-mannosidase, mannose-rich oligosaccharides accumulate in tissue and urine.

Affected persons may demonstrate coarse facies, prominent metopic suture, cardiac dysfunction, hepatosplenomegaly, and gibbus deformity. There may be multiple connective tissue defects, such as herniae, diastases, and testicular hydroceles.

Typically, these patients are hypotonic as infants with delayed motor development and with defects in conductive and sensory hearing.

Superficial corneal opacities have been reported in a few cases; however, spokelike posterior cortical cataracts have been suggested as a pathognomonic sign of this entity. These cataracts consist of numerous punctate vacuoles arranged in a wheellike or spokelike configuration. No retinopathy, ERG changes, or glaucoma has been reported.

FUCOSIDOSIS

The patients may suffer from a severe form with progressive psychomotor retardation and moderate chondrodystrophy reminiscent of mucopolysaccharidoses. Angiokeratoma corporis diffusum is seen in patients with fucosidosis who survive to adolescence, and tortuous conjunctival vessels occur in the conjunctiva.[3]

Snyder and associates[14] have reported the ocular findings in fucosidosis. They observed a central corneal opacity in Bowman's membrane and the posterior superficial corneal epithelium, dilated tortuous conjunctival vessels with local fusiform and saccular microaneurysms, and tortuous retinal veins that were beaded and sausage shaped.

REFERENCES

1. Arbisser, A.I., Murphree, A.L., Garcia, C.A., and Howell, R.R.: Ocular findings in mannosidosis, Am. J. Ophthalmol. **82:**465, 1976.
2. Berman, E.R., Livni, N., Shapira, E., Merin, J., and Levij, S.: Congenital corneal clouding with abnormal systemic storage bodies: a new variant of mucolipidosis, J. Pediatr. **84:**519, 1974.
3. Borrone, C., Gatti, R., Trias, X., et al.: Fucosidosis: clinical, biochemical, immunologic, and genetic studies in two new cases, J. Pediatr. **84:**727, 1974.
4. Bout, A., Sugarman, G.I., and Spencer, W.H.: Ocular involvement in I-cell disease (mucolipidosis II) light and electron-microscopic findings, Albrecht von Graefes Arch. Klin. Ophthalmol. **198:**25, 1976.
5. Emery, J.M., Greene, W.R., Wyllie, R.G., et al.: GM$_1$-gangliosidosis: ocular and pathological manifestations, Arch. Ophthalmol. **85:**177, 1971.
6. Goebel, H.H., Fix, J., and Zeman, W.: Retinal pathology in GM$_1$ gangliosidosis type II, Am. J. Ophthalmol. **75:**434, 1973.
7. Libert, J., Van Hoof, F., Farreaux, J.P., and Tousseaut, D.: Ocular findings in I-cell disease (mucolipidosis type II), Am. J. Ophthalmol. **83:**617, 1977.
8. Lightbody, J., Weesmann, U., Hadow, B., and Herschkowitz, N.: I-cell disease: multiple lysosomal-enzyme defect, Lancet **1:**451, 1971.
9. Luchsinger, U., Buhler, E.M., Menes, K., and Hirt, H.R.: I-cell disease, N. Engl. J. Med. **282:**1374, 1970.
10. Newell, F.W., Matalon, R., and Meyer, S.: A new mucolipidosis with psychomotor retardation, corneal clouding and retinal degeneration, Am. J. Ophthalmol. **80:**440, 1975.
11. O'Brien, J.: Generalized gangliosidosis, J. Pediatr. **75:**167, 1969.
12. Quigley, H.A., and Goldberg, M.F.: Conjunctival ultrastructure in mucolipidosis 3 (pseudo-Hurler polydystrophy), Invest. Ophthalmol. **10:**568, 1971.
13. Quigley, H.A., and Green, R.W.: Clinical and ultrastructural ocular histopathologic studies of

adult onset metachromatic leukodystrophy, Am. J. Ophthalmol. **82:**471, 1976.

14. Snyder, R.O., Carlow, T.J., Ledman, J., and Wenger, D.A.: Ocular findings in fucosidosis, Birth Defects **12:**241, 1976.

15. Spranger, J.W., and Wiedemann, H.R.: The gen- etic mucolipidoses: diagnosis and differential diagnosis, Humangenetik **9:**113, 1970.

16. Weiss, M.J., Krill, A.E., Dawson, G., Hindman, J., and Cotlier, E.: GM$_1$ gangliosidosis type I, Am. J. Ophthalmol. **76:**999, 1973.

CHAPTER

20 Sphingolipidoses

Fabry's disease (angiokeratoma corporis diffusum)
  Ocular involvement
Gaucher's disease (cerebroside lipidosis, glucocerebrosidosis)
Other diseases

FABRY'S DISEASE (ANGIOKERATOMA CORPORIS DIFFUSUM)*

This disease is one of the sphingolipidoses resulting from deficiency of ceramide trihexoxidase (an α-galactosidase) with accumulation of ceramide trihexoside principally in the cardiovascular and renal systems.

This disease may be transmitted as a sex-linked recessive trait. The hemizygous male is much more seriously affected. The heterozygous female may be asymptomatic or may manifest some of the same symptoms as does the hemizygous male. Skin eruptions are noted particularly on the breast, gluteal regions, and upper extremities. These are pinhead-sized vascular dilations (Fig. 20-1) that later become hyperkeratotic (Fig. 20-2). In addition to these skin findings, one might see fever and hypertension.

Amniocentesis can be performed after 17 weeks' gestation to make an in utero diagnosis. In a suspected case of Fabry's disease the detection of deficiency of ceramide and trihexosidase in the plasma, lymph nodes, leukocytes, and cultured skin fibroblasts is a reliable method.

Ocular involvement

Periorbital edema (25% of cases), papilledema, retinal edema, macular edema, optic atrophy, dilation and tortuosity of the retinal vessels, conjunctival aneurysm (60% of cases) (Fig. 20-3), and posterior spoke-like structural cataracts consisting of 9 to 12 spokes (Fig. 20-4) (50% of patients) occur. Probably glycolipid is deposited in the adult lens suture line. Visual acuity is not affected. The clinical course and prognosis in the heterozygotes is more favorable than that in the hemizygotes.

---

*References 1, 2, 4, 10, 13.

Text continued on p. 514.

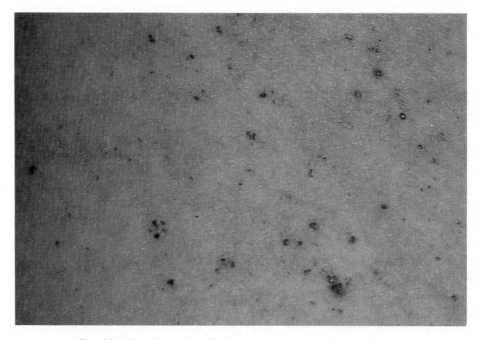

Fig. 20-1. Small vascular dilations noted in skin in Fabry's disease.

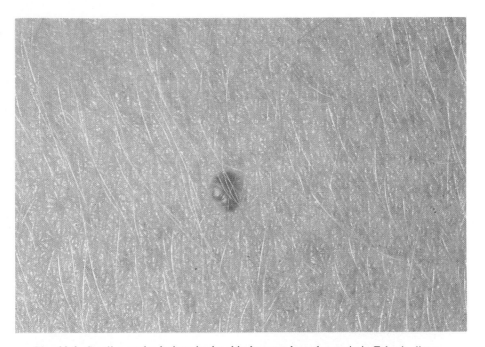

Fig. 20-2. Small vascular lesions in the skin become hyperkeratotic in Fabry's disease.

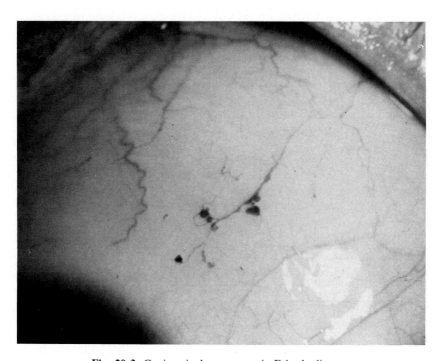

Fig. 20-3. Conjunctival aneurysms in Fabry's disease.

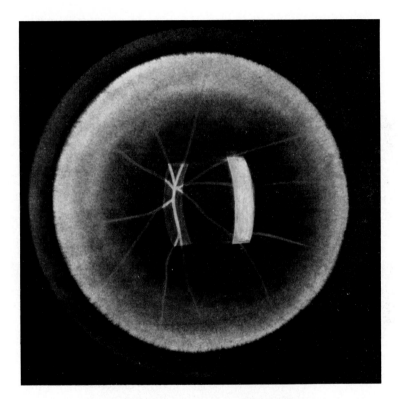

Fig. 20-4. Spokelike cataract in Fabry's disease.

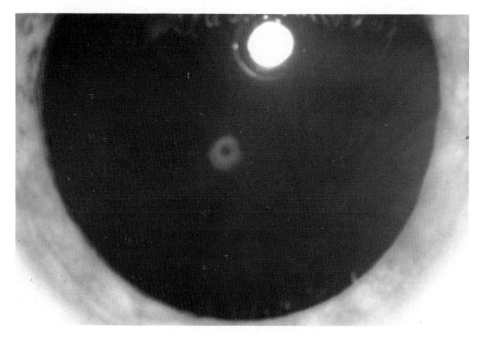

Fig. 20-5. Whorllike lesions in epithelium of cornea in Fabry's disease.

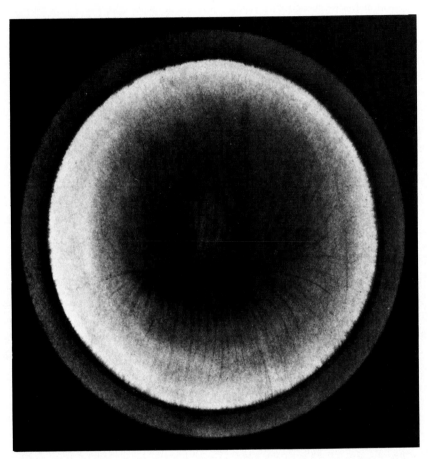

Fig. 20-6. Diagrammatic representation of whorllike lesion in epithelium in Fabry's disease.

In addition, a granular anterior capsular or subcapsular deposit can be found in 35% of the hemizygotes but not in any heterozygote. Lenticular opacities are inferior in position, and they may appear wedge shaped with bases near the lenticular equator. The density of the deposits varies widely.[9]

The corneal findings are extremely interesting and consist of fine, whorllike, superficial corneal opacities seen only with the slit lamp (Fig. 20-5). It is believed that hazy cornea is caused by the abnormal accumulation of sphingolipid in the deep corneal epithelium. These deposits take on a curvilinear or wavy configuration, radiating from a position below the corneal center, and occur in all affected males and in 90% of female carriers (Fig. 20-6). They have been seen in patients 6 months of age. No deposits are found in the stroma and corneal endothelium. Visual acuity is usually not affected.

Whorllike opacities have also been found with chloroquine deposition, indomethacin deposition, phenothiazine deposition, Tangier disease, fingerprint lines, healing corneal epithelium, striate melanokeratosis, and Melkersson-Rosenthal syndrome.

Whorllike opacities have also been described as a distinct and separate corneal dystrophy and named cornea verticillata or vortex dystrophy. This "dystrophy" is now believed to be a manifestation of Fabry's disease in systemically asymptomatic female carriers of X-linked Fabry's disease.

Small, saccular, conjunctival aneurysmal dilations are seen in Fabry's disease as well as in diabetes mellitus, arteriosclerosis, sickle-cell anemia, Degos' syndrome, hemorrhagic telangectasia, Olser-Weber-Rendu disease, and polycythemia rubra vera.

GAUCHER'S DISEASE (CEREBROSIDE LIPIDOSIS, GLUCOCEREBROSIDOSIS)[6,7]

Gaucher's disease is one of the sphingolipidoses and is transmitted as an autosomal recessive or as a dominant trait. Deficiency of β-glucosidase, the cerebroside-clearing enzyme, is found in the liver, spleen, and white blood cells. The patient may have yellow skin, anemia, enlargement of the spleen and liver, and thrombocytopenia.

Occasionally a cherry-red spot may be seen in the macula. Perimacular degeneration and ring granular opacities around the fovea occasionally occur. Retinal hemorrhages, edema, and nystagmus are seen in juveniles.

The adult form of the disease may exhibit prominent, dark-yellow pingueculae, usually located nasally, in 25% of the cases. Histologically these contain foamy epitheloid cells (Gaucher's cells) instead of the elastosis seen in the usual pingueculum.

OTHER DISEASES

Infantile metachromatic leukodystrophy, Sandhoff's disease [11] (GM$_2$ gangliosidosis II), and Niemann-Pick disease[3,5,7,12] may rarely exhibit cloudy corneas along with the appearance of the cherry-red spot.

Tables 20-1 and 20-2 organize the sphingolipidoses with regard to ocular signs and enzymatic defects.

Table 20-1. Sphingolipidoses with anterior segment findings

	Fabry's disease	Gaucher's disease[8]	Late infantile MLD	Sandhoff's disease (GM₂ gangliosidosis II)	Niemann-Pick disease
Heredity	Sex-linked recessive	Autosomal recessive*	Autosomal recessive	Autosomal recessive	Autosomal recessive
Enzyme defect	Ceramide trihexosidase (α-galactosidase)	β-Galactosidase	Arylsulfatase A	Hexosaminidase A and B	Sphingomyelinase
Tissue storage	Ceramide trihexoside	Ceramide glucoside (glucocerebroside)	Cerebroside sulfate	GM₂ ganglioside	Sphingomyelin and cholesterol
Corneal clouding	+	−	+	+†	+‡?
Macular grayness or cherry-red spots	−	±	+	+	
Optic atrophy	−	−	+	−	+‡?

*An adult type may have autosomal dominant inheritance. Pigmented pingueculae may be seen.
†One case reported.[1]
‡A peculiar corneal clouding was reported by Robb and Kuwabara.[7] Inclusions were also seen in keratocytes and endothelium.[3,4,11]

Table 20-2. Sphingolipidoses without anterior segment findings

	Juvenile GM₂ gangliosidosis II	Tay-Sachs disease (GM₂ gangliosidosis I)	Krabbe's disease	Lactosyl ceramidosis
Heredity	Autosomal recessive	Autosomal recessive	Autosomal recessive	Autosomal recessive
Enzyme defect	Partial deficiency of hexosaminidase A	Hexosaminidase A	Galactocerebroside β-Galactosidase	β-Galactosidase
Tissue storage	GM₂ ganglioside	GM₂ ganglioside	Galactosyl ceramide	Lactosyl ceramide
Corneal clouding	−	−		−
Macular grayness or cherry-red spots	+	+	+	?

REFERENCES

1. Grace, E.V.: Diffuse angiokeratosis (Fabry's disease), Am. J. Ophthalmol. **62:**139, 1966.
2. Hashimoto, K., Lieberman, P., and Lamkin, N.: Angiokeratoma corporis diffusum (Fabry disease), Arch. Dermatol. **112:**1416, 1976.
3. Howes, E.L., Wood, I.S., Golbus, M., and Hagan, M.: Ocular pathology of infantile Niemann-Pick disease: study of fetus of 23 weeks' gestation, Arch. Ophthalmol. **93:**494, 1975.
4. Karr, W.J., Jr.: Fabry's disease (angiokeratoma corporis diffusum universale), Am. J. Med. **27:** 829, 1959.
5. Hibert, J., Toussaint, D., and Guiselings, R.: Ocular findings in Niemann-Pick disease, Am. J. Ophthalmol. **80:**991, 1975.
6. Petrochelos, M., Tricoules, D., Kotseras, T., and Vouzoukos, A.: Ocular manifestations of Gaucher's disease, Am. J. Ophthalmol. **80:**1006, 1975.
7. Robb, R.M., and Kuwabara, T.: The ocular pathology of type A Niemann-Pick disease: a light and electron microscopic study, Invest. Ophthalmol. **12:**366, 1973.
8. Schettler, G., and Kohlke, W.: Gaucher's disease. In Schettler, G., editor: Lipids and lipidoses, New York, 1967, Springer-Verlag New York, Inc.
9. Sher, N.A., Letson, R.D., and Desnick, R.J.: The ocular manifestations in Fabry's disease, Arch. Ophthalmol. **97:**671, 1979.
10. Spaeth, G.L., and Frost, P.: Fabry's disease, Arch. Ophthalmol. **74:**760, 1965.
11. Tremblay, M., and Szots, F.: GM_2 Type 2— gangliosidosis (Sandhoff's disease)—ocular and pathological manifestations, Can. J. Ophthalmol. **9:**338, 1974.
12. Walton, D.S., Robb, R.M., and Crocker, A.C.: Ocular manifestations of group A Niemann-Pick disease, Am. J. Ophthalmol. **84:**174, 1978.
13. Weingeist, T.A., and Blodi, F.C.: Fabry's disease: ocular findings in a carrier female, Arch. Ophthalmol. **85:**169, 1971.

21 Nutritional defects

Vitamin A deficiency (keratomalacia)
    Pathogenesis
    Clinical signs
    Management
Riboflavin

VITAMIN A DEFICIENCY (KERATOMALACIA) (Table 21-1)

The clinical picture of vitamin A deficiency, which is a worldwide problem and associated with nutritional deficiencies, has been referred to by many authors.* Bilateral blindness is a frequent consequence of keratomalacia. Vitamin A deficiency may, by itself, result in death unless treated. It is seen in association with other problems such as multiple vitamin deficiency,[6] protein deficiency,[1, 8] and kwashiorkor.[22]

Pathogenesis

Factors that cause the rapid worsening of xerophthalmia with involvement of the cornea and its sudden perforation resulting in blindness are not all understood.

The serum levels of vitamin A and carotenes in patients with xerophthalmia and keratomalacia are decreased at least 50% from the normal levels.[16] However, since a considerable range of normal values exists for vitamin A and carotenes, the importance of these serum levels is open to question.

Vitamin A circulates as retinol bound to a specific transport protein—retinol-binding protein (RBP)—which forms a complex with prealbumin.[7, 13] Protein plays a very important role in the conversion of β-carotene to retinol in the intestine. The absorption, storage, and ultimate use of retinol by the tissues is extremely important. It has been shown[18] that vitamin A provokes no response in vitamin A–deficient children who are also deficient in protein unless milk is given as well. Giving vitamin A–deficient children skim milk, which is devoid of vitamin A, increases the level of vitamin A in their blood. This increase of serum vitamin A when the children are given protein (skim milk) suggests that the decreased vitamin A in their blood is secondary to a decrease in a protein carrier substance.

---

*References 3, 4, 11, 12, 14, 15, 19, 22.

Table 21-1. Corneal and conjunctival changes in defective nutritional states

Altered status	Defect
Vitamin A deficiency	Long eyelashes
	Lack of luster to conjunctiva
	Wrinkling of conjunctiva
	Pigmentation of conjunctiva
	Bitot's spots (meibomian secretions adhere to keratinized areas)
	Decrease in tear volume
	Xerophthalmia
	Punctate keratopathy
	Corneal infiltration
	Loss of stromal substance
	Keratomalacia
	Scarring of cornea
	Decreased corneal sensation
	Bilateral blindness
	Night blindness (occurs before corneal changes)
Severe malnutrition (protein-calorie deficiency)	Keratomalacia
Vitamin B complex deficiency	Vascularization of limbus and stroma (doubted by some to be positive finding)
Hypervitaminosis D^2	Band keratopathy
Ulcerative and regional enteritis	Marginal melting and corneal ulcers

The idea of an RBP and a prealbumin, the transport protein for vitamin A, in the serum has demonstrated the relationship between vitamin A and protein. A direct relationship exists among the levels of retinol, RBP, and prealbumin in the blood. If children who are deficient in vitamin A and also malnourished are given vitamin A parenterally, the level of RBP in their blood does not increase for 24 hours.[18] When protein alone without vitamin A is given to children with malnutrition, the levels of RBP, prealbumin, and vitamin A increase.[17] These findings suggest that the low levels of vitamin A in severe malnutrition (kwashiorkor) largely reflect a functional impairment in the hepatic release of vitamin A rather than vitamin A deficiency alone. Hepatic release of vitamin A is apparently impaired because of defective production of plasma transport protein for retinol, resulting from the limited supply of substrate for protein synthesis. When substrate is provided by protein, the hepatic production of plasma proteins increased, plasma RBP and prealbumin rise, and hence plasma vitamin A concentrations increase.[17]

Clinical signs

The early clinical signs in vitamin A deficiency are night blindness (seen earlier than corneal keratinization), conjunctival xerosis and keratinization, blepharitis, meibomitis with foamy discharge, lengthening of eyelashes, hyperkeratosis of the forehead, and hyperkeratotic skin rash. The conjunctiva is wrinkled, red, opaque, and pigmented and may exhibit a Bitot's spot.[9-11] Bitot's spots (Fig. 21-1) can occur in various nutritional de-

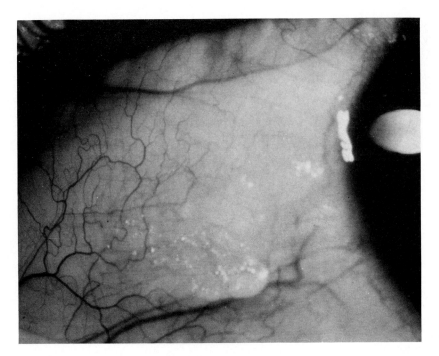

Fig. 21-1. Bitot's spot.

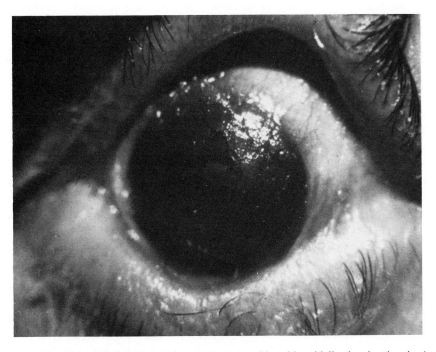

Fig. 21-2. Lusterless and dry conjunctiva and cornea with epidermidalization in vitamin A deficiency.

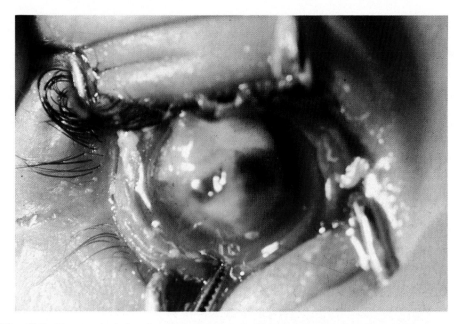

Fig. 21-3. Keratomalacia in vitamin A deficiency. (Courtesy D. Paton, M.D., Houston, Tex.)

ficiencies other than vitamin A deficiency and are therefore not pathognomonic of vitamin A deficiency. Lusterlessness of the conjunctiva is caused by epidermidalization and the lack of mucin caused by the paucity of goblet cells[5, 10, 14] (Fig. 21-2).

The occurrence of xerosis or xerophthalmia in vitamin-protein deficiency is not universal. Xerophthalmia accompanied by corneal ulceration of varying degrees occurs more frequently than does keratomalacia.[9]

When it occurs, keratomalacia (Fig. 21-3) may result in serious visual consequences.[3, 10, 19, 22] In this condition, the cornea may undergo swelling followed by melting and perforation with loss of intraocular contents. It has been suggested that a collagenase mechanism may account for the corneal melting.[5] Therefore keratomalacia is a diffuse noninflammatory melting of the cornea in vitamin-protein deficiency. It has been referred to as a discrete colliquative necrosis. Keratomalacia can occur in cachectic hospitalized patients secondarily to lethal disease.

The serum levels of vitamin A and carotenes in patients with xerophthalmia and keratomalacia are usually decreased, but it must be emphasized that no regular correlation exists between serum vitamin A levels and corneal manifestations of this vitamin deficiency.[11, 16] It is nonetheless established that vitamin A–deficient diets in humans and animals cause night blindness.[9, 12, 16]

In general therefore vitamin A deficiency may exhibit the pathologic conditions of conjunctival epidermidalization and pigmentation, atrophy and loss of goblet cells, keratinization, Bitot's spots, corneal drying, stromal necrosis, keratomalacia, corneal ulceration accompanied by vascularization and secondary infections, and corneal perforation. However, punctate epithelial keratopathy is a very early corneal manifestation of xerophthalmia. Topical retinoic acid has been used in vitamin A–deficient rabbits, and this reversed the corneal changes in 3 days. It appears that retinoic acid is more effective than systemic vitamin A alone in reversing moderately advanced keratinization caused by vitamin A deficiency.[21]

In well-fed populations of developed countries, xerophthalmia and keratomalacia, although rare, may occur because of systemic disease or dietary indiscretions. In clinical situations the picture of vitamin A deficiency is also complicated by dietary defects of protein and other vitamins; in fact, low serum albumin levels almost always accompany xerophthalmia and keratomalacia.[8, 9] The development of bilateral corneal ulcers in an uninflamed eye should suggest a diagnosis of keratomalacia. Measles, which is usually benign, may become a severely opacifying process of the cornea in a patient with nutritional deficiencies.

Dark adaptation tests may be a sensitive index for diagnosing subclinical vitamin A deficiency in patients with small bowel disease without any overt evidence of nutritional defect.[3]

Management

Therapy with parenteral and topical vitamin A, protein supplement, and soft contact lens should be instituted. Oral or intramuscular administration of 50,000 units of vitamin A and application of vitamin A ophthalmic ointment are advocated.

RIBOFLAVIN

Riboflavin deficiency[20] appears to cause cheilosis, which is fissuring and ulceration of the mucous membrane of the mouth, especially the corners. A fine desquamation occurs in the nasolabial folds and along the sides of the nose. In addition, one finds a glossitis. The tongue has a purplish hue with the filiform papillae flattened out.

The lid margins and conjunctivae are injected, and the patient complains of photophobia and twitching and burning of the eyes.

The corneal stroma may become invaded by new blood vessels; on occasion a superficial epithelial keratitis may be seen.

REFERENCES

1. Arroyave, G.G., Wilson, D., Contreras, C., et al.: Alterations in serum concentrations of vitamin A associated with hypoproteinemia, J. Pediatr. 62:920, 1963.
2. Baner, J.M., and Freybert, R.H.: Vitamin D intoxication, JAMA 130:1204, 1946.
3. Baum, J.L., and Gullipalli, R.: Keratomalacia in the cachectic hospitalized patient, Am. J. Ophthalmol. 82:435, 1976.
4. Damiean-Gillet, M.: Conjunctival lesions in avitaminosis A, Trop. Geogr. Med. 10:233, 1958.
5. Dohlman, C.H., and Kalevar, V.: Cornea in hypovitaminosis A and protein deficiency, Isr. J. Med. Sci. 8:1179, 1972.
6. Gifford, E., and Maguire, E.: Band keratopathy in vitamin D toxicity, Arch. Ophthalmol. 52:106, 1954.
7. Kanai, N.A., Raz, A., and Goodman, D.S.: Retinol-binding protein: the transport protein for vitamin A in human plasma, J. Clin. Invest. 47:2025, 1968.
8. Kie-Tong, Y.: Protein deficiency in keratomalacia, Br. J. Ophthalmol. 40:502, 1950.
9. Kuming, B.S., and Politzer, W.M.: Xerophthalmia and protein malnutrition in Bantu children, Br. J. Ophthalmol. 51:649, 1967.
10. Paton, D.: Keratomalacia: a review of its relationship to xerophthalmia and its response to treatment, Eye Ear Nose Throat Mon. 46:186, 1967.

11. Paton, D., and McLaren, D.S.: Bitot spots, Am. J. Ophthalmol. **50:**568, 1974.

12. Petersen, R.A., Petersen, V.S., and Robb, R.M.: Vitamin A deficiency with xerophthalmia and night blindness in cystic fibrosis, Am. J. Dis. Child. **116:**662, 1968.

13. Peterson, P.A., and Beggård, I.: Isolation and properties of a human retinol-transporting protein, J. Biol. Chem. **246:**25, 1971.

14. Pirie, A.: Xerophthalmia, Invest. Ophthalmol. **15:**417, 1976.

15. Rodger, F.C.: The ocular effects of vitamin A deficiency in man in the tropics, Exp. Eye Res. **3:**367, 1964.

16. Rodger, F.C., Saiduzzafar, H., Grover, A.D., and Fazal, A.: Nutritional lesions of the external eye and their relationship to plasma levels of vitamin A and the light thresholds, Acta Ophthalmol. **42:**1, 1964.

17. Smith, F.R., Goodman, D.S., Zaklama, M.S., et al.: Serum vitamin A, retinol-binding protein in PRM, a functional defect in hepatic release, Am. J. Clin. Nutr. **26:**973, 1973.

18. Smith. F.R., Suskind, R., Thalanangkul, O., et al.: Plasma vitamin A, retinol-binding protein and prealbumin concentration in PCM. III. Response to varying dietary treatment, Am. J. Nutr. **28:**732, 1975.

19. Smith, R.S., Farrell, T., and Bailey, T.: Keratomalacia, Surv. Ophthalmol. **20:**213, 1975.

20. Syndenstricker, V.P., Sebrell, W.H., Cleckley, H.M., and Krause, H.D.: The ocular manifestations of ariboflavinosis, JAMA **114:**2437, 1940.

21. Van Horn, D.L., DeCarlo, J.D., Schutten, W.H., and Hyndiuk, R.A.: Topical retinoic acid in the treatment of experimental xerophthalmia in the rabbit, Arch. Ophthalmol. **99:**317, 1981.

22. Venkataswamy, G.: Ocular manifestations of vitamin A deficiency, Br. J. Ophthalmol. **51:**854, 1967.

ADDITIONAL READING

Beaver, D.L.: Vitamin A deficiency in germ-free rat, Am. J. Pathol. **38:**335, 1961.

Beitch, I.: The induction of keratinization of the corneal epithelium, Invest. Ophthalmol. **9:**827, 1970.

Dingle, J.T., Fell, H.B., and Goodman, D.S.: The effect of retinol and of retinol-binding protein on embryonic skeletal tissue in organ culture, J. Cell. Sci. **11:**393, 1972.

Roy, F.H.: Xerophthalmia, Ann. Ophthalmol. **11:**84, 1974.

Sommer, A., Toureau, S., Cornet, P., Midy, C., and Pettiss, S.T.: Xerophthalmia and anterior segment blindness, Am. J. Ophthalmol. **82:**439, 1976.

Valenton, M.J., and Tan, R.V.: Secondary ocular bacterial infection in hypovitaminosis A and xerophthalmia, Am. J. Ophthalmol. **80:**673, 1975.

22 Neurologic diseases

The neurologic diseases discussed in this chapter are significant entities that may result in anterior segment changes. The cornea is often involved.

HEPATOLENTICULAR DEGENERATION (WILSON'S DISEASE)

Pathogenesis

Hepatolenticular degeneration is an inherited disorder characterized by the abnormal metabolism of copper[11] and associated with nodular cirrhosis of the liver, which usually precedes the degeneration of the central nervous system, especially the basal ganglia.[35] The pathogenesis of Wilson's disease and the basic genetic defect remain obscure; although excess copper clearly exists in the tissues, the mechanism of its deposition is unknown. In some way it may be associated with a failure to synthesize the serum copper protein, ceruloplasmin, normally. There is low serum copper and elevated tissue and urinary copper levels. Another theory suggests that an abnormal protein with a high affinity for copper may bind the metal and tissues.[11] The onset of the disease is during the first decade of life but may be seen in the teens and twenties. It is usually transmitted as a simple recessive trait. The carrier condition may be detected by the presence of aminoaciduria.

Clinical signs

One may see jaundice and hepatomegaly. Coarse tremors develop that are associated with the sclerotic changes seen in the basal ganglia of the brain. Other neurologic manifestations may be seen.

Ocular involvement

Pigment in or immediately under the lens capsule has been noted, but this occurs rarely. The cataract also occurs rarely and has been described as the ''sunflower cataract.''[4] Pigmentation of the cornea is a finding to arouse suspicion of Wilson's disease. The ring is seen earlier in the 6 and 12 o'clock position meridians.

The Kayser-Fleischer ring is situated peripherally in Descemet's membrane* (Fig. 22-1) and appears gray-brown, but the inner parts change from golden to green or blue. On slit-lamp examination the ring may appear to be a narrow band up to 3 to 4 mm in width. The ring extends to the limbus without any lucid interval. A lucid interval will be seen only if a posterior embryotoxon is present.

When the Kayser-Fleischer ring is suspected, gonioscopic examination is imperative, since the ring may be obscured by a wide limbus. The pigmentation extends to the extreme periphery of Descemet's membrane or at least to Schwalbe's ring even when there has previously seemed to be a narrow, clear peripheral area. On occasion, one may see a double ring, wherein one finds a ruby red ring concentric with the limbus and green

*References 13, 17, 19, 24, 28, 33, 34.

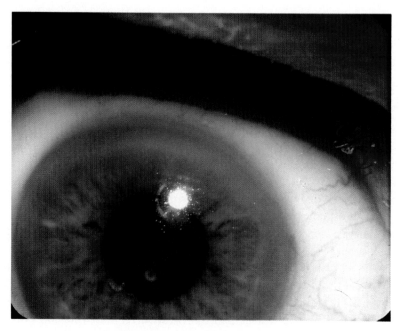

Fig. 22-1. Kayser-Fleischer ring.

inner ring.[13] The Kayser-Fleischer ring is often absent under the age of 10.[13, 24]

Copper appears to be the metal responsible for the ring. The clinically visible copper, which accounts for the Kayser-Fleischer ring, is probably present in a protein copper complex, a copper chelate.[34] Clinically invisible copper throughout the stroma has been described and the observation made that this copper is not bound to protein.

Differential diagnosis

Pigmented rings clinically identical to Kayser-Fleischer rings have been reported in primary biliary cirrhosis, progressive intrahepatic cholestasis of childhood, and chronic active hepatitis.[12] These diseases have in common an elevated level of copper in the blood, urine, and liver. Wilson's disease has subnormal levels of ceruloplasmin. Pigmented corneal rings in hepatic disease are therefore not pathognomonic of Wilson's disease; however, Kayser-Fleischer rings in combination with neurologic disease with or without evidence of hepatic disease remains a good indication of Wilson's disease.

Other conditions that may have to be taken in consideration as far as pigmentation of the posterior surface of the cornea is concerned and that may be mistaken for Wilson's disease are multiple myeloma, extensive copper treatment for trachoma (corneal and lenticular changes), and pseudo-Kayser-Fleischer rings in carotenemia. In the latter condition, golden-yellow rings are present at the site of a corneal arcus; in addition, night blindness can be seen. Table 22-1 lists clinical states in which copper is found in the cornea.

Table 22-1. Clinical conditions that involve copper in the cornea

Disease	Copper involvement	Cerulo-plasmin	Serum copper	Corneal and lenticular findings
Wilson's disease	Defective synthesis of ceruloplasmin (abnormal storage protein in hepatocyte with affinity for copper)	Decreased	Decreased	Kayser-Fleischer ring Deposition in anterior lens capsule
Menkes' kinky hair disease[6]*	Poor gastrointestinal absorption	Decreased	Decreased	None
Multiple myeloma	Myeloma protein binds copper	Marginal increase	Increased	Central deposition in Descemet's membrane, Bowman's layer, and trabeculum Anterior and posterior lens capsules
Chronic liver disease	Intrahepatic or extra-hepatic biliary obstruction	Increased	Increased	"Kayser-Fleischer" ring

*Menkes' kinky hair disease is a sex-linked neurodegenerative disorder characterized by slow growth, psychomotor retardation, seizures, and abnormalities of hair structure. It is suggested that the disease is caused by copper malabsorption; low copper serum, ceruloplasmin, and copper oxidase levels in children are seen. Visual function deteriorates. Late in the disease the electroretinogram (ERG) and visual evoked response (VER) may be abnormal. Death occurs before 3 years of age. The biochemical defect involves the intracellular transport of copper within the intestines.[6, 7]

Diagnosis

The following facts might be important in reference to the diagnosis of Wilson's disease. The serum ceruloplasmin is less than 20 mg/dl in the majority of patients. However, it should be noted that a low level of ceruloplasmin in an asymptomatic individual does not establish the diagnosis, since 20% of the heterozygous relatives will have such a level and never develop the disease.[31] Urinary copper is usually less than 50 μg/day. Serum copper levels are suggestive but variable; they may be as low as 50 μg/dl (the normal range is 90 to 130 μg/dl).[35] It is necessary to screen all relatives of patients afflicted with Wilson's disease. Asymptomatic individuals may be homozygous for the abnormal gene and will eventually manifest the disease, or they may be heterozygous and will never be affected. The former group should be treated prophylactically, whereas the latter group should not be treated.[31] A deficiency of ceruloplasmin requires a liver biopsy. Normal concentration of hepatic copper indicates that this is a heterozygote; concentration greater than 250 μg/gram establishes the diagnosis of Wilson's disease.[30]

Management

Treatment of hepatolenticular degeneration has been most effective with penicillamine,[32] which prevents, as well as reverses, the clinical manifestations. The dramatic response is in the neurologic symptoms, but some patients show improvement in their primary liver disease, too. Therapy involves a lifetime medication, since these patients will also return to a positive copper balance without chelating agents. It is emphasized that the most symptomatic patients may show the most remarkable improvement.[25, 32] In addition to the penicillamine treatment, it is necessary to avoid high copper intake. This usually results in marked clinical improvement if irreversible tissue damage has not occurred.

FAMILIAL DYSAUTONOMIA (RILEY-DAY SYNDROME)[14, 15, 18]

In this syndrome there is a deficiency of plasma dopamine-β-hydroxylase (DBH). This enzyme is localized in storage vesicles in the sympathetic nerve endings and in the adrenal medulla; it is released into the plasma together with catecholamines when these tissues are stimulated. Therefore patients excrete greatly elevated levels of homovanillic acid (HVA) and decreased amounts of vanillylmandelic acid (VMA) and 3-methoxy-4-hydroxyphenylethyleneglycol (HMPG). The excess HVA arises from the accelerated breakdown of dopa and dopamine, whereas the decreased VMA and HMPG indicate the lack of production of norepinephrine and epinephrine.

In normal individuals, the plasma level of DBH is highly age dependent, increasing during the first 4 years of life and more slowly for the next decade. In this disease the level is decreased at all ages in most but not all patients. Tests for detection of heterozygotes have not been developed.

Familial dysautonomia is inherited as an autosomal recessive trait[3] and seems to be confined to Jews whose families originate in eastern Europe. However, recently there has been a report of a black girl with autonomic dysfunction of this type.

Clinical findings

Patients with familial dysautonomia usually have a history of feeding difficulty from birth and show a definite emotional lability. They also demonstrate an abnormal esophageal motility, excessive sweating, and a blotching of the skin on excitement or stress. Postural hypotension and indifference to pain are part of the syndrome. On general examination, one may see absent or hypoactive deep tendon reflexes and an absence of fungiform papillae on the tip of the tongue (Fig. 22-2). Patients with familial dysautonomia also exhibit alacrima, corneal hypesthesia, exodeviation, and methacholine-induced miosis. These comprise an identifying set of findings with which a diagnosis can be made.[2, 22, 23]

Prompt and marked pupillary constriction following the instillation of dilute 2.5% methacholine is characteristic of familial dysautonomia and Adie's tonic pupil.[29] Following are several conditions to remember when making a diagnosis of the pupillary problems and the dry eye seen in Riley-Day syndrome:

1. Adie's pupil
2. Congenital alacrima
3. Congenital anhidrotic ectodermal dysplasia
4. Neuroparalytic keratitis
5. Keratitis sicca
6. Keratomalacia
7. Congenital insensitivity and indifference to pain

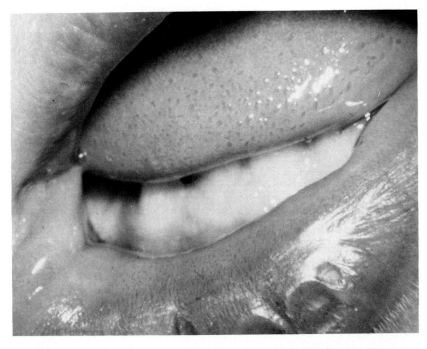

Fig. 22-2. Absence of fungiform papillae of tongue in Riley-Day syndrome.

Denervation supersensitivity of the iris sphincter to parasympathomimetics appears to be the explanation for the pupillary alteration in familial dysautonomia and Adie's syndrome. Although aniscoria and myopia have been seen in some patients, there seems to be little significance attached to these findings. The occurrence of retinal vascular tortuosity in some of the patients indicates that this finding may present another characteristic of dysautonomic syndrome.

The occurrence of corneal ulceration in more than 50% of these cases is seen associated with hypolacrima (Fig. 22-3). It should be noted that there is a failure to produce overflow tears with the usual stimuli, so that these patients have a definite dry eye problem.[8] Corneal anesthesia results in neurotrophic keratitis. There might be a wide variation in the severity of the corneal problems in dysautonomic syndrome; as a result, the degree of corneal damage varies greatly. Certain cases may be free of any corneal abrasions, whereas others may result in infiltration, vascularization, ulceration, and perforation.[2, 10, 22, 23]

Management

Early diagnosis of Riley-Day syndrome in infancy and childhood will permit routine care of the patient's cornea so that the complications are minimized. Therapy includes use of artificial tears as needed, punctum occlusion, and tarsorrhaphy. Parenteral administration of pilocarpine or neostigmine will produce tearing and significant increase in Schirmer paper wetting[21, 27, 29]; however, the side effects prevent parenteral therapeutic use of these drugs.

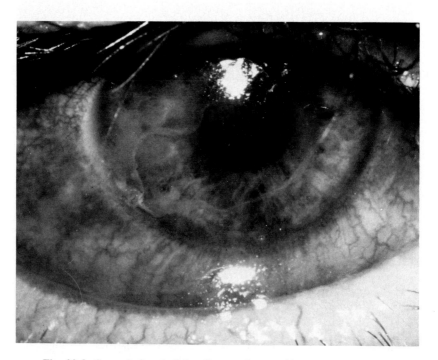

Fig. 22-3. Corneal ulcer in Riley-Day syndrome with severe hypolacrima.

SHY-DRAGER SYNDROME

This acquired failure of autonomic function involves orthostatic hypotension, urinary incontingence, and impotence.

The general eye findings may include iris atrophy, convergence defect, and anisocoria.

The cornea and conjunctiva may become involved because of keratoconjunctivitis sicca.

CONGENITAL ALACRIMA

The lack of tears at birth or shortly thereafter may be seen, but this is an unusual entity. One may divide the problem into several groups:

1. Persistent lack of tears in the newborn
2. Neurogenic hyposecretion
3. Absence of hypoplasia of the lacrimal gland
4. Association with Riley-Day syndrome
5. Associated congenital and anhidrotic ectodermal dysplasia

With congenital alacrima one finds epidermidalization of the corneal epithelium; keratinization is noted in the more advanced states. In addition, corneal vascularization may be a significant finding. The cornea is dry, and symblepharons may occur in the lower cul-de-sac.

NEUROTROPHIC KERATITIS

This complication of corneal denervation is frequently seen from surgical lesions of the trigeminal ganglion, the sensory route, or the descending trigeminal tract in the brain stem. Conditions that manifest decreased corneal sensation are summarized in Table 22-2.

Table 22-2. Conditions exhibiting decreased corneal sensation

Dystrophies	**Iatrogenic**
Lattice	Poorly fitting contact lens
Granular (rare)	Trauma to ciliary nerves with cryotherapy or diathermy
Functional	
Hysteria	**Virus**
	Herpes zoster*
Central nervous system	Herpes simplex
Cerebellopontine angle tumors	
Cavernous sinus disease	**Trauma**
Orbital apex and superior orbital apex syndromes	Lye burns
Brain stem lesions involving descending tract of fifth cranial nerve	Acid burns
	Perforation of cornea
	Corneal graft and cataract†
Posterior inferior cerebellar or vertebral artery occlusion	**Toxic**
Pontine lesions	Systemic intoxication with carbon disulfide‡

*Involves nasociliary nerve—sensation is never returned to normal.
†Temporary until regeneration occurs (6 to 8 months).
‡Pathologic condition is in the myelin sheaths of the peripheral nerves.

Ocular involvement

Early signs of corneal involvement are the development of a corneal haze and injection of the conjunctiva. These changes may be apparent within 24 hours after section of the trigeminal ganglion. Punctate keratopathy and widespread loss of epithelium are also seen. Decrease in luster, increased haziness, erosions, ulceration, hypopyon, and even perforation of the cornea are found. Rose bengal red provides a valuable aid for demonstrating the effects of desiccation in the desensitized eye. Although various external factors contribute to the production of desiccation, the primary cause is alteration of the adhesive forces between the ocular surface and the tear film. Desiccation is considered to be one of the principal factors responsible for the changes of neurotrophic and neuroparalytic keratitis.[8]

Etiologic factors

The neurotrophic disturbance that exists in these cases is not caused by the lack of trophic impulses or the presence of abnormal irritative impulses, but, because of the lack of normal peripheral antidromic activity of sensory nerves and the essential abnormality, an accumulation of tissue metabolites increases tissue edema. This edema, together with impaired vitality, leads to degeneration, desiccation, and exfoliation, allowing more trauma, which leads to gross defects and perhaps to access of organisms to the cornea.

Management

Early treatment, which is of the utmost importance, includes an airtight shield over the involved eye, which in effect creates a moist chamber. Epithelialization of eroded areas usually occurs after the establishment of adequate surface moisture to the cornea. Tarsorrhaphy is of benefit and may be necessary. If a tarsorrhaphy is performed, it should be complete; the first indication for this procedure is persistent epithelial punctate staining. After several weeks, the tarsorrhaphy may be partially opened to observe if the epithelium can tolerate exposure. Occasionally the tarsorrhaphy may have to be repeated, but usually the eye can be opened gradually. The eye may require partial closure for as long as a year.

EXPOSURE KERATITIS
Etiologic factors

Exposure keratitis causes improper moistening of the corneal surface. Any factor, local or systemic, that leads to the interference of the blink reflex or constant exposure of a particular area of the cornea caused by lid defects may result in an exposure keratitis. Systemic problems such as Parkinson's disease, neurologic disease causing a failure of Bell's phenomenon, coma with exposure of part of the cornea, facial paralysis, and thyroid disease with marked exophthalmos may cause exposure keratitis. Other local ophthalmic problems such as cicatricial ectropion, orbital tumors with proptosis, and exposure during sleep may result in exposure keratitis.[20]

Clinical findings

Chronic punctate keratitis of the central or lower cornea usually occurs. Occasionally, the entire lower half of the cornea is involved, or more frequently a horizontal superficial epithelial band across the involved corneal area is present. There is usually a lack of corneal luster as well as diffuse haziness and desiccation of the involved area.[9]

A high index of suspicion exists for corneal exposure during sleep, and, unless sought, this commonly occurring situation may be missed. When exposure changes from sleep (nocturnal) lagophthalmos occur, one may see mild change in the morning, which may heal later in the day. However, one can observe in this inferior area of the cornea map-dot-fingerprint lines, spheroidal degeneration, nodules similar to small deposits of Salzmann's nodular dystrophy, and, most common of all, a horizontal brown line—the Hudson-Stähli line—which signifies chronic epithelial damage and irritation.[20] The cornea may exhibit, in long-standing cases, infiltration, vascularization, ulceration, and melting.

Management

The management of exposure keratitis is treatment of the underlying condition, whatever the problem may be, either local or systemic. However, the immediate condition can be treated with the simple night application of ointment and taping the lid shut at night when the etiologic agent is one of mild lid nonclosure.

ALPORT'S SYNDROME

This disease is associated with hemorrhagic nephritis and aminoaciduria,[5] as well as with progressive nerve deafness and vestibular disturbances.

Progressive anterior and posterior lenticonus and spherophakia are seen. Subcapsular cataract, macular changes, albipunctate fundus, and optic nerve drusen also occur.

The cornea may exhibit an arcus juvenilis[5] and keratoconus. Pigment dispersion is noted in some cases with deposition of pigment in the cornea (Krukenberg's spindle) and in the lens capsule.[8]

In some cases severe corneal ulcers have been observed that were resistant to treatment.

COGAN'S SYNDROME

This nonluetic interstitial keratitis, which exhibits vestibuloauditory problems, is discussed in Chapter 4.

MYOTONIC DYSTROPHY

Myotonic muscular dystrophy is inherited as an autosomal dominant trait and manifested early or late in life, with the first signs of weakness occurring in the feet and hands. The dystrophy progresses slowly; occasionally facial and pharyngeal weaknesses are noted. Cardiomyopathy may occur with conduction block defects. The patient has an expressionless face, frontal balding, testicular or ovarian atrophy, and mental changes.

The eye signs include ocular hypotony, enophthalmos, depressed ERG, ophthalmoplegia, and ptosis. A multicolored, anterior and posterior, subcapsular, dotlike lens change is also seen.

Exposure keratitis is noted in the inferior portions of cornea. Orbicularis muscle weakness and atrophy and a poor Bell phenomenon contribute to the corneal exposure.

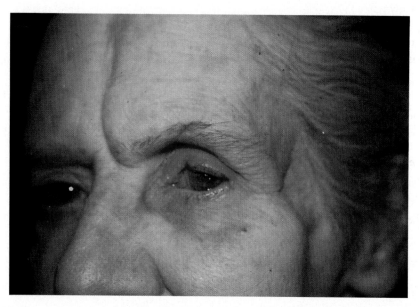

Fig. 22-4. Parry-Romberg syndrome of progressive hemifacial atrophy showing severe depression of zygomatic and temporal area. (From Grayson, M., and Pieroni, D.: Am. J. Ophthalmol. **70:**42, 1970.)

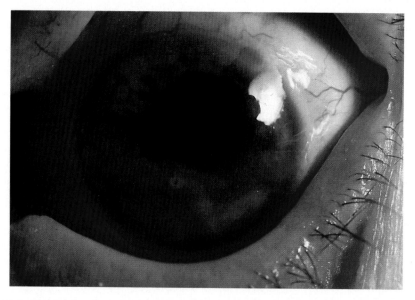

Fig. 22-5. Corneal involvement consisting of early corneal edema and early band keratopathy in Parry-Romberg syndrome. (From Grayson, M., and Pieroni, D.: Am. J. Ophthalmol. **70:**42, 1970.)

PARRY-ROMBERG SYNDROME[16]

This progressive hemifacial atrophy is sometimes associated with localized or linear scleroderma. Very early cases may appear simply with progressive asymptomatic unilateral enophthalmos and a depression and pigmentation of the zygomatic area (Fig. 22-4).

Horner's syndrome, mydriasis, alteration in lacrimation, heterochromia iritis, and paresis of extraocular muscles are also noted, as well as chronic degenerative uveitis and scleritis. The cornea may exhibit an exposure keratitis caused by ectropion and neuroparalytic keratitis, bullous keratopathy with guttata, and a band keratopathy[16] (Fig. 22-5).

GOLDENHAR-GORLIN SYNDROME[1]

Unilateral or bilateral neurotrophic keratitis has been seen in Goldenhar-Gorlin syndrome,[26] which is a complex consisting of oculoauriculovertebral dysplasia and hemifacial microsomia. The classic triad of Goldenhar's syndrome consists of epibulbar dermoids, preauricular tags, blind fistules, vertebral anomalies, associated ocular defects, facial anomalies, and skeletal deformities. Gorlin has demonstrated that Goldenhar's syndrome is a mild form of hemifacial microsomia; this contribution has been recognized by calling the complex Goldenhar-Gorlin syndrome.

Corneal ulcer production in some cases is caused by deficient tear production and corneal anesthesia; the resulting corneal anesthesia is caused by a defect in the ophthalmic division of the fifth nerve. The level at which this occurs is probably nuclear and the result of nuclear aplasia.

REFERENCES

1. Baum, J.L., and Feingold, M.: Ocular aspects of Goldenhar syndrome, Am. J. Ophthalmol. **75:**250, 1973.
2. Boruchoff, S.A., and Dohlman, C.H.: The Riley-Day syndrome: ocular manifestations in a 35-year-old patient, Am. J. Ophthalmol. **63:**523, 1967.
3. Brunt, P.W., and McKusick, V.A.: Familial dysautonomia: a report of genetic and clinical studies with a review of the literature, Medicine **49:**343, 1974.
4. Cairns, J.E., Williams, H.P., and Walshe, J.M.: Sunflower cataract in Wilson's disease, Br. Med. J. **3:**95, 1969.
5. Chavis, R.M., and Groshong, T.: Corneal arcus in Alport's syndrome, Am. J. Ophthalmol. **75:**793, 1973.
6. Danks, D.M., Cartwright, E., and Stevens, B.J.: Menkes' steely-hair (kinky hair) disease, Lancet **1:**891, 1973.
7. Danks, D.M., Campbell, P.E., Stevens, B.J., et al.: Menkes's kinky-hair syndrome: an inherited defect in copper absorption with widespread effects, Pediatrics **50:**188, 1972.
8. Davies, P.D.: Pigment dispersion in a case of Alport's syndrome, Br. J. Ophthalmol. **54:**557, 1970.
9. DeHass, E.B.H.: Desiccation of the cornea and conjunctiva after sensory denervation, Arch. Ophthalmol. **67:**439, 1962.
10. Dunnington, J.H.: Congenital alacrima in familial autonomic dysfunction, Arch. Ophthalmol. **52:** 925, 1954.
11. Evans, G.W., Dubois, R.S., and Hambidge, K.M.: Wilson's disease: identification of an abnormal copper binding protein, Science **21:**1175, 1973.
12. Fleming, C.R., Dickson, E.R., Wahner, H.W., Hollenhorst, R.W., and McCall, J.T.: Pigmented rings in non-Wilsonian liver disease, Ann. Intern. Med. **86:**285, 1977.
13. Froment, J., Bonnet, P., and Paufique, L.: Anneau pigmenté de Kayser-Fleischer dans la pseudosclérose, Bull. Soc. Ophthalmol. Fr. **2:**713, 1937.
14. Ginsberg, S.P., Polack, F.M., and Ravin, M.B.: Autonomic dysfunction syndrome, Am. J. Ophthalmol. **74:**1121, 1972.
15. Goldberg, M.F., Payne, J.W., and Brunt, P.W.: Ophthalmologic studies of familial dysautonomia, Arch. Ophthalmol. **80:**732, 1968.
16. Grayson, M., and Pieroni, D.: Progressive facial hemiatrophy with bullous and band-shaped keratopathy, Am. J. Ophthalmol. **70:**42, 1970.

17. Harry, J., and Tripathi, R.: Kayser-Fleischer ring: a pathological study, Br. J. Ophthalmol. **54:**794, 1970.

18. Howard, R.O.: Familial dysautonomia (Riley-Day syndrome), Am. J. Ophthalmol. **64:**392, 1967.

19. Johnson, B.L.: Ultrastructure of the Kayser-Fleischer ring, Am. J. Ophthalmol. **76:**455, 1973.

20. Katz, J., and Kaufman, H.E.: Corneal exposure during sleep (nocturnal lagophthalmos), Arch. Ophthalmol. **95:**499, 1977.

21. Kroop, I.G.: The production of tears in familial dysautonomia: preliminary report, J. Pediatr. **48:**328, 1956.

22. Liebman, S.D.: Ocular manifestations of Riley-Day syndrome, Arch. Ophthalmol. **56:**719, 1956.

23. Liebman, S.D.: Riley-Day syndrome, Arch. Ophthalmol. **58:**188, 1957.

24. Manschot, W.A.: Ring of Kayser and Fleischer, Ophthalmologica **132:**164, 1956.

25. Mitchell, A.M., and Heller, G.L.: Changes in Kayser-Fleischer ring during treatment of hepatolenticular degeneration, Arch. Ophthalmol. **80:**622, 1968.

26. Mohandessan, M.M.: Neuroparalytic keratitis in Goldenhar-Gorlin syndrome, Am. J. Ophthalmol. **85:**111, 1978.

27. Pilger, I.S.: Familial dysautonomia: report of case with stimulation of tear production by prostigmine, Am. J. Ophthalmol. **43:**285, 1957.

28. Slovis, T.L., Dubois, R.S., Rodgerson, D.O., and Silverman, A.: The varied manifestations of Wilson's disease, J. Pediatr. **78:**578, 1971.

29. Smith, A.A., Dancis, J., and Breinin, G.: Ocular responses to autonomic drugs in familial dysautonomia, Invest. Ophthalmol. **4:**358, 1965.

30. Sternliev, I., and Scheinberg, I.H.: The diagnosis of Wilson's disease in asymptomatic patients, JAMA **183:**747, 1963.

31. Sternliev, I., and Scheinberg, I.H.: Prevention of Wilson's disease in asymptomatic patients, N. Engl. J. Med. **278:**352, 1968.

32. Sussman, W., and Scheinberg, I.H.: Disappearance of Kayser-Fleischer rings: effects of penicillamine, Arch. Ophthalmol. **82:**738, 1969.

33. Tso, M.O.M., Fine, B.S., and Thorpe, H.E.: Kayser-Fleischer ring and associated cataract in Wilson's disease, Am. J. Ophthalmol. **79:**479, 1975.

34. Uzman, L.L., and Jakus, M.A.: The Kayser-Fleischer ring: a histochemical and electron microscope study, Neurology **7:**341, 1957.

35. Walshe, J.M.: Wilson's disease: its diagnosis and management, Br. J. Hosp. Med. **4:**91, 1970.

CHAPTER

23 Diseases of the skin

A number of dermatologic problems may indirectly or directly affect the conjunctiva and cornea. The ophthalmic findings and associations are often missed, since the patient is usually not examined on a systemic basis and is being seen by the ophthalmologist more often than not in a darkened room. Thus important diagnoses are not made. The corneal and conjunctival manifestations may be extremely subtle or very extensive. The ophthalmologist must bear in mind that skin diseases are an important and integral part of external ophthalmic disease.

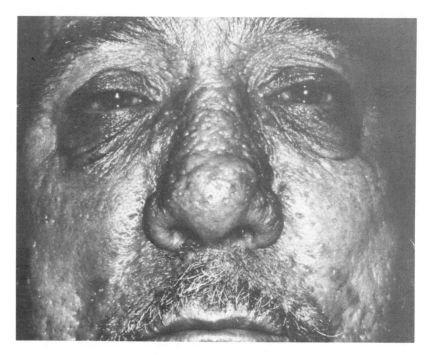

Fig. 23-1. Rhinophyma caused by rosacea.

ROSACEA

This skin disease occurs primarily in the area of the forehead, nose, cheeks, and chin. It is a chronic papular and pustular dermatitis with cutaneous erythema, as well as hypertrophy of the sebaceous glands, which is seen as rhinophyma (Fig. 23-1). Many small telangiectatic spots are noticed on the skin of the face and nose (Fig. 23-2). No comodones are seen. Rosacea occurs often in women and in the age group between 25 and 55 years. Abnormal vascular stability and activity exist, since rosacea and migraine[75] are associated.

Ocular involvement

The skin condition in rosacea is often missed, and certainly the problem is more common than realized; ocular manifestations may result in severe visual impairment. The ocular signs may appear before the skin manifestations on the face are noticed. Ophthalmic remissions and exacerbations may occur independently of the skin problem. Staphylococcal lid infections are high in incidence.

A chronic nonulcerative blepharitis associated with conjunctival hyperemia may occur. One of the main findings is that the blood vessels of the conjunctiva are dilated in a manner similar to that of the blood vessels of the eyelids and of the skin of the nose and face. The dilated blood vessels occur most often in the interpalpebral areas of the medial and lateral epibulbar conjunctivae. These conjunctival vessels are large and tortuous. Rosacea may be mistaken for an infectious conjunctivitis, and the patient is often medicated unnecessarily. In some instances, a nodular conjunctivitis is part of the picture. It is the persistent redness of the eye that is most disturbing to the patient.

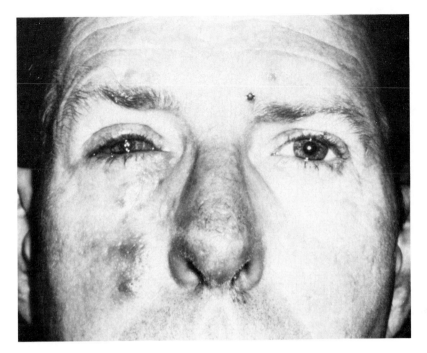

Fig. 23-2. Rosacea telangiectasia of skin of face and nose.

The cornea can be extensively involved with scarring and vascularization. Involvement of the inferior cornea with pannus formation is more frequently seen. When the cornea becomes involved, epithelial keratitis in combination with subepithelial infiltration may occur (Fig. 23-3), causing dense, white, leukomatous scars with heavy vascularization. Marginal corneal melting (Fig. 23-4) with progressive thinning may lead to perforation, especially if steroid therapy has been introduced and injudiciously used.

Treatment

The patient with rosacea should be under the joint care of a dermatologist and ophthalmologist.

Tetracycline, 250 mg to 1000 mg a day for 6 weeks, is recommended for cutaneous rosacea. However, patients with ocular rosacea require more prolonged treatment with gradual tapering of the daily dosage of the tetracycline. The reason that rosacea responds to tetracycline is really not known. Tetracycline does not appear to have an effect on the lipid composition of the meibomian secretions of the rosacea patient, and rosacea patients do not have a difference in the lipid composition of the meibomian secretions from apparently normal people.

Attempts at relating the cutaneous disease to the presence of mannitol-positive *Staphylococcus* organisms have not been successful, and organisms are still present on the eyelids and conjunctiva in most cases that respond to long-term treatment with tetracycline.[44]

The secondary infection can also be treated by the use of topical antibiotics such as

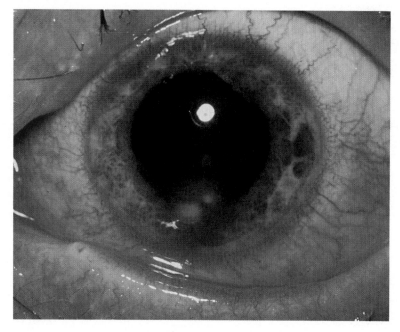

Fig. 23-3. Severe keratitis may be seen in rosacea. Dense white opacities and vascularization are not uncommon in rosacea.

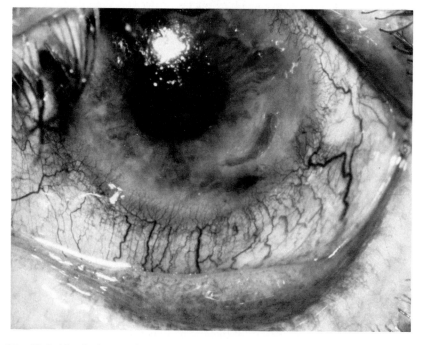

Fig. 23-4. Marginal corneal melting with progressive thinning may be seen in rosacea.

erythromycin or bacitracin ointment.[64] As was noted, if steroid therapy is introduced, care must be exercised as to the length of time it is used and the dose given, since severe side effects from treatment have occurred in the form of increased intraocular tension, cataract formation, and perforation of the cornea.

It may be necessary to perform a corneal graft if the cornea is extensively scarred, but the long-term results are not satisfactory. In addition to the measures already mentioned, it has been advised that intake of carbohydrates, tea, and coffee should be decreased; elimination of alcohol is also advised.

SEBORRHEIC DERMATITIS

The eyebrow, eyelids, nasolabial folds, ears, chest, and back may be involved in this oily skin eruption. The lid margins are also involved with a blepharitis, and one may see a conjunctivitis. Rarely, the cornea may exhibit an epithelial keratitis.

PSORIASIS

Increased epidermal cell proliferation occurs in certain conditions such as lamellar ichthyosis, epidermolytic hyperkeratitis, and psoriasis. The psoriatic patient exhibits a tendency to accelerated epidermopoiesis in response to external and internal stimuli. The nature of the stimuli is controversial, although it has been shown that in warmer climates the patient seems to be improved. Trauma may be an initiating factor in some cases. Streptococcal infection seems to be a particularly provoking agent in children.[82] It appears that cyclic AMP is decreased in the involved epidermis of patients with psoriasis as compared with both uninvolved and controlled epidermis.[79] Psoriasis occurs in about 4% of all patients with arthritis.

Psoriasis is a chronic, papulosquamous disorder (Fig. 23-5) with geographic, demarcated, erythematous patches on the skin that are covered with silvery-white scales. The disease may be seen in any age group extending from 10 to as late as the sixties or seventies. It is more common in whites and women.

Ocular involvement

Ocular signs occur in approximately 10% of cases. The eyelids are frequently involved, and scaling may be seen at the base of the lashes. Trichiasis and madarosis may occur in severe cases. If the lid margins become involved, they may be swollen, red, and scaly.

The bulbar conjunctiva may become injected and exhibit yellow plaquelike lesions. Phlyctenular-like lesions occur at the corneal limbus.

The corneal lesions are somewhat polymorphic and may consist of superficial and deep opacities and vascularization. In addition, one may find corneal erosions and melting (Fig. 23-6).

Treatment

The treatment of the systemic and dermatologic problems should be undertaken by the internist and the dermatologist. It has been suggested that methotrexate be used in conjunction with folinic acid in the treatment of psoriasis.[4, 42]

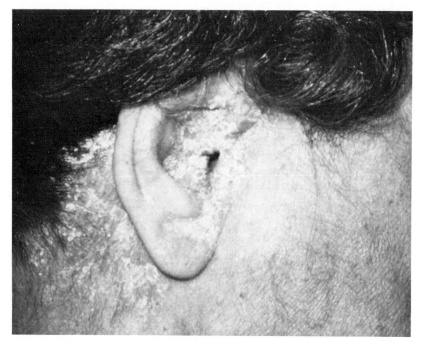

Fig. 23-5. Psoriasis is a chronic papulosquamous skin disorder.

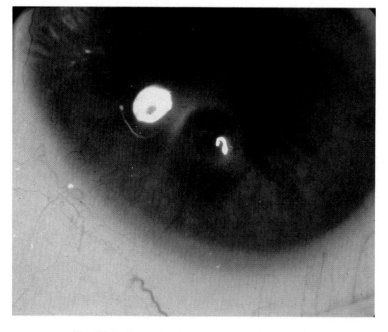

Fig. 23-6. Corneal melting may occur in psoriasis.

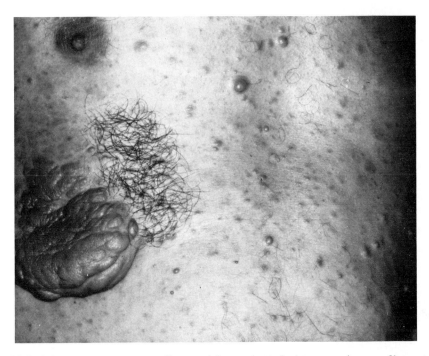

Fig. 23-7. Subcutaneous tumors are firm, nodular, and attached to nerve in neurofibromatosis.

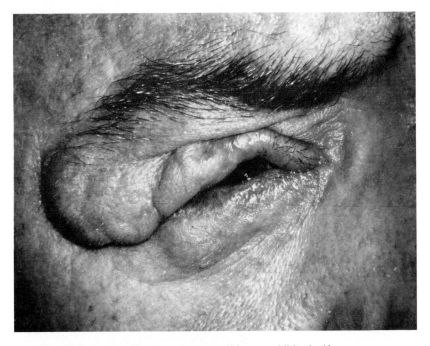

Fig. 23-8. In neurofibromatosis, upper lid may exhibit plexiform neuroma.

NEUROFIBROMATOSIS

This disease may be present at birth. Cutaneous lesions may occur during childhood and adolescence. The characteristic hyperpigmented lesions of the skin—café au lait spots—occur in 25% to 100% of the cases. These lesions increase in size and number and may precede cutaneous nodules. One may see discrete soft or firm cutaneous tumors, which may number a few to many hundreds. Subcutaneous tumors may be firm, discrete nodules that are often attached to a nerve (Fig. 23-7). Tumors of the central and peripheral nervous systems occur. Cranial nerve involvement may produce deafness, facial pain, numbness of the extremities, and any number of signs, depending on the nerve affected. Malignant degeneration occurs in 2% to 5% of these lesions. Some patients with neurofibromatosis may manifest an increase in intracranial pressure and proptosis.

Ocular involvement

Retinal and optic nerve gliomas result in varying clinical pictures. Plexiform neuromas of the upper lid occur and simulate a "bag of worms" (Fig. 23-8). One side of the face only may be involved (Fig. 23-9). The corneal nerves are increasingly visible. Decreased corneal sensation and neurotrophic keratitis may be found if the fifth cranial nerve is involved.

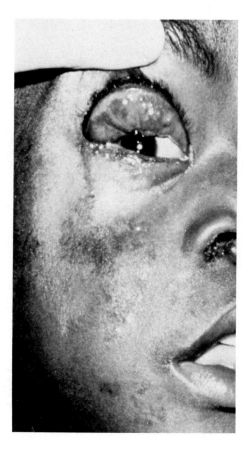

Fig. 23-9. Involvement of one side of face in neurofibromatosis.

ICHTHYOSIS

Ichthyosis is an inherited disorder of the skin and is characterized by thickening, fissuring, and scaling of the skin. Four main groups exist (Table 23-1): (1) ichthyosis vulgaris, inherited as an autosomal dominant trait; (2) X-linked ichthyosis, transmitted as a sex-linked character; (3) lamellar ichthyosis, an autosomal recessive trait; and (4) congenital ichthyosiform erythroderma.[26]

X-linked ichthyosis primarily affects the sons of heterozygous females, or *carriers*. The woman does not develop the full-blown dermatosis but will manifest certain X-linked ichthyosis clinical features.

Scaling is present at birth or hours afterward and is seen on the neck, trunk, buttocks, and extremities.[45] The palms and soles are normal in the dystrophic form, which distinguishes it from lamellar ichthyosis. Sweating and sebaceous functions are poor in ichthyotic areas. Scaling of arms and legs (Fig. 23-10) can be seen in heterozygote women and is more apparent in dry weather.

Ocular involvement

Lid entropion may be seen with lamellar ichthyosis.[71]

Slit-lamp examination of boys and carriers reveals punctate dots or striate opacities on Descemet's membrane or immediately anterior to it* (Fig. 23-11). Larger white or gray stromal opacities are deeply located.[27] Small refractile bodies in the epithelium, superficial stroma, and endothelium have also been reported. Prominent corneal nerves and band keratopathy may be the only corneal findings.[24, 43] Superficial nodular corneal

---

*References 22, 23, 68, 70, 77.

Table 23-1. Forms of ichthyosis

Features	Ichthyosis vulgaris	X-linked ichthyosis	Lamellar ichthyosis	Congenital ichthyosiform erythroderma
Time	Childhood	Birth or infancy	Birth	Birth
Inheritance	Dominant	X-linked	Autosomal recessive	Dominant
Scales on skin	Fine scales	Prominent scales on trunk, buttocks, and neck	Prominent scales over most of body	Scaling and redness of skin
Associated clinical findings	Atopy Keratosis of palmar and plantar areas	Findings in heterozygous women important in diagnosis	Hyperkeratosis of palms and soles	Hyperkeratosis of palms and soles
Eye findings	None	Superficial nodular lesions Band keratopathy Increased corneal nerve visibility Pre-Descemet opacities	Ectropion	Ectropion Conjunctivitis Keratitis

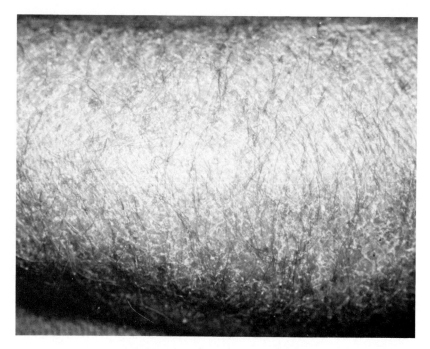

Fig. 23-10. Scaling of skin in ichthyosis.

degeneration, although rare, may be a part of the picture (Fig. 23-12).

Table 23-1 lists eye signs that occur in some forms of ichthyosis.

Differential diagnosis

Several systemic syndromes manifest scaling of the skin, for example, Sjögren-Larssen,[29] Conradi's, and Refsum's syndromes. In the former diseases, the condition resembles lamellar ichthyosis. However, spastic paralysis, macular pigmentary degeneration, aminoaciduria, and mental retardation may be seen in the Sjögren-Larssen syndrome. In Conradi's syndrome the scales form whorllike patterns. Superficial corneal opacities, lens opacities, high-arched palate, skeletal defects, and stippled epithesis are also seen. Refsum's syndrome, in addition to ichthyosis, exhibits bilateral eighth-nerve deafness, pigmentary retinal degeneration, chronic polyneuritis, electrocardiographic changes, and increased protein in the spinal fluid. Ichthyosis is also seen in Rud's syndrome.

KERATOSES

Richner-Hanhart syndrome

Richner-Hanhart syndrome is now considered a definite entity and was formerly known as keratosis plantaris et palmaris.[25,36] Historically the latter problem exhibited painful keratotic lesions on the hands and feet (Fig. 23-13) in addition to leukoplakia of the buccal mucosa (Fig. 23-14). Herpetical lesions of the cornea were described.[81] I[36] described a case of what was then known as keratosis plantaris et palmaris in which the corneal lesions were dustlike intraepithelial lesions randomly distributed in the lower

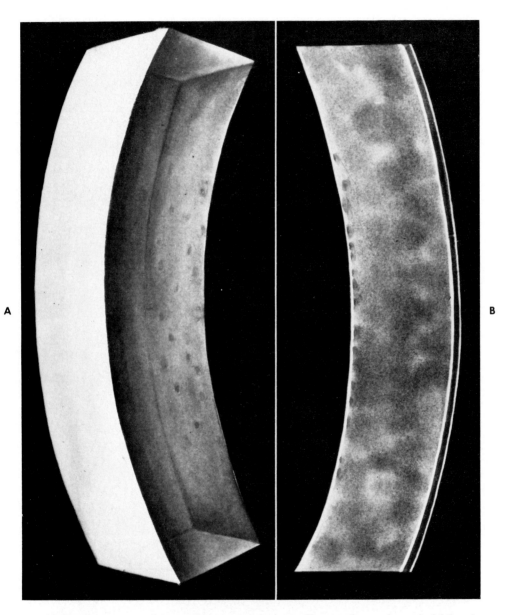

Fig. 23-11. Punctate or striate opacities on or anterior to Descemet's membrane in ichthyosis. **A,** Parallelepiped section. **B,** Optical section.

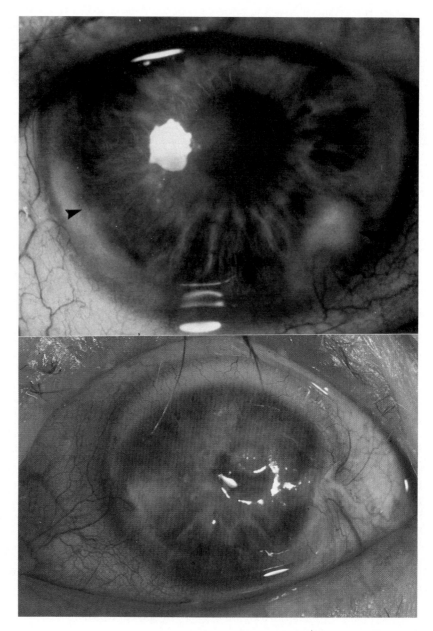

Fig. 23-12. Nodular corneal degenerations in ichthyosis.

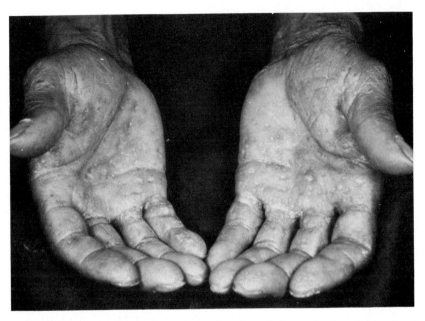

Fig. 23-13. Painful keratotic lesions on hands and feet in keratosis plantaris et palmaris.

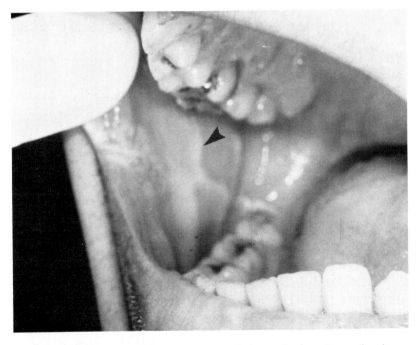

Fig. 23-14. Leukoplakia of buccal mucosa in keratosis plantaris et palmaris.

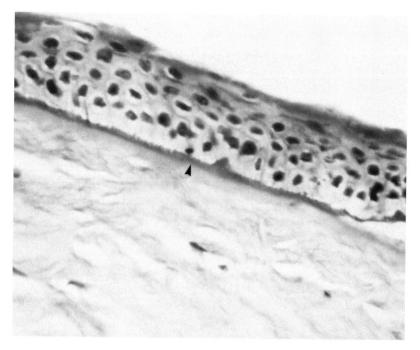

Fig. 23-15. Tiny fingerlike projections into basal layer of corneal epithelium in keratosis plantaris et palmaris.

aspect of the cornea. Histologic examination revealed thickening of the basement membrane with tiny fingerlike projections extending into the basal layer of the epithelium (Fig. 23-15).

Differential diagnosis. Hyperkeratosis of palms and soles with corneal disorders is involved in the following diseases:

1. Richner-Hanhart syndrome (keratosis plantaris et palmaris)
2. Pityriasis rubra pilaris
3. Hypohidrotic ectodermal dysplasia
4. Ichthyosis
5. Pachyonychia congenita
6. Papillon-Lefèvre syndrome
7. Keratosis follicularis (Darier's disease)

The Richner-Hanhart syndrome[5, 9, 34] embodies the features of hyperkeratotic lesions of the hands and feet,* thickening of the conjunctival epithelium, and corneal opacities and is related to an inborn error of tyrosine and metabolism.[31, 32] Improvement of these lesions can occur after introduction of a diet low in phenylalanine and tyrosine.

The conjunctiva appears less translucent than normal, but the important findings are seen in the corneal epithelium. Embedded in the corneal epithelium of each eye is a fine, branched opacity. These lesions give a herpetoid appearance. The opacity in some cases

---

*References 33, 36, 38, 65, 81.

may involve the anterior stroma and take on a sunburst effect.[9] They do not, however, stain with fluorescein.

It appears that there is a deficiency of tyrosine aminotransferase[18] or an absence of parahydroxyphenylpyruvic acid oxidase in this disease.

Keratosis follicular spinulosa decalvans (Sieman's disease)[22]

This disease is transmitted as an intermediate sex-linked factor or in a dominant fashion. Skin disease consists of hyperkeratotic follicular spines at the hair follicle opening, which give the skin a coarse texture.[20] Sites of predilection are the face, scalp, eyebrows, neck, arms, and dorsal fingers. In addition, some loss of hair occurs at the lateral portion of the eyebrow and occipital area of the head. Skeletal hypoplasia is also seen. Failure to thrive, deafness, and recurrent infections have been reported in infants.[7]

Ocular involvement. The cornea is affected in rare cases of Sieman's disease and may show circumferential pannus with diffuse, superficial, farinaceous opacities (Fig. 23-16, *A*). Female carriers may show recurrent erosions, epithelial or subepithelial opacities, and prominent corneal nerves. The epithelium may be thick and irregular, contain irregularly shaped nuclei, and show vacuoles and keratotic spines (Fig. 23-16, *B*) with projections of the basement membranes into the basal epithelium. The patient will complain of photophobia and epiphora as a result of erosions of the corneal epithelium (Fig. 23-16, *C*).

Kyrle's disease

Kyrle's disease[76] is a dermatologic disorder characterized by multiple, follicular keratoses. The flesh-colored, hard horny papules can be located in any part of the body except the mucous membranes and the palms and soles. The papule eventually acquires a central keratotic plug, which leaves a central cone-shaped crater that matches the shape of the plug when the plug is removed. The lesions, which are asymptomatic, come in crops, persist for several weeks, eventually disappear with no scarring, and may or may not involve the hair follicle. The plugs appear as red-brown, 2 to 4 mm papillary lesions over the limbs or trunks and may coalesce, forming hyperkeratotic plaques. The plugs penetrate deeply into the dermis, setting up an inflammatory reaction.

Ocular involvement. The corneal lesions of Kyrle's disease appear unique. They consist of minute, yellow-brown, subepithelial opacities (Fig. 23-17). Their greatest density and deepest penetration occur at the limbus; the least, at the corneal center.[76] In addition to the corneal lesions, one may find posterior subcapsular cataracts.

Keratosis follicularis (Darier's disease)[84]

In Darier's disease[6] one notes firm, brown scaly papules, which can be distributed over the forehead, scalp, and intertrigenous areas of the skin (Fig. 23-18). The disease is not limited to the hair follicles but also involves the interfollicular epidermis. Mucous membranes can also be affected, especially in the larynx and pharynx.[14] The papules may take on various forms such as linear, hemorrhagic, or hypertrophic forms. Hyperkeratotic lesions are seen on the soles and palms.

Text continued on p. 554.

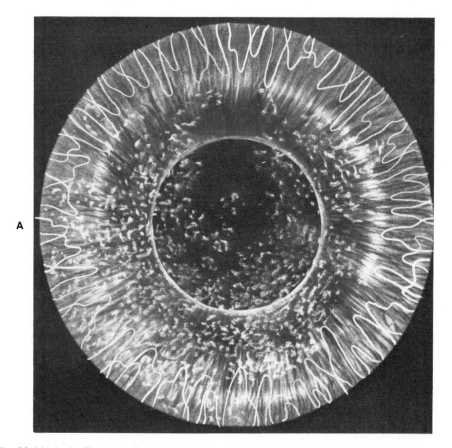

Fig. 23-16. A, In Sieman's disease one may see circumferential pannus with diffuse superficial farinaceous opacities. (**A** to **C** courtesy A. Franceschetti, M.D., Geneva, Switzerland.)

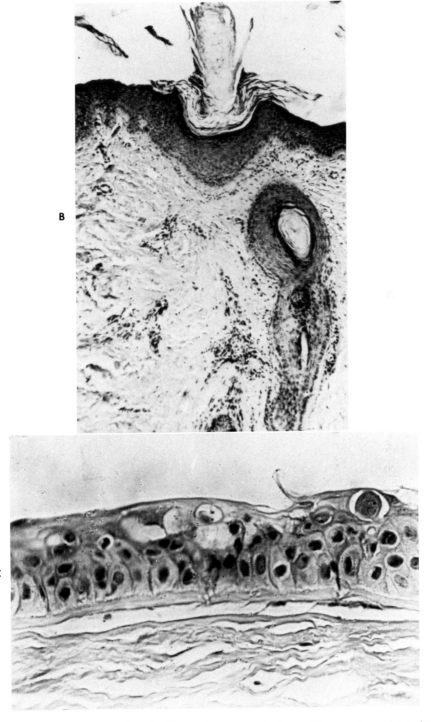

Fig. 23-16, cont'd. B, Epithelium is thick and shows projections of basement membrane into basal epithelium. **C,** Erosion of epithelium.

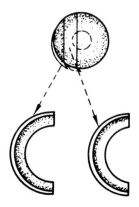

Fig. 23-17. Kyrle's disease shows minute, yellow-brown subepithelial opacities in subepithelial and anterior stroma. (From Tessler, H.H., Apple, D.J., and Goldberg, M.: Arch. Ophthalmol. **90:**278; copyright 1973, American Medical Association.)

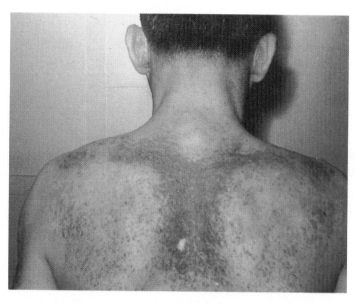

Fig. 23-18. Darier's disease, showing thick vegetative plaques and papulomatous growths covered with greasy crusts. (From Grayson, M., and Keates, R.H.: Manual of diseases of the cornea, Boston, 1969, Little, Brown & Co.)

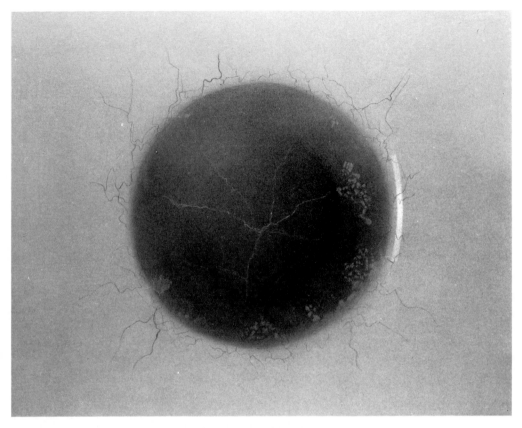

Fig. 23-19. Schematic illustration of peripheral opacities and central radiating lines in corneal epithelium of 43-year-old woman. (From Blackman, H.J., Rodrigues, M.M., and Peck, G.L.: Ophthalmology **87:**931, 1980.)

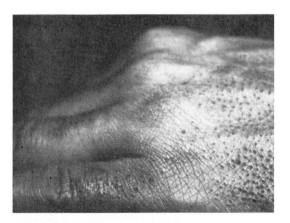

Fig. 23-20. Pityriasis rubra pilaris lesions exhibit spiny, keratotic, scaly, acuminate follicular papules on erythematous base. (From Grayson, M., and Keates, R.H.: Manual of diseases of the cornea, Boston, 1969, Little, Brown & Co.)

Ocular involvement. Corneal involvement is varied, but peripheral opacities and central epithelial irregularity in a radiating cobweb pattern are most often seen (Fig. 23-19). In addition, dense yellow peripheral pannus and a central stromal opacity can be noted.

The eyelids may exhibit keratotic plaques, and sometimes staphylococcal blepharitis and trichiasis are seen.

Corneal lesions do not change during 13-cis-retinoic acid therapy, but the eyelid and cutaneous lids do respond well.

PITYRIASIS RUBRA PILARIS

In this condition, keratotic lesions of the palms and the soles occur. There is no involvement of the mucous membrane like that seen in keratosis plantaris and palmaris.

Pityriasis rubra pilaris is autosomal dominant and exhibits spiney, keratotic, scaly, fine, acuminate follicular papules on an erythematous base[20] (Fig. 23-20). They appear mostly on the dorsal aspect of the proximal phalanges and wrist but may be seen on the entire body. Scales may develop, resembling ichthyosis.

Ocular involvement. Conjunctival and corneal keratinization are seen in this condition. A fibrovascular pannus, interstitial scarring, vascularization of the cornea, and epithelial erosions may also occur.

Management. Vitamin A therapy sometimes brings about a remission in pityriasis rubra pilaris. Marked vitamin A deficiency, from any cause, may result in the association of keratotic skin changes with corneal disease.

ROTHMUND'S SYNDROME (ROTHMUND-THOMSON SYNDROME)[17,51]

This condition is a recessively inherited disorder with the development of a photosensitivity rash within the first 6 months of life. This is later replaced by skin changes of atrophy, hyperpigmentation, depigmentation, telangiectasia, and keratosis.[72] Fingernail, bone, and tooth developmental anomalies occur, as well as a loss of hair. In addition to these characteristics, one may see a prominent forehead and a depressed nasal bridge. Systemic problems such as hypogonadism and short stature occur in 25% of patients with Rothmund's syndrome.

Ocular involvement

Cataracts, usually appearing at 3 to 6 years, occur in 47% of the patients.[17] They are usually rapidly progressive, bilateral, and posterior stellate cataracts.

Corneal involvement may reveal band keratopathy.[51]

WERNER'S SYNDROME[16,59]

Werner's syndrome is in essence a process of premature aging, with the onset between 20 and 30 years of age. It is transmitted as a recessive trait.[67] A cessation of growth occurs, followed by signs of premature aging.[60] Atrophy of the skin, sweat glands, nails, subcutaneous tissues, and muscles is seen. Other signs of premature aging are graying of the hair and loss of body hair. The face exhibits a beak-shaped nose, and the skin of the face as well as other areas becomes thin; alveolar ulcers may even develop. Painful hyperkeratotic lesions of the skin also occur. The voice becomes hoarse and high pitched.

Systemic involvement with bone changes, hypogonadism, diabetes mellitus, arthritis, arteriosclerosis, and soft tissue calcification occurs. In addition, neoplasms often appear.

Ocular involvement

Bilateral, posterior stellate cataracts occur between the ages of 20 and 35 in Werner's syndrome. Blue sclera,[76] telangiectasia, iritis, and retinitis pigmentosa,[46,78] have been reported.

Bullous keratopathy after cataract surgery is not infrequent.[24,60,67]

PACHYONYCHIA CONGENITA (JADASSOHN-LEWANDOWSKY SYNDROME)

This rare and dominant skin condition shows nails that are thick and upcurved; apparently they are overgrown nails. One also sees skin bullae, mucous membrane leukokeratosis, and keratosis and hyperhidrosis of the palms and soles. Pachyonychia congenita is transmitted as an autosomal dominant disease.

Corneal dyskeratoses and cataracts can be seen in this disease.[15]

ECTODERMAL DYSPLASIA[83]
Hereditary hypohidrotic ectodermal dysplasia

Hereditary hypohidrotic ectodermal dysplasia is generally transmitted in a sex-linked fashion, but females sometimes show partial forms of the disease.[21,79] In rare instances, it has been known to be transmitted as a dominant trait. Patients with hypohidrotic type of disease exhibit a facial appearance resembling that seen in congenital syphilis, with frontal bossing, prominent superficial orbital ridges, recession of the chin, and wrinkling of the skin about the eyelids and mouth.[79] Persons with this disease will also show absence of sweat glands and sebaceous glands. As a result they will have heat intolerance and diffuse dryness, roughness of the skin, and dental anomalies.[69] Toenail dysplasia occurs, as well as palmar and plantar hyperkeratosis. Alopecia, loss of eyebrows, acne, and comodones demonstrating facial and scalp sebaceous dysfunction are also noted.[79] Baldness is not uncommon.

Mammary glands are poorly developed and in some instances may be absent. Some patients have bilateral eighth-nerve deafness.[39,52]

A decrease occurs in lacrimal secretion and mild xerosis. Punctate epithelial keratopathy and a superficial pannus extending approximately 360 degrees are seen. The superficial, circumferential, peripheral vascularization may be accompanied by many tiny intraepithelial cysts; corneal thinning and stromal opacification also occur.

Hidrotic ectodermal dysplasia

In the hidrotic form, which is of autosomal dominant inheritance, there are usually no ocular abnormalities. However, the sweat glands are essentially unaffected, although the skin is dry, and hyperkeratosis of the palms and soles occurs, as does nail malformation. There is loss of hair and a tendency for the outer two thirds of the eyebrows to be absent. Neither dental abnormalities nor unusual facial characteristics are typical occurrences in this group of cases.

KERATITIS, ICHTHYOSIS, AND DEAFNESS SYNDROME (KID SYNDROME)[2,73]

The cause of this syndrome is unknown. It probably is transmitted as an autosomal recessive trait or a spontaneous mutation of a dominant gene. Several patients have decreased serum carotene, vitamin A, or zinc levels, suggesting a malabsorption problem.

Ichthyosis is usually present at an early age. Hyperkeratosis of the palms and soles with characteristic dotted and wavy pattern in bas-relief is noted. A reticulated pattern of hyperkeratosis of the palms and soles is seen in Figs. 23-21 and 23-22. Perioral furrowing is noted in this condition.

Some patients may exhibit leukoplakia of the buccal mucosa. Deep lingual fissuring along the dorsal midline of the tongue and rugae of the buccal mucosa can be seen.

Deafness is severe and is of the neurosensory type. It is seen at birth or develops in the first 2 years of life.

Scanty or absent hair, eyebrows, and eyelashes and follicular plugging are noted (Figs. 23-23 and 23-24).

Punctate epithelial keratopathy and vascularizing keratitis (Fig. 23-25) are prominent features. The pannus is superficial and may extend 360 degrees. The superficial circumferential peripheral vascularization may be accompanied by many intraepithelial cysts; corneal thinning and stromal opacification also occur.

Leukonychia, or thick dystrophic nails (Fig. 23-21), is noted.

Many patients may have decreased sweating caused by hyperkeratosis and plugging of the eccrine glands. Other conditions such as dental caries, skin infections, and squamous cell carcinoma of the tongue have been reported.

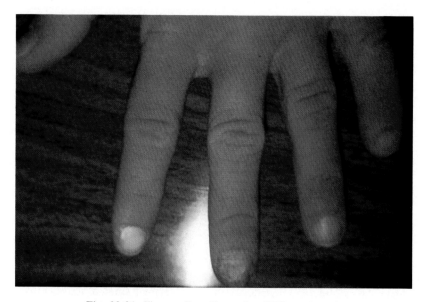

Fig. 23-21. Fingernail malformation (KID syndrome).

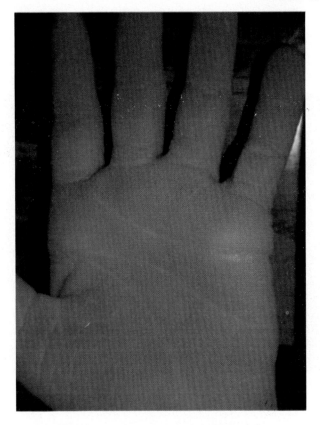

Fig. 23-22. Palmar hyperkeratosis in KID syndrome.

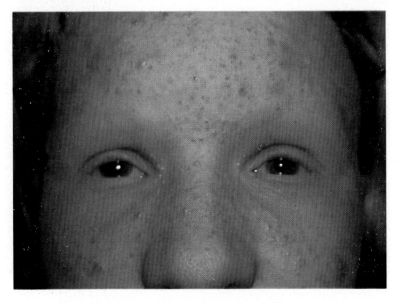

Fig. 23-23. Facial sebaceous dysfunction (KID syndrome).

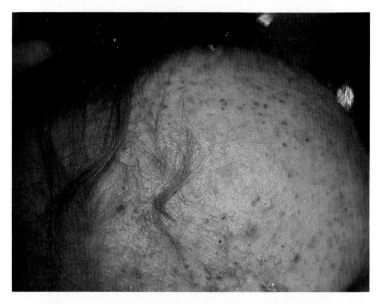

Fig. 23-24. Skin lesions as noted on scalp. Note loss of hair (KID syndrome).

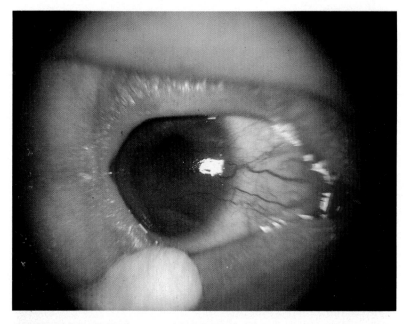

Fig. 23-25. Superficial, circumferential vascularization of cornea in KID syndrome, as well as corneal thinning and opacification.

This condition resembles hereditary hypohydrotic ectodermal dysplasia,* and some cases of KID syndrome have been incorrectly reported as hereditary hypohydrotic ectodermal dysplasia.

PAPILLON-LEFÈVRE SYNDROME[37]

This extremely rare syndrome is manifested by hypertrophic periodontopathy causing extrusion of teeth. In addition, one sees a hyperkeratosis of the palms and soles.

Occasionally, the cornea can be involved with peripheral vascularization and epithelial hypertrophy.

ACRODERMATITIS ENTEROPATHICA[80]

This rare familial disease[50] usually appears in infancy and is mostly seen in infant girls.[30] The illness follows a characteristic clinical course, and one sees a rash symmetrically distributed over the face, ears, back of the scalp, buttocks, elbows, knees, hands, and feet (Fig. 23-26), as well as periorally. The rash first goes through a vesicular,

---

*References 21, 39, 52, 69, 79, 83.

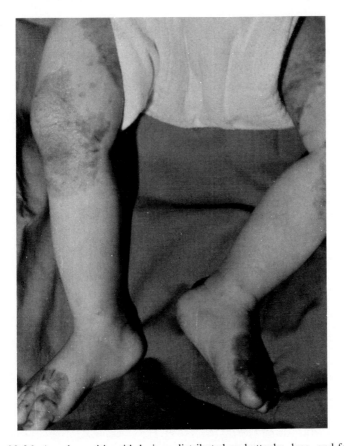

Fig. 23-26. Acrodermatitis with lesions distributed on buttocks, legs, and feet.

bullous stage, then dries and assumes a more erythematous, squamous, psoriasiform type. Dystrophy of the nails is part of the picture. Alopecia with loss of eyelashes and eyebrows is seen. The patient exhibits a poor general condition with low growth rate and gastrointestinal disturbances with diarrhea. Psychiatric disturbances of a schizoid nature can occur. If untreated, the majority of patients die before the age of 10. Frequently a secondary bacterial infection or infection with *Candida albicans* occurs. The patient exhibits a failure to thrive, as well as a low serum zinc level.

Ocular involvement

Blepharitis, photophobia, and conjunctivitis are some of the ocular findings present in cases of acrodermatitis enteropathica.

Superficial bilateral punctate lesions and nebulous subepithelial opacities of the cornea mainly located in the upper paralimbal cornea are seen.[53] These are radiating, linear, white to light brown, slightly whorllike opacities passing from the limbus about two thirds of the distance to the corneal center (Fig. 23-27). In some cases, a central corneal opacity occurs at the tips of these radiating lines. Following are other corneal conditions causing radiating lines in the corneal epithelium:

1. Fabry's disease
2. Toxicity to chloroquine phosphate and related drugs
3. Indomethacin toxicity
4. Healing erosions
5. Melkersson-Rosenthal syndrome
6. Striate melanokeratosis
7. Aminodarone toxicity
8. Chlorpromazine toxicity
9. Clofazimine toxicity

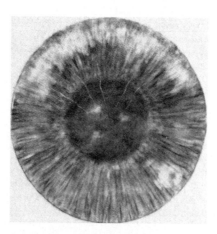

Fig. 23-27. Corneal lesions seen in some cases of acrodermatitis enteropathica are radiating, linear, white to light-brown, slightly whorllike opacities passing from limbus to about two thirds of distance to corneal center. (From Matta, C.S., Felker, G.V., Ide, C.H.: Arch. Ophthalmol. **93:**140; copyright 1975, American Medical Association.)

Management

Diiodohydroxyquin (Diodoquin) and zinc sulfate have been used to great advantage in treating acrodermatitis enteropathica; a daily regimen of 250 mg of zinc sulfate is most adequate.[11,40] Dandelions are known to be a source of zinc; as a result, the patient responds to the diet supplemented with dandelion.

CUTIS VERTICIS GYRATA (ROSENTHAL-KLOEPFER SYNDROME)[66]

The skin and periosteum are thick. The skin is thrown into convoluted folds, especially on the scalp. There is an acromegaloid habitus. The disease is transmitted as an autosomal dominant trait.

These findings plus the corneal leukomas that have been reported by Rosenthal and Kloepfer[66] constitute this syndrome. The condition occurred in a black family, wherein 13 persons in three generations were affected.

MALIGNANT ATROPHIC PAPULOSIS OF DEGOS[41]

Malignant atrophic papulosis is a rare systemic disease that exhibits vaso-occlusive disorders of unknown origin. The initial sign of the disease is a pathognomonic cutaneous lesion. The lesion varies from a small pink papule with crusting to a well-developed papule with an atrophic, porcelain-white center covered with thin white scales (Fig. 23-28). The lesions sometimes demonstrate pink telangiectatic borders. They develop through various stages from tiny, erythematous papules to those of fine scarring.[55]

Symptoms of abdominal pain are seen; the gastrointestinal involvement, which may rarely precede skin lesions, may result in bowel perforation, peritonitis, and death. A

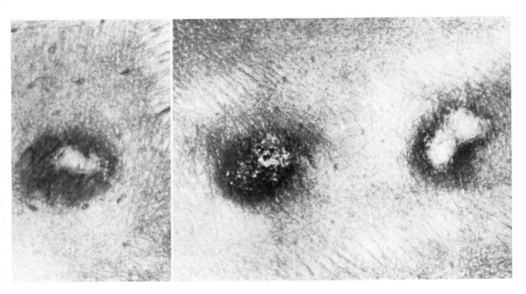

Fig. 23-28. Skin lesions with atrophic porcelain white centers are characteristic of malignant atrophic papulosis. (From Howsden, S.M., Hodge, S.J., Herndon, J.H., et al.: Arch. Dermatol. **112:** 1582; copyright 1976, American Medical Association.)

number of organ systems are involved and show similar vascular lesions that have been described as an obliterating arteriolitis or endovascularitis with secondary thrombosis and slow tissue necrosis.

Ocular involvement

Weakness of conjugate gaze and diplopia are frequently seen.

Conjunctival lesions, which can occur near the limbus, may be mistaken for a Bitot spot.

MELKERSSON-ROSENTHAL SYNDROME

This syndrome consists of recurrent swelling of the lip or the face, intermittent facial nerve paralysis, and furrowed tongue. Hodgkin's disease has been found in some patients.[56]

Ocular involvement

The corneal lesions are interesting in that they consist of thickening and opacification in Bowman's membrane. On retroillumination, the lesions correspond to a dense, central horizontal core with graceful swirling rods in the nature of horse hair (Fig. 23-29). The corneal epithelium may exhibit a diffuse punctate keratopathy in the interpalpebral fissure with focal thickening and opacification adjacent to the areas of opaque Bowman's layer. In addition, keratoconjunctivitis sicca occurs.

INCONTINENTIA PIGMENTI

Incontinentia pigmenti is a hereditary disorder of the skin that exhibits central nervous system involvement and ocular, dental, and skeletal alterations. It is more common in the female and lethal in the male. It is transmitted as an autosomal dominant or sex-linked trait.

Skin lesions, which are bullous in nature, are seen congenitally or at the end of the

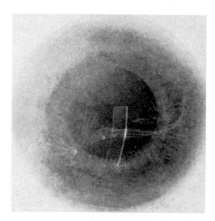

Fig. 23-29. Corneal lesions in Melkersson-Rosenthal syndrome show graceful swirling lines. (From Mulvihill, J.J., Echman, W.W., Fraumeni, J.F., Jr., Dryden, R.M., and Young, R.C.: Arch. Intern. Med. **132:**116; copyright 1973, American Medical Association.)

first week of life. They may, however, rarely be seen after the second month. Small, red nodules appear on the limbs, followed by warty lesions on the hands, feet, and toes. Pigmentation develops so that these areas of verrucous and hypertrophic change are followed by pigmented patches, striae, whorls, maculae, and atrophic skin areas (Fig. 23-30).

The Block-Sulzberger type of incontinentia pigmenti affects almost exclusively females and manifests the cutaneous pigmentation without other abnormalities.

The Naegeli type affects both sexes, is not congenital, and appears at about 2 years of age. The associated systemic disorders are central nervous system, skeletal, and dental changes, as well as ocular defects. In some instances, one may find a pheochromocytoma.[19] Other defects include abnormalities of the nails and patchy alopecia.

Ocular involvement

Ocular involvement has been seen with atrophy of the globe, retinal dysplasia,[85] pseudoglioma, optic atrophy, papillitis,[48] cataracts, and strabismus. Pigmentation of the conjunctiva and retina have also occurred.[54]

The cornea may be opaque as a result of developmental changes; interstitial keratitis can occasionally be found.

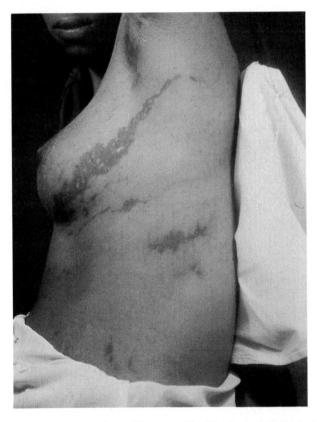

Fig. 23-30. Pigmented, whorllike striae and hypertrophic skin changes are typical of incontinentia pigmenti.

XERODERMA PIGMENTOSUM

Xeroderma pigmentosum is a recessive hereditary disorder associated with intolerance of the skin and eyes to light. Persistent erythema, pigmentation, scarring, and premature aging of the skin occur. Epithelial neoplasms and melanomas are often seen as part of the disease process. The disease is not often seen in blacks, but reports of a black family have been noted in the literature.[3]

There is a defective repair replication of DNA.[12,13,61] Normal skin fibroblasts are able to repair ultraviolet radiation damage to DNA by inserting new bases into DNA; fibroblasts obtained from patients with xeroderma pigmentosum show a much-reduced or absent repair replication of DNA in comparison to normal fibroblasts.[58] The diagnosis may be made prenatally.[61]

The skin is erythematous and pigmented, atrophic, telangiectatic, and neoplastic (Fig. 23-31). Before the second year of life, persistent erythema of the exposed areas of the face, neck, and arms is seen.

Progression occurs with the appearance of pigmented freckles, which become dark and coalesce. The skin atrophies, and telangiectasia and neoplastic degeneration occur. The process reaches its height at about 7 to 8 years of age. The malignant changes have a predilection for the circumoral and circumorbital areas.

Nervous system changes may be seen, such as mental deficiency, epilepsy, spastic paralysis, and deafness. Hypogonadism has also been noted.

Ocular involvement

Most patients with xeroderma pigmentosum have blepharospasm, and conjunctivitis is common. The conjunctivae are dry and hyperemic. Telangiectasia and pigmented

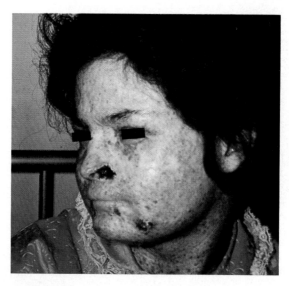

Fig. 23-31. Xeroderma pigmentosum with corneal vascularization and squamous and basal cell carcinomas of skin. (Courtesy D. Paton, M.D., Houston, Tex.)

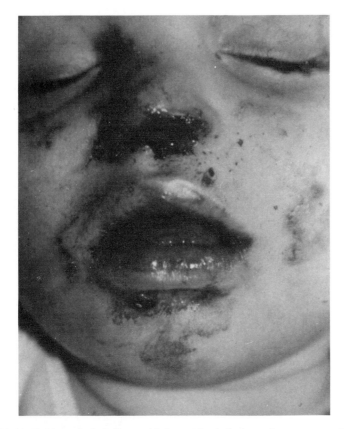

Fig. 23-32. Epidermolysis bullosa with hemorrhagic lesions of mucous membranes.

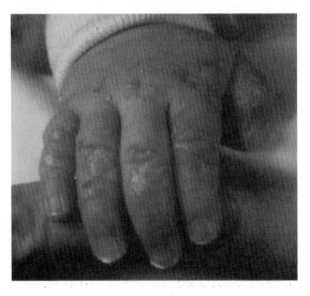

Fig. 23-33. Typical bullous lesions of hand in epidermolysis bullosa.

lesions occur on the bulbar conjunctiva. Symblepharons result from repeated incidences of inflammation. Atrophy of the lids with loss of cilia and ectropion and entropion are not uncommon (Fig. 23-31) and will result in conjunctival and corneal exposure lesions.[63]

The cornea shows an extensive vascularization and opacification in advanced cases (Fig. 23-31). Secondary corneal ulceration may occur. Malignant neoplasms frequently develop in the corneal limbal area.

ACANTHOSIS NIGRICANS[8]

This rare condition is manifested by pigmented, papillomatous, hyperkeratotic lesions of the oral mucosa, face, neck, groin, axillae, and periumbilical area. Acanthosis nigricans is distributed equally between males and females and may occur at any age.

The benign form of acanthosis nigricans may be present at birth and is transmitted as an autosomal dominant trait. A secondary form of this disease is known as *pseudoacanthosis nigricans* and occurs in association with endocrine disorders. The malignant form usually occurs when the person is over 20 years of age. No heredity has been established. Usually the malignant type is associated with adenocarcinomas of the gastrointestinal tract.

Coloration of the skin results from hyperkeratosis and not from melanosis. Out of 90 patients studied, mucosal involvement occurred only in individuals who had the malignant type of acanthosis nigricans. A third of them had mucosal disease, but the conjunctiva was not involved in any of the cases.

Ocular involvement

Corneal and conjunctival lid changes have been reported in the benign form of acanthosis nigricans.[47] In this particular instance the lids of both eyes were thick and pigmented, and the conjunctiva appeared clinically to be nonpigmented. Hypertrophic changes have been seen in very few cases in the palpebral conjunctiva.[57]

The cornea can become involved with infiltration and vascularization. The pathologic condition may become so advanced that a central perforation can occur. The conjunctiva can reveal marked epithelial hypertrophy, with hyperkeratosis and some melanin deposition in the basal corneal layer.

EPIDERMOLYSIS BULLOSA DYSTROPHICA[49]

Epidermolysis bullosa refers to a group of skin and mucous membrane diseases characterized by the formation of bullous lesions (Figs. 23-32 and 23-33). Dystrophic nail problems also occur (Fig. 23-34). Table 23-2[28,35] demonstrates the classification and mode of inheritance of this disease group. It is seen that nearly all forms of epidermolysis bullosa can in one way or another cause some eye changes.

The symptoms appear after birth or in early childhood and have a tendency to recur during the patient's life. Males and females are equally affected. Patients with epidermolysis bullosa dystrophica tend to develop epidermal neoplasms: usually low-grade squamous cell carcinoma of the skin and, less commonly, that of the mouth.[62]

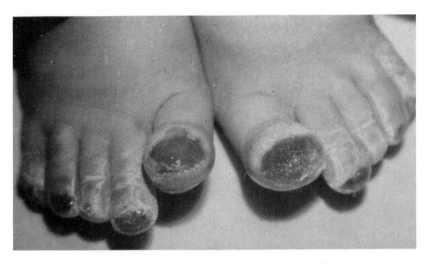

Fig. 23-34. Dystrophic nails in epidermolysis bullosa.

Table 23-2. Epidermolysis bullosa

Type	Mode of inheritance	Ophthalmic involvement
Non scarring		
Epidermolysis bullosa simplex (EBS)	Dominant	Bilateral and peripheral small cystic lesion at depth of epithelial basal cell layer; rupture of bullae
Recurrent bullous eruption of hands and feet (Cockayne's disease) (RBEHF)	Dominant	Mucosa not involved
Junctional bullous epidermolysis (Herliz disease) or epidermolysis bullosa letalis (JBE)	Recessive	Severe form with mucosal involvement; conjunctival disease and corneal disease; edematous changes in the cornea; also involvement of the uvea, pigment epithelium, lens, and optic nerve can be seen
Scarring		
Dystrophic hyperplastic (DBD-D)	Dominant	Granular clouding in the epithelium, erosive keratopathy, bullous keratopathy, corneal ulcers, opacification, and perforation; similar scleral involvement; cicatrization and drying, symblepharons also noted
Dystrophic polydysplasia (DBD-R)	Recessive	

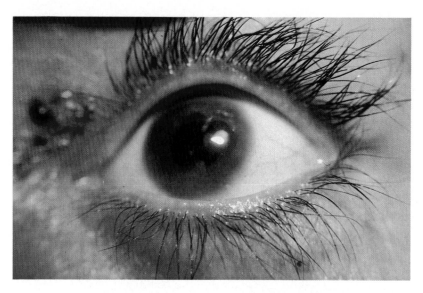

Fig. 23-35. Corneal involvement in epidermolysis bullosa.

Ocular involvement

The conjunctival involvement in epidermolysis bullosa most often occurs with pseudomembrane and vesicle formation. Ulceration and symblepharon formation are not unusual.[74]

Corneal involvement with epithelial erosion may lead to vascularization and opacification of the epithelium and Bowman's layer[1] (Fig. 23-35).

HYDROA VACCINIFORME

This condition results from a congenitally abnormal sensitivity to sunlight. The skin is involved with papulovesicular lesions. Since the face and eyelids are the areas of exposure, they are primarily involved (Fig. 23-36).

A hypertrophic conjunctivitis may occur. Conjunctival epithelial thickening and cyst formation are seen. The conjunctiva may also be hyperemic and may exhibit vesicles, ulceration, and scarring. These findings contribute to the photophobia.

Scarring and vascularization of the cornea may also occur.

The necrotizing and cicatrizing type of hydroa vacciniforme occurs with congenital porphyria.

DERMATITIS HERPETIFORMIS

This condition is an inflammatory dermatosis with erythematous, papillary, vesicular or pustular lesions occurring in groups and in polymorphic distribution accompanied by intense itching. The patient is in good health. However, blood eosinophilia may be seen.

Jejunal enteropathy may accompany this disease. Dermatitis herpetiformis may be

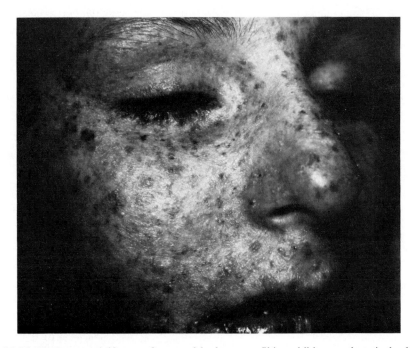

Fig. 23-36. Hydroa vacciniforme of exposed body areas. Skin exhibits papulovesicular lesions.

Table 23-3. Skin diseases with corneal findings that may show systemic malignant disease

Skin disease	Systemic malignant disease
Consistent findings of malignancy	
Acanthosis nigricans	Gastrointestinal cancer
Pachydermoperiostosis	Respiratory malignancy
Acquired ichthyosis	Lymphomatous
Palmar and plantar keratosis	Esophageal cancer
Less consistent findings of malignancy	
Dermatitis herpetiformis	Lymphomatous disease
Herpes zoster	Lymphomatous disease
Scleroderma	Lymphomatous disease
Erythema multiforme	Lymphomatous disease
Epidermolysis bullosa dystrophica	Squamous cell carcinoma of skin and mucous membranes
Xeroderma pigmentosum	Squamous cell carcinoma
Ectodermal dysplasia	Melanoma
	No systemic disease

confused with erythema multiforme and pemphigoid, but bullae are not present in dermatitis herpetiformis, which is characterized by small, tense vesicles whose size does not exceed 5 mm. Also, mucous membrane lesions are not seen in dermatitis herpetiformis but commonly occur in erythema multiforme and pemphigoid.

Eye involvement in dermatitis herpetiformis is not very common, but shrinkage of the conjunctiva as seen in mucous membrane pemphigoid may be noted. Conjunctival eosinophilia may occur.

SYSTEMIC MALIGNANT DISEASES

A number of the dermatologic conditions associated with corneal disease that have been described may be associated with malignant processes and are listed in Table 23-3.

REFERENCES

1. Aurora, A., Madhavan, M., and Rao, S.: Ocular changes in epidermolysis bullosis letalis, Am. J. Ophthalmol. **79:**464, 1975.
2. Baden, H.P., and Alper, J.C.: Ichthyosiform dermatosis, keratitis, and deafness, Arch. Dermatol. **113:**1701, 1977.
3. Bellows, R.A., Lahav, M., Lepreau, F.J., Deschapelle (Haiti), and Albert, D.M.: Ocular manifestations of xeroderma pigmentosum in a black family, Arch. Ophthalmol. **92:**113, 1974.
4. Bienfang, D.C., Kuwabara, T., and Pueschel, S.M.: Richner-Hanhart syndrome: report of a case associated with tyrosinemia, Arch. Ophthalmol. **94:**1133, 1976.
5. Black, R.L., O'Brien, W.M., Van Scott, E.J., et al.: Methotrexate therapy in psoriatic arthritis: double-blind study on 21 patients, JAMA **189:**743, 1964.
6. Blackman, H.J., Rodrigues, M.M., and Peck, G.L.: Corneal epithelial lesions in keratosis follicularis (Darier's disease), Ophthalmology **87:**941, 1980.
7. Britton, H., Lustig, J., Thompson, B.J., et al.: Keratosis follicularis spinulosa decalvans: an infant with failure to thrive, deafness and recurrent infections, Arch. Dermatol. **114:**761, 1978.
8. Brown, J., and Winkelmann, R.: Acanthosis nigricans: a study of 90 cases, Medicine **47:**33, 1968.
9. Buist, N.R.M., Kennaway, N.G., and Fellman, J.H.: Disorders of tyrosine metabolism. In Nyhan, W.L., editor: Heritable disorders of amino acid metabolism, New York, 1974, John Wiley & Sons, Inc.
10. Burns, R.P.: Soluble tyrosine aminotransferase deficiency: an unusual cause of corneal ulcers, Am. J. Ophthalmol. **73:**400, 1972.
11. Campo, A.G., and McDonald, C.J.: Treatment of acrodermatitis enterpathica with zinc sulfate, Arch. Dermatol. **112:**687, 1976.
12. Cleaver, J.E.: Defective repair replication of DNA in xeroderma pigmentosum, Nature **218:**652, 1968.
13. Cleaver, J.E.: DNA damage and repair in light sensitive human skin disease, J. Invest. Dermatol. **54:**181, 1970.
14. Dellon, A.L., Peck, G.L., and Chretien, P.B.: Hypopharyngeal and laryngeal involvement of Darier disease, Arch. Dermatol. **111:**744, 1975.
15. Diasio, F.: Pachyonychia congenita Jadassohn: variety of ichthyosis (pachyonychia ichthyosiformis) involving chiefly the nails, Arch. Dermatol. Syph. **30:**218, 1934.
16. Ellison, D.J., and Pugh, D.W.: Werner's syndrome, Br. Med. J. **2:**237, 1955.
17. Falls, H.F.: Poikiloderma congenitale, Trans. Am. Ophthalmol. Soc. **54:**308, 1956.
18. Fellman, J.H., Vanbellinghen, P.J., Jones, R.T., et al.: Soluble and mitochondrial forms of tyrosine aminotransferase: relationship to human tyrosinemia, Biochemistry **8:**615, 1969.
19. Fischbein, F., Schub, M., and Lesko, W.: Incontinentia pigmenti, pheochromocytoma and ocular abnormalities, Am. J. Ophthalmol. **73:**961, 1972.
20. Forgács, J., and Franceschetti, A.: Histologic aspect of corneal changes due to hereditary metabolic and cutaneous affections, Am. J. Ophthalmol. **47:**191, 1959.
21. Franceschetti, A.: Les dysplasies ectodermiques et les syndromes héréditaires apparentés, Dermatologica **106:**129, 1953.
22. Franceschetti, A.: Hereditary skin disease (genodermatosis) and corneal affections. In Beard, C., Falls, H.F., Franceschetti, A., et al., editors: Symposium on surgical and medical management of congenital anomalies of the eye, St. Louis, 1968, The C.V. Mosby Co.
23. Franceschetti, A., and Maeder, G.: Dystrophie profonde de la cornée dans un cas d'ichtyose congénitale, Bull. Mem. Soc. Fr. Ophtalmol. **67:**146, 1954.

24. Franceschetti, A., and Schlaeppe, V.: Dégénérescence en bandelette et dystrophie, prédescemétique de la cornée dans un cas d'ichtyose congénitale, Dermatologica 115:217, 1957.
25. Franceschetti, A., and Thiel, C.J.: Ueber Hornhautdystrophien bei Genodermatoser unter besonderer Berücksichtigung der Palmoplantarkeratosen, Albrecht von Graefes Arch. Klin. Ophthalmol. 162:610, 1961.
26. François, J.: Skin diseases. In Heredity in ophthalmology, St. Louis, 1961, The C.V. Mosby Co.
27. Friedman, B.: Corneal findings in ichthyosis, Am. J. Ophthalmol. 39:575, 1955.
28. Geddle, D.T., Jr.: Epidermolysis bullosa: a clinical, genetic and epidermiological study, Baltimore, 1971, The Johns Hopkins University Press.
29. Gilbert, W., and Smith, J.L.: Sjögren-Larssen syndrome, Arch. Ophthalmol. 80:308, 1968.
30. Ginsburg, R., Robertson, A., Jr., and Michel, B.: Acrodermatitis enteropathica: abnormalities of fat metabolism and integumental ultrastructures in infants, Arch. Dermatol. 112:653, 1976.
31. Gipson, I.K., Burns, R.P., and Wolfe-Lande, J.D.: Crystals in corneal epithelial lesions of tyrosine fed rats, Invest. Ophthalmol. 14:937, 1975.
32. Goldsmith, L.A.: Hemolysis and lysosomal activation by solid-state tyrosine, Biochem. Biophys. Res. Commun. 64:558, 1975.
33. Goldsmith, L.A., Kang, E., and Bienfang, D.C., et al.: Tyrosinemia with plantar and palmar keratosis and keratitis, J. Pediatr. 83:798, 1973.
34. Goldsmith, L.A., and Reed, J.: Richner-Hanhart syndrome: a treatable genetic syndrome, JAMA 236:382, 1976.
35. Granek, H., and Baden, H.P.: Corneal involvement in epidermolysis bullosa simplex, Arch. Ophthalmol. 98:469, 1980.
36. Grayson, M.: Corneal manifestations of keratosis plantaris and palmaris, Am. J. Ophthalmol. 59:483, 1965.
37. Haim, S., and Munk, J.: Keratosis palmoplantaria congenita with peridontosis, arachnodactyly and a peculiar deformity of the terminal phalanges, Br. J. Dermatol. 77:42, 1965.
38. Hanhart, E.: Neue Sonderformen von Keratosis palmoplantaris, u. a. eine regelmässig-dominante mit systematisierten Lipomen, ferner 2 einfachrezessive mit Schwachsinn und z. T. mit Hornhautveränderungen des Auges (Ektodermalsyndrom), Dermatologica 94:286, 1947.
39. Helweg-Larsen, H.F., and Ludvigsen, K.: Congenital familial anhidrosis and neurolabyrinthitis, Acta Derm. Vener. 26:489, 1946.
40. Hirsch, F.S., Michel, B., and Strain, W.H.: Gluconate zinc in acrodermatitis enteropathica, Arch. Dermatol. 112:475, 1976.
41. Howsden, S.M., Hodge, S.J., Herndon, J.H., and Freeman, R.G.: Malignant atrophic papulosis of Degos: report of a patient who failed to respond to fibrinolytic therapy, Arch. Dermatol. 112:1582, 1976.
42. Ive, F.A., and De Saram, C.F.W.: Methotrexate and the citrovorum factor in treatment of psoriasis, Trans. St. John's Hosp. Dermatol. Soc. 56:45, 1970.
43. Jay, B., Black, R.K., and Wells, R.S.: Ocular manifestations of ichthyosis, Br. J. Ophthalmol. 52:217, 1968.
44. Jenkins, M.S., Brown, S.I., Lempert, S.L., and Weinberg, R.J.: Ocular rosacea, Am. J. Ophthalmol. 88:618, 1979.
45. Katowitz, J., Yolles, E., and Yanoff, M.: Ichthyosis congenita, Arch. Ophthalmol. 91:208, 1974.
46. Kleeberg, J.: Werner's syndrome, Acta. Med. Orient. 8:145, 1949.
47. Lamba, P., and Lal, S.: Ocular changes in benign acanthosis nigricans, Dermatologica 140:356, 1970.
48. Leib, W., and Guerry, D.: Fundus changes in incontinentia pigmenti, Am. J. Ophthalmol. 45:265, 1958.
49. Lemmengson, W.: Epidermolysis bullosa, Klin. Monatsbl. Augenheilkd. 122:350, 1953.
50. Lynch, W.S., and Roenigk, H.H.: Acrodermatitis enteropathica, Arch. Dermatol. 112:1304, 1976.
51. Maeder, G.: Le syndrome de Rothmund et le syndrome de Werner (étude clinique et diagnostique), Ann. Ocul. 182:809, 1949.
52. Marshall, D.: Ectodermal dysplasia: report of a kindred with ocular abnormalities and hearing defect, Am. J. Ophthalmol. 45:143, 1958.
53. Matta, C.S., Felker, G.V., and Ide, C.H.: Eye manifestations in acrodermatitis enteropathica, Arch. Ophthalmol. 93:140, 1975.
54. McCrary, J., and Smith, J.L.: Conjunctival and retinal incontinentia pigmenti, Arch. Ophthalmol. 79:417, 1968.
55. Muller, S.A., and Landry, M.: Malignant atrophic papulosis (Degos disease): a report of two cases with clinical and histological studies, Arch. Dermatol. 112:357, 1976.
56. Mulvihill, J.J., Eckman, W.W., Fraumeni, J.F., Dryden, R.M., and Young, R.C.: Melkersson-Rosenthal syndrome, Hodgkin disease, and corneal keratopathy, Arch. Intern. Med. 132:116, 1973.
57. Newman, G., and Carsten, M.: Acanthosis nigricans: conjunctival and lid lesions, Arch. Ophthalmol. 90:259, 1973.
58. Newsome, D.A., Kraemer, K.H., and Robbins, J.H.: Repair of DNA in xeroderma pigmentosum conjunctiva, Arch. Ophthalmol. 93:660, 1975.

59. Oppenheimer, B.S., and Kugel, U.H.: Werner's syndrome: report of first necropsy and of findings in a new case, Am. J. Med. Soc. **202:**629, 1941.

60. Petrohelos, M.A.: Werner's syndrome: a survey of 3 cases with review of the literature, Am. J. Ophthalmol. **56:**941, 1956.

61. Ramsay, C.A., Coltart, T.M., Blunt, S., et al.: Prenatal diagnosis of xeroderma pigmentosum: report of the first successful case, Lancet **2:**1109, 1974.

62. Reed, W.B., Collega, J., Francis, M.J.O., et al.: Epidermolysis bullosa dystrophica with epidermal neoplasms, Arch. Dermatol. **110:**894, 1974.

63. Reese, A., and Wilber, J.: The eye manifestations of xeroderma pigmentosum, Am. J. Ophthalmol. **26:**901, 1943.

64. Resh, W., and Stoughton, R.B.: Topically applied antibiotics in acne vulgaris, Arch. Dermatol. **112:**182, 1976.

65. Richner, H.: Hornhautaffektion bei Keratoma palmare et plantare hereditarium, Klin. Monatsbl. Augenheilkd. **100:**580, 1938.

66. Rosenthal, J.W., and Kloepfer, H.W.: An acromegaloid, cutis verticis gyrata, corneal leukoma syndrome: a new medical entity, Arch. Ophthalmol. **68:**772, 1962.

67. Rud, E.: Werner's syndrome in 3 siblings, Acta Ophthalmol. **34:**255, 1956.

68. Savin, L.H.: Corneal dystrophy associated with congenital ichthyosis and allergic manifestations in male members of a family, Br. J. Ophthalmol. **40:**82, 1956.

69. Schirren, C., Hoffman, D.H., Kunhan, J., et al.: Ektodermale Dysplasie mit Hypohidrosis und Hypodontie, Hautarzt **11:**70, 1960.

70. Sever, R.J., Frost, P., and Weinstein, G.: Eye changes in ichthyosis, JAMA **206:**2283, 1968.

71. Shindle, R., and Leone, C.: Cicatricial entropion associated with lamellar ichthyosis, Arch. Ophthalmol **89:**62, 1973.

72. Silver, H.K.: Rothmund-Thomson syndrome: an oculocutaneous disorder, Am. J. Dis. Child. **111:**182, 1966.

73. Skinner, B.A., Greist, M.C., and Norins, A.L.: The keratitis, ichythosis, and deafness (KID) syndrome, Arch. Dermatol. **117:**285, 1981.

74. Sorsby, A., Frazer-Roberts, J.A., and Bran, R.T.: Essential shrinking of the conjunctiva in a hereditary affection allied to epidermolysis bullosa, Doc. Ophthalmol. **5:**118, 1951.

75. Tan, S.G., and Cunliffe, W.J.: Rosacea and migraine, Br. Med. J. **1:**21, 1976.

76. Tessler, H.H., Apple, D.J., and Goldberg, M.F.: Ocular findings in a kindred with Kyrle disease: Hyperkeratosis follicularis et parafollicularis in cutem penetrans, Arch. Ophthalmol. **90:**278, 1973.

77. Vail, D.: Corneal involvement in congenital ichthyosis, Arch. Ophthalmol. **24:**215, 1940.

78. Valero, A., and Gellei, B.: Retinitis pigmentosa, hypertension and uremia in Werner's syndrome, Br. Med. J. **2:**351, 1960.

79. Vorrhus, J.J., Duell, E.A., Bass, L.J., et al.: Decreased cyclic AMP in the epidermis of lesions in psoriasis, Arch. Dermatol. **105:**695, 1972.

80. Warshawsky, R.S., Hill, C.W., Doughman, D.J., and Harris, J.E.: Acrodermatitis enteropathica, Arch. Ophthalmol. **93:**194, 1975.

81. Westmore, R., and Billson, F.A.: Pseudoherpetic keratitis, Br. J. Ophthalmol. **57:**654, 1973.

82. Whyte, H.J., and Baughman, R.D.: Acute guttata psoriasis and streptococcal infection, Arch. Dermatol. **89:**350, 1964.

83. Wilson, F.M., II, Grayson, M., and Pieroni, D.: Corneal changes in ectodermal dysplasia: case report, histopathology, and differential diagnosis, Am. J. Ophthalmol. **75:**17, 1973.

84. Wright, J.C.: Darier's disease, Am. J. Ophthalmol. **55:**134, 1963.

85. Zweifach, P.: Incontinentia pigmenti: its association with retinal dysplasia, Am. J. Ophthalmol. **62:**712, 1966.

ADDITIONAL READING

Baden, H.P., and Alper, J.C.: Ichthyosiform dermatosis, keratitis and deafness, Arch. Ophthalmol. **113:**1701, 1977.

Brown, S.I., and Shahinian, L., Jr.: Diagnosis and treatment of ocular rosacea, Am. Acad. Ophthalmol. Otolaryngol. **85:**779, 1978.

Cram, D.L., Resneck, J.S., and Jackson, W.B.: A congenital ichthyosiform syndrome with deafness and keratitis, Arch. Dermatol. **115:**467, 1979.

Dodd, M.J., Pusin, S.M., and Green, W.R.: Adult cystinosis, Arch. Ophthalmol. **96:**1054, 1978.

Reed, J.W., Cashwell, F.L., and Klintworth, G.K.: Corneal manifestations of hereditary intraepithelial dyskeratosis, Arch. Ophthalmol. **97:**297, 1979.

Silvestri, D.L.: Ichthyosiform dermatosis and deafness. Arch. Dermatol. **114:**1243, 1978.

24 Drugs, metals, and pigmentations

This chapter deals with the deposition of metals and drugs in the conjunctiva and the cornea. The lesions caused by these agents must be recognized, since in many instances their effects may aggravate the initial disease.

A discussion of pigmented lesions of the cornea and conjunctiva is also included in this section because so many of the metals and drug depositions are pigmented. Thus it is essential to differentiate and become aware of all possible problems resulting in pigment deposition.

METAL DEPOSITIONS
Gold

Gold can accumulate in the cornea after systemic administration of gold compounds.[22] This condition of gold deposition in the cornea is known as *ocular chrysiasis*. The deposition is often related to the total dose of gold and to the amount of drug injected weekly. The deposition in the cornea may disappear after gold therapy is discontinued.

Slit-lamp examination reveals that the corneal stroma contains fine, dustlike, gold to purple-violet[34] granules. The granules are not present in the epithelium or the endothelium but are seen in the deep stroma. On transillumination, the slit-lamp appearance of the cornea is purple. Some fine gold granules in the conjunctiva may also be seen.

A second type of corneal reaction is a severe one, consisting of marginal ulcera-

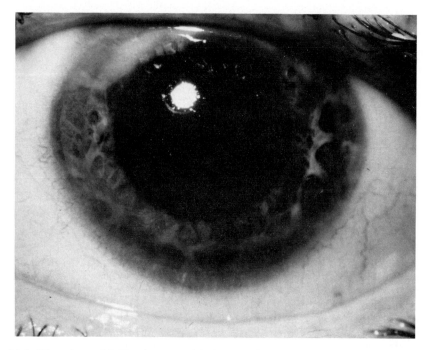

Fig. 24-1. Ulcerative and infiltrative corneal lesion seen in gold therapy for rheumatoid arthritis.

tive keratitis (Fig. 24-1) and iritis, caused by an allergy to the gold.[35] The ulcerative keratitis is seen as a white, crescent-shaped ulcer bordering the limbus and associated with conjunctival hyperemia, pain, and no evidence of bacterial infection. In addition to the ulcerative keratitis, one may see a corneal infiltration. The infiltration may start as a flat, distinct, superficial white opacity at one side of the cornea, with no line of normal cornea between the opacity and the scleral limbus. The white ulceration and infiltration tend to remain in the anterior layers of the cornea but spread from the periphery over the cornea and along the limbus.

If the gold treatment is stopped, the keratitis heals, but a vascularized area may remain. Penicillamine appears to be effective for the toxic reaction.

Mercury

Mercury toxicity causes changes in the lens and cornea.[19,27] Chronic absorption of mercury by people who work with this product can occur.

Mercurialentis consists of a rose-brown or pinkish homogeneous opacity that may involve the whole anterior surface of the lens but sometimes is entirely limited to an anterior subcapsular disc.[6] Not only is mercurialentis seen occupationally with chronic exposure to mercury vapor and mercury compounds, but it can occur as a result of chronic local application of medication containing mercurial compounds such as mercuric oxide and organic mercury preservatives such as phenylmercuric salts.

When phenylmercuric salts are employed as antimicrobial preservatives in eye drops,

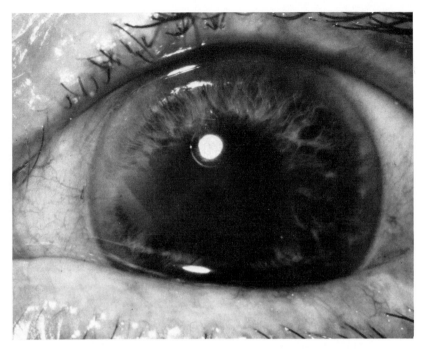

Fig. 24-2. Band keratopathy caused by phenylmercuric nitrate.

very low concentrations should be used so that they do not cause eye injury and are generally well tolerated. It appears that the phenylmercuric nitrate and acetate penetrate the eye readily and bind persistently to sulfhydryl groups in the lens. These actions occur more readily than with other mercurial antimicrobial preservatives such as thimerosal. In addition, thimerosal (Merthiolate) may cause a delayed hypersensitivity reaction in some patients who use it to sterilize soft contact lenses. In such patients lens storage in sterile, unit-dose, preservative-free saline with thermal disinfection should be instituted.[44]

Patients chronically exposed to metallic mercury vapor or the long-term use of medications containing the aforementioned preservatives can develop calcific band keratopathy (Fig. 24-2). In a few cases fine glistening particulate opacities have been seen located centrally in the corneal stroma with the periphery remaining clear.

Penicillamine has been reported to be effective in treatment of mercury poisoning.[25]

Copper[30]

Chalcosis is the term used for discoloration and impregnation of ocular tissue by copper, which is usually from intraocular foreign bodies. Pure copper tends to cause a violent purulent reaction that usually leads to panophthalmitis and loss of the eye. Alloy metals with high concentrations of copper tend to cause chalcosis.

Copper has an affinity for basement membranes, such as Descemet's, and the lens capsule. Bowman's layer may also be affected.

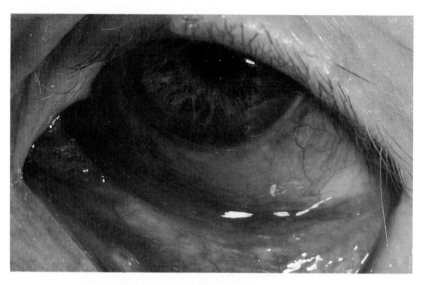

Fig. 24-3. Silver pigmentation of lids in argyrosis.

The discoloration of the eye in chalcosis from intraocular copper is noted in the iris, lens, vitreous, and cornea.[36] The iris is seen as a slightly greenish color; the vitreous, yellowish green-blue. Iridescent, multicolored reflection principally appears beneath the anterior lens capsule and may take on the form of a sunflower.[30]

In the cornea, discoloration from intraocular copper[36] is observed as a blue-green color between the endothelium and Descemet's membrane, perhaps more intensely in the peripheral areas.

The ERG has been shown to be a valuable means for detection of significant injury to the retina from intraocular copper as well as from iron. Once abnormalities in the ERG begin, vision is believed to be in serious danger unless the foreign body is removed or medical treatment such as penicillamine therapy is instituted. If the ERG is already abnormal, it is probably too late to expect benefit from surgical or medical treatment.

The deposition of copper in the cornea in systemic diseases such as Wilson's disease and in nonwilsonian hepatic disease has been described in Chapter 22.

Silver

Argyrosis occurs after long-term therapeutic use of silver-containing medications. In recent years, the nonuse of silver-containing medications has decreased the incidence of argyrosis. If argyrosis occurs at all today, it is a result of an industrial injury with exposure to organic salts of silver.

The chronic use of silver-containing medications may result in a slate-gray discoloration of the mucous membranes, including the conjunctiva. A slate-gray hue is also imparted to the skin, possibly including the eyelids (Fig. 24-3). The discoloration may also be seen in the nasolacrimal apparatus and the nails.[47]

Anterior subcapsular lens discoloration may also occur.[2]

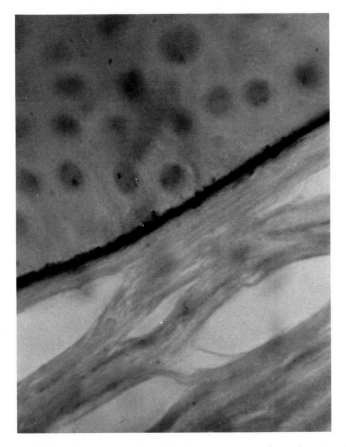

Fig. 24-4. Silver impregnation of epithelial basement membrane in argyrosis.

Histologically, the silver is deposited in loose collagenous fibrils of the subepithelial tissue and in basement membranes of the epithelium (Fig. 24-4) and endothelium. Thus a gray-blue-green or even golden sheen is imparted to Descemet's membrane (Fig. 24-5) and the deep corneal stroma.

Electron-microscopic examinations of the conjunctiva and cornea in ocular argyrosis have been studied.[21] The minute silver deposits were located intracellularly in the connective tissue of the conjunctiva and extracellularly in Descemet's membrane of the cornea.

Solutions of high concentrations of silver nitrate can result in opacification of the cornea that may be permanent.[20] However, in less severe instances, despite initial ground-glass or blue-gray appearance of the cornea from high concentrations of silver nitrate dropped into the eye, the cornea does have a tendency to clear spontaneously. Severe corneal injuries have been produced when solid silver nitrate was used to cauterize a chalazion or conjunctival lesion. The situation can be severe enough as a result of this cauterization so that dense opacification (Fig. 24-6) and cataract can occur. Histologic

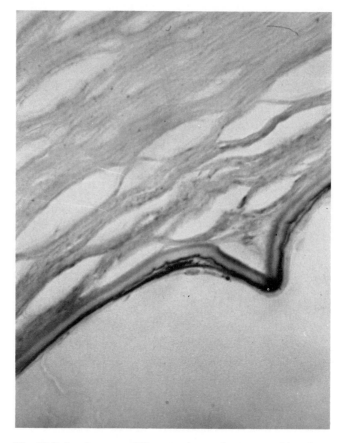

Fig. 24-5. Involvement of Descemet's membrane caused by silver.

examination will show silver present in the tissues 5 years after the injury.

A sterile solution containing 6% sodium thiosulfate and 0.25% potassium ferricyanide, prepared within 30 minutes of use, can be injected into the skin to solubilize and remove the dark deposits of silver. The solution can be injected subconjunctivally and has been observed to remove the gray discolorization of argyrosis without causing inflammation or injury. In the cornea, the solution has been observed to remove discoloration from the anterior layers of the stroma, but the treatment has not been observed to alter the discoloration in the deepest layers of the cornea. The argyrosis in the deeper layers of the cornea does not interfere with vision in any way.

Iron[11]

The impregnation of the tissues of the eye with iron such as that which may be derived from a foreign body is known as *siderosis*. The tissues surrounding the iron become a rust-brown color regardless of whether the iron is in the cornea, sclera, iris, vitreous, lens, or retina. Iron may then become transported in some soluble form to a more distant part of the eye, which discolors in a selected manner and is functionally disturbed in various ways.

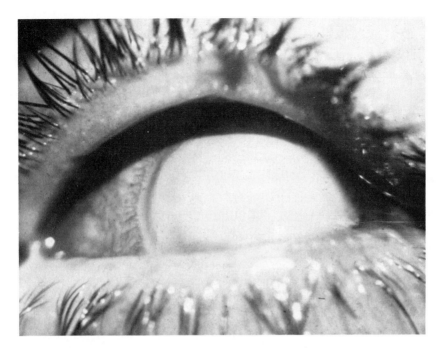

Fig. 24-6. Diffuse opacity of cornea resulting from concentrated silver solution.

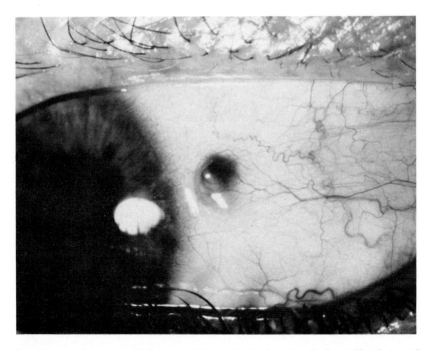

Fig. 24-7. Pigmented spot near limbus caused by retained subconjunctival metallic (ferrous) foreign body.

Iron particles in the cornea or sclera principally have local effects, and particles in the anterior chamber slowly form diffusible iron compounds that are washed away by the flow of aqueous and do not cause siderosis except in tissues in which they are in immediate contact. Metallic iron in the lens causes siderosis of the lens but may have little effect on the posterior portion of the eye. The most widespread and serious distribution of iron comes from particles in the posterior part of the globe and the vitreous or in the neighborhood of the ciliary body. The larger the particle and the less encapsulated it is, the more rapid the distribution of the siderosis.

Although seldom discolored by intraocular iron, the cornea can have a rust-brown color consisting of fine dots in the deepest layers. The cornea can show a granular staining of the keratocytes, and epithelial change can occur late. The corneal deposition is characteristic in that the granule will show an affinity for elastic tissue; as a result, Descemet's membrane and deep stroma may show a gray, dirty appearance that on oblique illumination appears greenish blue or golden. Encapsulation of an iron foreign body by organized hemorrhage may prevent development of siderosis; thus one sees great variability in the amount of siderosis produced by intraocular iron foreign bodies. A localized intracorneal iron foreign body may cause a localized brownish-red pigmentation of the cornea or conjunctiva (Fig. 24-7); however, if it is allowed to remain long and is large enough, the foreign body can cause a pigmentation of the cornea by spreading into the epithelium, stroma, and endothelium.[49] Many rust rings cause no trouble.

In siderosis discoloration of the iris occurs early, and the activity of the pupil is commonly affected, resulting in poor reaction to light and accommodation. The lens develops

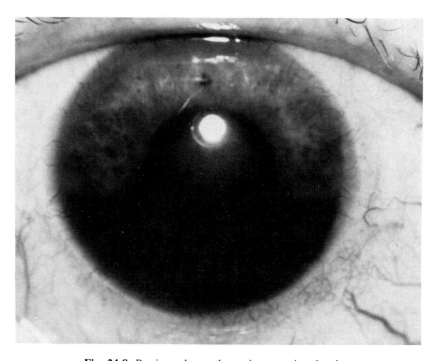

Fig. 24-8. Persistent hemorrhages into anterior chamber.

a special type of discoloration, either from a particle of iron embedded in the lens or from iron in the posterior segment without mechanical injury to the lens. Many fine brown dots may be seen by slitlamp examination immediately beneath the anterior capsule, each dot being a discolored epithelial cell. The vitreous becomes liquified and contains floating foreign bodies; glaucoma occurs in some cases of ocular siderosis. The retina shows change and alteration in the ERG. Ultimately, complete degeneration of the retina, atrophy of the optic nerve, and gliosis result.

After persistent hemorrhage in the anterior chamber (Fig. 24-8), the corneal endothelium may become affected, and siderin granules may be found in the corneal stromal cells, resulting in the so-called hematogenous pigmentation of the cornea (hemosiderosis)[11] (Fig. 24-9). Hemosiderosis occurs after intraocular hemorrhage with long persistence of iron-containing siderin or hemosiderin granules; the changes in the eye and the distribution of the iron have been found to be the same as in siderosis caused by intraocular metallic iron.

A bilateral circular pigmented line of the cornea is seen in hereditary spherocytosis (Dalgleisch's line). This line resembles the Hudson-Stähli line and other iron-containing subepithelial lines of the cornea[16] (Table 24-1).

Systemic hemochromatosis[10] does not usually involve the cornea, although it may involve the sclera, which is usually evident only histologically. Rusty discolorization anterior to the horizontal rectus muscles, however, has been seen. A localized corneal hemochromatosis consisting of a diffuse gray corneal haze of tiny dots or droplets in the anterior third of the cornea has been described.

Deferoxamine, a chelator of iron, has been used for treatment of siderosis.[14,41,46]

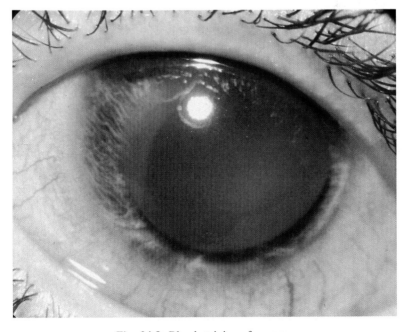

Fig. 24-9. Blood staining of cornea.

Deferoxamine has been given systemically and has reportedly resulted in some improvement. It may also be given as an application of 5% ointment in the eye. In the treatment of rust ring in the cornea, 5% solution and 10% ointment have been applied repeatedly to the surface of the eye in patients without evidence of adverse effects.[15] The rust ring may be removed with a foreign body spud at the slit lamp or with an appropriate electric drill.[5]

Table 24-1. Corneal deposits

Deposition	Color	Location	Pattern
Systemic drugs and metals			
Phenothiazines	Yellow	Deep stroma	Deep ones are diffuse
	Gray-brown	Endothelium Epithelium	Superficial deposits are linear and spiral
Chloroquine	Gray-white Brown	Deep epithelium Superficial stroma	Vortex or whorllike occasional clumps
Clofazimine	Brown	Epithelium	Fine brown lines
Indomethacin	Gray-brown	Deep in epithelium Superficial stroma	Vortex or whorllike
Aminodarone	Yellow-brown	Epithelium	Whorllike pattern
Epinephrine	Black-brown	Between epithelium and Bowman's layer	No pattern
Copper	Brown-green-red	Peripheral Posterior half of Descemet's membrane	Kayser-Fleischer ring
Silver	Gray-blue-green or golden	Descemet's membrane Deep stroma	Diffuse
Pigment lines			
Systemic problems			
Localized hemochromatosis	Gray corneal haze	Anterior third of stroma	Diffuse distribution of dots
Systemic hemochromatosis	—	No corneal involvement	—
Hereditary spherocytosis (Dalgleisch's line)	Brown	Subepithelium	Linear
Local problems			
Coat's white ring	White	Epithelium	Small circular pattern
Hudson-Stähli line	Brown	Epithelium	Linear
Fleischer's ring	Brown	Epithelium	Base of cone in keratoconus
Stocker's line	Brown	Epithelium	Linear curve in front of pterygium
Ferry's line	Brown	Epithelium	Linear in front of filtering bleb
Blood staining	Yellow-brown-red	Breakdown products of erythrocytes and hemosiderin between corneal lamellae, keratocytes, and in Bowman's layer	Diffuse

DRUG DEPOSITIONS

Chlorpromazine

This drug is one of the phenothiazines, which are used for treatment of mental illness.

Chlorpromazine is often employed in high doses (300 to 1500 mg daily) for long periods of time (1 to 5 years) in treating psychiatric patients. Generalized toxic effects, which can be serious, should be looked for and include such problems as diseases of the liver, nervous system involvement such as extrapyramidal affections, and blood dysplasias. The skin, especially areas exposed to light, may also show a purplish discoloration similar to that seen in the conjunctiva and cornea.[28]

The cornea is less often affected than the lens and demonstrates very fine granules within the deepest layers of the stroma next to Descemet's membrane and endothelium. The granules are yellow-brown-white dots similar to those seen beneath the anterior lens capsule.[29] They tend to occupy the interpalpebral fissure area and are accompanied by similar granules in the palpebral fissure area of the conjunctiva. In the cornea, in addition to fine granular deposits deep in the stroma, one may see pigmented streaks or lines located in the corneal epithelium in the palpebral fissure[23] (Fig. 24-10). These epithelial changes have been observed in patients who have received very large doses of chlorpromazine. The changes, however, will subside with discontinuance of the drug.

The distribution in the palpebral fissure area of the cornea and conjunctiva and the association in some patients with photosensitization of the skin suggests that exposure to light may be a factor in producing these deposits.

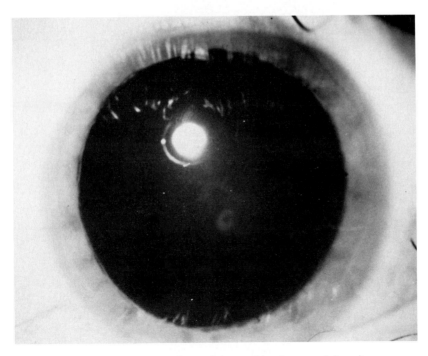

Fig. 24-10. Chlorpromazine toxicity resulting in corneal deposits.

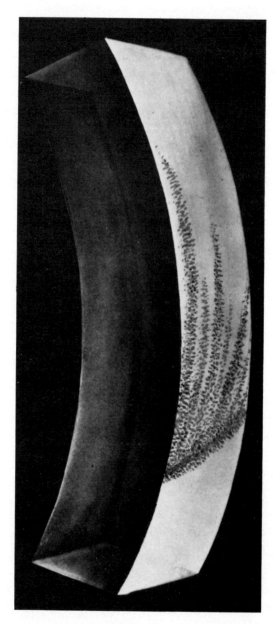

Fig. 24-11. Chloroquine toxicity resulting in whorllike corneal deposits in epithelium.

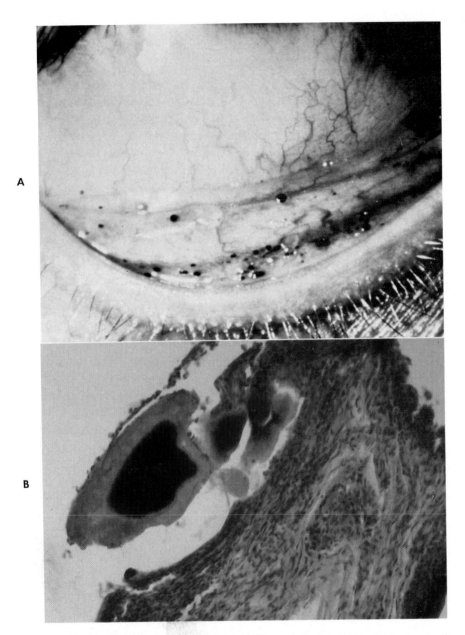

Fig. 24-12. A, Dark deposits in conjunctiva resembling melanin are result of chronic use of eye drops containing epinephrine. **B,** Histologic appearance of conjunctival adrenochrome, with solid, homogeneous black aggregate. (From Wilson, F.M., II: Surv. Ophthalmol. **24:**57, 1979.)

Chloroquine and related medications

Chloroquine diphosphate (Aralen Diphosphate) and hydroxychloroquine sulfate (Plaquenil) are quinoline derivatives used as antimalarials and in treating lupus erythematosus and several other systemic diseases. Chronic administration of chloroquine can produce deposits in the cornea that are seen with the biomicroscope; however, a serious retinopathy can develop, which may result in deprivation of vision.

Corneal deposits from chronic oral use of chloroquine occur and consist of many fine yellowish or white dots in the epithelium, particularly in the palpebral fissure area, and arranged in patterns of curved lines forming a whorllike or vortex figure[4,8,9,26] (Fig. 24-11). The deposits usually do not disturb the surface of the epithelium. Corneal deposits can be seen in individuals who work in industries manufacturing chloroquine; the changes are analogous to the changes in the cornea of individuals exposed to large quantities of quinacrine hydrochloride (Atabrine, mepacrine hydrochloride). The corneal deposits do not harm and disappear after the medication is discontinued or if the dose is reduced. They are not considered a contraindication to continued use of the drug. Development of the deposits in the cornea have no known relationship to the occurrence of retinopathy; one apparently develops entirely independently of the other. The deposits seem to be similar to those produced by quinacrine hydrochloride and hydroxychloroquine. Deposits may be present in the skin, and the hair may whiten.

The most serious complication that may occur is involvement of the retina; the dose of chloroquine appears to be the most fundamentally important factor determining the development of retinopathy.[8,24] Retinal involvement appears as serious retinopathy in almost all instances that have been caused by taking more than 250 mg of chloroquine to a total amount greater than 100 g.

When retinopathy is recognized early and chloroquine is discontinued, in most cases the vision that has been lost is not recovered; however, in a small portion of cases there has been significant recovery. In a particularly unfortunate small portion, loss of vision has been progressive despite discontinuance of the drug.

Quinacrine hydrochloride is used in treatment of malaria and rheumatoid arthritis as well as lupus erythematosus. Yellow discolorization of the cornea and sclera and complaint of seeing yellow, green, or violet, presumably because of changes in the cornea, can be seen. Yellow-brown particles in the corneal epithelium may cause the patient to see blue halos or multicolored rings around lights.

Indomethacin[7]

This drug is an anti-inflammatory, antipyretic agent used particularly in the treatment of arthritis. Fine, speckled opacities in the epithelium and anterior stroma resembling chloroquine keratopathy have been reported, but these disappeared when the medication was stopped. The true nature of the deposits has not been determined.

In addition to the corneal problems, retinopathy and pallor of the optic disc have been reported; however these findings are not believed to be true effects of the medication.

Epinephrine

Dark deposits in the conjunctiva and cornea are produced by chronic use of epinephrine drops[32] (Fig. 24-12). These consist of melanin-like oxidation products of epinephrine accumulated in the conjunctival cysts and sometimes on the cornea. These deposits are innocuous and require no treatment.

Corneal discoloration, seemingly by the same material that accumulates in the conjunctival cysts, develops as dark deposits in the cornea. The discolored cornea appears brown or black, apparently depending on the amount of pigment. This accumulation has been mistaken for a malignant melanoma. Obstruction of nasal lacrimal ducts by the accumulation of oxidation products of epinephrine can occur.[40]

Mascara may cause a black pigmentation at the superior border of the upper tarsus. These deposits may be mistaken for adrenochromes.

Clofazimine[43]

Clofazimine is a phenazine derivative that is active against mycobacteria. It has been used for leprosy treatment and recently for treatment of psoriasis. Clofazimine can cause red-brown discoloration of the skin and pigmentation of the conjunctiva and cornea. Fine brown lines similar to those of chloroquine keratopathy were observed in psoriatic patients given clofazimine. The changes are reversible.

Aminodarone

This drug,[1,45] a coronary dilator benzofuran derivative, has been reported to produce deposits in the epithelium of the cornea similar to those produced by chloroquine. The deposits are yellowish-brown and take on a whorllike figure. No aftereffects occur, and the deposits disappear after the drug is discontinued.

Table 24-1 summarizes the condition of corneal deposits as to color of deposit, location, and pattern.

PIGMENTED LESIONS

The melanocytes in the conjunctiva are analogous to those of the epidermis.[48] They are located within the basal layer of the epithelial cells and have delicate branching and dendritic processes that contain little or no pigment. Even when stimulated to produce excess amounts of melanin, the melanocytes typically secrete the pigment into the adjacent epithelial or underlying stromal cells. Therefore the melanin, which is responsible for limbal pigmentation as observed in many blacks, is found in the epithelial cells rather than in the melanocytes that produce the pigment.

The conjunctival melanocyte is derived, most agree, from the neural crest cells. In histologic sections stained with hematoxylin and eosin, conjunctival melanocytes are solitary dendritic cells with clear cytoplasm. The cells vary in size, number, and melanin content, as well as by race. Although the melanocytes never undergo reactive proliferation, they may undergo neoplastic change. In addition, pigmented cells in the conjunctiva may come from the basal cell or a melanocytic nevus.

The following list of conditions involving pigmentation of the cornea, limbus, and neighboring conjunctiva, as well as related conditions, is useful in differential diagnosis of pigmented lesions:

A. Benign pigmented lesions, congenital
B. Congenital melanosis oculi
C. Congenital oculodermal melanocytosis (nevus of Ota)

D. Benign conjunctival nevus
   1. Junctional
   2. Subepithelial
   3. Compound
E. Acquired melanosis
   1. Stage I: benign
      a. With minimal junctional activity
      b. With marked junctional activity
   2. Stage II: cancerous
      a. With minimal invasion
      b. With marked invasion
   3. Melanocytoma[42]
F. Secondary pigmentation
   1. Chronic conjunctival disorders
      a. Trachoma
      b. Vernal conjunctivitis
      c. Vitamin A deficiency
   2. Skin lesions
      a. Xeroderma pigmentosum
      b. Acanthosis nigricans
   3. Chemicals
      a. Arsenic
      b. Phenothiazines
      c. Epinephrine products
   4. Metabolic and systemic problems
      a. Addison's disease
      b. Folic acid–deficiency anemias[18]
      c. Pregnancy
      d. Thyroid disease
      e. Alkaptonuria—ochronosis
      f. Alport's syndrome
   5. Endothelial pigmentation*
      a. Diabetes mellitus
      b. Pigmentary glaucoma and dispersion syndrome (Krukenberg's spindle)
      c. Cornea guttata
      d. Trauma—anterior chamber hemorrhage
      e. Uveitis with pigmented keratic precipitates

---

*Retrocorneal pigmentation is seen with Krukenberg's spindle (endothelial phagocytosis of free melanin pigment), with the presence of iris melanocytes, with iris pigment epithelial cells, and with pigment-containing macrophages on the posterior corneal surface.

With transmission electron microscopy and scanning electron microscopy, the melanocytes demonstrate endothelial properties. The iris melanocytes can cover the posterior surface of the cornea and contribute to a fibrous tissue located between themselves and Descemet's membrane. Ultrastructural features of these hyperplastic iris melanocytes suggest that they have undergone fibrous metaplasia, with resultant synthesis and deposition of basement membrane and fibrillar collagen. This process can extend on to the trabecula and result in secondary glaucoma.[39]

6. Other conditions causing pigmentation in the general area of the limbus and neighboring conjunctiva
   a. Striate melanokeratosis[12]
   b. Mascara particle inclusions
   c. Scleral plaque
   d. Uveal tissue, for example, staphyloma
   e. Hematogenous pigmentation

Benign pigmented lesions, congenital

Pigmentation can occur subepithelially. A scleral uveal spot, Axenfeld's loop, is a pigmented area along the intrascleral nerve loop. It is seen as a pigmented area 4 mm from the limbus (Fig. 24-13). The spots occur regularly in blacks and with less frequency in whites, especially those with lightly pigmented irides. Pigment may also be seen around the anterior ciliary vessel. It must be remembered that these areas may be possible routes for extraocular melanoma extension. Episcleral gray patches may also occur that are groups of melanocytes in the sclera and episclera.

These benign lesions are present from birth and do not exhibit any malignant potential. They are always stationary and as noted are more frequently seen in pigmented races.

Benign conjunctival nevus

The benign conjunctival nevus, a congenital lesion that may be seen at the limbal area, may or may not be pigmented. Nevus cells have variable morphologic features,

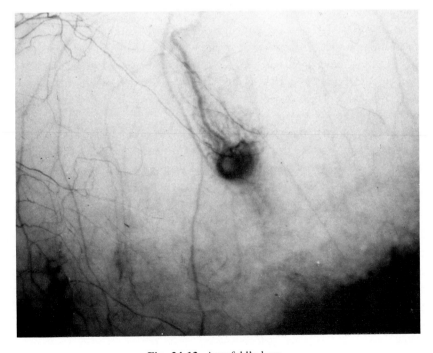

Fig. 24-13. Axenfeld's loop.

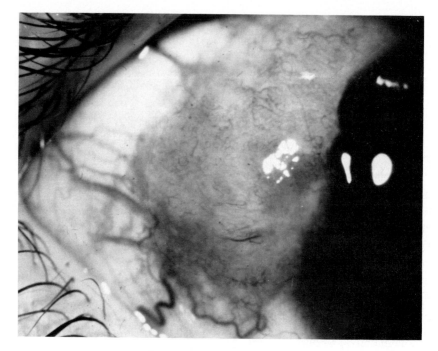

Fig. 24-14. Pigmented nevus.

but most are polyhedral cells that form nests in the conjunctival epithelium or in the underlying connective tissue.

About 70% of benign nevi are fully pigmented (Fig. 24-14); the rest show a variation in pigmentation. About 50% are apparent in childhood, and 75% become apparent by 30 years of age. There is a tendency for the nevi to involute late in life. The nevus may be unrecognized because of a lack of pigmentation, but pigmentation may occur later, especially at puberty. These lesions should always be photographed and carefully evaluated and followed up pictorially.

Nevi are divided into three types. The *junctional nevus* is located in the basal epithelial area. It may remain stationary, regress, or spread into the subepithelial tissues and become malignant. The *subepithelial nevus* is seen in the stroma and tends to involute with age. It never undergoes malignant change. There is no junctional activity. The *compound nevus* is located in the epithelium and stroma. The conjunctival nevus may have a cystic appearance resulting from epithelial inclusions. Goblet cells may be present.

The nevus is not necessarily pigmented and is essentially benign. It is potentially dangerous; it should be remembered that nevi are very common, but malignant melanomas are rare. In addition to its presence at the limbus, the benign conjunctival nevus may also be seen on the caruncle. As noted, however, the pigmentation may be brown, black, or pink-yellow in color, and often the use of ultraviolet light may be used to note the extent of the tumor. The pigmentation may increase under hormonal influence, as in pregnancy.

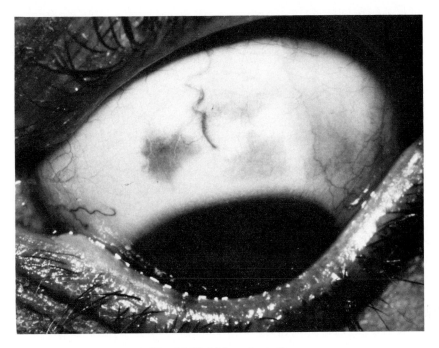

Fig. 24-15. Melanosis oculi.

Another pigmented lesion seen in childhood that may appear at the limbus is the spindle cell A juvenile melanoma, a special form of compound nevus occurring in children. At one time it was thought that these lesions were malignant, but they are in reality benign.

The treatment of nevi of the conjunctiva is quite varied. However, it may be wise to remove the nevi before puberty; the excision should be wide and total. One may employ ultraviolet light to note the extent of the borders. In general nevi are radioresistant.

Congenital melanosis oculi

Subepithelial melanin-containing lesions are not malignant. Included in this area is the condition of melanosis oculi[16] (Fig. 24-15), in which one finds an increase in melanocytes in the uveal tract and episclera. These cases are usually unilateral, congenital, and stationary. However, associated choroidal melanoma occurs and must be considered for the duration of the patient's life.

Congenital oculodermal melanocytosis

Congenital oculodermal melanocytosis (nevus of Ota)[17] is a blue nevus of the skin about the orbit (distribution of the first and second divisions of the fifth cranial nerve) with melanosis oculi. It is usually unilateral, occurring mainly in the dark races (blacks and Orientals). Bilateral cases have been recently reported.[37] Malignant melanoma of choroid is seen only rarely (Fig. 24-16). Thus a young patient with unilateral melanosis

LESION

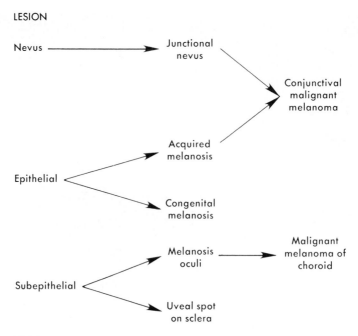

Fig. 24-16. Possible pathways for development of pigmented malignant tumors.

oculi should have lifelong fundus examinations. In addition, deficiencies of hearing,[31] Takaysu's arteritis, and cataracts have been reported.[33, 38]

Acquired melanosis

Bilateral. Bilateral acquired racial melanosis, seen commonly in blacks, is limbal in location and brown in color. There is neither associated pigmentation nor malignant tendency. No treatment is essential.

Unilateral. Benign melanoma occurs as an isolated pigmented spot on the bulbar conjunctiva. It may arise in later age groups, that is 20 years and older, and has the potential of becoming malignant. The spots can be excised.

Acquired melanosis of the conjunctiva may be benign, precancerous, or cancerous. It is patchy or diffuse and may be tan, black, or brown (Fig. 24-17). The conjunctiva, cornea, and lids may be involved. The onset usually occurs in the thirties.[10, 11] The time span between onset and malignant change is 5 to 10 years. The frequency of malignant change is 17%, and mortality is reasonably high: 40% (Fig. 24-16).

In the benign cases an orderly increase occurs in the amount of melanin in the basal cell layer, but cellular activity is not disturbed.

In the precancerous lesions the conjunctival epithelium is disorganized by a profuse overgrowth of melanocyte cells. The underlying stroma may show inflammatory cells. No actual cytologic disturbance is noted. Confusion can occur in interpretation of these cases; thus pathologists would call situations of this nature malignant.

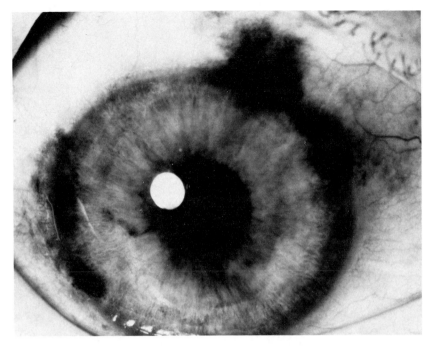

Fig. 24-17. Adult acquired melanoma of limbal area.

In cancerous melanosis malignant change is usually evident within the conjunctival epithelium over a broad area. Tumor cells completely efface normal architecture and infiltrate underlying tissue, abnormal mitotic figures, and multinucleated cells.

Certain concepts and philosophies have evolved regarding these pigmented lesions:

1. Always perform adequate photographic follow-up.
2. In precancerous melanosis the principal treatment is to do nothing.
3. Never hesitate to perform biopsies.
4. Perform excisional biopsy if possible; if not, obtain a biopsy specimen of central or elevated areas in certain cases.

Management. The various procedures to observe after a biopsy follow.

Stage I: benign acquired melanosis

With minimal junctional activity. In some cases, the tissue shows only hyperpigmentation of the epithelium, whereas in others, a few clusters of nevus cells may also be seen in the affected cells. Most conjunctival melanomas arise from junctional activity, which must therefore be watched carefully. Treatment is usually not advised; however, some believe that simple corneal excision can be effective.

With marked junctional activity. In addition to hyperpigmentation, there are many nests of nevus cells, some of which appear somewhat disturbing, and engorged vessels and inflammatory cells occur in the substantia propria. No treatment is usually advised, but local excision can be done. The patient should be observed carefully, photographs of the lesion taken, and perhaps anti-inflammatory drugs given if one chooses not to excise the lesion.

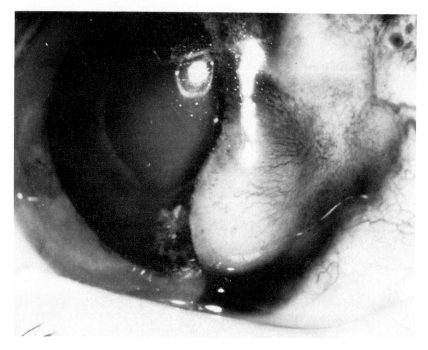

Fig. 24-18. Malignant melanoma of limbus arising from acquired melanoma.

Stage II: cancerous acquired melanosis[3] (Fig. 24-18)

With minimal invasion. Atypical melanocytes with mitotic activity are seen. Foci of invasion of the substantia propria may be found. Recommended treatment is wide excision with preservation of the eye and eyelids.

With marked invasion. Frank-invasion malignant melanoma occurs in addition to other changes listed in stages I and II. Exenteration may be necessary.

The pigment location and cell type in a tumor do not relate to predicting the survival rate. The overall 5-year survival rate for malignant melanoma of the conjunctiva is 75%.

Radiation is usually not advised in precancerous melanosis, since the melanosis may not be radiosensitive. A precancerous condition needs as much treatment as a cancerous one that may subsequently arise. Once this is done, the risks of treatment must be accepted; in addition, the ophthalmologist may later be in an unhappy position, since the treatment of this condition and its apparent cure are no guarantee whatsoever against further recurrence in a cancerous form at a later stage, when the condition of the patient is infinitely worse. Patients in this later stage will be deprived of further radiotherapy at the time they may need it most. Many persons may be treated unnecessarily, since in treating precancerous melanosis much depends on the definition and concept of what a precancerous state is. This is a pathologic probability: no one truly knows how many persons actually may develop cancerous melanosis. Therefore the melanosis must be watched and repeat biopsies should be performed. It must be realized that a definite mortality rate exists and some people die. This rate can be as high as 40%, but the patients die of me-

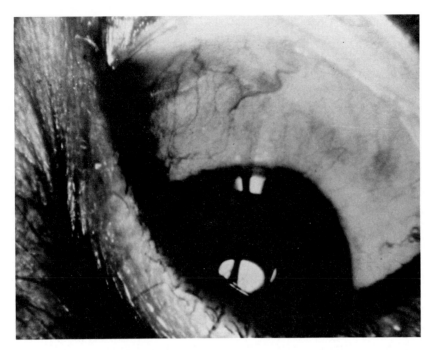

Fig. 24-19. Pigmentation caused by Addison's disease.

tastasis regardless of the treatment, whether irradiation or exenteration.

The type of tumor in which the greatest disasters occur is the bulky tumor in the fornix with invasion of the lid. This tumor is not suitable for radiation. The closer the tumor is to the limbus, the better the response to radiation. The nearer it is to the lid margin and skin surface of the lid, the worse the response is, on the whole. This bulky tumor should be treated by surgery.

Melanocytoma. This congenital, slowly progressive pigmented tumor of the conjunctiva is composed of normal-appearing dendritic melanocytes. This tumor can occur in the limbal area and be mistaken for a malignant melanoma.[42] It occurs in the subepithelial tissues and in some instances may be referred to as a *blue nevus,* since it arises subepithelially.

Other causes of melanosis

Melanosis can occur secondarily after excessive radiation; in metabolic disorders such as Addison's disease (Fig. 24-19); in chemical toxicity, for example, epinephrine, arsenic, and thorazine toxicity; and in chronic conjunctival disorders such as trachoma, vernal conjunctivitis, and vitamin A deficiency. In xeroderma pigmentosum and acanthosis nigricans, pigmentation can also be seen. The pigmentation of alkaptonuria must always be considered in a differential diagnosis.

Striate melanokeratosis[12] consists of lines traversing the corneal epithelium in continuation with the normal limbal pigmentation. This infiltration of melanocytes between the epithelium and Bowman's layer is seen in blacks, as well as after severe inflammation and injury in nonblacks.

In older individuals, one may see brownish-yellow flecks of melanin pigment scattered over the endothelium without any specific pattern. This is the result of migration of uveal pigment from the iris ciliary body to the back of the cornea; in all probability it is physiologic pigmentation occurring with age.

In some instances, of course, pigmentation of the endothelium can occur in dystrophic, atrophic, or inflammatory conditions. This is pathologic pigmentation.

Deposition of pigment can be influenced by the convection current of the anterior chamber fluid. The conditions that most frequently cause pigmentation of this particular nature are cornea guttata, myopia, diabetes, chronic open-angle glaucoma, trauma, and intraocular surgery.

A fine pigment dispersion with dusting of the posterior corneal surface is seen in Alport's syndrome.[13] A fine brownish granular pigmentation occurs inferiorly on the endothelial surface. Alport's syndrome is a rare hereditary disease with nephritis, deafness, lenticonus, microspherophakia, and lens opacities.[13]

Secondary causes of pigmentation

Hematogenous pigmentation. Hemorrhage into the cornea may occur in association with subconjunctival hemorrhage, but usually the hemorrhage does not penetrate farther than a few millimeters into the corneal substance. Intracorneal hemorrhage can also occur from new vessels present in the cornea as a result of traumatic and inflammatory conditions. These usually resolve with no permanent change.

Corneal blood staining (Fig. 24-9) is a much more serious problem and is seen in individuals who have hyphema usually associated with the increased intraocular pressure. The intraocular pressure remains elevated, and hemorrhages persist. The products of blood disintegration will cross the endothelial barrier into the corneal stroma; as a result, the cornea takes on a reddish-brown color, which over a period of months becomes yellow. Often this staining may be mistaken for a displacement of the lens into the anterior chamber (Fig. 24-9), and one has to look very carefully with the slit lamp to make the differentiation. Permanent opacification of the cornea may result; of course, over a period of years the iron-containing pigment and proteinaceous debris are often resolved. Blood staining may occur even in the face when the intraocular pressure is normal and when there is an extensive anterior chamber hemorrhage.

Keratic precipitates. This cellular material is deposited on the posterior surface of the cornea and is visible by direct or retroillumination on slit-lamp examination. The distribution of the precipitates depends on convection currents in the anterior chamber, the size and type of particle, the nature of the lesion, and gravity. Precipitates that lie in the lower portion of the cornea in a fine, vertical line form Turk's line. A classic distribution pattern of a triangle with the apex above is known as Arlt's triangle. These terms are not used often and are primarily of historical interest.

Keratic precipitates can accumulate over the entire posterior surface, as is often seen in severe uveitis. "Mutton-fat" keratic precipitates, which consist of plasma cells and monocytes and are the result of clumping and aggregation of inflammatory cells on the posterior corneal surface, appear as large, greasy-looking, circular or ovoid masses. It is not unusual to see physiologic precipitates that are scattered, have no definite pattern, and represent leukocytes or pigmentary positions. Keratic precipitates from iritis or uveitis may become pigmented in the latter course of the disease. Later they may become "hyalinized" and appear as raised water droplets on the posterior aspect of the cornea.

Erythrocytes may appear in parallel columns or streaks on the posterior surface of the cornea after hyphema.

Occasionally neoplastic precipitates may be seen. These tumor cells may be derived from an intraocular melanoma or a retinoblastoma. Lens material may appear on the posterior surface of the cornea after traumatic cataract extraction or discission. White flakes may be seen on the posterior surface of the cornea, as well as in the pupillary area and other parts of the chamber, as seen in pseudoexfoliation of the lens capsule.

REFERENCES

1. Babel, J., and Stangos, N.: Lésions oculaires iatrogènes; l'action d'un nouveau médicament contre l'angor pectoris, Arch. Ophthalmol. **30:** 197, 1970.
2. Bartlett, R.E.: Generalized argyrosis with lens involvement, Am. J. Ophthalmol. **38:**402, 1954.
3. Bernardino, B.V., Jr., Naidoff, M.A., and Clark, W.H.: Malignant melanomas of the conjunctiva, Am. J. Ophthalmol. **82:**383, 1976.
4. Bernstein, H.N.: Chloroquine ocular toxicity, Surv. Ophthalmol. **12:**415, 1967.
5. Brown, N., Clemett, R., and Grey, R.: Corneal rust removal by electric drill: clinical trial by comparison with manual removal, Br. J. Ophthalmol. **59:**586, 1975.
6. Burn, R.A.: Mercurialentis, Proc. R. Soc. Med. **55:**322, 1962.
7. Burns, C.A.: Indomethacin, reduced retinal sensitivity, and corneal deposits, Am. J. Ophthalmol. **66:**825, 1968.
8. Burns, R.P.: Delayed onset of chloroquine retinopathy, N. Engl. J. Med. **275:**693, 1966.
9. Carr, R.E., Henkind, R., Rothfield, N., and Siegel, I.M.: Ocular toxicity of antimalarial drugs, Am. J. Ophthalmol. **66:**738, 1968.
10. Cibis, P.A., Brown, E.B., and Hong, S.M.: Ocular aspects of systemic siderosis, Am. J. Ophthalmol. **44:**158, 1957.
11. Cibis, P.A., Yamashita, T., and Rodrigues, F.: Clinical aspects of ocular siderosis and hemosiderosis, Arch. Ophthalmol. **62:**180, 1959.
12. Cowan, T.: Striate melanokeratitis in Negroes, Am. J. Ophthalmol. **57:**443, 1964.
13. Davies, P.D.: Pigment dispersion in a case of Alport's syndrome, Br. J. Ophthalmol. **54:**557, 1970.
14. Falbe-Hanse, I.: Treatment of ocular siderosis and haemochromatosis with desferrioxamine, Acta Ophthalmol. **44:**95, 1966.
15. Galin, M.A., Harris, L.S., and Papariello, G.J.: Nonsurgical removal of corneal rust stains, Arch. Ophthalmol. **74:**674, 1965.
16. Gass, J.D.M.: The iron lines of the superficial cornea, Arch. Ophthalmol. **71:**348, 1964.
17. Gewirtzman, G., and Rasmuseen, J.E.: Nevus of Ota with ipsilateral congenital cataract, Arch. Dermatol. **112:**1284, 1976.
18. Gilliam, J.N., and Cox, A.J.: Epidermal changes in vitamin B_{12} deficiency, Arch. Dermatol. **107:** 231, 1973.
19. Gourlay, J.S.: Mercurialentis, Trans. Ophthalmol. Soc. U.K. **74:**441, 1954.
20. Grayson, M., and Pieroni, D.: Severe silver nitrate injury to the eye, Am. J. Ophthalmol. **70:** 227, 1970.
21. Hanna, C., Fraunfelder, F.T., and Sanchez, J.: Ultrastructural study of argyrosis of the cornea and conjunctiva, Arch. Ophthalmol. **92:**18, 1974.
22. Hashimoto, A., Maeda, Y., Ito, H., Okozaki, M., and Hora, T.: Corneal chrysiasis: a clinical study in rheumatoid arthritis receiving gold therapy, Arthritis Rheum. **15:**309, 1972.
23. Johnson, A.W., and Buffaloe, W.J.: Chlorpromazine epithelial keratopathy, Arch. Ophthalmol. **76:**664, 1966.
24. Henkind, P., Carr, R.E., and Siegel, I.M.: Early chloroquine retinopathy: clinical and functional findings, Arch. Ophthalmol. **71:**157, 1964.
25. Kark, R.A.P., Poskanzer, D.C., Bullock, J.D., and Boylen, G.: Mercury poisoning and its treatment with N-acetyl-D,L-penicillamine, N. Engl. J. Med. **285:**10, 1971.
26. Lawwill, T., Appleton, B., and Alstatt, L.: Chloroquine accumulation in human eyes, Am. J. Ophthalmol. **65:**530, 1968.

27. Locket, Z., and Nazroo, I.A.: Eye changes following exposure to metallic mercury, Lancet **1:** 528, 1952.
28. Mathalone, M.B.R.: Eye and skin changes in psychiatric patients treated with chlorpromazine, Br. J. Ophthalmol. **51:**86, 1967.
29. McClanahan, W.S., Harris, J.E., and Knoblock, W.H., et al.: Ocular manifestations of chronic phenothiazine derivative administration, Arch. Ophthalmol. **75:**319, 1966.
30. Rao, N.A., Tso, M.O.M., and Rosenthal, R.: Chalcosis in the human eye, Arch. Ophthalmol. **94:**1379, 1976.
31. Reed, W.B., and Sugarman, G.I.: Unilateral nevus of Ota with sensorineural deafness, Arch. Dermatol. **109:**881, 1974.
32. Reinecke, R.D., and Kuwabara, T.: Corneal deposits secondary to topical epinephrine, Arch. Ophthalmol. **70:**170, 1963.
33. Reinki, R.T., Haber, K., and Josselson, A.: Ota nevus, multiple hemangiomas, and Takayasu arteritis, Arch. Dermatol. **110:**447, 1974.
34. Roberts, W.H., and Wolter, J.R.: Ocular chrysiasis, Arch. Ophthalmol. **56:**48, 1956.
35. Rodenhäuser, J.H., and von Behrend, T.: Type 2 incidence of eye involvement after parenteral gold therapy, Dtsch. Med. Wochenschr. **94:**2389, 1969.
36. Rosenthal, A.R., Appleton, B., and Hopkins, J.L.: Intraocular copper foreign bodies, Am. J. Ophthalmol. **78:**671, 1974.
37. Skalka, H.W.: Bilateral oculodermal melanocytosis, Ann. Ophthalmol. **8:**565, 1976.
38. Smith, T.R., and Brockhurst, R.J.: Cellular blue nevus of the sclera, Arch. Ophthalmol. **94:**618, 1976.
39. Snip, R.C., Green, W.R., Kreutzer, E.W., et al.: Posterior corneal pigmentation and fibrous proliferation by iris melanocytes, Arch. Ophthalmol. **99:**1232, 1981.
40. Spaeth, G.L.: Nasolacrimal duct obstruction by topical epinephrine, Arch. Ophthalmol. **77:**355, 1967.
41. Valvo, A.: Desferrioxamine B in ophthalmology, Am. J. Ophthalmol. **63:**98, 1967.
42. Verdaguer, J., Valenzuela, H., and Strozzi, L.: Melanocytoma of the conjunctiva. Arch. Ophthalmol. **91:**363, 1974.
43. Wålinder, P.E., Gip, L., and Stempa, M.: Corneal changes in patients treated with clofazimine, Br. J. Ophthalmol. **60:**526, 1976.
44. Wilson, L.A., McNatt, J., and Reitschel, R.: Delayed hypersensitivity to thimerosal in soft contact lens wearers, Ophthalmology **88:**804, 1981.
45. Wilson, F.M., Schmitt, T.E., and Grayson, M.: Aminodarone-induced cornea verticillata, Ann. Ophthalmol. **12:**657, 1980.
46. Wise, J.B.: Treatment of experimental siderosis bulbi, vitreous hemorrhage, and corneal blood staining with deferoxamine, Arch. Ophthalmol. **75:**698, 1966.
47. Yanoff, M., and Scheie, H.G.: Argyrosis of the conjunctiva and lacrimal sac, Arch. Ophthalmol. **72:**57, 1964.
48. Zimmerman, L.E.: Melanocytes, melanocytic nevi and melanocytomas, Invest. Ophthalmol. **4:**11, 1965.
49. Zuckerman, B.D., and Lieberman, T.W.: Corneal rust ring, Arch. Ophthalmol. **63:**254, 1960.

CHAPTER

25 Chromosomal aberrations

TRISOMY 21 (DOWN'S SYNDROME, MONGOLISM)[13]

This condition is the most common of all chromosomal disorders and is primarily caused by a trisomy of chromosome 21. Nondisjunction of chromosome 21 results in 47 chromosomes instead of 46. In a small number of cases, however, a translocation defect of chromosome 21 occurs, and thus the number of chromosomes is 46.

The risk of occurrence is 16/10,000 live births, but, as the maternal age increases after 40 years, the incidence of Down's syndrome increases to 200/10,000 births. The life expectancy in these cases is shortened.

The mentally retarded patient has a characteristic facies with small nose, depressed nasal bridge, epicanthal folds, mongoloid slant, and hypertelorism. The stature is short with low-set deformed ears and short stubby hands with a prominent transverse palmar crease. Often the abdomen is protuberant. Visceral anomalies are also present. The skin is dry and scaly, and the hair is dry and soft.

Patients with trisomy 21 frequently exhibit motility problems such as esotropia; epicanthal folds, mongoloid slant, and ectropion also occur. Refractive error of hyperopia and myopia are frequent, as are cataracts (Fig. 25-1). An increase occurs in the number and spoke-wheel effect of blood vessels crossing the margin of the optic disc,[14] and Brushfield's spots (Fig. 25-2) and pale gray spots in the midperiphery of the iris appear. Retinal dysplasia may also be seen.[3]

Keratoconus and acute hydrops occur with reasonable frequency.

599

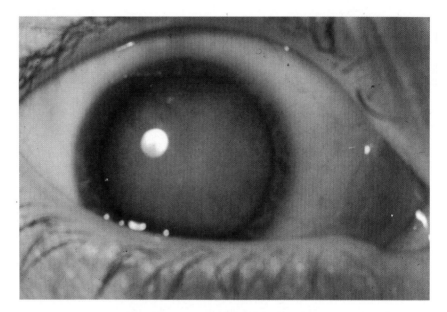

Fig. 25-1. Cataract of Down's syndrome.

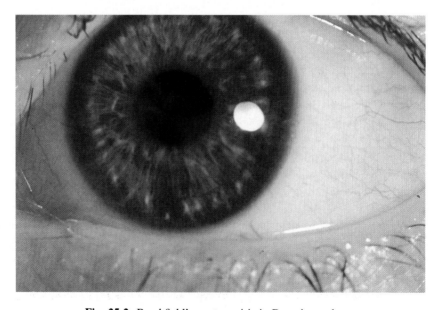

Fig. 25-2. Brushfield's spots on iris in Down's syndrome.

TRISOMY 17-18 (EDWARDS' SYNDROME)[5,9]

The cause of this trisomy is thought to be nondisjunction during gametogenesis, resulting in 47 chromosomes. It occurs in 2/10,000 births and more often in females. The fatality rate in the first month is 30%; in the first year, 90%.

Patients with this disorder exhibit stunted stature, round face, short neck, low-set ears, hypoplastic supraorbital ridge, hypertelorism, harelip, cleft palate, clenched fist with index finger overlapping the third finger, syndactyly, and rocker-bottom feet. They have systemic visceral anomalies of the renal, skeletal, intestinal, and cardiac systems.

Shallow orbits, epicanthal folds, cataracts, and pupillary anomalies are noted. In addition, dysplasia, hyperpigmentation, and hypopigmentation of the retina occur.[12]

Corneal opacities and hyperplastic corneal endothelium are present in trisomy 17-18.

TRISOMY 13 (BARTHOLIN-PATAU SYNDROME)[1,10]

The abnormality is caused by a triplicated chromosome 13 resulting in 47 chromosomes as a result of a nondisjunction in gametogenesis in most cases. It occurs in about 1/5000 births, equally distributed between both sexes. The prognosis for life is poor; 95% of patients succumb by 3 years of age. Neurologic, hematologic, cardiac, renal, and intestinal anomalies are frequent and serious.

External ocular anomalies occur such as epicanthal folds, absent brows, and hypertelorism.

Microphthalmia and large colobomas are frequently seen. Cartilage is found in the colobomatous regions of the eye. Retinal dysplasia and folds are noted[4] (Fig. 25-3).

Dysgenesis of the cornea, iris, and anterior chamber angle is seen. The cornea can be poorly defined with opacification and even may resemble sclera. Nonspecific spotty corneal opacities may be found.

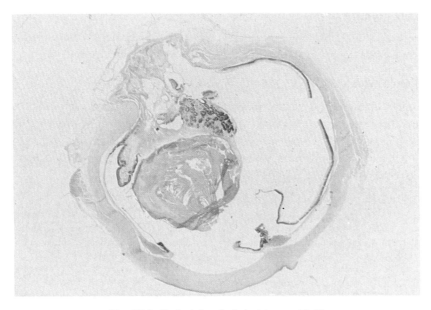

Fig. 25-3. Retinal dysplasia in trisomy 13-15.

XO SYNDROME (TURNER'S SYNDROME)[7,8]

This results from the loss of one X chromosome in the patient during gametogenesis, producing the pattern of 45 XO. The incidence is near 1/5000 births.

Patients with XO syndrome usually have a normal life span and are phenotypically female with webbed neck and a low posterior hairline. Anomalies of the extremities, face, and ears and visceral anomalies of the heart, kidneys, and gonads occur.

Ocular anomalies include ptosis, epicanthal folds, hypertelorism, strabismus and abnormal retinal pigmentation,[8] blue sclera, and cataracts.

Oval corneas and corneal opacities occur in some patients.

CHROMOSOME 18 DELETION DEFECTS[15]

Abnormalities of chromosome 18 include short-arm deletion, long-arm deletion, and ring chromosome.

Short-arm deletion

In short-arm deletion females are affected more frequently than males, and life expectancy is normal. Individuals with this defect are short and mentally retarded; some are microcephalic.

Hypertelorism, epicanthal folds, ptosis, strabismus, and cataracts are found. Posterior keratoconus and corneal opacities are noted.

Long-arm deletion

In long-arm deletions females outnumber males, and mental retardation is great.

The ocular findings include hypertelorism, epicanthal folds, strabismus, retinal degenerations, and optic atrophy. Although rarely found, corneal opacities and microcornea can be seen.

Ring chromosome

The general and ophthalmic findings in ring chromosome 18 are the same as those in deletion of the long and short arms. Corneal opacities are rarely seen.

OTHER CHROMOSOMAL DEFECTS

In other chromosomal abnormalities the corneal signs are extremely rare, but the condition may be worth mentioning. In ring D chromosome,[2] retrocorneal membranes have been reported; in the cri du chat syndrome, deletion of the short arm of chromosome 5[6] and epibulbar dermoids occur. In unbalanced translocation (17p, 10q), sclerocornea has been reported.[11]

REFERENCES

1. Apple, D.J., Holden, J.D., and Stallworth, B.: Ocular pathology of Patau's syndrome with unbalanced O-D translocation, Am. J. Ophthalmol. 70:383, 1970.
2. Bilchik, R.C., Zockai, E.H., Smith, M.E., and Williams, J.D.: Anomalies with ring D chromosome, Am. J. Ophthalmol. 73:83, 1972.
3. Ginsberg, J., Bofinger, M.K., and Roush, J.R.: Pathologic features of the eye in Down's syndrome with relation to other chromosomal anomalies, Am. J. Ophthalmol. 83:6, 874, 1977.
4. Ginsberg, J., and Bove, K.E.: Ocular pathology or trisomy 13, Ann. Ophthalmol. 6:113, 1974.
5. Ginsberg, J., Perin, E.V., and Sueoka, W.T.:

Ocular manifestations of trisomy 18, Am. J. Ophthalmol. **66:**59, 1968.

6. Howard, R.O.: Ocular abnormalities in cri-du-chat syndrome, Am. J. Ophthalmol. **73:**949, 1972.

7. Khodadoust, A., and Paton, D.: Turner's syndrome in a male, Arch. Ophthalmol. **77:**630, 1967.

8. Lessell, S., and Forbes, A.P.: Eye signs in Turner's syndrome, Arch. Ophthalmol. **77:**211, 1966.

9. Mullaney, J.: Ocular pathology in trisomy 18 (Edwards' syndrome), Am. J. Ophthalmol. **76:**246, 1973.

10. Roch, L.M., Petrucci, J.V., and Varber, A.B.: Studies on the development of the eye in 13-15 trisomy syndrome, Am. J. Ophthalmol. **60:**1067, 1965.

11. Rodrigues, M.M., Calhoun, J., and Weinreb, S.: Sclerocornea with unbalanced translocation (17p, 10q), Am. J. Ophthalmol. **78:**49, 1974.

12. Rodrigues, M.M., Punnett, H.A., Valdes-Dapena, M., and Martryn, L.J.: Retinal pigment in a case of trisomy 18, Am. J. Ophthalmol. **76:**265, 1973.

13. Schub, M.: Corneal opacities in Down's syndrome with thyrotoxicosis, Arch. Ophthalmol. **80:**618, 1968.

14. Williams, E.J., McCormick, A.Q., and Tischler, B.: Retinal vessels in Down's syndrome, Arch. Ophthalmol. **89:**269, 1973.

15. Yanoff, M., Rorke, L.B., and Niederer, B.S.: Ocular and cerebral abnormalities in chromosome 18 deletion defect, Am. J. Ophthalmol. **70:**391, 1970.

26 Toxic reactions

IDU and gentamicin
Topical anesthetics
IDU
Amphotericin B
Phenylmercuric nitrate
Topical epinephrine

Topical antibiotics and steroids have been of great help in the treatment of diseases of the cornea and conjunctiva; however, they have been abused, resulting in serious problems affecting the cornea and conjunctiva (Table 26-1).

The use of long-term topical antibiotics, as well as steroids,[3,4,16] can result in colonization and superinfection with saprophytic pathogenic and opportunistic microorganisms.[3] The natural gram-positive flora of the conjunctival sac can be converted to a gram-negative one. Steroids may also result in enhancement of the virulence of fungi[2]; it should be remembered that steroids also result in increased virulence and proliferation of bacteria and viruses. Since the steroids are immunosuppressive in nature, this reaction is understandable.[18] Other immunosuppressive topical medications such as IDU can provoke secondary opportunistic *Staphylococcus aureus* and α-hemolytic streptococci infection when used for a long period of time in corneas devoid of intact epithelium.[25,30] Steroids also may heighten the activity of collagenase, thus enhancing a melting problem of the cornea, which may result in perforation of the cornea.[5]

Alteration of the flora of the conjunctiva can occur by inoculation of the sacs with overwhelming numbers of organisms, as seen in contaminated eye drops and cosmetics.[1]

Contact dermatokeratoconjunctivitis can result from the prolonged use of such topical medications as atropine, gentamicin, neomycin, miotics, penicillin, tetracyclines, chloramphenicol, and topical anesthetic agents. Mucopurulent discharge and follicular conjunctivitis are also seen. Prolonged use of IDU, atropine, and miotics may result in follicular conjunctival reactions.[29,31] Nonspecific papillary conjunctival reactions can also occur. In addition, I have seen cases of epidermidalization, symblepharon formation, keratinization, cicatrization of the conjunctiva, and punctal stenosis, all of which resulted from prolonged use of pilocarpine (Fig. 26-1) or IDU (Fig. 26-2). I have also observed other instances of ocular pemphigoid-like conjunctival reactions that have been reported

Table 26-1. Adverse reactions of drugs on conjunctiva and cornea

Follicular	Cicatrizing	Punctate keratopathy	Allergic dermatokerato-conjunctivitis
IDU	IDU	Preservatives such as	IDU
Atropine	Pilocarpine	benzalkonium and	Miotics
Physostigmine (Eserine)	Echothiophate iodide	thimerosal	Atropine
Echothiophate iodide	(Phospholine Iodide)	IDU	Gentamicin
Diisopropyl fluorophos-	Practolol (systemic	Neomycin	Chloramphenicol
phate (DFP)	drug used for angina	Gentamicin	(Chloromycetin)
Neostigmine	pectoris)	Tetracycline	Neomycin
Pilocarpine		Chloramphenicol	Tetracycline
Atropine		Atropine*	
		Miotics*	

*Products of drug degradation.

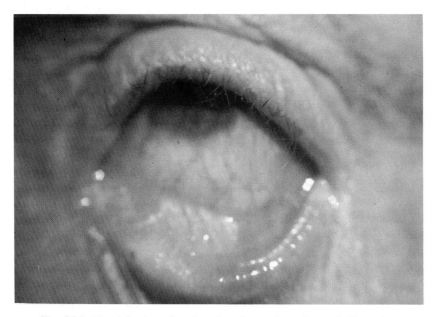

Fig. 26-1. Keratinization of conjunctiva after prolonged use of pilocarpine.

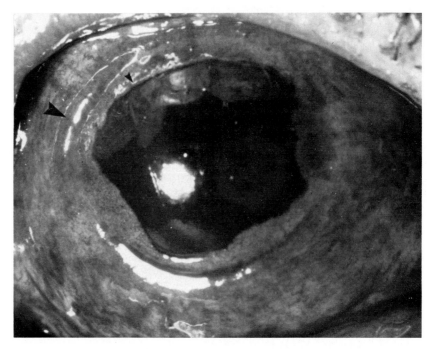

Fig. 26-2. Toxic reaction of conjunctiva and cornea to prolonged IDU and gentamicin topical medication. *Large arrow,* Limbal hypertrophy; *small arrow,* rolled-up thick epithelium with wavy border. Large ulcer base stains with rose bengal red.

with the use of echothiophate iodide (Phospholine Iodide).[26] Systemically administered practolol, a beta-adrenergic blocking agent for cardiac problems, has been reported to cause a pseudopemphigoid picture, corneal ulceration, and opacification.

IDU AND GENTAMICIN

The cornea may exhibit an epithelial keratopathy. The chronic use of IDU (Fig. 26-2) and gentamicin can result in epithelial degeneration with heaping up of epithelium and extensive areas of erosion. Fig. 26-2 demonstrates limbal hypertrophy (follicle formation), thickened rolled-up epithelium, and an extensive area of corneal erosion, the base of which stains with rose bengal red. Although this illustration demonstrates an extreme reaction to the 5-month use of IDU and gentamicin, one may see lesser involved cases with the heaped-up epithelium that may resemble a dendritic figure. One must interpret this pseudodendritic finding correctly; otherwise one may be prompted to increase the antiviral agent, which would only aggravate the condition. Toxic effects on the epithelium may be manifest as fine or coarse lesions. A number of references have been cited regarding this effect,[12,27] especially when 0.01% benzalkonium is the drug or preservative under discussion.[12] Changes in the epithelial cells consist of loss of microvilli, disruption of plasma membranes, and desquamation of the top two layers of cells. To a lesser degree 4% cocaine and Neo-Polycin were also found to be offenders. Neostigmine, carbachol, epinephrine, and echothiophate also have toxic effects on the epithelium.[21]

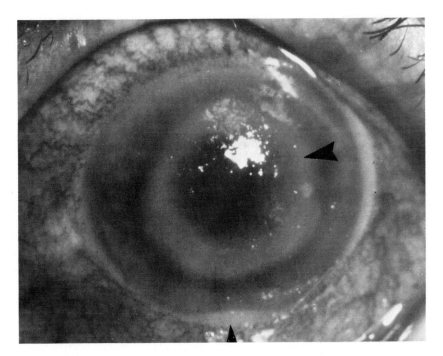

Fig. 26-3. Wessely-immune ring *(large arrow)* and hypopyon *(small arrow)*.

TOPICAL ANESTHETICS

Prolonged use of topical anesthetic agents causes ultramicroscopic changes in the mitochondria, endoplasmic reticulum, tonofibrils, desmosomes, and microvilli of the corneal epithelial cells.[15,22] All membrane physiologic conditions are adversely altered.[6,17] The findings may reveal one of the following: a conjunctival injection, toxic epithelial defect with typical rolled-up edges, stromal infiltration, or Wessely's ring (Fig. 26-3) in the stroma and endothelium,[7] as well as a hypopyon (Fig. 26-3) in some cases. If the agent is continued, greater stromal infiltration of the cornea will occur with extensive vascularization.

IDU

IDU is a widely used medication that, if its use is abused, will cause a severe keratopathy. It will not retard healing of the epithelium[13,14] but will cause a retardation of stromal healing.[14] It will produce an epithelial keratopathy with coarse punctate staining.[9,24] The large noninfectious ulcer as seen in Fig. 26-1 shows the characteristic thick epithelial edge, which is rolled under. The edges are smooth and wavy, and the base of the ulcer stains with rose bengal red. Preauricular adenopathy, corneal pannus (Fig. 26-4), conjunctival follicles (Fig. 26-5), limbal follicles (Fig. 26-6), and scarring can be seen in severe toxicity. This picture resembles one of trachoma and is thus called pseudotrachoma.[26,31] IDU, when incorrectly used to treat superficial punctate keratitis of

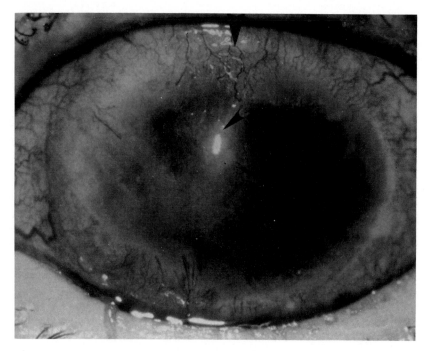

Fig. 26-4. "Pseudotrachoma." *Large arrow,* Pannus; *small arrow,* corneal infiltrate. (Courtesy F.M. Wilson II, M.D., Indianapolis, Ind.)

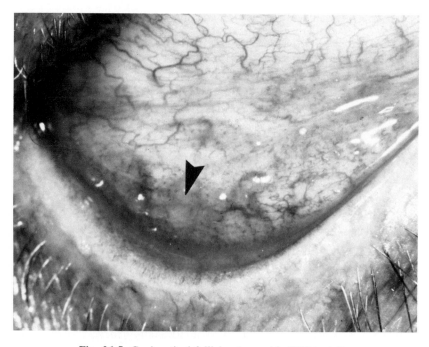

Fig. 26-5. Conjunctival follicles *(arrow)* in IDU toxicity.

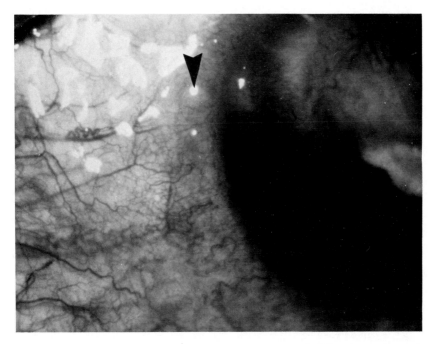

Fig. 26-6. Limbal follicles *(arrow)* in IDU toxicity. (Courtesy F.M. Wilson II, M.D., Indianapolis, Ind.)

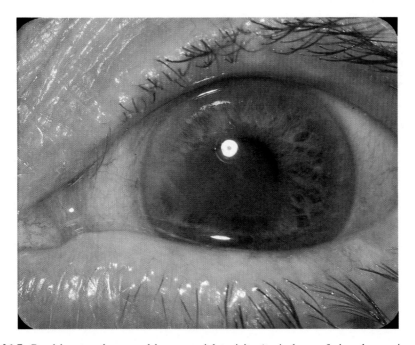

Fig. 26-7. Band keratopathy caused by mercurial toxicity (topical use of phenylmercuric nitrate as preservative).

Thygeson, may result in subepithelial infiltrate. The same type of infiltrate can be seen occasionally beneath herpetic dendrites so treated.[25]

AMPHOTERICIN B

When amphotericin B is used to treat fungal keratopathy, irritation of the conjunctiva and cornea may occur. This has been attributed to the sodium desoxycholate that is used to increase the drug's solubility in water.[32] I have observed this reaction in most cases of *Aspergillus fumigatus* keratitis treated with topical amphotericin B. It is advised that amphotericin B never be given subconjunctivally, since it is extremely irritating and will cause a conjunctival slough.

PHENYLMERCURIC NITRATE

Phenylmercuric nitrate that is used as a preservative for some topical ophthalmic medications for a long period of time can cause a calcific band keratopathy[10,19,20] (Fig. 26-7). The protein of the cornea is believed to be denatured by the mercury, resulting in calcific degeneration.[10] Pilocarpine and sulfisoxazole (Gantrisin) are drugs in which this preservative was used. As a result of this mercurial toxic reaction, the anterior capsule of the lens may also exhibit a light-brown discoloration known as *mercurialentis*.[11]

TOPICAL EPINEPHRINE

Pigmentations were discussed in Chapter 24, but it should be emphasized that conjunctival deposits may occur from chronic use of topical epinephrine. These deposits, which are in reality melanin,[8,23,28] can also occur on the cornea and cause "black cornea"; this should not be mistaken for a melanoma.

REFERENCES

1. Abel, R., Jr.: The danger of accidental corneal trauma from cosmetic applicators: mascara use and abuse, Ann. Ophthalmol. **9:**348, 1977.
2. Basu, P.K.: Experimental oculomycosis. Abstract of paper presented at University of Toronto Annual Research Meeting, May, 1971, Am. J. Ophthalmol. **72:**653, 1971.
3. Bettman, J.W., Aronson, S.B., Kagawa, C.M., and Hinson, D.B.: The incidence of adverse reactions from steroid/anti-infective combinations, Surv. Ophthalmol. **20:**281, 1976.
4. Binder, P.S., Abel, R.A., Jr., and Kaufman, H.E.: The effect of chronic administration of a topical antibiotic on the conjunctival flora, Ann. Ophthalmol. **7:**1429, 1975.
5. Bloomfield, S.E., and Brown, S.I.: Treatment of corneal ulcers with collagenase inhibitors, Int. Ophthalmol. Clin. **13:**225, 1973.
6. Bryant, J.A.: Local and topical anesthetics in ophthalmology, Surv. Ophthalmol. **13:**263, 1969.
7. Epstein, D.L., and Paton, D.: Keratitis from misuse of corneal anesthetics, N. Engl. J. Med. **279:**296, 1968.

8. Ferry, A.P., and Zimmerman, L.E.: Black cornea: a complication of topical use of epinephrine, Am. J. Ophthalmol. **58:**205, 1964.
9. Fraunfelder, F.T.: Drug-induced ocular side effects and drug interactions, Philadelphia, 1976, Lea & Febiger.
10. Galin, M.A., and Obstbaum, S.A.: Band keratopathy in mercury exposure, Ann. Ophthalmol. **6:**1257, 1974.
11. Garron, L.K., Wood, I.S., Spencer, W.H., and Hayes, T.L.: A clinical pathologic study of mercurialentis medicamentosus, Trans. Am. Ophthalmol. Soc. **74:**295, 1966.
12. Gasset, A.R., Ishii, Y., Kaufman, H.E., and Miller, T.: Cytotoxicity of ophthalmic preservatives, Am. J. Ophthalmol. **78:**98, 1974.
13. Gasset, A.R., and Katzin, D.: Antiviral drugs and corneal wound healing, Invest. Ophthalmol. **14:**628, 1975.
14. Grant, W.M.: Toxicology of the eye, ed. 2, Springfield, Ill., 1974, Charles C Thomas, Publisher.
15. Harnisch, J.P., Hoffmann, F., and Dumitrescu, L.: Side-effects of local anesthetics on the corneal

epithelium of the rabbit eye, Albrecht von Graefes Arch. Klin. Ophthalmol. **197:**71, 1975.

16. Havener, W.H.: Ocular pharmacology, ed. 4, St. Louis, 1978, The C.V. Mosby Co.
17. Hermann, H., Moses, S., and Friedenwald, J.S.: Influence of Pontocaine hydrochloride and chlorobutanol on respiration and glycolysis of cornea, Arch. Ophthalmol. **28:**652, 1942.
18. Kass, E.H., and Finland, M.: Corticosteroids and infections, Adv. Intern. Med. **9:**45, 1958.
19. Kennedy, R.E., Roca, P.D., and Landers, P.H.: Atypical band keratopathy in glaucomatous patients, Am. J. Ophthalmol. **72:**917, 1971.
20. Kennedy, R.E., Roca, P.D., and Platt, D.S.: Further observations on atypical band keratopathy in glaucoma patients, Trans. Am. Ophthalmol. Soc. **72:**107, 1974.
21. Krejci, L., and Harrison, R.: Antiglaucoma drug effects on corneal epithelium: a comparative study in tissue culture, Arch. Ophthalmol. **84:**766, 1970.
22. Leuenberger, P.M.: Ultrastructure of corneal epithelium after topical anesthetics, Albrecht von Graefes Arch. Klin. Ophthalmol. **186:**73, 1973.
23. McCarthy, R.W., and LeBlanc, R.: A black cornea secondary to topical epinephrine, Can. J. Ophthalmol. **11:**336, 1976.
24. McGill, J., Fraunfelder, F.T., and Jones, B.R.: Current and proposed management of ocular herpes simplex, Surv. Ophthalmol. **20:**358, 1976.
25. Ostler, H.B.: The management of ocular herpesvirus infections, Surv. Ophthalmol. **21:**136, 1976.
26. Patten, J.T., Cavanagh, H.D., and Allansmith, M.R.: Induced ocular pseudopemphigoid, Am. J. Ophthalmol. **82:**272, 1976.
27. Pfister, R.R., and Burstein, N.: The effects of ophthalmic drugs, vehicles, and preservatives on corneal epithelium: a scanning electron microscope study, Invest. Ophthalmol. **15:**246, 1976.
28. Reinecke, R.D., and Kuwabara, T.: Corneal deposits secondary to topical epinephrine, Arch. Ophthalmol. **70:**170, 1963.
29. Theodore, F.H., and Schlossman, A.: Ocular allergy, Baltimore, 1958, The Williams & Wilkins Co.
30. Thygeson, P.: Historical observations on herpetic keratitis, Surv. Ophthalmol. **21:**82, 1976.
31. Thygeson, P., and Dawson, C.R.: Pseudotrachoma caused by molluscum contagiosum virus and various chemical irritants, Exc. Med. Int. Cong. Ser. **222:**1894, 1970.
32. Wood, T.O., and Williford, W.: Treatment of keratomycosis with amphotericin B 0.15%, Am. J. Ophthalmol. **81:**847, 1976.

27 Acid and alkali injuries

Lye burn
Management

A chemical burn of the external eye from a strong acid or alkali is an acute ophthalmic emergency. It must be recognized as an emergency, since acids and alkalies may result in blinding sequelae. The severe effects of these agents result from an alteration of the concentration of hydrogen and hydroxide ions. If ionization in solution is weak, the agent will be relatively harmless. An example of this is the potentially acidic substance carbon dioxide, which is lipoid soluble and penetrates the epithelial layer of the cornea. The carbolic acid is not harmful, since its ionization is weak.

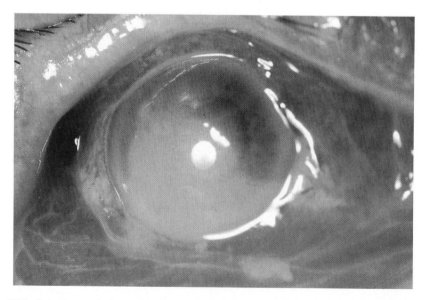

Fig. 27-1. Injection and chemosis of conjunctiva with small areas of necrosis. Note increased relucency of cornea.

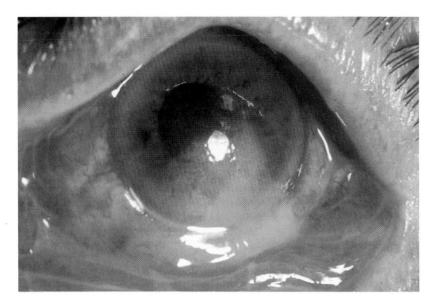

Fig. 27-2. Small area of limbal ischemia.

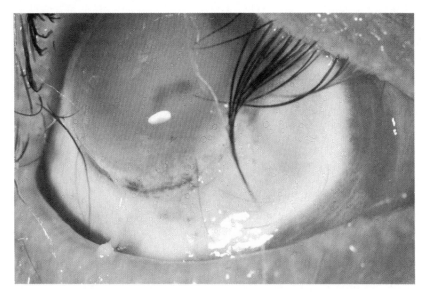

Fig. 27-3. Marbleization of cornea and severe limbal ischemia.

LYE BURN

When the eye is first involved in a lye burn, injection of the conjunctiva occurs; indeed, areas of the conjunctiva may become necrotic. Strong alkaline chemicals result in disruption of cells, since the high pH results in saponification and dissociation of fatty acids in the cell membranes. If the pH exceeds 11.5 in any area of the affected cornea, one may see loss of mucopolysaccharide and swelling of collagen fibers. It is well known that acids bind tissue protein, which in effect tends to limit further penetration. There is less tendency in acid burns for any such comparable loss of collagen. However, the alkali burn to the cornea can be a tragedy because of its propensity to penetrate into the anterior chamber.[9] It should be noted that if the cation has a tendency to penetrate rapidly through the epithelium, such as occurs with the ammonia ion, severe and rapid damage to the stroma may occur, which is more rapid and severe than is seen with calcium hydroxide or sodium hydroxide.

The cornea exhibits epithelial denudation and increased relucency. There is a reaction of the lye on the stromal keratocytes, ground substance, and endothelium.[1] The keratocytes are coagulated, and the mucopolysaccharide ground substance is severely altered. In the more severe cases, in addition to the findings listed previously, severe marbleization of the cornea and limbal ischemia are seen (Figs. 27-1 to 27-3). The latter finding offers an extremely unfavorable prognosis.

After the immediate acute phase (1 to 3 days), the patient is subjected to a prolonged period in which the eye exhibits poor epithelial healing and stromal ulceration. This may progress to actual perforation of the eye (Fig. 27-4). The burn may involve a localized area of the cornea, but in spite of this a spreading area of neovascularization, which scars connective tissue, may be seen. The vascularization may also contribute to lipid deposition in the cornea. The loss of epithelium of the conjunctiva results in a severe inflammation reaction; cicatrization may occur, which results in symblepharon formation and loss of the cul-de-sacs (Fig. 27-5). It can be readily seen that the sequela of a lye burn may be a vascularized and opacified cornea associated with a frozen globe caused by scarring and cicatrization.

In addition to the preceding, one may, in extremely severe cases, encounter cataracts, iris necrosis, secondary glaucoma, and phthisis. Acid burns produce denaturation and coagulation of corneal proteins with precipitation of soluble acid proteinates. No great penetration of the tissues occurs, since continued activity is neutralized by the buffering action of the tissues. The precipitated protein also sets a barrier to penetration.

MANAGEMENT

It is vital that the chemically injured eye be copiously irrigated as soon as possible.[1,2,7] The caustic matter must be irrigated away.[7] Removal of solid lye, lime, and the like is essential and may require double eversion of the lid to properly ensure that this area is free of chemical. Topical anesthetic agents or lid block may be required for this initial treatment. In some instances it may be necessary to apply continuous irrigation for 12 to 24 hours to aid in countering the chemical action, especially in severe lye burns. An intravenous catheter is inserted into the conjunctival fornix for continuous infusion.

Topical antibiotic and debridement of necrotic conjunctiva may prevent a severe infection, since this area is now in a compromised state and subject to bacterial infection. In addition, since there may be a severe iritis reaction, cycloplegics (1% atropine) many times a day are advised. If there is an increased intraocular pressure, oral acetazolamide, 500 mg twice a day, should be given. It has been recently shown that the pH of the anterior chamber is significantly lowered by paracentesis, and, if possible and performed early enough, anterior chamber reformation with sterile solution[7] may be a procedure to reduce the ravages of the high pH on the lens, iris, and chamber angle. Grant,[6] however, in 1950 did not believe this was so. Corticosteroids must be used with caution if used at all, since they suppress repair. It is to be recalled that in almost all these cases epithelial stroma defects and limbal ischemia are already present. The steroids may have a disastrous effect on the eye if used in the face of these findings.

A critical period in the treatment of these corneas is in the 7- to 10-day period after the injury. The use of collagenase inhibitors such as cysteine may minimize the effect of the collagenase.[1-3] The regenerating epithelium and circulating lymphocytes and neutrophils may release collagenase and other enzymes that digest the stroma.* Evidence exists to implicate collagenases as a possible cause of the corneal ulceration and perforation. In addition, the dryness, exposure, and corneal anesthesia must be considered and dealt with as they arise.

Treatment must be continued until the corneal epithelium has completely covered the denuded surface. Healing of the epithelium, which must be achieved as soon as possible, may be enhanced by patching or by the use of a therapeutic soft contact lens. The soft contact lens also protects the cornea when trichiasis, insufficient tears, incomplete lid closure, and recurrent erosion are problems. Work has been done with subconjunctival dibutyryl adenosine 3':5'-cyclic monophosphoric acid (DBCAMP); it is suggested that this may reduce the incidence of ulceration in alkali-burned rabbit corneas.[4,8] However, this is yet to be proved. The following treatments may have an effect on corneal healing: 10% ascorbate in Adsorbotear, administered as eye drops hourly every day, and high doses of ascorbic acid, given orally. Medroxyprogesterone may decrease the inflammation without decreasing the repair of collagen, which takes place with prednisone.

In the severely scarred corneas and conjunctival sacs one may resort to keratoplasty and reconstructive plastic surgery. Although results with penetrating corneal transplantation have been encouraging in some instances, the overall prognosis for the marbleized corneas from alkali burns is still guarded. The treatment may be improved when special emphasis is placed on the associated findings of exposure, drying, and the guarded and judicious use of steroid drugs.

Encouraging results have been obtained from conjunctival transplantation associated with lamellar keratectomy after chemical or thermal burns. Conjunctival resection and lamellar keratectomy are followed by grafting of healthy conjunctival patches.[12] This procedure aids in the epithelialization of the cornea from the small grafts; it is most effective in superficially vascularized corneas and may be a preliminary step to keratoplasty later.

*References 2, 3, 5, 10, 11.

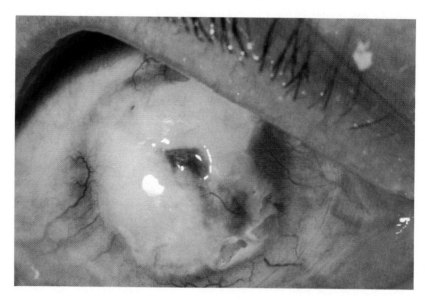

Fig. 27-4. Perforation of cornea as result of lye burn.

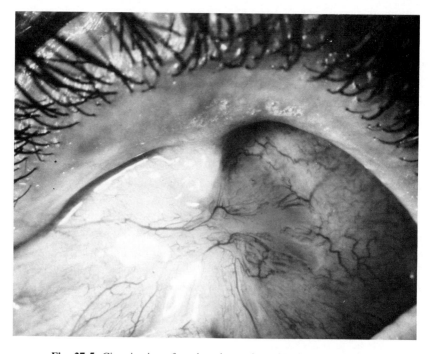

Fig. 27-5. Cicatrization of conjunctiva and symblepharon formation.

REFERENCES

1. Brown, S.I., Tregakis, M.P., and Pearce, D.B.: Treatment of the alkali burned cornea, Am. J. Ophthalmol. **74:**361, 1972.
2. Brown, S.I., and Weller, C.A.: Pathogenesis and treatment of collagenase induced diseases of the cornea, Trans. Am. Acad. Ophthalmol. Otolaryngol. **74:**375, 1970.
3. Brown, S.I., Weller, C.A., and Wasserman, H.E.: Collagenolytic activity of alkali burned corneas, Arch. Ophthalmol. **81:**370, 1969.
4. Crabb, C.V.: Endocrine influences on ulceration and regeneration in alkali burned cornea, Arch. Ophthalmol. **95:**1866, 1977.
5. Gnädringer, M.C., Ioti, M., Slansky, H.H., and Dohlman, C.H.: The role of collagenase in alkali burned cornea, Am. J. Ophthalmol. **68:**478, 1969.
6. Grant, W.M.: Experimental investigation of paracentesis in the treatment of ocular ammonia burns, Arch. Ophthalmol. **44:**399, 1950.
7. Hughes, W.F., Jr.: Alkali burns of the eye: review of the literature and summary of present knowledge, Arch. Ophthalmol. **35:**423, 1946.
8. Miller, J.D., Eakino, K.E., and Atwal, M.: The release of PGE-2 like activity into aqueous humor after paracentesis and its prevention by aspirin, Invest. Ophthalmol. **12:**939, 1973.
9. Paterson, C.A., Pfister, R.R., and Levinson, R.A.: Aqueous humor pH changes after experimental alkali burns, Am. J. Ophthalmol. **79:**414, 1975.
10. Slansky, H.H., and Dohlman, C.H.: Collagenase and the cornea, Surv. Ophthalmol. **14:**402, 1970.
11. Slansky, H.H., Dohlman, C.H., and Berman, M.B.: Prevention of corneal ulcers, Trans. Am. Acad. Ophthalmol. Otolaryngol. **75:**1208, 1971.
12. Thoft, R.A.: Conjunctival transplantation, Arch. Ophthalmol. **95:**1475, 1977.

ADDITIONAL READING

Brown, S.I., Bloomfield, S.E., and Pearce, D.B.: A follow-up on transplantation of the alkali-burned cornea, Am. J. Ophthalmol. **77:**538, 1974.

Brown, S.I., Tragakis, M.P., and Pearce, D.B.: Corneal transplantation for severe alkali burns, Trans. Am. Acad. Ophthalmol. Otolaryngol. **76:**1266, 1972.

Duke-Elder, S., and MacFaul, P.A.: Mechanical injuries. In Duke-Elder, S., editor: System of ophthalmology, vol. XIV. Injuries, pt. 1, St. Louis, 1972, The C. V. Mosby Co.

Sommer, A., and Muhilal: Nutritional factors in corneal xerophthalmia and keratomalacia, Arch. Ophthalmol. **100:**399, 1982.

Sommer, A., and Sugana, T.: Corneal xerophthalmia and keratomalacia, Arch. Ophthalmol. **100:**404, 1982.

28 Limbal lesions

Congenital lesions
Lymphomas
Epithelial tumors
Papillomata
Hereditary benign intraepithelial dyskeratosis
Precancerous lesions
Carcinoma in situ
Squamous cell carcinoma
Fibrous histiocytoma

The limbal area is an important part of the anterior segment and is often associated with disease manifestations. It is necessary to consider the tumors of the conjunctiva and cornea, since in many instances the lesions may involve both structures in this area.

The etiologic factors of limited lesions include toxic conditions, surgical and traumatic problems, congenital masses, systemic diseases, inflammatory disease, and degenerative and neoplastic conditions, including papillomata, keratoses, malignant and premalignant lesions, and pigmented tumors (Table 28-1).

Tumors and related conditions are discussed in this chapter.

CONGENITAL LESIONS

The congenital lesions include dermoids and dermatofibromas[17] of fibrous tissue, hair follicles, and sebaceous glands, all covered by conjunctival epithelium. The dermal lipoma contains structures similar to those of the dermoid but may show larger amounts of normal fat. Goldenhar's syndrome is a congenital anomaly that exhibits limbal dermoids, preauricular skin tags, aural fistulae, mandibulofacial dystrophies, vertebral abnormalities, and other musculoskeletal abnormalities.

Dermoids may be removed if cosmetically objectionable; however, care must be exercised in their removal so as not to cut into the anterior chamber. A corneal graft of superficial nature may have to be employed to reinforce the area of the cornea from which the tumor was removed.

In addition one may see rarer congenital masses of the limbus such as ectopic lacrimal gland[8] and episcleral osseous choristomas.[2] The latter are usually found in the upper temporal quadrant and are not usually seen with any other congenital changes, as are seen with dermoids.

Table 28-1. Limbal lesions

Inflammatory
Trachomatous follicles

Immune allergic
Phlyctenule
Vernal catarrh (Fig. 28-1)

Degenerative
Pterygium
Pingueculae
Amyloid

Neoplastic
Epithelial
  Benign papillomata
    Viral (Fig. 28-2)
    Noninfectious (Fig. 28-3)
  Benign hereditary intraepithelial dyskeratosis
  Malignant and premalignant
    Precancerous
    Carcinoma in situ
    Invasive carcinoma
Lymphoma
  Benign
  Malignant (Fig. 28-4)
Fibrous histiocytoma
Pigmented lesions
  Nevi (Fig. 28-5)
  Benign acquired melanomas (Fig. 28-6)
  Malignant melanoma (Figs. 28-7 and 28-8)
Lipomas

Toxic
Limbal follicles: IDU
Epidermidalization and keratinization (Fig. 28-9): pilocarpine

Surgical and traumatic
Granulomas (Fig. 28-10)
Foreign bodies
Inclusion cysts (Fig. 28-11)
Filtering blebs (Fig. 28-12) for glaucoma or after cataract
Uveal prolapse (Fig. 28-13)
Keloid
Air injected into limbal area (Fig. 28-14)

Congenital
Dermoids
Ectopic lacrimal gland[10]
Episcleral osseous choristomas[4]
Vascular hamartomas

Systemic
Gaucher's disease (pigmented pingueculae)
Neurofibromatosis
Alkaptonuria (pigmented deposit)

Vitiligo[5]
Perilimbal vitiligo (Sugiura's sign) (Vogt-Koyanagi-Harada syndrome)

LYMPHOMAS (Fig. 28-4)

Subconjunctival locus is one of the sites where lymphomatous eye masses may occur as single or multiple elevated masses that generally assume the contour of the site involved. They invariably are salmon-colored, exhibit sharply demonstrated borders, lack gross blood vessels, are not tender or ulcerated, and have smooth overlying conjunctiva. The usual histologic appearance of lymphoid tumors is that of a sheet of small lymphocytes lying in a delicate fibrovascular stroma.

The only constant features are that germinal follicles are of some predictive value in benign lesions, whereas lymphoblastic infiltration is consistent with lymphosarcoma. Lymphocytic tumors of indeterminate nature require long-term follow-up because many of these lesions lack distinguishing features enabling the pathologist to exclude a malignant process.

It now appears well established that the lymphoid system can be viewed as being made up of two functionally separate, though frequently morphologically similar, classes of lymphocytes. The B lymphocytes, particularly after further differentiation into plasma

Text continued on p. 628.

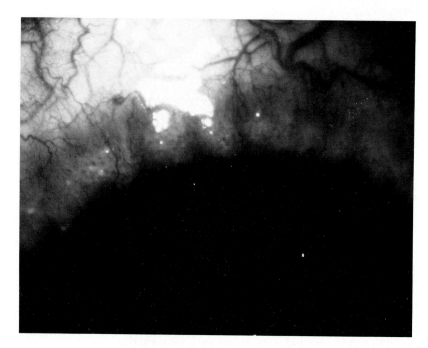

Fig. 28-1. Limbal vernal catarrh.

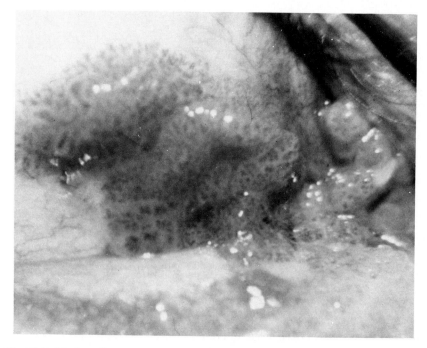

Fig. 28-2. Viral papilloma extending from limbal area to bulbar conjunctiva and caruncle.

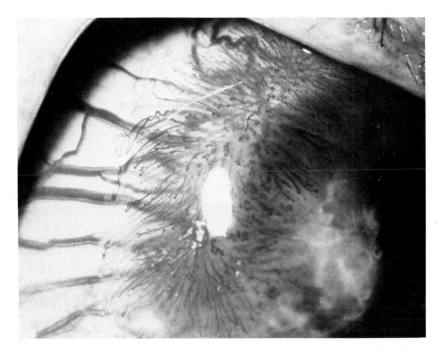

Fig. 28-3. Neoplastic papilloma.

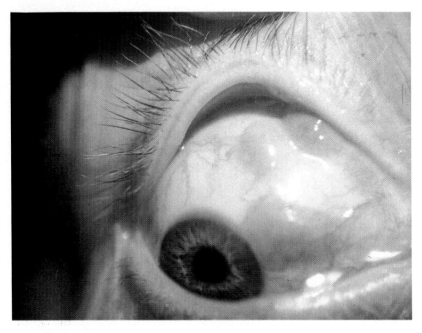

Fig. 28-4. Malignant lymphoma in limbal area showing smooth, raised, salmon-pink lesion.

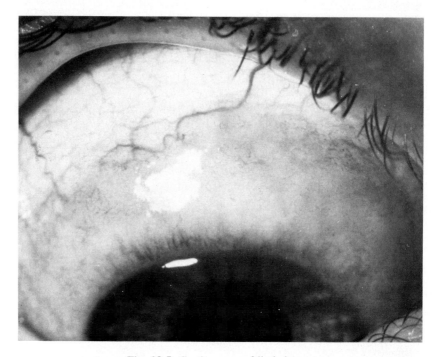

Fig. 28-5. Cystic nevus of limbal area.

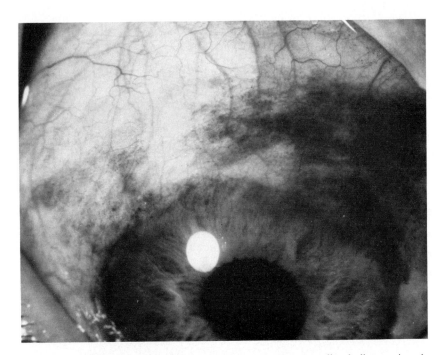

Fig. 28-6. Acquired benign melanosis of limbal area and surrounding bulbar conjunctiva.

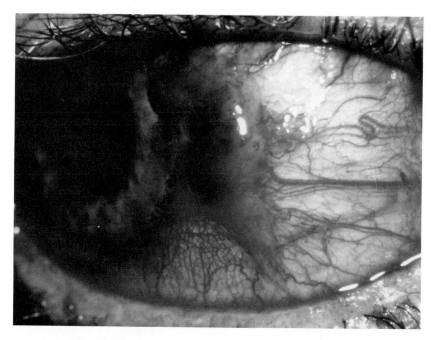

Fig. 28-7. Limbal melanoma with extensive vascularization.

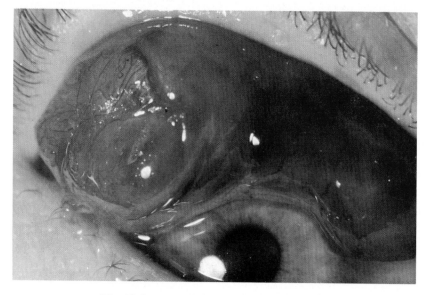

Fig. 28-8. Larger limbal malignant melanoma.

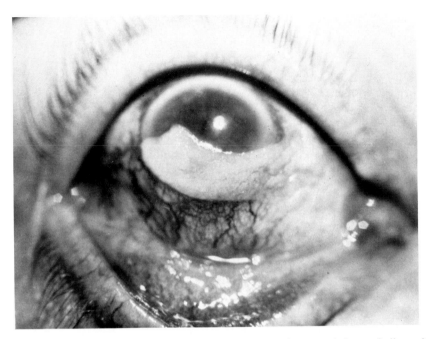

Fig. 28-9. Keratinization of limbus and bulbar conjunctiva after extended use of pilocarpine.

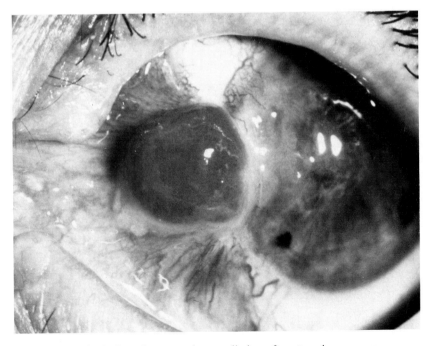

Fig. 28-10. Granulomatous tissue at limbus after pterygium surgery.

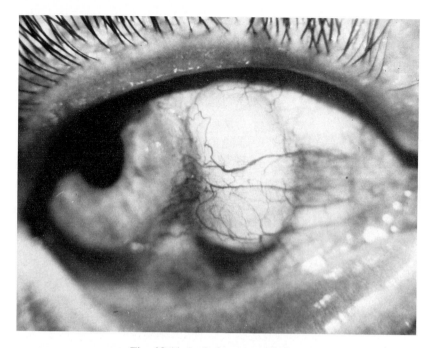

Fig. 28-11. Inclusion cyst at limbus.

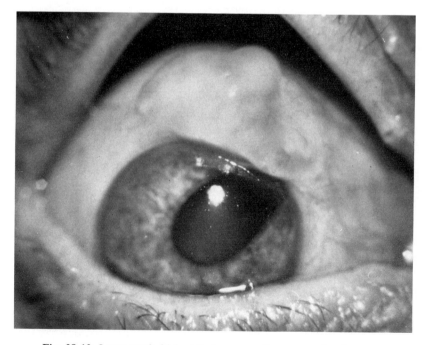

Fig. 28-12. Large cystic bleb at limbus seen after surgery for glaucoma.

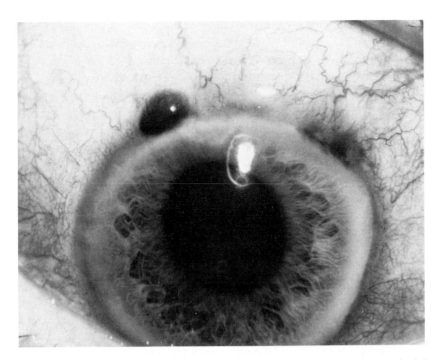

Fig. 28-13. Uveal exposure from perforation of cornea resulting from Terrien's marginal degeneration.

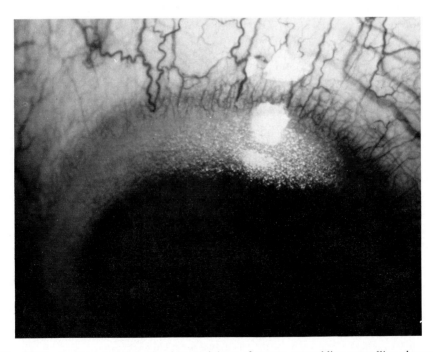

Fig. 28-14. Accidental air injection into periphery of cornea, resembling crystalline change.

cells, make immunoglobulins and constitute the humoral immunity system. The T lymphocytes provide control for the B cell response to antigens and act on their own in providing those functions traditionally included in cell-mediated immunity. B lymphocytes are characterized by the presence of easily detectable surface-bound immunoglobulin. Under normal conditions, one cell carries only one specific type of immunoglobulin. T lymphocytes do not have immunoglobulins detectable by conventional methods. However, they form spontaneous rosettes with sheep red blood cells and carry a surface antigen identifiable with the appropriate antisera. T and B lymphocytes may undergo blast transformation under proper stimulation. A group of lymphocytes without detectable membrane markers is also recognized and termed null cells.

Malignant lymphomas are now recognized as neoplasms of the immune system. Application of immunologic surface marker techniques to malignant lymphomas has demonstrated that most non-Hodgkin's malignant lymphomas can be typed as B or T cells.[13] In addition, particularly in B cell lymphomas, a monoclonal pattern of cell population can be identified, that is, cells bearing one specific type of immunoglobulin.

The prognostic value of surface markers on nonocular lymphoma cells have shown that nodular lymphomas are of the B cell type and that diffuse lymphomas are predominantly B cell, but T and null cells were found. Patients with nodular lesions survive significantly longer than those exhibiting a diffuse pattern. Interestingly, patients with B cell–marker diffuse lymphoma survive appreciably longer than those with alleged T and null cell lymphoma.

Essential to the evaluation of any patient with suspected ocular lymphoma is a thorough physical examination combined with radiologic and hematologic surveys to rule out systemic disease. Biopsy specimens should include touch imprints and snap-frozen tissue for immune studies in addition to routine histologic techniques.

EPITHELIAL TUMORS

Tumors of the epithelium include pingueculae, pterygia, cysts, papillomata, and keratoses. These are benign lesions. In the premalignant category one must consider the precancerous lesions and carcinoma in situ. Malignant tumors of epithelial origin include invasive carcinoma.[1]

Papanicolaou smear cytology is a simple procedure for the evaluation and management of external lesions of this nature. Cytology can prove useful in the management of squamous cell carcinoma and related tumors of the conjunctiva and limbus and malignant melanoma of the same areas. Cytology can be valuable in tumor recurrence or squamous cell carcinoma and carcinoma in situ and in meibomian gland carcinoma of the eyelid.[6] Following are terms that are often used to describe squamous neoplasia[14] and should be understood:

squamous metaplasia Reversion to a more primitive type of cell.
epidermidalization Dermislike.
acanthosis Thickening of the prickle cell layer.
hyperkeratosis Increased keratin in granular cell layer.
parakeratosis Nuclei present in the keratin layer.
dysplasia Cells show atypical size, shape, stain, and mitotic figures.
neoplasia Tumor formation.

Pingueculae are raised yellow or white limbal lesions that may occur in the bulbar conjunctiva in the interpalpebral area. The overlying conjunctival epithelium is usually thin but may exhibit dyskeratosis and acanthosis. The stroma exhibits collagen breakdown, which stains basophilically and also stains positively with elastic tissue stains but is not sensitive to elastase (elastotic degeneration).[8,17] If cosmetically objectionable, pingueculae may be simply excised.

Pterygia are seen with great frequency in tropical areas and may also be associated with chronic irritation caused by dryness, solar exposure, and inflammation. The thickened Bowman's layer of the epithelium is often absent and damaged where the pterygium invades the cornea. The epithelium may exhibit acanthosis and dyskeratosis. Pterygium, in addition, exhibits new blood vessel formation together with mild inflammatory changes. Pingueculae and pterygia represent degenerative changes of the tissue in and around the limbus. Pterygia may be resected. There is a definite tendency for recurrence.

PAPILLOMATA[15]

Conjunctival papillomata may be seen in young and old patients alike (Table 28-2). However, the lesions seen in the younger age group occur more often on a viral basis, whereas the lesion in older persons may be neoplastic. The viral lesion affects the palpebral, conjunctival, bulbar, and fornicate areas. It may also involve the limbus. These transmissable lesions may be multiple in nature (Fig. 28-2) and, if improperly removed, may even become alarmingly widespread in the conjunctiva and lid margin (Fig. 28-2).

In viral papillomata fine epithelial keratitis may be seen. The problem is best left untreated; a 2-year period of waiting is recommended, since many of the papillomata resolve by that time. However, if treatment becomes necessary, application of the cryo-

Table 28-2. Clinical characteristics of conjunctival papillomata

Infectious (viral)	Noninfectious (unknown cause)
Usually in children or young adults	Usually in older adults
May be bilateral	Nearly always unilateral
May be multiple	Nearly always single
Usually on palpebral conjunctiva, fornix, or caruncle, especially below; less commonly at limbus	Usually on bulbar conjunctiva or at limbus
Pedunculated	Sessile or diffuse
Smooth surface	More surface irregularity and thickening
May occur with verrucae on eyelid or elsewhere	No such association
Multiple lesions may appear after excision of single lesion	Each recurrence usually single
Transmissible	Not transmissible
Usually little or no conjunctivitis; rarely moderate conjunctivitis	Occasionally marked conjuctivitis ("masquerade syndrome")
Occasionally fine ("toxic") epithelial keratitis	Cornea involved only by direct extension or mechanical factors
Rarely, if ever, malignant	Benign, dysplastic, or malignant
Spontaneous resolution common	Spontaneous resolution uncommon

From Wilson, F.M., II, and Oster, H.B.: Am. J. Ophthalmol. **77**:103, 1974.

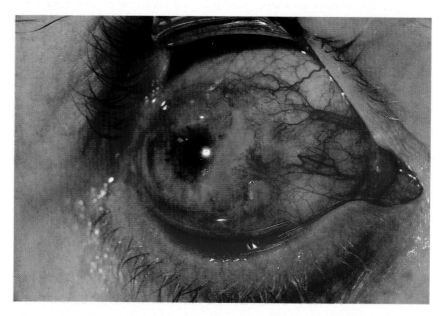

Fig. 28-15. Leukoplakic limbal lesions with large conjunctival feeder vessels and corneal pannus adjacent to lesions. (From McLean, I.W., et al.: Ophthalmology **88:**164, 1981.)

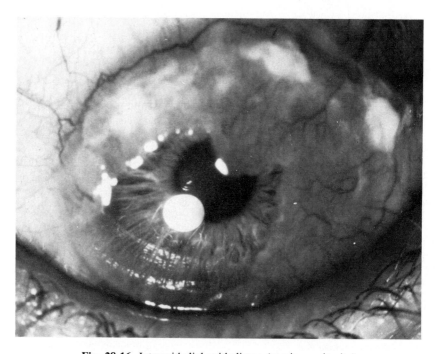

Fig. 28-16. Intraepithelial epithelioma (carcinoma in situ).

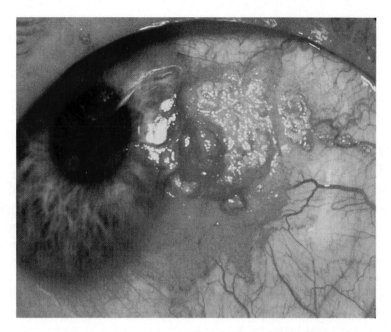

Fig. 28-17. Squamous neoplasia of limbus stained with rose bengal red.

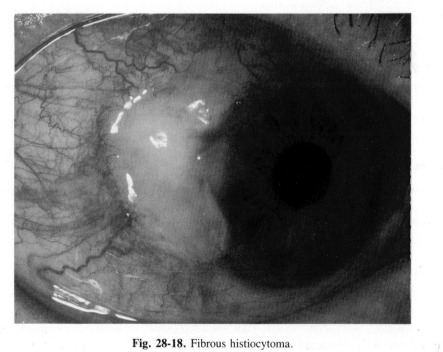

Fig. 28-18. Fibrous histiocytoma.

probe at $-70°$ to $-100°$ C is recommended. It may be necessary to excise the epithelial lesion and then apply the cryotherapy unit to the base of the lesion.

In the older individual a neoplastic papilloma may be seen at the limbus (Fig. 28-3). This diffuse lesion is not transmissible, and spontaneous resolution is not seen. The cornea is involved in a number of cases by extension onto and into it. Excision of these lesions is advised.

For differentiation of the infectious (viral) papillomata and noninfectious papillomata, see Table 28-2.

HEREDITARY BENIGN INTRAEPITHELIAL DYSKERATOSIS

Benign hereditary intraepithelial dyskeratosis, a rare condition, [16, 17] is transmitted in a dominant fashion. It is a benign keratotic lesion of the bulbar conjunctiva that extends to the limbus. The conjunctival lesions are elevated and show dyskeratosis and acanthosis, with which vascularization and a moderate inflammatory reaction in the conjunctival connective tissue is associated. The raised, granular, semitransparent, horseshoe-shaped plaque, which is apparent by the first year, extends to the superior and inferior limbus and is located in the palpebral tissue. Corneal opacities occur that are usually deep and are associated with vascularization. Corneal involvement is rare. Benign hereditary intraepithelial dyskeratosis is also often associated with oral mucosal dyskeratosis.

The malignant and premalignant lesions are categorized as precancerous lesions, carcinoma in situ, and invasive carcinoma.

Hereditary benign intraepithelial dyskeratosis (HBIO) has been traced to descendants from Halowar Indians of Halifax and Warren counties in North Carolina. Some cases have been seen in Texas.[11, 12]

One sees bilateral temporal and nasal limbal plaques (Fig. 28-15). These may encircle the cornea, encroach on the cornea, or remain as isolated nodules. In addition, one may see rubeosis iridis, papillary hypertrophy of the tarsal conjunctiva, iritis, and injected bulbar conjunctiva.

Oral lesions, such as white spongy lesions on the buccal and labial mucosa and the ventral aspect of the tongue, are seen.

The differential diagnosis can include actinic dyskeratosis, in situ or squamous cell carcinoma, pterygium, limbal vernal, and papillomata.[11, 12]

PRECANCEROUS LESIONS

The precancerous lesions are usually seen as white elevated plaques at the limbus. The epithelium shows acanthosis, dyskeratosis, and epidermidalization. Although usually benign, they may progress to malignant changes. The early lesions may be treated by excision or by cryotherapy.[3]

CARCINOMA IN SITU

Intraepithelial epithelioma (Fig. 28-16) (carcinoma in situ) appears as a raised, somewhat gelatinous-appearing lesion, which may be gray and slightly red, depending on the vascularity.[1] Carcinoma in situ begins in the conjunctiva at the limbus and then may spread over onto the cornea (Fig. 28-16). It may even take on a papillomatous appearance. The full thickness of the epithelium is involved and shows marked dyskeratosis and bizarre, pleomorphic epithelial cells with many mitotic figures and multinucleated giant cells. Polarity of the epithelium is lost, but the basement membrane of the epithelium is intact, and there is no invasion of the subepithelial tissue of the conjunctiva or of the corneal stroma.

Intraepithelial epithelioma responds to complete excision. However, there are recurrences.

SQUAMOUS CELL CARCINOMA (Fig. 28-17)

This may arise from preexisting carcinoma in situ and papillomata. In this disease, one may find an elevated, pearly-white lesion at the limbus caused by the keratin. The cells are anaplastic with irregular proliferation. Invasion has occurred by the malignant pleomorphic cells through the basement membrane into the subepithelial tissues of the conjunctiva or of the cornea. If left neglected, the invasion of deeper tissues of the cornea and sclera will occur. Squamous cell carcinoma may extend into the eye, although this is uncommon. Distant metastases may occur if the interior of the eye is involved.

Excision is the recommended treatment. The excision should be adequate in the conjunctiva and cornea to eradicate the disease.

The keratinized tumor and surrounding involved tissue can be visualized well with the application of rose bengal red[14] (Fig. 28-17). This area of stain affords an excellent guide to the extent of the area that should be excised.[14] Squamous cell carcinoma rarely metastasizes.

FIBROUS HISTIOCYTOMA[9]

These raised yellow limbal masses are usually solitary confined lesions[4,15] (Fig. 28-18), which consist of lipid-laden histiocytes in addition to fibrocytic cells. The lesions occurring at the limbal area are benign. It is not clear if the pathologic process is reactive or neoplastic. In the orbit these lesions may show malignant potential.

Fibrous histiocytoma appears to occur more frequently in females and may occur in patients with diseases involving the immune system and in those on immunosuppressives.[15]

The differential diagnosis must include amyloid, lymphoma of the limbus (Fig. 28-4), xanthoma of the limbus,[7] Gaucher's disease, juvenile xanthogranuloma, and the histiocytosis X group of tumors. These conditions may appear as a yellow or tan lipid-appearing lesion at the limbal area and must be considered in making a diagnosis of lesions of this area.

REFERENCES

1. Blodi, F.C.: Squamous cell carcinoma of the conjunctiva, Doc. Ophthalmol. **34**:93, 1973.
2. Boniuk, M., and Zimmerman, L.E.: Epibulbar osteoma (episcleral osseous choristoma), Am. J. Ophthalmol. **53**:290, 1962.
3. Brownstein, S., Jakobrec, F.A., Wilkinson, R.D., et al.: Cryotherapy for precancerous melanoma (atypical melanocytic hyperplasia) of the conjunctiva, Arch. Ophthalmol. **99**:1224, 1981.
4. Faludi, J.E., Kenyon, K., and Green, W.R.: Fibrous histiocytoma of the corneoscleral limbus, Am. J. Ophthalmol. **80**:619, 1975.
5. Friedman, A.H., and Deutsch-Sokol, R.H.: Sugiura's sign: perilimbal vitiligo in the Vogt-Koyanagi-Harada syndrome, Ophthalmology **88**:1159, 1981.

6. Gelender, H., and Forster, R.K.: Papanicolaou cytology in the diagnosis and management of external ocular tumors, Arch. Ophthalmol. **98:**909, 1980.

7. Grayson, M., and Pieroni, D.: Solitary xanthoma of the limbus, Br. J. Ophthalmol. **54:**562, 1970.

8. Hogan, M.J., and Zimmerman, L.E.: Ophthalmic pathology, ed. 2, Philadelphia, 1962, W.B. Saunders Co.

9. Jakobiec, F.A.: Fibrous histiocytoma of the corneoscleral limbus, Am. J. Ophthalmol. **78:**700, 1974.

10. Kessing, S.V.: Ectopic lacrimal gland tissue at the corneal limbus (glands of Manz), Acta Ophthalmol. **46:**398, 1966.

11. McLean, I.W., Riddle, P.J., Scruggs, J.H., and Jones, D.B.: Hereditary benign intraepithelial dyskeratosis, Ophthalmology **88:**164, 1981.

12. Reed, J.W., Cashwell, L.F., and Klintworth, G.K.: Corneal manifestations of hereditary benign intraepithelial dyskeratosis, Arch. Ophthalmol. **97:**297, 1979.

13. Udell, I.J., Ballen, P.H., Mir, R., and Perry, H.D.: Subconjunctival lymphoma: a review of six suspected cases and the use of immunologic surface markers, Ann. Ophthalmol. **13:**471, 1981.

14. Wilson, F.M., II: Rose bengal staining of epibulbar squamous neoplasms, Ann. Ophthalmol. **7:**21, 1976.

15. Wilson, F.M., II, and Ostler, H.B.: Conjunctival papillomas in siblings, Am. J. Ophthalmol. **77:**103, 1974.

16. Yanoff, M.: Hereditary benign intraepithelial dyskeratosis, Arch. Ophthalmol. **79:**291, 1968.

17. Yanoff, M., and Fine, B.S.: Ocular pathology, New York, 1975, Harper & Row, Publishers.

Suggestions for laboratory work and analysis of conjunctival and corneal smears and scrapings

Exudate smear
Follicular expression
Corneal smear
Scraping
Normal epithelial cells
Mucus
Fibrin
Polymorphonuclear leukocytes (PMNs)
Mononuclear cells (MNs) (lymphocytes,
    monocytes, plasma cells)
Basophils
Eosinophils
Plasma cells
Russell bodies
Leber's cells
Keratinized and keratinizing epithelial cells
Goblet cells
Multinucleated epithelial cells
Inclusions
Other inclusions
Nuclear chromatin
Phagocytosed cellular debris
Bacteria
Tumor cells
Molluscum bodies
Granulomatous inflammation
Granulation tissue
Gram's stain
Giemsa's stain

Cytology is frequently of value in helping one to determine the etiologic diagnosis of external disease problems of the eye. One may frequently see the organisms or from the cellular type of reaction get a good idea as to the etiologic agent and hence possible forms of treatment.

Exudate smear

This type of smear is easy to do and requires only the removal of the exudate present on the lid margin or within the conjunctival sac with a glass rod or the wooden end of an applicator stick and smearing it onto the microscopic slide.

The exudate smear shows only cells that have been sloughed from the conjunctiva such as keratinized or keratinizing epithelial cells, inflammatory cells, and occasionally organisms.

This technique is especially good for demonstrating eosinophils; occasionally one may find eosinophils in an exudate smear when they are not seen in a scraping.

One cannot see epithelial cells with an exudate smear.

Follicular expression

One may express follicles with the use of ring forceps. This is a valuable method to help differentiate the trachomatous follicles from nontrachomatous. The difference in "softness" is probably a result of the necrotizing action of the trachoma agent.

Corneal smear

One can readily obtain cells from the superficial epithelium of the cornea by raking a coverslip or a glass slide over the cornea after the instillation of an anesthetic. This is especially helpful in cases where one may be desirous of obtaining cells for examination for multinucleation. One should not use a glass coverslip for this because of the danger of breaking the thin glass and losing the glass particles in the conjunctival sac.

Scraping

Scraping of the conjunctiva or cornea is more difficult to do than the other usual methods for obtaining cells for cytologic examination, but this method is the most satisfactory in the majority of cases.

A topical anesthetic, such as 0.5% proparacaine, is required as well as an instrument to scrape the area to be examined. (I prefer a Kimura platinum spatula.)

Epithelial cells, inflammatory cells, and often organisms responsible for the disease may be visible with this method.

Normal epithelial cells

Normal epithelial cells have a large central nucleus that is oval and uniform in size. There is a slightly granular, pale-blue cytoplasm.

Epithelial cells from a normal conjunctiva come off in sheets, whereas in trachoma the cells are single. The nuclei are round and variable in size, are larger than usual, and stain irregularly and less intensely.

Nonkeratinized epithelial cells are parasitized by three types of bacteria: *Neisseria gonorrhoeae, N. meningitidis,* and *Haemophilus aegypticus.*

Degenerative changes in the epithelium are characteristic of a chronic conjunctivitis only. These changes are manifest by the cells appearing polymorphic with a poorly staining nucleus.

Mucus

Mucus stains blue with Giemsa's stain. It tends to be increased in keratoconjunctivitis sicca and in cases of chronic conjunctivitis or at the time an acute conjunctivitis begins to subside. Mucus is predominant in *H. influenzae* infections.

Fibrin

Fibrin appears red on Giemsa's stain. It is marked in conjunctivitis because of *N. catarrhalis* and diplobacillus infections.

Polymorphonuclear leukocytes (PMNs) (Table A-1)

The PMN is the main inflammatory cell in acute inflammations:
1. It may stain pink or blue with cytoplasmic granules (small cells with pigmented nuclei).
2. PMNs originate in the bone marrow.
3. PMNs are the most numerous of the circulating leukocytes, making up to 50% to 75% of the total.

4. The PMN functions at an alkaline pH.

5. It is attracted by chemotaxis to an involved area and acts by phagocytosis and lysosomal digestion. Lysosomes in the PMN are saclike cytoplasmic structures that contain digestive enzymes and other polypeptides.

6. PMNs are the most frequent cytologic reaction seen in acute and chronic infections (Table A-1). All bacterial infections, except those caused by *N. catarrhalis* and the diplobacillary organisms, result in a polymorphonuclear response.

In *N. catarrhalis* infections there is a marked abundance of bacteria; in infections from the *Moraxella* group there is a high fibrin content and a deficiency in mucus.

Variations in the intensity of polymorphonuclear reactions may occur according to the stage of the infection: for example, in acute granulocytic ophthalmia an intense polymorphonuclear reaction occurs with marked fibrin formation. In later stages of the

Table A-1. Ocular cytology

Polymorphonuclear cells

Bacteria, except:
  Moraxella species
  N. catarrhalis
Fungi
Chlamydiae
Membranes
Necrosis

Mononuclear cells (lymphocytes)

Viruses
Phlyctenules
Thyroid conjunctival hyperemia
Normals

Mixed (polymorphonuclear predominate)

Chlamydiosis (chronic)
Most chronic conjunctivitis
Catarrhal ulcers
Phlyctenules (resolving)
Superior limbic keratoconjunctivitis
Pemphigoid
Erythema multiforme
Reiter's syndrome
Rosacea
Chemical burns

Mixed (lymphocytes predominate)

Viruses with membranes
Most drug reactions
Keratoconjunctivitis sicca

Eosinophils and basophils

Vernal catarrh
Atopic eczema keratoconjunctivitis
Hay fever conjunctivitis
Occasionally in drug allergies
Erythema multiforme
Pemphigoid
Occasionally trachoma

Free eosinophilic granules

Most suggestive of vernal catarrh

Keratinized epithelial cells

Keratoconjunctivitis sicca
Pemphigoid
Chemical burns
Erythema multiforme
Superior limbic keratoconjunctivitis
Squamous neoplasia
Vitamin A deficiency
Trachoma
Radiation
Severe membranous conjunctivitis
Some drug reactions

Goblet cells

Keratoconjunctivitis sicca
Chronic conjunctivitis

Multinucleated giant epithelial cells

Herpes simplex
Varicella-zoster
Chlamydiosis
Measles
Squamous neoplasia
Radiation

same disease there is an increased number of mononuclear cells, although PMNs still predominate. In addition, there is an increase of mucus and a decrease of fibrin.

In chronic infections the PMNs will be predominant with mononuclear cells present in a moderate amount. The exception is staphylococcal conjunctivitis, in which the PMNs are present in marked numbers even in chronic conjunctivitis.

PMNs are also predominant in trachoma, inclusion conjunctivitis, lymphogranuloma venereum, and psittacosis, as well as in Reiter's disease, psoriasis, and erythema multiforme.

Phlyctenulosis of the conjunctiva characteristically shows little exudate unless it is caused by staphylococci, in which case PMNs will be the predominant type of cell.

Mononuclear cells (MNs) (lymphocytes, monocytes, plasma cells) (Table A-1)

1. The mononuclear cells are derived from circulating monocytes.
2. They make up 3% to 7% of circulating leukocytes, fixed-tissue histiocytes (reticuloendothelial system), and possibly defense lymphocytes and arrive after the PMN and depend on PMN release of a chemotactic factor for their arrival.
3. Monocytes live for weeks.
4. They can proliferate.
5. MNs are phagocytic and employ proteolytic digestion.
6. They cause less necrosis than PMNs and are more efficient phagocytes than are PMNs.
7. Monocytes have a fixed antigen on their surface to behave as an immunogenic substance.
8. MNs can change into epithelioid cells and inflammatory giant cells.
9. The monocytes have folded, large, kidney bean–shaped vesicular nuclei and only a moderate amount of cytoplasm. They are larger than PMNs. The lymphocyte is smaller than the epithelial cell.
10. MNs are the predominant cells in true viral disease of the conjunctiva such as adenovirus infection, herpes, verruca, Newcastle disease, and molluscum contagiosum.
11. MNs may rarely be the preponderant cells in tuberculosis, syphilis, and trachoma.
12. MNs may be seen in large numbers in chronic conjunctivitis, but they are not the predominant cells.
13. In herpes infection of the cornea the predominant cell may be the PMN if there is necrosis of the cornea or secondary bacterial infection.

Basophils (Table A-1)

These are small bluish cells containing basophilic granules.
1. Mast cells seem to be identical to basophils except for their location. Mast cells occur in fixed-tissue cells and have large nonsegmented nuclei. Basophils occur in circulation (1% of circulating leukocytes) and have segmented nuclei.
2. Mast cells (basophils) elaborate histamine and heparin and are important for the initiation of the acute inflammatory response.

3. The cytoplasm of mast cells stains with alcian blue stain for acid mucopolysaccharide; Unna's stain may be employed for staining the cell.
4. Basophils are characteristically seen in allergic inflammation, especially vernal conjunctivitis.
5. Basophils may also be seen in small numbers in trachoma.

Eosinophils (Table A-1)

Eosinophils and mast cells may be involved in the acute phase of inflammation. Following are characteristics of eosinophils:
1. They originate in bone marrow.
2. They comprise 1% to 2% of circulating leukocytes.
3. The number of eosinophils increases in parasitic and allergic reactions.
4. The number decreases with stress and steroid administration.
5. Eosinophils have bilobed nuclei and exhibit pink, granular cytoplasm.
6. The finding of one eosinophil in the conjunctival scraping is an abnormal finding.
7. Eosinophils are the characteristic cells of allergic inflammation and are usually readily demonstrated in this state.
8. Dispersed eosinophilic granules are suggestive of vernal catarrh. The eosinophilic granules may be seen during the quiescent period of the vernal catarrh, also.
9. A few eosinophils are seen in drug and cosmetic allergies such as atropine sensitivity. They do not occur in eserine or pilocarpine sensitivity.
10. Pemphigoid is characterized by the presence of a few eosinophils.
11. Eosinophils are seen in eosinophilia, parasite infestation of the conjunctiva, and phlyctenular conjunctivitis.

Plasma cells (Table A-1)

1. The plasma cell shows clumping of nuclear chromatin.
2. The spoked nucleus is eccentrically located.
3. A halo is seen adjacent to the nucleus and contains immunoglobulin.
4. The cytoplasm tapers.
5. Electron microscopic studies show a great deal of endoplasmic reticulum, which accounts for basophilic cytoplasm and also contains mitochondria.
6. Plasma cells are produced by bone marrow–derived lymphocytes.
7. They produce immunoglobulins (antibodies).

Russell bodies

1. Russell bodies are plasma cells changed so that their cytoplasm is filled with eosinophilic grapelike clusters in a morular form with eosinophilic crystalline structures.
2. The nucleus is eccentric or missing.
3. The eosinophilic material in plasma cells and Russell bodies seem to be inspissated immunoglobulins (alpha globulin).
4. Plasma cells are characteristically seen in trachoma. Plasma cells may be seen

frequently in the subepithelial infiltration in any type of conjunctivitis, but they do not occur in the scrapings or the exudate.

5. The cells are probably seen in trachoma as a result of the follicle rupturing readily on scraping and not because of the ability of the plasma cells to penetrate intact epithelium.

6. Plasma cells are never numerous.

Leber's cells

1. Leber's cells are merely very large macrophages. They are more numerous in trachoma than in other types of conjunctivitis. They are often several times the size of epithelial cells and contain phagocytized cellular debris that is primarily nuclear in origin.

2. The Leber cell seen in trachoma is usually much larger than the macrophage seen in other types of conjunctivitis.

Keratinized and keratinizing epithelial cells (Table A-1)

1. Partial keratinization is identified by the presence of faint red granules in the cytoplasm, as well as by a change of the color of the cytoplasm to a type of red. The nucleus begins to show degenerative changes.

2. Complete keratinization of the cell is characterized by a blue-staining cytoplasm with loss of the nucleus.

3. Keratinized and keratinizing epithelial cells may result from exposure of the conjunctiva, as with ectropion of the lid. They may occur from extreme cicatrization, as occurs with pemphigoid, trachoma, erythema multiforme, and other severe membranous and pseudomembranous conjunctivitides. Keratinized and keratinizing epithelial cells are also seen in vitamin A deficiency, keratoconjunctivitis sicca, limbic keratitis, and epithelial plaques and after irradiation of the conjunctiva. Bitot's spot is characteristic of a vitamin A deficiency and on scraping shows keratinizing or keratinized cells with numberous diphtheroids.

4. Normal conjunctival epithelial cells never show keratinization.

5. The epithelial cells of the lid margin, on the other hand, are keratinized.

Goblet cells (Table A-1)

1. The nucleus of the goblet cell is displaced by a large mass of mucoid material that stains pink. The nucleus is purple and is pushed aside to the cell wall. The color is readily cleared or removed when the slide is passed through an alcohol rinse.

2. Goblet cells may be found in a scraping taken from a normal conjunctiva if the scraping includes the conjunctiva toward the nasal or temporal side as well as at the edge of the tarsus (the part next to the cul-de-sac).

3. The number of goblet cells increases in keratoconjunctivitis sicca.

Multinucleated epithelial cells (Table A-1)

1. Multinucleated epithelial cells may be produced by either failure of the nucleus to completely divide during mitosis or a fusion of several cells.

2. Multinucleated cells may be seen in scrapings from the conjunctiva in herpes simplex and in herpes zoster as well as in varicella and vaccinia.
3. Tumor cells that are multinucleated usually have 3 to 5 nuclei and are often larger cells.
4. The multinucleated cells of trachoma usually have 5 to 6 nuclei. The cells look better preserved and are not necrotic in appearance.
5. Multinucleated cells seen after irradiation are variable in appearance.

Inclusions (Table A-2)

The likelihood of identifying cytoplasmic and intranuclear inclusions in an adult is remote.

1. Inclusion bodies in trachoma are seen only in the epithelium. The PMNs can show elementary bodies from phagocytosis. Inclusion bodies in trachoma are not seen in mononuclear cells as they are in psittacosis. Inclusion bodies in trachoma occur in the outer third of the epithelium and not in the basal cell layers. In herpes, the basal layer is more involved.
2. The elementary body is the infectious particle containing DNA. It enters the epithelial cell and forms the initial body (RNA). The initial body divides to form more elementary bodies. The elementary body is sharp edged, round, and reddish blue or purplish in color. The elementary body is uniform in size and gains access into the epithelial cell by phagocytosis. Inside the epithelial cell the granules are embedded in a clear matrix that is a glycogen-like substance easily stained with

Table A-2. Inclusions

Disease	Cytologic characteristics	Designation
Inclusion bodies		
Trachoma-inclusion conjunctivitis	Basophilic,* cytoplasmic	Halberstraedter-Prowazek
Vaccinia	Eosinophilic, cytoplasmic	Guarnieri
Variola	Eosinophilic, cytoplasmic, nuclear	Guarnieri
Molluscum	Eosinophilic, cytoplasmic	Molluscum bodies, Henderson-Paterson
Herpes simplex	Eosinophilic,† nuclear	Cowdry's type A
Varicella-zoster	Eosinophilic,† nuclear	Lipschütz
Adenovirus		
No inclusions at all		
Trachoma and inclusion conjunctivitis	PMNs predominate	
	Lymphocytes if chronic	
	Lymphoblasts	
	Plasma cells	
	Leber's cells	
	Inclusions	
	Giant cells	
	Sometimes keratinization	

*A knife-sharp border edge is noted with elementary bodies. The initial body is bipolar staining.
†A Papanicolaou stain is necessary for intranuclear inclusion bodies. Giemsa's stain does not show them.

iodine. The elementary body then swells to a bacillary body 1000 nm in size and takes on a blue stain.

3. The initial bodies are about the size of an individual coccus of the streptococci. The initial body varies in size, shape, and density, usually being round or oval in shape. This now divides by binary fission, giving a bipolar staining body that constricts to form two signet ring–like cells, which may be seen clumped in the epithelial cells in areas like a morula. These are the new elementary bodies, which fill the entire cell of the cytoplasmic area. The cell eventually ruptures, releasing the elementary bodies to begin the same cycle.

   Free initial bodies may be seen and are recognized by their blue stain and their bipolar staining tendency.

4. The inclusion body characteristically has a crescent shape.

Other inclusions

1. Melanin granules may be large initial or small elementary bodies. The melanin granules in an unstained slide are deep brown and when stained with Giemsa are greenish black.
2. Mascara can be phagocytosed by epithelial cells, giving granules of pigment.

Nuclear chromatin

The nucleus can rupture (nuclear membrane), producing a herniation of nuclear substance. This substance will have the same texture and color as the nucleus, whereas inclusion bodies are particulate and blue or blue-red.

Phagocytosed cellular debris

Nuclear debris stains uniform dark blue with a clear circumscribed border.

Bacteria

Staphylococci and other bacteria may occasionally be observed clumped on the surface of an epithelial cell. These may give the illusion of an intracellular body somewhat like an initial body, but the bacteria are larger than an initial body.

Tumor cells

Scrapings from tumors of the conjunctiva and cornea may exhibit several of the following findings:

1. Disproportionate enlargement of nucleus as compared to the size of the cytoplasm
2. Increase in chromatin content, producing a hyperchromasia (may also be seen in pyknosis and overstaining of the slide)
3. Aberrant chromatin pattern, with elongation and irregularity in outline
4. Enlarged nucleoli or increase in number (usually 4 or more)
5. Mitotic activity with abnormal mitotic figures
6. Multinucleation with associated nuclear changes
7. Marked thickening of the nuclear membrane

8. Degenerative changes such as abnormal vacuolation and fading or complete re-sorption of the nucleus
9. Cytoplasmic changes—vacuolation
10. Enlargement of cells beyond normal range
11. Extreme enlargement and bizarre shape
12. Irregularity of cells, irregularity of size of cells, and lack of distinct cell boundary

Molluscum bodies

The epithelial cells are greatly enlarged in molluscum bodies, with the nuclei pushed to the side and ultimately destroyed. The cytoplasm is replaced by an enormous eosinophilic inclusion body, which is composed of innumerable elementary bodies lying in a gelatinous carbohydrate matrix.

Granulomatous inflammation

A. Proliferative inflammation is characterized by a cellular infiltrate of epithelioid cells, which are a syncytium of cells formed by macrophages that lose their distinct boundaries. This syncytial arrangement of macrophages, which resembles epithelium, provides the name for epithelioid cells.
B. Giant inflammatory cells are formed by the fusion of macrophages or by a mitotic division of macrophages.
   1. Langerhans' cells: homogeneous eosinophilic center with peripheral rim of nuclei
   2. Touton giant cell: like a Langerhans giant cell with a rim of foamy cytoplasm peripheral to the nucleus; seen in lipid disorders
   3. Tuberculous giant cell: nuclei randomly distributed through eosinophilic cytoplasm
C. Three patterns of inflammatory reaction occur in granulomatous infections:
   1. *Diffuse:* epithelioid cells in random distribution against a background of lymphocytes and plasma cells, that is Vogt-Koyanagi-Harada syndrome, sympathetic uveitis, lepromatous leprosy and toxoplasmosis
   2. *Zonal:* nidus of necrosis surrounded by epithelioid cells, lymphocytes, and plasma cells seen in fungal infection, rheumatoid arthritis, scleritis, and caseating tuberculosis
   3. *Discrete:* accumulation of epithelioid cells in nodules, surrounded by lymphocytes and plasma cells (sarcoid, tuberculoid leprosy, miliary tuberculosis)

Granulation tissue

1. Granulation tissue is composed of leukocytes, proliferating blood vessels, and fibroblasts.
2. PMNs arrive first, then come MNs and capillaries. Fibroblasts arise from fibrocytes and other cells (monocytes) and lay down collagen and elaborate ground substance.
3. There is no resolution; the process becomes chronic.

Gram's stain

Material needed

1. Gentian violet
2. Gram's iodine solution
3. 95% Ethyl alcohol
4. Safranin

Stain

1. Fix the slide in methanol for 5 minutes.
2. Flood the slide with crystal violet for 30 seconds. Rinse with water.
3. Flood the slide with iodine for 30 seconds. Rinse with water.
4. Tilting the slide, allow the ethyl alcohol–acetone decolorizing solution to run over the slide until the purple color ceases to be washed off.
5. Counterstain by flooding the slide with safranin for 45 seconds. Rinse with water and gently blot dry.

NOTE

Each solution may be left on for a longer period of time (30 seconds) if you wish to preserve the slide (for example, for teaching purposes). For routine clinical use, however, 1 to 3 seconds is sufficient time for the cells to become properly stained.

Giemsa's stain

Material needed

1. Stock Giemsa's solution
2. Absolute alcohol
3. 95% Ethyl alcohol
4. Buffered water

Stain

1. Fix with methyl alcohol for 5 minutes. Allow to dry.
2. Place fixed slide in Giemsa's working stain for 30 minutes (working stain prepared by mixing 2 parts of Giemsa's stain with 50 parts of buffered water [pH 7.0 at 25° C]). The staining solution should be made up fresh each time.
3. Rinse the slide quickly in ethyl alcohol. Air dry.

Index

A

Abscess, ring, 49
Absidia, 78
Acanthamoeba, 49, 80
Acanthosis, 628
  nigricans, 566
Acetylcysteine, 345
  for herpetic keratitis, 175
  for vernal catarrh, 365
Acid injuries, 612-616
Acid mucopolysaccharides in stroma, 489
Acid-fast organisms in keratitis, 57-58
Acremonium, 78
Acrodermatitis enteropathica, 559-561
Actinomyces
  culture of, 53
  israelii, 26
    in keratitis, 46, 59
Acyclovir, 173
Addison's disease, melanosis in, 595
Adenine arabinoside
  for herpes simplex keratitis, 171-172, 175
  in herpes zoster, 187
  monophosphate, 172
Adenovirus, 8, 191, 431
  and superficial punctate keratitis of Thygeson, 333
Adhesion of regenerating epithelium, 242
Adhesive, surgical
  for corneal melting, 394
  for corneal perforation, 408
Adolescent, inclusion conjunctivitis in, 135-137, 138, 143
Adrenalin; *see* Epinephrine
Adult, inclusion conjunctivitis in, 135-137, 138, 143
Aerobacter, 57
Aerosporin; *see* Polymixin B
Aging, changes with, 210-212
Air injection, accidental, 627
Alacrima, congenital, 529

Alkali injuries, 612-616
Alkaptonuria, 441-443
Alkylating agents, 356
Allergic contact dermatoconjunctivitis, 357-358
Allergic reactions, immunoglobulin E in, 350
Allergy in catarrhal infiltrates and ulcers, 382
Alport's syndrome, 531, 596
Alternaria, 48
  in keratitis, 78
American Thyroid Association, 464
Amikacin, 65, 69, 71-72
Amino acid metabolism, diseases of, 441-461
Aminodarone, 587
Aminoglycosides for bacterial keratitis, 70-72, 75
Aminophylline, 356
Amorphous dystrophy, posterior, 256-257, 275
Amphotericin B
  for fungal keratitis, 84, 85-86
  toxic reactions to, 610
Ampicillin, 62, 63, 64, 67, 68, 69
Amyloid
  in lattice dystrophy, 262, 263-264
  staining of, 453
Amyloid degeneration, 222
Amyloidosis, 452-454
  lattice dystrophy as form of, 264
  primary familial, 265
  secondary localized, 222
Anaphylactoid hypersensitivity, 354, 355-356
Anatomy of cornea, 1-15
Anesthesia, corneal, 528, 529
  in Goldenhar-Gorlin syndrome, 533
Anesthetics, topical, toxic reactions to, 607
Aneurysms, conjunctival, 510
Angiokeratoma corporis diffusum, 507-514, 515
Ankylosing spondylitis, 353
Anomaly(ies)
  Axenfeld's, 28, 35
  congenital, 27-43
    from herpes infection, 153
  Peters', 32, 33, 36
  Rieger's, 29-31